Chronic Headache

Mark W. Green • Robert Cowan
Frederick G. Freitag
Editors

Chronic Headache

A Comprehensive Guide
to Evaluation and Management

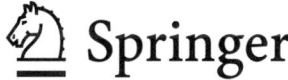 Springer

Editors
Mark W. Green, MD
Department of Headache and Pain
Medicine
Icahn School of Medicine at Mt. Sinai
Department of Headache and Pain
Medicine
New York
NY, USA

Robert Cowan, MD
Neurology & Neurological Sciences
Stanford School of Medicine Neurology
& Neurological Sciences
Stanford
CA, USA

Frederick G. Freitag, DO
Department of Neurology
Medical College of Wisconsin
Department of Neurology
Milwaukee
WI, USA

ISBN 978-3-030-08259-8   ISBN 978-3-319-91491-6   (eBook)
https://doi.org/10.1007/978-3-319-91491-6

Dedicated to many giants in the field of headache medicine:
Donald Dalessio
John Edmeads
Steven Graff-Radford
John Graham
Robert Kunkel
Marcia Wilkinson

Preface

Chronic daily headache occurs in 3 and 5% of the population worldwide. While not as common as many other primary headache disorders, the various chronic daily headaches are associated with greater healthcare utilization, loss of productivity, and relatively poor quality of life. In many forms of chronic daily headache, they represent the end stage of headache.

Chronic daily headache is not a diagnosis but a constellation of symptoms. The headache needs to be evaluated with a thorough understanding of the history, careful examination of the patient, appropriate diagnostic studies, consultation with colleagues, and ongoing assessment of the patient leading to the appropriate diagnosis and treatment.

This book hopes to clarify the diagnosis of chronic daily headache disorders, provide an understanding of the underlying biological substrates, provide guidance on the use of diagnostic testing and additional consultations, and develop treatment strategies with the greatest potential to alleviate the burden of these patients through the highest quality of care.

The book includes an examination of chronic daily headache, the role of behavioral medicine, and the important elements of the history. Following are the major forms of these disorders, the role of diagnostic testing and treatment. The underlying biology of these disorders is reviewed and the impact of these headaches in society is examined. The risk factors that lead patients to transform episodic primary headache disorders into the chronic form are examined. Invasive and neuromodulatory techniques are discussed. Somewhat by way of review and summary we close with a section on the classification of these disorders.

It is the belief of the authors that this logical approach to chronic daily headache will provide a greater understanding of these disorders leading to effective quality care for patients and reduces the burden they experience.

New York, NY   Mark W. Green
Stanford, CA   Robert Cowan
Milwaukee, WI   Frederick G. Freitag

Contents

Contributors

Iryna S. Aberkorn, MD Dartmouth-Hitchcock Medical Center, Lebanon, NH, USA

Jessica Ailani, MD, FAHS Department of Neurology, Medstar Georgetown Headache Center, Medstar Georgetown University Hospital, Washington, DC, USA

Rebecca C. Anderson, BS, MSE, PhD Department of Anesthesiology, Medical College of Wisconsin, Milwaukee, WI, USA

Xianghong Arakaki, MD, PhD Neurosciences, Huntington Medical Research Institutes (HMRI), Pasadena, CA, USA

Shannon Babineau, MD Pediatrics, Goryeb Children's Hospital, Morristown, NJ, USA

José Biller, MD, FACP, FAAN, FANA, FAHA Department of Neurology, Loyola University Chicago Stritch School of Medicine, Maywood, IL, USA

Marius Birlea, MD, FAHS Neurology, University of Colorado Denver School of Medicine, Aurora, CO, USA

Cristina Cabret-Aymat, MD Central Texas Headache Fellowship, Headache Medicine, Baylor Scott and White, Temple, TX, USA

Robert Cowan, MD Department of Neurology and Neurological Sciences, Stanford Headache and Facial Pain Clinic, Stanford School of Medicine, Stanford, CA, USA

Weiwei Dai, DO Neurology, Presbyterian Hospital, Rio Rancho, NM, USA

Danielle D. DeSouza, MSc, PhD Neurology and Neurological Sciences, Stanford University, Palo Alto, CA, USA

Hans-Christoph Diener, MD, PhD Clinical Neurosciences, Department of Neurology, University Duisburg-Essen, Essen, Germany

Michael Doerrler, DO Department of Neurology, Loyola University Chicago Stritch School of Medicine, Maywood, IL, USA

Carrie Dougherty, MD, FAHS Department of Neurology, Medstar Georgetown Headache Center, MedStar Georgetown University Hospital, Washington, DC, USA

Salman Farooq, MD Neurology, Medical College of Wisconsin, Wauwatosa, WI, USA

Alfred N. Fonteh, PhD Neurosciences, Huntington Medical Research Institutes (HMRI), Pasadena, CA, USA

Frederick G. Freitag, DO Department of Neurology, Medical College of Wisconsin, Milwaukee, WI, USA

Laura Granetzke, MSN, FNP-C, NCHP Neurology, Wake Forest School of Medicine, Winston-Salem, NC, USA

Mark W. Green, MD Neurology, Icahn School of Medicine at Mt. Sinai, New York, NY, USA

Anesthesiology, Icahn School of Medicine at Mt. Sinai, New York, NY, USA

Rehabilitation Medicine, Icahn School of Medicine at Mt. Sinai, New York, NY, USA

Noah B. Gross, PhD Neurosciences, Huntington Medical Research Institutes (HMRI), Pasadena, CA, USA

Michael G. Harrington, MB, ChB, FRCP Neurosciences, Huntington Medical Research Institutes (HMRI), Pasadena, CA, USA

Andrew D. Hershey, MD, PhD, FAHS Department of Pediatrics, Division of Neurology, Cincinnati Children's Hospital Medical Center, University of Cincinnati College of Medicine, Cincinnati, OH, USA

Dagny Holle-Lee, MD, PhD Department of Neurology and Headache Center, University Hospital Essen, Essen, Germany

Sam Hooshmand, DO Department of Neurology, Froedtert and the Medical College of Wisconsin, Milwaukee, WI, USA

Emily J. Kalscheur, MS (Clinical Psychology) Department of Psychology, Rosalind Franklin University of Medicine and Science, North Chicago, IL, USA

Department of Anesthesiology, Medical College of Wisconsin, Milwaukee, WI, USA

Robert Kaniecki, MD Headache Division, Department of Neurology, UPMC Headache Center, University of Pittsburgh School of Medicine, Pittsburgh, PA, USA

Linda Kirby Keyser, MD Central Texas Headache Fellowship, Headache Medicine, Baylor Scott and White, Temple, TX, USA

Miguel J. A. Láinez, MD, PhD, FAAN, FANA, FAHS Department of Neurology, Neurology Service, University Clinical Hospital, Catholic University of Valencia, Valencia, Spain

Morris Levin, MD Department of Neurology, UCSF Headache Center, University of California San Francisco, San Francisco, CA, USA

Ane Mínguez-Olaondo, MD Neurology Service, University Clinical Hospital, Catholic University of Valencia, Valencia, Spain

Teshamae S. Monteith, MD Department of Neurology, Miller School of Medicine, University of Miami, Miami, FL, USA

Bridget Mueller, MD, PhD Department of Neurology, Icahn School of Medicine at Mount Sinai, New York, NY, USA

Lauren R. Natbony, MD Neurology, Center for Headache and Facial Pain, Icahn School of Medicine at Mount Sinai, New York, NY, USA

Barbara L. Nye, MD Dartmouth-Hitchcock Medical Center, Lebanon, NH, USA

Hope L. O'Brien, MD Division of Neurology, Department of Pediatrics, Cincinnati Children's Hospital Medical Center, University of Cincinnati College of Medicine, Cincinnati, OH, USA

Anna Pace, MD Department of Neurology, Icahn School of Medicine at Mount Sinai, New York, NY, USA

Brielle Paolini, MD, PhD Wake Forest School of Medicine, Winston-Salem, NC, USA

Duren Michel Ready, MD, FAHS Central Texas Headache Fellowship, Headache Medicine, Baylor Scott and White, Temple, TX, USA

Anton Rogachov, BSc (PhD Candidate) Institute of Medical Science, Krembil Research Institute, Toronto Western Hospital, Toronto, ON, Canada

John Farr Rothrock, MD Department of Neurology, GW-MFA Headache Center, George Washington University School of Medicine and Health Sciences, Washington, DC, USA

Soma Sahai-Srivastava, MD Clinical Professor of Neurology, Keck school of Medicine, Los Angeles, CA, USA

Benjamin J. Saunders, MD Commonwealth of Massachusetts, Boston, MA, USA

Fallon C. Schloemer, DO Department of Neurology, Froedtert and the Medical College of Wisconsin, Milwaukee, WI, USA

Matthew T. Seipel, MS Department of Psychology, Iowa State University, Ames, IA, USA

Huma U. Sheikh, MD Neurology, Mount Sinai, New York, NY, USA

Derrick Alan Shumate, DO Neurology, Medical College of Wisconsin, Milwaukee, WI, USA

Sara Siavoshi, MD Department of Neurosciences, University of California San Diego, San Diego, CA, USA

Shalonda S. Slater, PhD Division of Behavioral Medicine and Clinical Psychology, Department of Pediatrics, Cincinnati Children's Hospital Medical Center, University of Cincinnati College of Medicine, Cincinnati, OH, USA

Shweta Teckchandani, DO Department of Neurology, Stanford Headache and Facial Pain Clinic, Stanford Hospital and Clinics, Palo Alto, CA, USA

Amanda Tinsley, MD, MS Department of Neurology, GW-MFA Headache Center, George Washington University School of Medicine and Health Sciences, Washington, DC, USA

Sarah E. Trost, PhD Department of Anesthesiology, Medical College of Wisconsin, Milwaukee, WI, USA

Maggie W. Waung, MD, PhD Department of Neurology, University of California San Francisco, San Francisco, CA, USA

Rebecca Erwin Wells, MD, MPH Neurology, Wake Forest School of Medicine, Winston-Salem, NC, USA

Chronic Daily Headache: Do We Know It When We See It?

Shweta Teckchandani and Robert Cowan

Definition

According to Silberstein et al., Chronic daily headache (CDH) is a primary headache disorder, in which headaches occur at least 15 days out of the month for 3 months or more. This is further subdivided into short-duration (<4 h) headaches and long-duration (>4 h) headaches. The category includes chronic tension-type headache, chronic migraine, new daily persistent headache, chronic cluster headaches, and hemicrania continua. The vast majority of patients with CDH meet criteria for chronic migraine or chronic tension-type headache. More than half of these patients have associated medication overuse headache (MOH), which is a separate entity classified as a secondary headache, but commonly seen in patients with CDH [1].

Introduction

Supreme Court Justice Potter Stewart famously said (in another context) "I shall not today attempt further to define the kinds of material I under-

stand to be embraced within that shorthand description and perhaps I could never succeed in intelligibly doing so. But *I know it when I see it…*" Most doctors would agree that this statement is equally applicable to the topic of Chronic Daily Headache (CDH). However, in the International Headache Society's International Classification of Headache Disorders, CDH does not appear as a discrete primary or secondary headache disorder. Rather, for chronic migraine and tension-type headaches there exists an episodic presentation. This presumes that the episodic headaches precede their chronic presentation and that they share a common pathophysiology.

This chapter will explore the roles of treatment response, pathophysiology, epidemiology, comorbidity, and other factors in chronic daily headaches. This chapter is not intended to answer these questions. Other chapters in this book will look, in detail, at various aspects of CDH in headache practice. Here we will create a framework, a context, for this important discussion.

Epidemiology

The prevalence of CDH worldwide is approximately 3%, with a range in between 1 and 4% [2, 3]. In the United States, CDH is 33% more common in caucasions and in women [4]. CDH is more commonly found in patients with lower socioeconomic status, individuals with comorbid

S. Teckchandani (✉)
Department of Neurology, Stanford Headache and Facial Pain Clinic, Stanford Hospital and Clinics, Palo Alto, CA, USA

R. Cowan
Department of Neurology and Neurological Sciences, Stanford Headache and Facial Pain Clinic, Stanford School of Medicine, Stanford, CA, USA

© Springer International Publishing AG, part of Springer Nature 2019
M. W. Green et al. (eds.), *Chronic Headache*, https://doi.org/10.1007/978-3-319-91491-6_1

pain disorders, and patients who tend to overuse acute medications for headache management. According to Yancey et al., among patients with CDH, 63% use rescue medications for 14 days or more to treat headaches [5]. Patients with CDH are also more likely to have psychiatric comorbidities including depression, anxiety, and post-traumatic stress disorder (PTSD) [1, 6]. CDH is associated with poor quality of life and impaired functioning, as well as a decrease in work productivity. This results in an increased economic burden on society [6]. In the United States, direct and indirect costs from migraines are estimated to be $20 billion annually, most of which is due to chronic migraine [7]. As compared to an individual with episodic migraine, the yearly average cost per person with chronic migraine is more than four times greater [7].

Pathophysiology

The pathophysiology of CDH remains largely unknown but is likely multifactorial. The proposed mechanism involves genetic factors, in association with maladaptive neural plasticity of the nervous system that includes peripheral and central sensitization, defective pain modulation, and lack of habituation [1]. In addition, abuse of analgesics, significant comorbidity with psychiatric disorders (anxiety, depression, and panic), and sleep disorders may all be involved [8]. Epidemiological studies have identified several risk factors associated with chronification of headaches. These include medication overuse, obesity, female gender, caffeine overuse, psychiatric comorbidities (depression, anxiety, and somatization disorders), allodynia, high baseline headache frequency, old age and low socioeconomic status [9].

Diagnosis and Classification of Chronic Daily Headache

The first step in the evaluation of patients with chronic daily headache is to obtain a thorough history and physical examination to exclude a secondary cause. Diagnostic workup may include brain imaging and a laboratory evaluation, lumbar puncture, if indicated, physical examination to assess for postural dysfunction and muscle spasms, and a thorough psychiatric evaluation to discover underlying psychiatric comorbidities. In a study by Mercante et al., major depression was present in 58.7% of the patients with chronic migraine [8]. The prevalence of "some depression" was 85.8% in patients with CM, whereas it was only 28.1% in patients with episodic migraine [10]. It is also important to identify any underlying medication overuse, specifically if the patient takes barbiturates or opioid medications. The National Association of State Controlled Substances Authorities is working to provide a forum for the discussion and exchange of information and ideas to develop, implement, and monitor ongoing strategies to curtail the abuse, misuse, and diversion of controlled substances. The availability of such a report may help with the type of medication use, dosing, and timing of pharmacotherapy. Once a secondary cause is ruled out, treatment includes appropriate management therapy of the underlying primary headache with a multidisciplinary approach.

Chronic Migraine

As defined by the ICHD-3 criteria, chronic migraine is a headache occurring on 15 or more days per month for more than 3 months, with on at least 8 days per month, with features of episodic migraine with or without aura.

Diagnostic Criteria for Chronic Migraine

A. Headache (tension-type-like and/or migraine-like) on ≥15 days per month for >3 months [6] and fulfilling criteria B and C.
B. Occurring in a patient who has had at least five attacks fulfilling criteria B-D for 1.1 Migraine without aura and/or criteria B and C for 1.2 Migraine with aura.

C. On ≥8 days per month for >3 months, fulfilling any of the following [2]:
   1. Criteria C and D for 1.1 Migraine without aura.
   2. Criteria B and C for 1.2 Migraine with aura.
   3. Believed by the patient to be migraine at onset and relieved by a triptan or ergot derivative.
D. Not better accounted for by another ICHD-3 diagnosis.

Treatment

There is an attractive misconception in medicine that if treatment A is recommended for diagnosis X, then it follows that if the treatment is unsuccessful, the diagnosis is incorrect. Nowhere in medicine is treatment response less reliable as a diagnostic tool than in chronic daily headache diagnosed as Chronic Migraine. The best approach to treatment of chronic migraine is a combination of pharmacologic and non-pharmacologic therapies. Pharmacologic treatment typically involves daily preventative medication. It should be noted that only two agents (OnabotulinumtoxinA and topiramate) have strong evidence in chronic migraine [11], while a wide variety, with evidence only for episodic migraine, is commonly used.

First-line agents that have evidence of efficacy include medications from three broad classes: anti-epileptics, anti-depressants, and anti-hypertensives [12]. Medications that are commonly used in treating chronic migraine are listed in Table 1.1. In the United States only a few have FDA approval for migraine prophylaxis (propranolol, timolol, divalproex sodium, and topiramate) [13]. However, calcium-channel blockers including verapamil, flunarizine (not available in the United States), and some antidepressants (tricyclic antidepressants, serotonin reuptake inhibitors, serotonin norepinephrine reuptake inhibitors) are frequently used off-label [13]. Dosages should be increased gradually to avoid adverse effects

Table 1.1 Medications for the Treatment of Chronic Migraine

Drug	Daily dose range	Possible adverse effects
Beta blockers		
Propranolol	80–240 mg divided bid or tid	Hypotension, fatigue, asthma/COPD exacerbations
Timolol	10–50 mg bid or 20 mg daily	
Anti-epileptic drugs		
Valproate	250–500 mg bid	Alopecia, drowsiness, weight gain, tremors, liver abnormalities, fetal abnormalities
Valproate extended release	500–1000 mg daily	
Topiramate	50 mg bid	Paresthesias, word-finding difficulty, cognitive slowing, nephrolithiasis, acute angle-closure glaucoma
Gabapentin	300–3600 mg divided bid or tid	Edema, sedation, fatigue
Tricyclic antidepressants		
Nortriptyline	10–150 mg daily	Weight gain, dry mouth, drowsiness
Amitriptyline	30–150 mg daily	
Venlafaxine	75–150 mg daily	Nausea, vomiting
Calcium Channel blockers		
Verapamil	80–480 mg divided tid	Constipation, atrioventricular conduction disturbances
Extended-release-generic	240 mg daily	
Angiotensin–converting enzyme indicator		
Lisinopril, generic	5–40 mg daily	Hypotension
Angiotensin–Receptor blocker		
Candesartan	8–21 mg daily	Hypotension

Data from [58, 59]

and treated for an adequate period of time. Once an effective treatment is found, it should typically be continued for at least 3–12 months. An effective treatment is one without significant adverse effects and improvement in headache frequency by at least 50% [12]. Increasingly, improvement in disability measures is considered an important measure of overall improvement.

OnabotulinumtoxinA: Botox is FDA-approved for chronic migraine, rather than high frequency episodic migraine. It was approved in 2010 by the Food and Drug Administration (FDA) based on phase III research studies evaluating migraine prophylactic therapy (PREEMPT protocol). At a 24-week follow-up, researchers assessed whether patients had at least 50% reduction in their headache frequency. According to the study, at least 47.1% of the patients treated with onabotulinumtoxinA had achieved this degree of improvement as compared to 37.1% of the placebo group [14, 15].

Patients should also be cautioned regarding medication overuse headaches and advised to limit the use of acute medications. Non-pharmacologic strategies involve behavioral therapies and life-style changes, primarily and are discussed later [16].

Chronic Tension-Type Headache

Tension-type headache is the most prevalent type of headache, and affects 78% of people at some point in their life. Chronic tension-type headache (CTTH) affects 3% of the population in the United States and is more prevalent in women [17]. Those with TTH are less likely to come to medical attention compared to migraineurs.

According to ICHD-3 beta classification, chronic tension-type headache (CTTH) evolves from frequent episodic tension-type headache, with daily or very frequent episodes of headache. They are typically bilateral, pressing, or tightening in quality, and of mild to moderate intensity, lasting hours to days, or unremitting. The pain does not worsen with routine physical activity, but may be associated with mild nausea, photophobia, or phonophobia, but not more than one of these.

Diagnostic Criteria

A. Headache occurring on ≥15 days per month on average for >3 months (≥180 days per year), fulfilling criteria B-D.
B. Lasting hours to days, or unremitting.
C. At least two of the following four characteristics:
   1. Bilateral location.
   2. Pressing or tightening (non-pulsating) quality.
   3. Mild or moderate intensity.
   4. Not aggravated by routine physical activity such as walking or climbing stairs.
D. Both of the following:
   1. No more than one of photophobia, phonophobia, or mild nausea.
   2. Neither moderate or severe nausea nor vomiting
E. Not better accounted for by another ICHD-3 diagnosis.

Treatment of Chronic Tension-Type Headache

Anxiety and depression are common in patients experiencing CTTH. Therefore, management of CTTH may properly include pharmacotherapy, psychotherapy including cognitive behavioral therapy, biofeedback, and physical therapy to include trigger point focused massage. Evidence for pharmacologic therapies is limited and inconsistent, but strongest for tricyclic anti-depressants [18]. In a study by Jackson et al., it was noted that TCAs significantly reduced the number of days with tension-type headache and number of headache attacks compared to placebo. The effect of TCAs increased with longer duration of treatment and TCAs were also more likely to reduce the intensity of headaches by at least 50% compared to placebo or SSRIs [19]. Tricyclic antidepressants (TCAs) that are commonly used for prophylaxis include amitriptyline and nortriptyline. According to Cohen, protriptyline may be comparable in effectiveness to amitriptyline in CTTH without causing drowsiness and weight gain [20]. In a double-blind placebo-controlled trial conducted by Saper et al. of fluoxetine in patients with chronic daily headache and migraine, it was reported to be helpful, but in general the use of SSRIs in chronic tension-type headache has little evidence [21]. Small studies using venlafaxine and mirtazapine have been positive. There is little support for the use of muscle relaxants in CTTH. In a randomized controlled trial by Holroyd et al., combination therapy of antidepressants and stress management therapy had better outcomes than either treatment individually [22]. In addition to medications, individualized psychotherapy targeting stress and anxiety management, developing relaxation techniques, and biofeedback training play an important role in the management of CTTH. Other treatment modalities that are useful as adjunct therapies include physical therapy with heat, massages, transcutaneous electric nerve stimulation (TENS), and stretching exercises [23, 24]. Additionally, minimally invasive procedures such as trigger point injections, greater and occipital nerve blocks, and acupuncture can be helpful [25, 26].

Hemicrania Continua

Hemicrania continua (HC) is one of the trigeminal autonomic cephalalgias (TACs), and is an extremely disabling disorder. Exact prevalence of HC is unknown. The incidence is higher among females, with a ratio of approximately 2:1 and can occur at any age [27]. It commonly occurs in the third decade of life, but with a range from first to seventh decades [28]. As defined by the ICHD-3 beta, HC is a persistent, strictly unilateral side-locked headache, associated with ipsilateral conjunctival injection, lacrimation, nasal congestion, rhinorrhea, forehead and facial sweating, miosis, ptosis and/or eyelid edema, and/or restlessness or agitation. The headache is absolutely responsive to indomethacin.

Diagnostic Criteria

A. Unilateral headache fulfilling criteria B-D.
B. Present for >3 months, with exacerbations of moderate or greater intensity.
C. Either or both of the following:

1. At least one of the following symptoms or signs, ipsilateral to the headache:
   a) Conjunctival injection and/or lacrimation.
   b) Nasal congestion and/or rhinorrhea.
   c) Eyelid edema.
   d) Forehead and facial sweating.
   e) Forehead and facial flushing.
   f) Sensation of fullness in the ear.
   g) Miosis and/or ptosis.
2. A sense of restlessness or agitation, or aggravation of the pain by movement.
D. Responds absolutely to therapeutic doses of indomethacin.
E. Not better accounted for by another ICHD-3 diagnosis.

Treatment of Hemicrania Continua

As indicated in the diagnostic criteria, indomethacin is the first-line treatment for treating HC [2, 27]. It is recommended to start at 25 mg three times daily, with a gradual titration in dose until complete pain relief. Typically, therapeutic doses range from 150 mg to 225 mg daily [2]. Treatment failure is considered if the patient does not respond to a dose of 300 mg daily or develops significant adverse effects. Given the significant gastrointestinal adverse effects of Indomethacin, periodic attempts to decrease the dose should be made. Concurrent use of proton pump inhibitors is indicated to protect from gastrointestinal side effects of indomethacin [28]. It remains controversial whether alternative delivery (such as suppository) can circumvent the GI side effects. Although not commonly used, there have been case reports of other alternative therapies including melatonin, Boswellia, topiramate, verapamil, COX-2 inhibitors, gabapentin, and occipital nerve stimulation [27, 29–34].

Chronic Cluster Headache

Cluster headache belongs to a group of idiopathic headache entities, the trigeminal autonomic cephalalgias (TACs), all of which involve unilateral, often severe headache attacks and typical accompanying autonomic symptoms [2, 35].

About 10–15% of cluster headache patients have chronic cluster headache (CCH) [36].

ICHD 3-beta defines cluster headaches as attacks of severe, strictly unilateral pain which is orbital, supraorbital, temporal, or in any combination of these sites, lasting 15–180 min and occurring from once every other day to eight times a day. The pain is associated with ipsilateral conjunctival injection, lacrimation, nasal congestion, rhinorrhea, forehead and facial sweating, miosis, ptosis and/or eyelid edema, and/or with restlessness or agitation.

Diagnostic Criteria

A. At least five attacks fulfilling criteria B-D.
B. Severe or very severe unilateral orbital, supraorbital and/or temporal pain lasting 15–180 min (when untreated).
C. Either or both of the following:
   1. At least one of the following symptoms or signs, ipsilateral to the headache:
      a) Conjunctival injection and/or lacrimation.
      b) Nasal congestion and/or rhinorrhea.
      c) Eyelid edema.
      d) Forehead and facial sweating.
      e) Forehead and facial flushing.
      f) Sensation of fullness in the ear.
      g) Miosis and/or ptosis.
   2. A sense of restlessness or agitation.
D. Attacks have a frequency between one every other day and 8 per day for more than half of the time when the disorder is active.
E. Not better accounted for by another ICHD-3 diagnosis.

Chronic cluster headache is defined as having all the features mentioned above occurring without a remission period, or with remissions lasting <1 month, for at least 1 year.

Treatment of Chronic Cluster Headache

In general, treatment for cluster headache can be divided into acute therapy to abort individual headache attacks and prophylactic therapy aimed to prevent future attacks [37]. Cluster headache pain is intense and builds up rapidly. Therefore, for acute therapy, medications with a rapid onset are needed [38]. The most effective treatments for acute therapy include 100% oxygen or a rapidly-acting triptan [38]. A double-blind randomized trial evaluated 76 patients, each treating four cluster headache attacks, and compared 100 percent oxygen therapy (at 12 L/min for 15 min) with air placebo. By intention-to-treat analysis, pain-free status or adequate relief of attacks at 15 minutes was significantly more frequent with oxygen (78 percent of attacks, versus 20 percent with placebo) [39]. Randomized, double-blind, placebo-controlled trials have established that triptans, particularly sumatriptan (subcutaneous and intranasal) and zolmitriptan (intranasal), are effective for the acute treatment of cluster headache [40]. Another important consideration is the use of transitional medications while prophylactic medications are being increased to therapeutic levels. A tapering schedule of oral corticosteroids is frequently used to rapidly stop cluster attacks, usually within days [38]. However, in rare cases, corticosteroids may be used long-term if patients fail to respond to other prophylactic therapies [41, 42]. Prolonged systemic steroid use can cause weight gain, Cushingoid facies, easy bruising and skin fragility, cataracts, aseptic necrosis of the femoral or humeral heads, hypertension, diabetes, infection, and osteoporosis all of which need to be discussed with the patient prior to initiating therapy.

With respect to prophylactic therapy, verapamil has the best evidence in the treatment of chronic cluster headaches [35, 38]. In a double-blinded study by Leone et al., verapamil significantly reduced attack frequency and analgesic consumption as compared to placebo [43]. Verapamil is usually initiated at a dose of 240 mg daily (divided into three doses) and an adequate trial for most patients entails use of a total daily dose of 480 mg to 960 mg daily or as tolerated before the medication is regarded as a failure [35, 44]. At higher doses, verapamil can cause bradycardia and prolongation of PR interval. Therefore, regular electrocardiographic (ECG) monitoring is recommended [37]. Lithium carbonate is second-line therapy in cases where verapamil is contraindicated or ineffective, or as an add-on to verapamil. In a comparison study by Bussone et al., verapamil and lithium appeared to have similar efficacy but lithium was found to work slowly and had more adverse effects [45]. The initial dose for adults is usually 300 mg two or three times daily, with a gradual increase in dose based upon lithium levels and the response; the typical maintenance dose is 900–1200 mg/day given in three to four divided doses of the regular formulation, or in two divided doses of the sustained release formulation. The lithium plasma level should be monitored and should not exceed 1.2 mEq/L [35]. No therapeutic lithium level in cluster headache has been established. Major adverse effects of lithium include renal dysfunction, tremor, and endocrinologic abnormalities [38]. Other medications that have been used as adjunctive therapies include topiramate, melatonin, and divalproex sodium [42].

Although not yet approved, CGRP antibodies show promise in the treatment of cluster headache. External vagal nerve stimulation has been approved in the United States for the treatment of cluster headache.

New Daily Persistent Headache

New daily persistent headache (NDPH) presents as a prolonged, unremitting headache that is often refractory to treatment [3]. It starts out abruptly, sometimes following a particularly stressful event or a viral illness, but often times, without any specific triggering event. Up to 30% of individuals have had a viral illness prior to onset of the headache [46]. In one study, more than 50% of 186 NDPH patients tested positive for Epstein-Barr virus (EBV) serology [47]. However, more than 50% of the patients do not recall any triggering event. Once the headache starts, it is unremitting, persisting as a continuous headache [48]. Often, there is no previous history of headaches. As defined by ICHD-3, it is a persistent headache, daily from its onset, the time of which is often remembered. The pain lacks characteristic features, and may be migraine-like, or tension-type-like, or have elements of both.

Diagnostic Criteria

A. Persistent headache fulfilling criteria B and C.
B. Distinct and clearly-remembered onset, with pain becoming continuous and unremitting within 24 h.
C. Present for >3 months.
D. Not better accounted for by another ICHD-3 diagnosis.

NDPH can occur at any age, with an average onset at about 35 years. Clinically, NDPH may resemble migraine or tension-type headaches or have no distinguishing features. However, the key difference is that patients with NDPH remember the exact time of onset of headache [46]. The precise mechanism that underlies this condition is unknown. In a study by Rozen et al. it was noted that TNF-alpha levels were elevated in the CSF of 19 out 20 NDPH patients, but these findings have not been replicated [49]. Postsurgical events, stressful life events, and/or toxic exposures are also thought to be triggers for the development of NDPH. Patients who develop NDPH after a viral illness or a stressful event may develop glial activation and persistent cytokine production that triggers a chronic inflammatory response [46]. When evaluating a patient with a suspected diagnosis of NDPH, diagnostic workup should exclude secondary causes of headache prior to establishing the diagnosis of NDPH. Initial workup includes MRI of the brain with and without contrast, and MRV and MRA of the head and neck. Laboratory testing includes complete blood count, serum chemistry and electrolyte panel, thyroid studies, erythrocyte sedimentation rate, lupus antibody, and viral titers [50]. Finally, a lumbar puncture should be considered if the above-mentioned studies are within normal limits.

Treatment of NDPH

The challenges with NDPH are establishing this diagnosis, and the lack of evidence-based treatments [50]. A reasonable course of management is to combine a healthy lifestyle with exercise, a regular diet, and a regular sleep schedule in combination with preventative medications used for other headache disorders [50]. Given that there is little evidence for effective treatments for NDPH, a commonly used strategy by headache specialists is to select treatments based on the phenotype (migrainous vs tension-type). Potential treatments that have been studied for NDPH include doxycycline, low dose naltrexone, topiramate, and prazosin [51]. Naltrexone is commonly used for chronic pain disorders and is shown to inhibit the production of TNF-α which is a proposed mechanism for the development of NDPH [51, 52]. In a small study by Rozen, four patients with NDPH were treated with doxycycline 100 mg twice daily [49]. These patients had previously failed five other preventative agents. All of the patients had a significant improvement after 3 months. Two patients were pain-free, and the other two patients had more than 50% reduction in frequency of the headaches. These findings have not been replicated in larger studies.

Non-Pharmacologic Treatment for Chronic Daily Headache

CDH is a serious disease and results in a poor quality of life, impaired function, and disability. Pharmacologic therapies, both acute and preventative, are insufficient in the management of these patients [53, 54]. Therefore, CDH should be managed with an interdisciplinary approach. In conjunction with pharmacologic therapy, non-pharmacologic treatments such as cognitive behavioral therapy, physical therapy, biofeedback, and mindfulness training as a form of relaxation therapy may be useful [54]. The Cochrane review from 2014 showed that psychological treatments in children and adolescent patients are effective in reducing pain intensity and maintenance of therapeutic gains [55]. Cognitive behavioral therapy (CBT) can have short-term and long-term benefits in patients with migraines [12, 56]. Patients are taught to use imagery and distraction techniques as coping skills [55]. The other aspect

of CBT includes behavioral techniques that include differential reinforcement, progressive muscle relaxation, and pacing strategies [55]. Simultaneous use of different therapies may be needed for maximum benefit. In a study by Marcus et al., a combination of physical therapy and biofeedback was shown to provide greater relief than physical therapy alone [57].

Discussion

There are many challenges in the diagnosis and treatment of CDH. With respect to the diagnosis, an important question remains: Is CDH simply the chronic presentation of a primary episodic headache? In other words, does a patient with headache more days than not, of which 8 headache days monthly have migrainous features, have the same headache as a patient without daily headaches who also has 8 headache days with migrainous features? Considerable evidence suggests that one with CM has a different medical condition and pathophysiology compared to someone with episodic migraine. Other questions persist: Why is chronic migraine seen in only 4% of migraine sufferers while chronic cluster is present in 10–15% of patients with cluster headache? Why are treatments for episodic primary headache disorders poorly effective in their episodic counterparts, even in the absence of medication overuse? And finally, is NDPH, in which half of patients report some precipitating event, truly a primary headache disorder or simply a secondary headache disorder with a yet to be unidentified etiology?

Challenging the assumptions behind these classification decisions remains equally important. The underlying genetic and epigenetic features, comorbidities, and behavioral factors that determine whether a given individual will progress from either no headaches or episodic headaches to chronic headaches are yet to be identified. Future improved imaging, proteomic and genomic marker development, and novel therapies are likely to better elucidate the underlying pathophysiology and risk factors for the chronification of headache disorders [60].

Conclusion

CDH is widely viewed as arising from its episodic counterpart. It is clear from recent imaging and pathophysiologic studies that CDH differs from its episodic antecedents in a number of ways. In the future, careful phenotyping and investigative studies might help to predict which patients with episodic headache syndromes are at increased risk for developing CDH. Careful attention to the consensus-based diagnostic criteria presented here, in combination with the evidence-based treatment strategies, remains our best hope for diagnosing and managing CDH.

References

1. Tzu-Hsien L. Update of inpatient treatment for refractory chronic daily headache. Berlin: Springer Science; 2015. Read by QxMD Icon Web. 07 May 2017
2. Headache Classification Committee of the International Headache Society (IHS). The international classification of headache disorders, 3rd edn. (beta version). Cephalalgia. 2013;33(9):629–808. https://doi.org/10.1177/0333102413485658.
3. Lenaerts Marc EP, James R. Couch, Shweta Teckchandani, and Shuu-Jiun Wang. "Chronic daily headache". Medlink Neurol. 2016.
4. Silberstein, S. D., et al. "Classification of Daily and near-Daily Headaches: Field Trial of Revised IHS Criteria." Neurology. 1996;47(4):871–5.
5. Yancey J, Sheridan R, Koren KG. Chronic daily headache: diagnosis and management. Am Fam Physician. 2014;89(8):642–8.
6. Soo-Jin C. Outcome of chronic daily headache or chronic migraine. Berlin: Springer Science; 2015.
7. Murinova N, Krashin D. Chronic daily headache. Phys Med Rehabil Clin N Am. 2015;26(2):375–89.
8. Volcy-Gomez M Chronic daily headache: I. Diagnosis and pathophysiology. Read by QxMD Icon. N.p., 2005, Curr Neurol Neurosci Rep. Mar 2001;1(2):118–24.
9. Cho SJ, Chu MK. Risk factors of chronic daile headache or chronic migraine. Curr Pain Headache Rep. 2015;19:465.
10. Mercante JP, Peres MF, Guendler V, et al. Depression in chronic migraine: severity and clinical features. Arq Neuropsiquiatr. 2005;63(2A):217–20.
11. Chiang CC, Schwedt TJ, Wang SJ, Dodick DW. Treatment of medication-overuse headache: a systematic review. Cephalalgia. 2015;36(4):371–86.
12. Garza I, Schwedt TJ. Diagnosis and management of chronic daily headache. Semin Neurol. 2015;30(2):154–66.
13. Bloudek LM. Cost of healthcare for patients with migraine in five European countries: results from the international burden of migraine study (IBMS). J Headache Pain. 2012;13(5):361–78. https://doi.org/10.1007/s10194-012-0460-7. Published online 2012 May 29PMCID: PMC3381065
14. Silberstein S, Mathew N, Saper J, for the Botox Migraine Clinical Research Group. Botulinum toxin a as a migraine preventive treatment. Headache. 2000;40:445–50.
15. Tepper D, Traduzido por Marcelo MV. Onabotulinum A (Toxina OnabotulÂnica Do Tipo A, BotoxÂ®). Headache. 2014;54(4):791–2.
16. Barton PM, Schultz GR, Jarrell JF, Becker WJ. A flexible format interdisciplinary treatment and rehabilitation program for chronic daily headache: patient clinical features, resource utilization and outcomes. Headache. 2014;54(8):1320–36.
17. Jensen R. Diagnosis, epidemiology, and impact of tension-type headache. Curr Pain Headache Rep. 2003;7(6):455–9.
18. Verhagen AP. Lack of benefit for prophylactic drugs of tension-type headache in adults: a systematic review. Fam Pract. 2010;27(2):151–65.
19. Jackson JL, Shimeall W, Sessums L, DeZee KJ, Becher D, Diemer M, Berbano E, O'Malley PG. Tricyclic antidepressants and headaches: systematic review and meta-analysis. BMJ. 2010;341:c5222.
20. Cohen GL. Protriptyline, chronic tension-type headaches, and weight loss in women. Headache. 1997;37(7):433–6.
21. Saper JR. Chronic daily headache: transformational migraine, chronic migraine, and related disorders. Curr Neurol Neurosci Rep. 2008;8(2):100–7.
22. Holroyd KA, Labus JS, Carlson B. Moderation and mediation in the psychological and drug treatment of chronic tension-type headache: the role of disorder severity and psychiatric comorbidity. Pain. 2009;143(3):213–22.
23. Tella BA, Unubum EV, Danesi MA. The effect of tens on selected symptoms in the management of patients with chronic tension type headache: a preliminary study. Nig Q J Hosp Med. 2008;18(1):25–9.
24. Espí-López GV, Arnal-Gómez A, Arbós-Berenguer T, González ÁAL, Vicente-Herrero T. Effectiveness of physical therapy in patients with tension-type headache: literature review. J Jpn Phys Ther Assoc. 2014;17(1):31–8.
25. Karadas O, Gül HL, İnan LE. Lidocaine injection of pericranial myofascial trigger points in the treatment of frequent episodic tension-type headache. J Headache Pain. 2013;14:44.
26. Linde K. Acupuncture for the prevention of tension-type headache. Chichester, UK: Wiley. John Wiley & Sons, Ltd; 2016.
27. Dodick D. Hemicrania continua: diagnostic criteria and nosologic status. Cephalalgia. 2015;21(9):874–7.

28. Peres MFP, Silberstein SD, Nahmias S, Shechter AL, Youssef I, Rozen TD, Young WB. Hemicrania continua is not that rare. Neurology. 2001;57(6):948–51.
29. Rozen TD. Melatonin responsive hemicrania continua. Headache. 2006;46(7):1203–4.
30. Peres MF, Silberstein SD. Hemicrania continua responds to cyclooxygenase-2 inhibitors. Headache. 2002;42(6):530–1.
31. Schwedt TJ, Dodick DW, Hentz J, Trentman TL, Zimmerman RS. Occipital nerve stimulation for chronic headache—long-term safety and efficacy. Cephalalgia. 2007;27(2):153–7.
32. Camarda C, Camarda R, Monastero R. Chronic paroxysmal hemicrania and hemicrania continua responding to topiramate: two case reports. Clin Neurol Neurosurg. 2008;110(1):88–91.
33. Burns B, Watkins L, Goadsby PJ. Treatment of hemicrania continua by occipital nerve stimulation with a bion device: long-term follow-up of a crossover study. Lancet Neurol. 2008;7(11):1001–12.
34. Garza I, Cutrer F. Pain relief and persistence of dysautonomic features in a patient with hemicrania continua responsive to botulinum toxin type a. Cephalalgia. 2009;30:500–3.
35. Obermann M, Holle D, Naegel S, Burmeister J, Diener H-C. Pharmacotherapy options for cluster headache. Expert Opin Pharmacother. 2015;16(8):1177–84.
36. Ãzge A. Chronic daily headache in the elderly. Curr Pain Headache Rep. 2013;17:12.
37. May A, Leone M, Áfra J, Linde M, Sándor PS, Evers S, Goadsby PJ. EFNS guidelines on the treatment of cluster headache and other trigeminal-autonomic cephalalgias. Eur J Neurol. 2006;13(10):1066–77.
38. Becker WJ. Cluster headache: conventional pharmacological management. Headache. 2013;53(7):1191–6.
39. Cohen AS, Burns B, Goadsby PJ. High-flow oxygen for treatment of cluster headache. JAMA. 2009;302(22):2451.
40. Law S, Derry S, Andrew Moore R. Triptans for acute cluster headache. Cochrane Database Syst Rev. 2010;7:CD008042.
41. Ekbom K, Je H. Cluster headache: aetiology, diagnosis and management. Headache. 2003;43(3):307–8.
42. Dodick DW, Capobianco DJ. Treatment and management of cluster headache. Curr Pain Headache Rep. 2001;5(1):83–91.
43. Leone M, D'Amico D, Frediani F, Moschiano F, Grazzi L, Attanasio A. Verapamil in the prophylaxis of episodic cluster headache: a double blinded study versus placebo. Neurology. 2000;54(6):1382–5.
44. Goadsby PJ, Cittadini E, Burns B, Cohen AS. Trigeminal autonomic cephalalgias: diagnostic

and therapeutic developments. Curr Opin Neurol. 2008;21(3):323–30.
45. Bussone G, Leone M, Peccarisi C, Micieli G, Granella F, Magri M, Manzoni Gc, Nappi G. Double blind comparison of lithium and verapamil in cluster headache prophylaxis. Headache. 1990;30(7):411–7.
46. Nierenburg H, Newman LC. Update on new daily persistent headache. Curr Treat Options Neurol. 2016;18(6):25.
47. Mack KJ. What incites new daily persistent headache in children? Pediatr Neurol. 2004;31:122–5.
48. Sheikh HU. Approach to chronic daily headache. Curr Neurol Neurosci Rep. 2015;15(3):4.
49. Rozen T. New daily persistent headache: an update. Curr Pain Headache Rep. 2014;18(7):431.
50. Tepper D. New daily persistent headache. Headache. 2016;56(7):1249–50.
51. Joshi SG, Mathew PG, Markley HG. New daily persistent headache and potential new therapeutic agents. Curr Neurol Neurosci Rep. 2014;14(2):425.
52. San-Emeterio EP, Hurlé MA. Modulation of brain apoptosis-related proteins by the opioid antagonist naltrexone in mice. Neurosci Lett. 2006;403:276–9.
53. Chiappedi M, Mensi MM, Termine C, Balottin U. Psychological therapy in adolescents with chronic daily headache. Curr Pain Headache Rep. 2015;20:1.
54. Saper JR, Dodick D, Gladstone JP. Management of chronic daily headache: challenges in clinical practice. Headache. 2005;45(S1):S74–85.
55. Eccleston C, Fisher E, Craig L, Duggan GB, Rosser BA, Keogh E. Psychological therapies (internet-delivered) for the management of chronic pain in adults. Cochrane Database Syst Rev. 2014;2:CD010152.
56. Martin PR, Forsyth MR, Reece J. Cognitive-behavioral therapy versus temporal pulse amplitude biofeedback training for recurrent headache. Behav Ther. 2007;38(4):350–63.
57. Marcus DA, Scharff L, Mercer S, Turk DC. Nonpharmacological treatment for migraine: incremental utility of physical therapy with relaxation and thermal biofeedback. Cephalalgia. 1998;18(5):266–72.
58. Glauser J. Assessment and management of migraine headaches–Primary care reports–Oct 01, 2012. Emergency medicine reports, 2012.
59. Garza I, Swanson JW. Prophylaxis of migraine. Neuropsychiatr Dis Treat. 2006;2(3):281–91.
60. Tzu-Hsien L. Neural plasticity in common forms of chronic headache. Neural Plast. 2015;2015:205985.

Refractory Headache or Refractory Patient? Issues of Locus of Control in Chronic Daily Headache (CDH)

2

Sarah E. Trost, Matthew T. Seipel,
Emily J. Kalscheur, and Rebecca C. Anderson

Introduction

The treatment of chronic daily headache (CDH) can be a challenge for both patient and provider. While many patients find relief with available treatment options, some patients continue to experience intractable symptoms despite the best efforts of their treatment team. In this scenario, it is not uncommon for patients to become frustrated, expecting their provider to do more to treat their pain. In the same way, providers may become frustrated that a patient's pain remains unchanged and speculate how the patient may be contributing to the maintenance of the status quo. In short, treatment can become stuck. The psychological construct of locus of control has much to offer in understanding this dynamic between patient and provider and to help each move toward a more positive treatment outcome.

In this chapter, we present an overview of locus of control and the related concept of self-efficacy and discuss findings from the empirical literature relevant to the treatment of CDH. Next, we provide a broad overview of two psychosocial interventions, cognitive-behavioral therapy and motivational interviewing, both of which can be used to increase a patient's sense of control over the management of their headaches as well as the self-efficacy to make necessary behavioral changes. Common assessments and the use of biofeedback in the treatment plan are also discussed. We conclude by offering providers suggestions to increase both patient and provider locus of control and self-efficacy to optimize the course of treatment. Concepts are illustrated in a case study.

Locus of Control

Locus of Control Defined

The locus of control (LOC) construct was originally introduced in Rotter's social learning theory of personality [1] to characterize the extent to which people believe the outcomes of events in their lives are controlled by themselves or by external factors (e.g., other people, chance). Rotter emphasized that LOC is a continuum, ranging from internality to externality, rather than a

S. E. Trost (✉) · R. C. Anderson
Department of Anesthesiology, Medical College of
Wisconsin, Milwaukee, WI, USA
e-mail: strost@mcw.edu

M. T. Seipel
Department of Psychology, Iowa State University,
Ames, IA, USA

E. J. Kalscheur
Department of Psychology, Rosalind Franklin
University of Medicine and Science, North Chicago,
IL, USA

Department of Anesthesiology, Medical College of
Wisconsin, Milwaukee, WI, USA

© Springer International Publishing AG, part of Springer Nature 2019
M. W. Green et al. (eds.), *Chronic Headache*, https://doi.org/10.1007/978-3-319-91491-6_2

dichotomous typology. For example, a person with a more strongly internal LOC may attribute their ability to fall asleep to their own capacity to relax their body, yet they may also acknowledge the contribution of external factors such as room temperature and street noise. Additionally, each person can be thought to exhibit a global LOC orientation, as well as varying LOC for specific life domains (e.g., health, work, romantic relationships), with internal LOC generally associated with more positive outcomes [2]. The application of LOC theory and research has guided practice in a variety of domains, including health psychology, clinical psychology, and medicine.

Health LOC

The concept of LOC has been applied to health since Rotter introduced it, and a health-specific LOC construct emerged in the literature in the early 1970s. Wallston and Wallston provided a simple definition of health LOC (HLOC): "the degree to which individuals believe that their health is controlled by internal versus external factors" [3], p. 68. Initially HLOC was conceptualized as a unidimensional construct, with its first formal measure classifying individuals as either "health externals" or "health internals" [4]. Shortly thereafter, a new paradigm and associated measure emerged that conceptualized HLOC as multidimensional, involving internal LOC and two forms of external LOC. Specifically, it divided external HLOC into two distinct components: powerful others (e.g., physicians, family members) and chance [5]. Thus, an individual with external HLOC could to varying degrees believe their health is contingent upon the acumen of their medical providers as well as fate. This multidimensional measure has since been adapted to assess LOC relative to a specific illness or disease (as opposed to overall health), as well as to include a higher power (i.e., God) as a third type of external locus.

HLOC has demonstrated significant relationships with health behaviors and outcomes in various populations. The three predominant types of HLOC were significantly related to self-rated global health in a recent study: the relationship was positive for internal HLOC and negative for chance and powerful others HLOC [6]. Another recent study found chance HLOC to be associated with deficits in health promotion behaviors (e.g., physical activity, usage of preventative healthcare, health information-seeking) [7]. Higher levels of internal HLOC have also been associated with better treatment adherence in patients with type 2 diabetes [8], higher quality of life and physical functioning in recently hospitalized older adults [9], and adolescents' engagement in positive health behaviors [10]. Stronger internal HLOC, in addition to lower powerful others HLOC, was also associated with a greater likelihood of patients with coronary heart disease returning to work [11], as well as improved physical functioning in patients with chronic pain [12]. Conversely, in a sample of cancer patients, internal HLOC was associated with higher risk of depression, whereas powerful others HLOC was associated with lower risk of depression [13]. Examining newer conceptualizations of HLOC, a stronger belief that a higher power determined health outcomes has also been associated with lower treatment compliance (e.g., asthma medication adherence) [14]. Attention is now turned to a growing niche in this literature: headache-specific locus of control.

Headache-Specific LOC

General HLOC was naturally extended to research and treatment conceptualization in the headache domain, but experts in this area quickly began to question if chronic headache patients attributed control of their headache symptoms to the same source(s) as their overall heath, as well as whether simply imputing the word "headache" into existing HLOC measures would provide accurate and useful information. The construct of headache-specific LOC (HSLC) first appeared in the literature in 1990, with the publication of the headache-specific locus of control scale (discussed further in *Assessments* below) [15]. This measure was developed from new, expert-generated items, as well as adapted items from the multidimensional HLOC scale. A similar three-factor structure was upheld in the HSLC scale (i.e., internal LOC, chance LOC, and healthcare professionals LOC), and it demonstrated incremental validity by explaining significant variance in outcomes (e.g., headache frequency and intensity) beyond that accounted for by the general HLOC scale.

The initial validation of the HSLC scale yielded interesting results that illustrated the practical impact of HSLC for chronic headache patients [15]. Chance HSLC was positively associated with headache-related disability, physical complaints, depression, and maladaptive coping strategies. Healthcare professionals HSLC was positively associated with level of medication use and preference for medical treatment. Internal HSLC was positively associated with preference for self-regulation treatment. Additionally, all of these associations remained significant after controlling for headache frequency and intensity, which suggests that HSLC is a salient treatment consideration for chronic headache patients. The psychometric properties and predictive validity of the HSLC scale were independently validated shortly thereafter, with scores on the three subscales differentiating chronic headache patients from non-patients with less severe headache symptoms [16].

These early findings have been largely supported by ensuing research, with many studies highlighting additional nuances and complexity in the relationships between HSLC and headache-related outcomes [17–19]. However, the evidence has been particularly consistent that high chance and healthcare professionals HSLC are associated with poor headache-related outcomes. A recent study found both chance and healthcare professionals HSLC were related to lower quality of life [17]. Another recent study found higher chance HSLC was associated with greater symptom chronicity [20]. Healthcare professionals HSLC previously demonstrated a positive association with headache-related disability [21]. Another earlier study also found greater chance and healthcare professionals HSLC were predictive of greater pain intensity and subjective impairment [22]. Thus, research suggests that

patients who believe their headache pain is due to chance or the skill of their doctor fare more poorly than those who do not have such external attributions.

The direct relationship between internal HSLC and headache-related outcomes has been less clear. On the one hand, some researchers have found internal HSLC was related to impairments in quality of life and emotional functioning [17], as well as greater headache-related disability [18]. However, other researchers have found that internal HSLC was associated with lower levels of depression and that it moderated the relationship between headache pain severity and depression [23]. Additionally, some evidence suggests that internal HSLC may have an indirect positive association with quality of life by way of self-efficacy (discussed later in this chapter) [18], and researchers have noted that behavioral treatments (e.g., behavioral migraine management) that increase internal HSLC are effective in decreasing migraine-related impairment [19].

In a recent article, Grinberg and Seng offered the following attempt to reconcile the discrepant findings regarding internal HSLC:

It is possible that internal HSLC is multifactorial; perhaps internal HSLC is adaptive in relation to headache-related phenomena that are indeed controllable by the individual (e.g., stress management, migraine medication-taking behaviors), whereas, internal HSLC is less adaptive in relation to phenomena which the individual may exert little influence (e.g., the presence of migraine), partly due to the relationship with anxiety and emotional migraine-related quality of life impairments[…] Although effective behavioral treatments increase internal HSLC, higher internal HSLC in the absence of migraine management tools taught during behavioral treatment may be maladaptive [17] *pp. 140–1.*

Thus, the relationship between internal HSLC and headache-related outcomes appears to be context-dependent and is likely affected by the type of outcome measured, as well as the presence of symptom management tools and supports.

Overall, the dimensions of HSLC are clearly salient in headache patient outcomes. This makes

HSLC an important consideration in and potential target of medical and psychosocial interventions, with its utility optimized when regarded alongside other psychological constructs such as self-efficacy.

Self-Efficacy

Self-efficacy (SE), introduced in 1977 as a key construct in Bandura's social cognitive theory, is defined as a person's belief in his or her ability to complete a specific task or be successful in a specific situation [24]. Additionally, SE has also been regarded as a broader individual difference construct in which a person possesses a general belief regarding his or her ability to complete *any* task that they encounter. SE is typically considered to be moderately to strongly related to LOC, and some scholars have even suggested that the two may be markers of a higher-order psychological construct [25]. However, the relationship between these two constructs is not perfect, as someone could believe that a behavioral outcome is within their control (internal LOC), but not think that they have the ability to achieve the desired outcome (low self-efficacy). Further, Luszczynska and Schwarzer [26] noted an important distinction in that LOC beliefs do not necessarily imply subsequent action, whereas SE beliefs are by nature prospective and operative.

Like LOC, SE was quickly applied to medicine and behavioral health. An early review identified two pathways by which SE influenced health. First, SE was directly related to the adoption of health promotion behaviors (e.g., smoking cessation, condom use). Second, SE impacted the physiological stress response in bodily regions such as the endogenous opioid and immune systems, which in turn exerted an influence on health and illness [27]. Much research has applied SE to pain management, broadly defined. For example, in rheumatoid arthritis patients, SE was positively associated with active efforts to prevent and manage pain [28]. In fibromyalgia patients, SE was negatively associated with maladaptive pain behaviors [29]. SE has also been associated with increased pain tolerance in a non-clinical sample [30].

Unlike LOC, standardized measures of health-related SE have been less prevalent. A notable exception is the Arthritis Self-Efficacy Scale, which has been widely used since 1989 and has demonstrated good validity and reliability [31]. The first headache-specific SE scale appeared in the literature in 1993, and it focused on SE regarding the prevention of headaches [32]. The Headache Management Self-Efficacy (HMSE) scale (discussed further in *Assessments* below) was published in 2000 and continues to be the most cited measure of headache-specific SE today [18]. It extended beyond beliefs about preventing headaches to include beliefs about managing headaches and headache-related disability, which is noteworthy given that for most patients headaches are difficult to predict and prevent. Recently, a measure was also introduced that targets SE specifically for acute headache medication adherence, an important component of treatment for most chronic headache patients [33].

The initial validation of the HMSE scale illustrated the relationships of HMSE with HSLC and headache-related outcomes. HMSE was positively associated with internal HSLC, negatively associated with chance HSLC, and did not display a significant relationship with healthcare professionals HSLC. Patients' coping strategies were able to be discriminated based on HMSE, such that patients who used positive coping strategies (e.g., cognitive restructuring, coping self-statements) had significantly higher HMSE scores. HMSE was also associated with lower levels of headache-related disability and less severe headache symptoms, and it explained unique variance in headache-related disability beyond that accounted for by headache severity and HSLC. HMSE was not significantly related to level of depression [18].

The linkage between HMSE and headache-related disability was replicated in a recent study that found HMSE was negatively associated with disability and also that HMSE significantly mediated the relationship between pain severity and disability [34]. An earlier study also confirmed this linkage in primary care headache patients [35]. Additionally, a body of literature has also found SE to mediate or moderate outcomes of several headache treatments (e.g., biofeedback, pharmacological, cognitive-behavioral) [36].

Thus, while the direct relationships between HMSE and HSLC and headache-related outcomes are fairly clear, such that greater HMSE and internal HSLC are generally associated with positive functioning and treatment outcomes, the nature of indirect relations incorporating HMSE and HSLC is less clear. For example, Seng and Holroyd [19] discussed how "clinical wisdom" suggests that that HMSE moderates the relationship between HSLC and treatment outcomes, yet the question has received minimal empirical attention. Further, the directionality of a potential moderation effect remains disputed. That is, does higher baseline internal HSLC enable patients to make greater HMSE gains during treatment, or do patients with lower baseline internal HSLC see more improvement in HMSE because they simply have more room to change [19]? More research is needed to refine our understanding of how HSLC and HMSE jointly impact headache symptoms, impairment, and treatment outcomes.

Psychosocial Interventions for CDH: Cognitive-Behavioral Therapy and Motivational Interviewing

Illness, including chronic headache, can be conceptualized not only as a biological phenomenon but also as a social phenomenon. An individual suffering from illness can take on sickness as their social function, thereby adopting a "sick role" [37]. The sick role script reads that the patient is relieved of his or her usual responsibilities in order to focus on regaining health. The assumption is that the patient wants to achieve wellness as quickly as possible, condones the undesirability of their illness [38], and defers responsibility to the medical professional. These expectations set the stage for an externally based LOC and low SE in the management of the health condition, a combination commonly encountered clinically in chronic headache populations [19]. Within this framework, the patient may lack both (1) the

understanding that certain behaviors may cause or at least influence their headaches and (2) the confidence in their ability to modify behavior in order to ameliorate or reduce the severity of their headaches. Thus, enhancing internal LOC and increasing SE for modifiable health behaviors are targets of psychosocial interventions for the CDH population, including cognitive-behavioral therapy and motivational interviewing, discussed next.

Cognitive-Behavioral Therapy

Cognitive-behavioral therapy (CBT) is recognized as the leading psychological treatment for individuals with chronic pain, including CDH [39]. In short, CBT for chronic pain aims to reduce pain and psychological distress, as well as to increase functionality. Common goals include decreasing behaviors that adversely affect the pain condition (e.g., erratic sleep, medication overuse); increasing adaptive behaviors (e.g., regular exercise, implementation of stress management tools); identifying, challenging, and replacing unhelpful thoughts and beliefs (e.g., "I can't do anything with this headache"); and increasing SE that one can manage or influence pain [40].

As many patients will attest, headache symptoms are often triggered and/or exacerbated by stress. CBT teaches patients to notice how thoughts influence the stress response. In our own practice, we often ask patients whether there are things they could think about that might make their headaches worse. The answer is a resounding "yes" with work demands, financial strain, deadlines of various sorts, and marital and parenting difficulties as commonly identified stressors that exacerbate headache pain. Through use of a daily thought record, patients learn to notice thoughts relating to stress, pain, and the impact of pain on daily functioning. Often patients identify thoughts that can be characterized as catastrophizing: "I can't deal with this pain. Nothing helps. No one understands how I suffer." A goal of CBT is to help patients recognize such thoughts, gently challenge them, and to replace with thoughts that have less of a deleterious impact on a patient's mood, level of tension, and subsequent ability to function (e.g., "I've functioned with this level of pain before. I can do it again."). Patients learn that they have the ability to modify their thoughts and to thereby exert influence on their pain experience.

In addition to thought monitoring, relaxation training is an aspect of CBT that also teaches patients how to influence their experience of pain. Penzien et al. [41] identify *progressive muscle relaxation (PMR), autogenic training,* and *meditation/passive relaxation* as forms of relaxation training commonly used to treat chronic headaches. PMR has been used since the 1930s as a treatment to lower anxiety [42]. Patients practice tensing and relaxing muscle groups throughout the body. With continued practice, patients become skilled at recognizing the first signs of tension in the body and to effectively and quickly relax. Autogenic training involves patients using the suggestions of heaviness, warmth, calmness, and ease to promote a sense of deep relaxation in the body. For example, a patient will subvocally or mentally repeat the suggestion, "My arms are heavy and warm," before moving to another part of the body. Put simply, meditation and passive relaxation involve focusing on an anchor (e.g., breath, words) to calm both mind and body. When thoughts wander, they are redirected to the anchor. Relaxation training as a whole aims to enhance patients' sense of control over physiological responses, in particular sympathetic arousal [41]. In other words, patients learn they are capable of exerting influence over the level of tension in the body and their subsequent experience of pain.

Biofeedback and Assessments

Biofeedback is used alongside CBT techniques to teach headache patients how to reduce physiological arousal. For the treatment of chronic headaches, thermal biofeedback (measuring finger temperature) and electromyographic (EMG) biofeedback (measuring muscle tension) are often used [41]. Heart rate variability biofeedback can also be employed. Patients learn to use breathing and cognitive strategies in real time to calm the body, and audial or visual feedback allows patients to know when sympathetic arousal is reduced. Over time, patients learn to recognize tension in the body and lower arousal before tension levels become high.

The effectiveness of biofeedback for headaches has been documented for decades (see, e.g., [43, 44]), and two recent meta-analyses [45, 46] found sound evidence supporting the effectiveness of biofeedback training for the treatment of headache pain. In addition, multiple studies demonstrate that when coupled with medical therapy, biofeedback enhances outcomes for headache patients [47–49]. A recent study in our own clinic found biofeedback to be an effective strategy to manage headache and other forms of pain [50]. Participants ($N = 72$) reported a significant reduction in self-reported pain and distress immediately following biofeedback sessions, with pain and distress ratings decreasing more than a point on a 0–10 rating scale. While decreases in pain and distress were not maintained from session to session, patients' scores on a measure of catastrophizing significantly decreased across biofeedback sessions, suggesting that beliefs in one's ability to cope with pain can be enhanced over time through a biofeedback intervention.

Cognitive factors such as LOC and SE influence the patient's participation in headache management, including medical adherence and the monitoring and management of triggers [51]. The assessment of these cognitive constructs in the context of CBT and other psychosocial interventions serves a number of purposes: (1) to better understand the patient's beliefs about chronic headache before beginning treatment, (2) to inform the treatment plan by including targeted interventions aimed at such beliefs and bolstering confidence in the patient's skills to prevent and manage headaches (i.e., increasing SE and internal LOC), and (3) to examine changes throughout the treatment process. A number of standardized assessments have been developed, three of which are described below. The first two directly assess the concepts of LOC and SE, while the final assesses LOC indirectly through the construct of catastrophizing.

Headache-Specific Locus of Control (HSLC) Scale

The HSLC scale is a 33-item measure consisting of three subscales: (1) healthcare professionals LOC (e.g., "Following my doctor's medication regimen is the best way for me not to be laid-up with a headache"), (2) internal LOC (e.g., "My actions influence whether or not I have headaches"), and (3) chance LOC (e.g., "My headaches are beyond all control"). Participants respond to each item using a 5-point Likert scale where 1 = strongly disagree and 5 = strongly agree. For each subscale, higher values indicate greater LOC ascribed [15, 16].

As discussed earlier in the chapter, the subscales have demonstrated good internal consistency (α's ranging from 0.80 to 0.89) and adequate 3-week test-retest reliability (rs ranging from 0.72 to 0.78) [15]. Additionally, expected relationships have been demonstrated with other related measures: the chance LOC subscale is associated with catastrophizing ($r = 0.44$), the internal LOC subscale is associated with preference for self-regulation treatments ($r = 0.21$), and the healthcare professionals LOC subscale is associated with preference for medical treatment ($r = 0.45$) [15]. Versions of the HSLC have been validated for Spanish-speaking populations [52].

Headache Management Self-Efficacy (HMSE) Scale

The HMSE scale consists of 25 items measuring the patient's confidence in his or her ability to apply behavioral skills to prevent or manage recurrent headaches [18]. Participants respond to items (e.g., "I can reduce the intensity of a headache by relaxing") on a 7-point Likert scale where 1 = strongly disagree and 7 = strongly agree with higher scores indicating greater headache management SE. The HMSE has shown good internal consistency ($\alpha = 0.90$)[18] and predictive validity (described previously in this chapter).

Pain Catastrophizing Scale (PCS)

The PCS is a 13-item scale assessing thoughts and feelings associated with pain. Three dimensions of pain catastrophizing are measured and constitute subcategories of the scale: rumination (4 items), magnification (3 items), and helplessness (6 items) [53]. Participants respond to each item using a 5-point Likert scale (where 0 = not at all and 4 = all the time) in reference to the degree to which they have specific thoughts and feelings when experiencing pain (e.g., "There's nothing I can do to reduce the intensity of the pain"; "I can't seem to keep it out of my mind"). Total PCS scores are calculated by summing the scores of all items, with higher scores representing a higher tendency to catastrophize pain. The items included in each subcategory are also summed to provide subscale scores. Scores ≥ 30 indicate clinically significant levels of catastrophizing [53].

The PCS has been validated for a many different languages, including Arabic [54], Korean [55], Hindi [56], Turkish [57], Brazilian [58], Sinhala [59], and Italian [60]. The scale has also been validated for use in children, including German- [61] and Catalan-speaking [62] children. Additionally, a short form of the PCS has been validated for English-[63] and Japanese-speaking populations [64].

In sum, assessments can be an effective tool to measure client LOC and SE, providing objective data to observe the process of change. Additionally, they can serve as a useful springboard for conversation about the patient's capacity to influence headache pain, one that may increase motivation to make necessary behavioral changes.

Motivational Interviewing

Motivational interviewing (MI), a therapeutic intervention that specifically explores and addresses the difficulties inherent in trying to modify behavior, has powerful potential to move CDH patients toward lasting behavioral change. A growing body of literature demonstrates that MI can be effectively delivered in medical settings by a range of providers with minimal investment of time [65]. Reviewed in a recent meta-analysis, MI was successfully employed to address a variety of diverse health concerns including body weight, alcohol and tobacco use, dental outcomes, sedentary behavior, HIV viral load, and optimal utilization of physical therapy [65]. Few empirical studies exist that examine MI exclusively with the CDH population (although see [66] for a study on telephone-based MI for adolescent chronic headache). However, the behavioral changes often needed by individuals with CDH (e.g., prioritizing sleep, exercise, nutrition, and daily relaxation) – and the associated ambivalence in making such changes—lend themselves well to modification via MI. While a thorough review of MI is beyond the scope of this chapter, Rollnick et al. [67] provide an excellent resource on MI in healthcare settings.

In short, MI is "a client-centered, directive method for enhancing intrinsic motivation to change by exploring and resolving ambivalence" [68], p. 25. It is client-centered in the sense that it is an open, respectful, and nonjudgmental way of being with clients. It is directive in that the provider chooses what to attend to and therefore is gently guiding the session to elicit from patients their own motivations for behavior change.

MI is based in part on the Stages of Change model developed by Prochaska and DiClemente [69]. According to this model, change happens gradually, in stages. In the first stage of change, *precontemplation*, a client does not acknowledge that they have a problem with a given behavior. The task of the provider is to raise awareness through education and feedback. In the realm of CDH, education can be on the contributory roles of medication overuse, missed meals, poor hydration, or inadequate sleep to headache risk, for example. Feedback can be given in the form of assessment results (discussed above), which allows the patient to see how their pain behaviors and beliefs compare to others as well as to themselves across time. In the second stage of change, *contemplation*, a person experiences ambivalence about changing a given behavior. A patient may want to make time to exercise most days, and she may know it will help her headaches, but she also does not believe she has enough time to exercise and views exercise as taking away from other work and home responsibilities. The provider's role is to help the patient explore her ambivalence and ultimately to resolve it such that she is ready to make the first steps toward behavior change.

When a person is leaning toward making a behavior change, he or she is said to be in *preparation*. Here is where the provider works with the patient to explore and identify change strategies by offering a menu of options. In the *action* stage of change, a person chooses a strategy and makes a clear commitment to behavior change. *Maintenance* follows, whereby the provider checks in to see if what the patient is doing is still working, in order to maintain gains and continue skill building. Lastly, an integral component of the model is *relapse*, when a person stops a healthy behavior and/or resumes an unhealthy behavior. Relapse is reframed as a more forgiving "slip," and the patient and provider evaluate what went wrong, with the patient ultimately recommitting to change.

The underlying philosophy of MI is to meet patients where they are in the Stage of Change model and to work with them to increase their motivation for change. The question is "for what is this person motivated?" (e.g., to contemplate, to take action). MI understands that pushing a person toward change when they are not committed will result in resistance [67, 70].

A core clinical principle in MI is that of developing discrepancy [70]. The provider works with the patient to develop the discrepancy between their current behavior and current values. Put another way, the patient is prodded to discuss the difference between what they say they want and what they are actually doing. The goal of developing discrepancy is to maximize opportunities for the patient to present reasons for change (also called "change talk"; see [67, 70]). In other words, the aim is for the patient to engage in problem recognition (e.g., "I guess my stress level makes my headaches worse"), express concern about problem ("I can see that staying up late to work is literally hurting me"), state advantages of change ("My children would like it if I exercised with them"), express SE ("I think I could make self-care a priority if I decided to"), and/or verbalize intention to change ("I've got to do something").

While it is the patient that presents reasons to change, the provider can help to evoke change talk via simple questions such as, "What is truly important to you? How does this fit with behaviors that contribute to CDH?" For example, a client might state that being a good parent is of primary importance. The provider can [gently] wonder how a lack of self-care—that ultimately leads to lost time with family—fits with such a value. Ultimately, the goal is for the patient to see that self-care supports the priority of being a good parent. Other useful questions include, "What worries you about your behavior? What do you think will happen if you don't change your behavior? What encourages you that you can change if you want to?" Discussing the positive as well as the negative aspects of change is also an important conversation to have, so that the patient makes a choice to engage in behavior change having thought about all sides of the issue.

Other core clinical principles include providing empathy for the patient's situation, treading carefully when clients show resistance to change (e.g., by responding "the choice is up to you. You can decide to do what you like"), and supporting a patient's SE to make changes by asking them to reflect on other times in their lives where they made a difficult change and followed through with it.

In MI, motivation for change comes from within and is not imposed from without. Through meaningful conversation, MI cultivates internal resources for change, leaving the client with the sense that change is within his or her own control and not something the provider can make happen for him or her. In this way, MI is a tool to support SE and increase internal HSLC.

LOC and SE: Suggestions for the Provider

Healthcare providers treating headache patients may face frustrations of their own. The provider may be caught between wanting to help the patient find a means to manage headaches and struggling when nothing appears to be working. Sometimes the refractory headache patient is considered by the provider to be difficult. Indeed, they may be difficult to manage medically, especially if all reasonable options have

been trialed, and providers may feel helpless in the face of dwindling options to offer. Refractory patients are often high utilizers of services. Some are seeking answers, treatments, and cures, while others may experience anxiety, mood disorders, substance abuse issues, and personality disorders. Provider workload may increase the perception of a patient being difficult, with healthcare system pressures such as reduction of costs and increased productivity playing a role [71].

Just as patient SE is important for the effective treatment of CDH, so is provider SE. Understanding the needs of headache patients can bolster a provider's SE to effectively treat this population. Cottrell and associates [72] conducted a focus group to identify the perceptions and needs of migraine patients. The results suggested that patients seek better understanding of their migraines and information as well as pain relief. They would like a collaborative relationship with their physicians combined with a team approach to treatment. Participants identified areas of concern, which included the impact of their headaches on family, relationships/social functioning, and employment, as well as issues related to physician care. Physician care factors involved the provider's willingness to consider alternative treatments, the ability of the provider to listen, and a sense of feeling dismissed by providers who failed to take them seriously. Ability to obtain insurance coverage of prescribed medications was also a concern. Patients in the focus group recognized that tools related to technology may be available to them and appreciated physicians who understood this fact. Providers who acknowledge such patient concerns are in a better position to more effectively meet the needs of their patients.

There appear to be specific patient and physician characteristics that contribute to the perception that a given headache patient is difficult to manage [72, 73]. Challenging patients include those with refractory headaches, psychiatric pathology, multiple unexplained symptoms, and substance abuse difficulties. Interestingly, there are physician characteristics associated with the provider perception that a patient is difficult. Those physicians who are younger, under greater stress, and who do not utilize collaborative treatment models are more likely to perceive a patient as challenging. General principles that might prove helpful in the management of the refractory patient include evaluating for possible mental health or substance abuse problems followed by specific treatment if identified as useful. A shift from the treatment philosophy of searching for a cure in favor of the goal of management and the use of written agreements that outline conditions of treatment can prove valuable in the approach to refractory patients. Lastly and importantly, use of an integrated, multimodal treatment approach that includes behavioral and nonpharmacological treatment options is suggested.

In the treatment of headaches, there are modifiable risks and those over which the patient has less capability to change [74]. Those risks over which the patient has the ability to exercise some element of control or may modify include such factors as sleep-related difficulties, obesity, medication overuse, allodynia or increased pain sensitivity, and nausea or prolonged headache duration. Non-modifiable risks include age, sex, genetic background, head and/or neck injury, socioeconomic status, and uncontrollable major life events (e.g., job loss). Headache providers should encourage patients to gain a sense of SE for modifiable risks. As discussed above, CBT or MI can prove useful in reframing the patient's sense of control over modifiable risks and increasing efficacy to make positive changes.

Once headaches have transitioned from episodic to chronic and daily, they become more difficult to manage. Management of the risk factors prior to that happening is very important. Risk factors for transition from episodic to chronic daily headaches include obesity, headache frequency, medication overuse, and psychiatric comorbidity [75]. Often these patients are difficult to treat due to multiple factors, not the least of which is nonadherence. They should be seen frequently and educated about the mechanisms of headache. Treatment favors a collaborative relationship between patient and provider and the use of behavioral strategies to help the patient take an active role in managing their headache disorder and the therapeutic program [75].

Rains and colleagues [76] identify four important dimensions of care in the management of the migraine patient, which include administration, psychoeducation, behavioral factors, and social support. In the area of administration, they suggest scheduling regular contact and rapport building, providing verbal and written recommendations, screening for psychiatric comorbidities, tracking compliance, encouraging participation of significant others, and assessing and treating psychiatric comorbidities. Psychoeducation encompasses providing patient education about migraines, use of printed materials, patient involvement in planning, and education related to adherence and health-related behavior change. The behavioral piece includes providing a simple daily health regimen, training the patient in self-monitoring of compliance, understanding and managing stimulus control (such as known headache triggers), using medication contracts, enhancing SE, and reinforcing successes. Lastly, social support factors such as provider communication and support, a collaborative therapeutic alliance, and spouse and family support offer potential benefit for headache management.

With these factors in mind, take the illustrative case of Dr. Nikou and Ms. Connelly to see how each might alter their approach or belief systems to effect a better patient outcome.

Case Study

Ms. Connelly, a 40-year-old female, presents to the clinic complaining of sharp pain at the base of her neck that radiates behind and over her head. She meets with Dr. Nikou, a young physician who just began his practice at the clinic less than a year ago. Besides having a heavy clinical load each week, Dr. Nikou is also developing a research program within the clinic and is finding the day he sees Ms. Connelly to be an especially busy day. Dr. Nikou introduced himself to the patient and began taking her medical history. Ms. Connelly rated her pain today as 8/10 (with 10 being the worst). She reported a 3-year history of severe daily headaches and has found little to no relief with previous prescription trials. Ms. Connelly is a mother of three elementary school-aged children who are involved in many after-school activities. She previously worked as a real estate agent but is currently unemployed due to her daily headaches. While she has a history of anxiety dating back to high school, for which she took a short-term anxiolytic, her anxiety has recently increased due to changes in her husband's work schedule. She shared this with Dr. Nikou, but she did not feel that he was listening because he was typing on the computer. Ms. Connelly reported drinking three to four cups of coffee daily and is a regular Diet Coke drinker. She does not sleep well: she averages 4–5 h per night and reports difficulty with early morning awakenings. She also regularly skips meals because she "forgets" which has resulted in a loss of 10 lbs. unintentionally over the past several months. Dr. Nikou inquired about headache triggers, but Ms. Connelly was unable to identify any: "They just happen. I can't predict it." She feels helpless, as no medications have helped and no one has been able to identify the cause of her headaches. This has become very unsettling to her, leading her to seek out medical advice from a number of specialists who have helped to reduce her pain to a 5/10 temporarily (via injections, physical therapy, and chiropractic care), but have not been able to cure her from her headache pain. She has begun to identify as a sick person, and she spends much of her day lying on the couch or looking up her symptoms online to try to find a cause and possible cure for her pain. She reported she has failed to keep a headache diary because she does not have time. She also has little energy to engage in relaxation strategies. Dr. Nikou, with little time left before needing to meet the next patient, said he would change the dose of an existing medication and told her to make a follow-up visit for 6 weeks later. Ms. Connelly left the clinic to get her prescription, but found herself feeling dejected and wanting a plan to address her headaches so that she can return to work.

There may be ways for Dr. Nikou to better meet the needs of this patient and the patient may benefit from an adjustment in both behavior and expectations. First, Dr. Nikou might do well to adjust the location of his computer so that he can make eye contact with the patient and enter data into the medical record at the same time. He could use reflective listening strategies such as "I hear you saying that …" or "I understand that when … you…." Summarizing what the patient says will help them to feel heard, and ending the visit by asking if there are any remaining questions gives the patient a last opportunity to get clarification. Additionally, Dr. Nikou might ask a nurse or medical assistant to come back in to offer patient education. He might want to talk to the patient about her expectations and explore what realistic outcomes for treatment might look like. In addition, he might identify if there is a psychologist, therapist, or social worker serving the clinic who could work with Ms. Connelly to manage her pain nonpharmacologically, given that the patient is open to doing so.

Ms. Connelly appears to expect Dr. Nikou to have the answers to her headaches, and she has not taken an active role in her treatment such as keeping a headache diary (i.e., external LOC). Additionally, she appears to want a cure, which might not be a realistic expectation for her. Utilizing strategies such as guided imagery, biofeedback, breathing approaches, avoiding headache triggers, and trying yoga or Tai Chi might build a sense of internal LOC in the management of her pain. For example, in the biofeedback study presented earlier, Wilson, Melchert, and Anderson [77] discovered that when patients noted a reduction in pain and distress during biofeedback, they reported a sense of gaining greater control of their pain. Successfully employing stress management strategies and verbalizing the importance of self-care will help her to build a greater sense of SE.

Generally speaking, a team approach where the provider listens and works together with the patient to establish reasonable and attainable expectations leads to a better outcome. When patients accept that there may be no magic bullet for their headaches and recognize they can actually influence their headaches through the use of self-care strategies, they tend to report greater satisfaction with their care.

Conclusion

When patients continue to struggle with CDH despite multiple interventions, treatment can become stuck, with both patient and provider wondering what the other is doing (or not doing) to fix the problem. The construct of LOC, and its application to the treatment and management of CDH, offers fruitful avenues to explore to help both patient and provider move forward toward positive treatment outcomes.

In this chapter, we reviewed literature on LOC and the related concept of SE as they relate to health and headaches specifically. As a whole, the literature suggests that internal LOC, as opposed to chance or healthcare professionals LOC, is associated with favorable treatment outcomes for modifiable health behaviors, such as sleep, exercise, nutrition/weight management, relaxation, and stress management. High SE can enable a patient to make necessary behavioral changes to influence their experience of and susceptibility to pain.

Psychological treatments can be employed to modify LOC and SE. In particular, CBT and MI show patients that they have the capacity to influence health outcomes. CBT teaches skills and strategies to reduce pain and psychological distress, with patients learning that they can use such strategies in real time to make a lasting impact on their functioning. MI has much to offer both patients and providers alike in moving patients closer toward internally driven change. Even a refractory patient has the potential to shed this label when they are able to verbalize the importance of self-care behaviors and actualize their commitment to change.

Lastly, we encourage providers to recognize the potential difficulty in working with CDH patients. By understanding the perspectives and beliefs common to this population, and recognizing that there are modifiable psychological variables that can benefit treatment, providers can increase their own LOC and SE to work collaboratively with CDH patients to achieve a favorable outcome.

Acknowledgments The authors wish to thank Annette Wilson, Ph.D., for her contributions to the chapter, in particular the results of her biofeedback study.

Correspondence regarding this chapter should be addressed to Sarah E. Trost, Pain Management Center, Department of Anesthesiology, Medical College of Wisconsin, 959 N. Mayfair Rd., Wauwatosa, WI 53226.

References

1. Rotter JB. Social learning and clinical psychology. New York (NY): Prentice-Hall; 1954.
2. Rotter JB. Generalized expectancies for internal versus external control of reinforcement. Psychol Monogr. 1966;80(1):1–28.
3. Wallston KA, Wallston BS. Who is responsible for your health? The construct of health locus of control. In: Sanders GS, Suls JM, editors. Social psychology of health and illness. Hillsdale (NJ): Lawrence Erlbaum; 1982. p. 65–95.
4. Wallston BS, Wallston KA, Kaplan GD, Maides SA. Development and validation of the health locus of control (HLC) scale. J Consult Clin Psychol. 1976;44(4):580–5.
5. Wallston KA, Wallston BS, DeVellis R. Development of the multidimensional health locus of control (MHLC) scales. Health Educ Monogr. 1978;6(1):160–70.
6. Berglund E, Lytsy P, Westerling R. The influence of locus of control on self-rated health in context of chronic disease: a structural equation modeling approach in a cross sectional study. BMC Public Health. 2014;14(1):492–500.
7. Grotz M, Hapke U, Lampert T, Baumeister H. Health locus of control and health behaviour: results from a nationally representative survey. Psychol Health Med. 2011;16(2):129–40.
8. O'Hea EL, Grothe KB, Bodenlos JS, Boudreaux ED, White MA, Brantley PJ. Predicting medical regimen adherence: the interactions of health locus of control beliefs. J Health Psychol. 2005;10(5):705–17.
9. Milte CM, Luszcz MA, Ratcliffe J, Masters S, Crotty M. Influence of health locus of control on recovery of function in recently hospitalized frail older adults. Geriatr Gerontol Int. 2015;15(3):341–9.
10. Cassidy T, Hilton S. Family health culture, health locus of control and health behaviours in older children. J Pediatric Med Care. 2017;1(1):4–9.
11. Bergvik S, Sørlie T, Wynn R. Coronary patients who returned to work had stronger internal locus of control beliefs than those who did not return to work. Br J Health Psychol. 2012;17(3):596–608.
12. Keedy NH, Keffala VJ, Altmaier EM, Chen JJ. Health locus of control and self-efficacy predict back pain rehabilitation outcomes. Iowa Orthop J. 2014;34:158–65.
13. Aarts JW, Deckx L, Abbema DL, Tjan-Heijnen VC, Akker M, Buntinx F. The relation between

depression, coping and health locus of control: differences between older and younger patients, with and without cancer. Psychooncology. 2015;24(8):950–7.

14. Ahmedani BK, Peterson EL, Wells KE, Rand CS, Williams LK. Asthma medication adherence: the role of god and other health locus of control factors. Ann Allergy Asthma Immunol. 2013;110(2):75–9.

15. Martin NJ, Holroyd KA, Penzien DB. The headache-specific locus of control scale: adaptation to recurrent headaches. Headache. 1990;30(11):729–34.

16. VandeCreek L, O'Donnell F. Psychometric characteristics of the headache-specific locus of control scale. Headache. 1992;32(5):239–41.

17. Grinberg AS, Seng EK. Headache-specific locus of control and migraine-related quality of life: understanding the role of anxiety. Int J Behav Med. 2017;24(1):136–43.

18. French DJ, Holroyd KA, Pinell C, Malinoski PT, O'donnell F, Hill KR. Perceived self-efficacy and headache-related disability. Headache. 2000;40(8):647–56.

19. Seng EK, Holroyd KA. Dynamics of changes in self-efficacy and locus of control expectancies in the behavioral and drug treatment of severe migraine. Ann Behav Med. 2010;40(3):235–47.

20. Seng EK, Buse DC, Klepper JE, J Mayson S, Grinberg AS, Grosberg BM, et al. Psychological factors associated with chronic migraine and severe migraine-related disability: an observational study in a tertiary headache center. Headache. 2017;57(4):593–604.

21. Nash JM, Williams DM, Nicholson R, Trask PC. The contribution of pain-related anxiety to disability from headache. J Behav Med. 2006;29(1):61–7.

22. Scharff L, Turk DC, Marcus DA. The relationship of locus of control and psychosocial-behavioral response in chronic headache. Headache. 1995;35(9):527–33.

23. Heath RL, Saliba M, Mahmassani O, Major SC, Khoury BA. Locus of control moderates the relationship between headache pain and depression. J Headache Pain. 2008;9(5):301–8.

24. Bandura A. Self-efficacy: toward a unifying theory of behavioral change. Psychol Rev. 1977;84(2):191–215.

25. Judge TA, Erez A, Bono JE, Thoresen CJ. Are measures of self-esteem, neuroticism, locus of control, and generalized self-efficacy indicators of a common core construct? J Pers Soc Psychol. 2002;83(3):693–710.

26. Luszczynska A, Schwarzer R. Multidimensional health locus of control: comments on the construct and its measurement. J Health Psychol. 2005;10(5):633–42.

27. O'Leary A. Self-efficacy and health: behavioral and stress-physiological mediation. Cognit Ther Res. 1992;16(2):229–45.

28. Lefebvre JC, Keefe FJ, Affleck G, Raezer LB, Starr K, Caldwell K, et al. The relationship of arthritis self-efficacy to daily pain, daily mood, and daily pain coping in rheumatoid arthritis patients. Pain. 1999;80:425–35.

29. Buckelew SP, Parker JC, Keefe FJ, Deuser WE, Crews TM, Conway R, et al. Self-efficacy and pain behavior among subjects with fibromyalgia. Pain. 1994;59(3):377–84.

30. Litt MD. Self-efficacy and perceived control: cognitive mediators of pain tolerance. J Pers Soc Psychol. 1988;54(1):149–60.

31. Wilcox S, Schoffman DE, Dowda M, Sharpe PA. Psychometric properties of the 8-item english arthritis self-efficacy scale in a diverse sample. Arthritis. 2014;2014:1–8.

32. Martin NJ, Holroyd KA, Rokicki LA. The headache self-efficacy scale: adaptation to recurrent headaches. Headache. 1993;33(5):244–8.

33. Seng EK, Nicholson RA, Holroyd KA. Development of a measure of self-efficacy for acute headache medication adherence. J Behav Med. 2016;39(6):1033–42.

34. Peck KR, Smitherman TA. Mediator variables in headache research: methodological critique and exemplar using self-efficacy as a mediator of the relationship between headache severity and disability. Headache. 2015;55(8):1102–11.

35. Nicholson RA, Smith TR. Predicting self-efficacy, satisfaction with care, and headache impact among migraine sufferers in a primary care setting. Headache. 2006;46(5):874.

36. Nicholson RA, Houle TT, Rhudy JL, Norton PJ. Psychological risk factors in headache. Headache. 2007;47(3):413–26.

37. Parsons T. The sick role and the role of the physician reconsidered. Milbank Mem Fund Q Health Soc. 1975;53(3):257–78.

38. Heidarnia MA, Heidarnia A. Sick role and a critical evaluation of its application to our understanding of the relationship between physicians and patients. Novel Biomed. 2016;4(3):126–34.

39. Ehde DM, Dillworth TM, Turner JA. Cognitive-behavioral therapy for individuals with chronic pain: efficacy, innovations, and directions for research. Am Psychol. 2014;69(2):153–66.

40. Turner JA, Romano JM. Cognitive-behavioral therapy for chronic pain. In: Loeser JD, Bonica JJ, editors. Bonica's management of pain. 3rd ed. Philadelphia (PA): Lippincott Williams & Wilkins; 2001. p. 1751–8.

41. Penzien DB, Andrasik F, Freidenberg BM, Houle TT, Lake AE, Lipchik GL, et al. Guidelines for trials of behavioral treatments for recurrent headache, first edition, American headache society behavioral clinical trials workgroup. Headache. 2005;45(S2):S110–32.

42. Jacobson E. Progressive relaxation: a physiological and clinical investigation of muscular state and their significance. Chicago (IL): University of Chicago Press; 1938.

43. Blanchard EB, Andrasik F. Biofeedback treatment of vascular headache. In: Hatch JP, Fisher JG, Rugh J, editors. Biofeedback studies in clinical efficacy. New York (NY): Plenum Press; 1987. p. 1–79.

44. Blanchard EB, Andrasik F, Ahles TA, Teders SJ, O'Keefe D. Migraine and tension headache: a meta-analytic review. Behav Ther. 1980;11(5):613–31.

45. Nestoriuc Y, Martin A, Rief W, Andrasik F. Biofeedback treatment for headache disorders: a comprehensive efficacy review. Appl Psychophysiol Biofeedback. 2008;33(3):125–40.

46. Nestoriuc Y, Reif W, Martin A. Meta-analysis of bio-feedback for tension-type headache: efficacy, specificity, and treatment moderators. J Consult Clin Psychol. 2008;76(3):379–96.

47. Grazzi L, Andrasik F, D'Amico D, Leone M, Usai S, Kass SJ, et al. Behavioral and pharmacologic treatment of transformed migraine with analgesic overuse: outcome at 3 years. Headache. 2002;42(6):483–90.

48. Andrasik F. Behavioral treatment of migraine: current status and future directions. Expert Rev Neurother. 2004;4(3):403–13.

49. Holroyd KA, France JL, Cordingley GE, Rokicki LA, Kvaal SA, Lipchik GL, et al. Enhancing the effectiveness of relaxation-thermal biofeedback training with propranolol hydrochloride. J Consult Clin Psychol. 1995;63(2):327–30.

50. Wilson AM. Heart rate variability biofeedback training as an intervention for chronic pain. PhD [dissertation]. Milwaukee (WI): Marquette University; 2017.

51. Nicholson R, Nash J, Andrasik F. A self-administered behavioral intervention using tailored messages for migraine. Headache. 2005;45(9):1124–39.

52. Cano-Garcia FJ, Rodriguez-Franco L, Lopez-Jimenez AM. A shortened version of the headache-specific locus of control scale in Spanish population. Headache. 2010;50(8):1335–45.

53. Sullivan M, Bishop SR, Pivik J. The pain catastrophizing scale: development and validation. Psychol Assess. 1995;7(4):524–32.

54. Terkawi AS, Sullivan M, Abolkhair A, Al-Zhahrani T, Terkawi RS, Alasfar EM, et al. Development and validation of Arabic version of the pain catastrophizing scale. Saudi J Anaesth. 2017;11(S1):S63–70.

55. Cho S, Kim HY, Lee JH. Validation of the Korean version of the pain catastrophizing scale in patients with chronic non-cancer pain. Qual Life Res. 2013;22(7):1767–72.

56. Bansal D, Gudala K, Lavudiya S, Ghai B, Arora P. Translation, adaptation, and validation of Hindi version of the pain catastrophizing scale in patients with chronic low back pain for use in India. Pain Med. 2016;17(10):1848–58.

57. Suren M, Okan I, Gokbakan AM, Kaya Z, Erkorkmaz U, Arici S, et al. Factors associated with the pain catastrophizing scale and validation in a sample of the Turkish population. Turk J Med Sci. 2014;44(1):104–8.

58. Lopes RA, Dias RC, Queiroz BZ, Rosa NM, Pereira Lde S, Dias JM, et al. Psychometric properties of the Brazilian version of the pain catastrophizing scale for acute low back pain. Arq Neuropsiquiatr. 2015;73(5):436–44.

59. Pallegama RW, Ariyawardana A, Ranasinghe AW, Sitheeque M, Glaros AG, Dissanayake WP, et al. The Sinhala version of the pain catastrophizing scale: validation and establishment of the factor structure in pain patients and healthy adults. Pain Med. 2014;15(10):1734–42.

60. Meroni R, Piscitelli D, Bonetti F, Zambaldi M, Cerri CG, Guccione AA, et al. Rasch analysis of the Italian version of pain catastrophizing scale (PCS-I). J Back Musculoskelet Rehabil. 2015;28(4):661–73.

61. Kroner-Herwig B, Maas J. The German pain catastrophizing scale for children (PCS-C) - psychometric analysis and evaluation of the construct. Psychosoc Med. 2013;10:Doc07.

62. Sole E, Castarlenas E, Miro J. A Catalan adaptation and validation of the pain catastrophizing scale for children. Psychol Assess. 2016;28(6):e119–26.

63. McWilliams LA, Kowal J, Wilson KG. Development and evaluation of short forms of the pain catastrophizing scale and the pain self-efficacy questionnaire. Eur J Pain. 2015;19(9):1342–9.

64. Nishigami T, Mibu A, Tanaka K, Yamashita Y, Watanabe A, Tanabe A. Psychometric properties of the Japanese version of short forms of the pain catastrophizing scale in participants with musculoskeletal pain: a cross-sectional study. J Orthop Sci. 2017;22(2):351–6.

65. Lundahl B, Moleni T, Burke BL, Butters R, Tollefson D, Butler C, et al. Motivational interviewing in medical care settings: a systematic review and meta-analysis of randomized controlled trials. Patient Edu Couns. 2013;93(2):157–68.

66. Stevens J, Hayes J, Pakalnis A. A randomized trial of telephone-based motivational interviewing for adolescent chronic headache with medication overuse. Cephalalgia. 2014;34(6):446–54.

67. Rollnick S, Miller WR, Butler CC. Motivational interviewing in health care: helping patients change behavior. New York (NY): Guilford Press; 2008.

68. Miller W, Rollnick S. Motivational interviewing: preparing people for change. New York (NY): Guilford Press; 2002.

69. Prochaska JO, DiClemente CC. Transtheoretical therapy: toward a more integrative model of change. Psychother Theor Res Pract. 1982;19(3):276–88.

70. Miller W, Rollnick S. Motivational interviewing: preparing people to change addictive behavior. New York (NY): Guilford Press; 1991.

71. Haas LJ, Leiser JP, Magill MK, Sanyer ON. Management of the difficult patient. Am Fam Physician. 2005;72(10):2063–8.

72. Cottrell CK, Drew JB, Waller SE, Holroyd KA, Brose JA, O'Donnell FJ. Perceptions and needs of patients with migraine: a focus group study. J Fam Pract. 2002;51(2):142–7.

73. Loder E. The approach to the difficult patient. Handb Clin Neurol. 2010;97:233–8.

74. Cho SJ, Chu MK. Risk factors of chronic daily headache or chronic migraine. Curr Pain Headache Rep. 2015;19(1):465.

75. Grazzi L. Behavioural approach to the "difficult" patient. Neurol Sci. 2008;29(S1):S96–8.

76. Rains JC, Lipchik GL, Penzien DB. Behavioral facilitation of medical treatment for headache–part 1: review of headache treatment compliance. Headache. 2006;46(9):1387–94.

77. Wilson AM, Melchert T, Anderson RC. Biofeedback facilitates greater pain control in a diverse sample of patients with chronic pain. Unpublished manuscript. 2018.

Collecting the History in the CDH Patients

Marius Birlea and Mark W. Green

Chronic daily headache (CDH), while being a great public health challenge and the "bread and butter" of specialized headache clinics, represents a symptom rather than a diagnosis. Although the classification remains intensely debated, the consensus is that the term CDH refers to headache disorders which are experienced 15 or more days a month [1]. Correct identification of the underlying headache etiology is necessary for treatment planning. The vast majority of CDH is attributable to "benign" primary headache disorders, not related to a structural or systemic illness. Nonetheless, practitioners need to be vigilant for secondary causes of headaches, and elimination of those causes is always the first step when a patient with CDH presents in the office of the physician [2]. A thorough history is the most critical aspect of the evaluation and provides the diagnosis in the vast majority of cases [3]. It is possible to classify virtually all chronic headache patients using the International Headache Society Classification of Headache Disorders (ICHD), currently third edition, with the final version in development, not available at the time of current publication [4]. Chapter 27 undertakes to review and summarize the classification of the chronic daily headache disorder. Patients with chronic headache may have multiple headache diagnoses, and correct application of the IHS classification implies that every type of headache in each patient should be classified. When retrospectively answering questions about their various headaches, patients often cannot distinguish between the types of headaches, and structured questionnaires, i.e., Bon Triage questionnaire, may be useful before the first clinic appointment [5]. The distinction between headache types is possible only through a carefully performed clinical interview, supplemented, when needed, by a headache diary [6]. The question "How long do the patient's individual headaches last if left untreated?" narrows the main primary CDH subtypes into two categories: (1) headaches that are short lasting (<4 h if untreated) and (2) those that are long lasting (>4 h if left untreated) [3]. Targeted questions to establish an anchor in time and subsequent temporal profile may help diagnose secondary headaches.

M. Birlea (✉)
Neurology, University of Colorado Denver School of Medicine, Aurora, CO, USA
e-mail: Marius.Birlea@ucdenver.edu

M. W. Green
Neurology, Icahn School of Medicine at Mt. Sinai, New York, NY, USA

Anesthesiology, Icahn School of Medicine at Mt. Sinai, New York, NY, USA

Rehabilitation Medicine, Icahn School of Medicine at Mt. Sinai, New York, NY, USA

© Springer International Publishing AG, part of Springer Nature 2019
M. W. Green et al. (eds.), *Chronic Headache*, https://doi.org/10.1007/978-3-319-91491-6_3

Classification of Chronic Daily Headache (CDH)

1. **Primary** Chronic Daily Headaches.
   - Primary CDH of long duration: Chronic migraine, chronic tension-type headache, new daily persistent headache, hemicrania continua, and nummular headache.
   - Primary CDH of short duration: Chronic cluster headache, chronic paroxysmal hemicrania, chronic short-lasting unilateral neuralgiform headache attacks (chronic SUNCT/SUNA), hypnic headache, and primary stabbing headache.
2. **Secondary** Chronic Daily Headaches.
   - CDH attributed to trauma: Persistent headache attributed to traumatic injury to the head.
   - CDH attributed to cervical or cranial vascular disorders.
   - CDH attributed to nonvascular intracranial disorder.
   - CDH attributed to high cerebrospinal fluid pressure.
   - CDH attributed to low cerebrospinal fluid pressure.
   - CDH attributed to intracranial neoplasia and other intracranial disorders.
   - CDH attributed to a substance or its withdrawal. Medication-overuse headache.
   - CDH attributed to infection: Intracranial and systemic infection.
   - CDH attributed to disorders of homeostasis.
   - CDH attributed to disorders of the cranium, neck, eyes, ears, nose, sinuses, teeth, mouth, or other facial or cervical structures.
   - CDH attributed to psychiatric disorders.
   - CDH attributed to painful cranial neuropathies and other facial pains.
   - CDH not elsewhere classified and chronic headache unspecified.

Chronic Primary Headaches

Primary CDH of Long Duration

Chronic Migraine (CM)

The most common primary (or secondary) chronic daily headache encountered in the practitioner's office or in emergency rooms is chronic migraine (CM). This is a headache occurring on ≥15 days per month for >3 months, which has the features of migraine headache for at least 8 days per month and there is no other explanation for it [4]. It is still underdiagnosed and undertreated [7]. In a recent representative study [8], the diagnosis of CM among those consulting was most likely to obtain be the correct diagnosis if symptoms were severe. Rates of diagnosis among consulters were far lower for CM (25%) than for episodic migraine, EM (87%). This difference suggests an unmet need for better CM diagnosis, particularly in primary care settings. Barriers associated with diagnosis may be addressed by encouraging HCPs to use screening tools for migraine and CM, such as the Identify (ID)-Migraine and ID-Chronic Migraine (ID-CM) [7, 8]. Patients with CM usually have a history of episodic migraine that began in their teens or 20s and has lasted for 10–20 years. In the majority, the "transformation" from episodic to CM is gradual, although the transition can be abrupt in ~ 30% of cases [3]. It is important to mention that, with treatment or spontaneously, patients with chronic migraine often reverts back to episodic migraine. Two forms of CM can be encountered in clinical practice: CM with continuous headache and CM with pain-free periods (near-daily headache); these two forms are not separately classified but are proposed in the Appendix of the ICHD-3 beta classification. There may also be constant fluctuating subtypes [9].

Chronic Tension-Type Headache (CTTH)

This is a disorder that usually, but not always, evolves from frequent episodic tension-type headache, gradually developing daily or almost daily episodes of headache, typically bilateral, pressing or tightening in quality and of mild to moderate intensity, lasting hours to days or unremitting. The pain does not worsen with routine physical activity, but may be associated with mild nausea, photophobia, or phonophobia [4]. A diagnosis of CM excludes the diagnosis of chronic tension-type headache (CTTH, "featureless headache") although there can be significant overlap and controversies regarding proper separation of these two conditions exist. CTTH can be associated or unassociated with pericranial tenderness, classified separately based on this criterion.

Hemicrania Continua (HC)

This is one of the trigeminal autonomic cephalalgias and is discussed with other conditions in the same group below.

New Daily Persistent Headache (NDPH)

This is a persistent headache for more than 3 months that became continuous and unremitting within 24 h from its onset, which is distinct and clearly recalled, and if the patient cannot do so, another diagnosis should be considered. The pain lacks pathognomonic features and may be migraine-like or tension-type-like or have elements of both. It typically occurs in individuals without a prior headache history. Nevertheless, patients with prior headache (episodic migraine or tension-type headache) are not excluded from this diagnosis, but they should not describe increasing headache frequency prior to onset. New daily persistent headache (NDPH) has two subforms: a self-limiting subform that typically resolves within several months without therapy and a refractory form that is resistant to aggressive treatment regimens. The diagnosis of new daily persistent headache is one of exclusion [10]. Secondary headaches such as headache attributed to infection, headache attributed to increased cerebrospinal fluid pressure, headache attributed to low cerebrospinal fluid pressure, and headache attributed to traumatic injury to the head and medication-overuse headache should be excluded by appropriate investigations.

Nummular Headache (NH)

This is a head pain of highly variable duration but is chronic (more than 3 months) in up to 75% of published cases, continuous or intermittent, present in a small circumscribed area of the scalp (1–6 cm diameter), and fixed in size and shape. The painful area can be localized in any part of the scalp but is most common in the parietal region. Rarely, nummular headache is bi- or multifocal, each symptomatic area retaining all the characteristics of nummular headache. The pain intensity is generally mild to moderate but occasionally severe. Superimposed on the background pain, spontaneous or triggered exacerbations may occur. Other causes, in particular meningeal, bone, scalp, and skin lesions, must be excluded by history, physical examination, and appropriate investigations [4].

Primary CDHs of Short Duration

Chronic trigeminal autonomic cephalalgias (TACs) share historical and other diagnostic features that also includes with several additional entities of like hypnic headache and primary stabbing headache. Primary cranial neuralgias that consist of short-lasting recurrent attacks of head/face pain without autonomic symptoms are described at the end of the chapter. Chronic trigeminal autonomic cephalalgias (TACs) represent a group of unilateral headache disorders, associated with autonomic symptoms, separated from each other by criteria of frequency and duration with the exception of hemicrania continua; they generally consist of attacks of severe strictly unilateral pain which is orbital, supraorbital, temporal, or any combination of these sites. The pain is associated with at least one of the following: ipsilateral conjunctival injection, lacrimation, nasal congestion, rhinorrhea, forehead and facial sweating, miosis, ptosis and/or eyelid edema, and/or restlessness or agitation (cluster headache). Episodic forms of TACs exist and may be more frequent than the chronic ones. The TACs are sufficiently rare that any time a TAC is encountered clinically, secondary causes need to be considered and appropriately investigated [11].

Chronic Cluster Headache (CCH)

Patients with chronic cluster headache present with head pain attacks that last 15–180 min and occur from once every other day to eight times a day. The pain, which is strictly unilateral, is associated, ipsilaterally, with at least one of the autonomic symptoms described above. Chronic cluster headache attacks occur for more than 1 year without remission or with remission periods lasting less than 1 month. Chronic cluster headache may arise de novo (previously referred to as "primary chronic cluster headache") or evolve from episodic cluster headache (previously "secondary chronic cluster headache") [4]. In some patients, chronic cluster headache can revert to episodic cluster headache, with remissions longer than 1 month.

Chronic Paroxysmal Hemicranias (CPH)

The CPH attacks last 2–30 min, occur several or many times a day, and are associated with at least one of the autonomic symptoms described for chronic cluster headache above. They occur without a remission period, or with remissions lasting <1 month, for at least 1 year. Characteristically, indomethacin prevents the attacks. There are rare patients who present with both CPH and trigeminal neuralgia (sometimes referred to as CPH-tic syndrome). This recognition is important since both disorders may require treatment [4].

Chronic Short-Lasting Unilateral Neuralgiform Headache Attacks

There are two chronic trigeminal autonomic cephalalgias characterized by high frequency, short duration, and not more than two autonomic symptoms – conjunctival injection and tearing – chronic short-lasting unilateral neuralgiform headache with conjunctival injection and tearing (SUNCT) and chronic short-lasting unilateral neuralgiform headache with cranial autonomic symptoms (SUNA).

SUNCT is characterized by pain attacks lasting between 1 and 600 s, at least once a day for at least half the time, and at least 20 such attacks have occurred. Attacks of chronic SUNCT occur for more than 1 year without remission or with remission periods lasting less than 1 month. Often such attacks occur tens to hundreds per day, as single stabs, series of stabs, or in a saw-tooth pattern.

SUNA resembles SUNCT except either conjunctival injection or lacrimation (tearing) or both are absent.

Hemicrania Continua (HC)

This is a trigeminal autonomic cephalalgia presenting with a persistent, strictly unilateral headache for at least 1 year, rather than separate attacks. The headache, like in chronic cluster headache or chronic paroxysmal hemicrania with which HC can overlap, is associated with at least one of the following ipsilateral autonomic symptoms: conjunctival injection, lacrimation, nasal congestion, rhinorrhea, forehead and facial sweating, miosis, ptosis and/or eyelid edema, and/or restlessness or agitation. HC can have pain that is not continuous but is interrupted by remission periods of at least 1 day, or it can be daily and continuous [4]. The headache in HC is highly sensitive to indomethacin, which should be initiated anytime when the diagnosis of HC is suspected; the response to indomethacin should be absolute, 100% [2].

The differentiating clinical characteristics of the TACs are presented in Table 3.1.

Table 3.1 Chronic trigeminal autonomic cephalalgias: clinical characteristics

Disorder	Duration	Frequency	Location	Character
Chronic cluster headache (CCH)	15–180 min	Every other day to 8/day	Orbital, frontal, temporal, extracephalic	Very severe, boring
Chronic paroxysmal hemicrania (CPH)	2–30 min	1–40/day	Orbital, frontal, temporal	Very severe, boring, throbbing
Chronic SUNCT SUNA	1–600 s	Dozens to hundreds per day	Orbital, frontal	Very severe, burning, stabbing
Hemicrania continua (HC)	Continuous	Continuous	Orbital, frontal	Moderate, with spikes in severity

Hypnic Headache (HH)

HH presents with recurring headache attacks, occurring on at least 10 days/month for more than 3 months, developing only during sleep, causing wakening. Attacks usually last from 15 to 180 min, although longer than 4 h duration has also been described. Most cases are persistent, with daily or near-daily headaches, but an episodic subform (less than 15 days per month) may occur. HH usually begins after age 50 years but may be encountered in younger people. The pain is usually mild to moderate, although severe pain is reported by one-fifth of patients and some patients experienced nausea during attacks. Pain is bilateral in about two-thirds of cases. Other possible causes of headache developing during and causing wakening from sleep should be excluded, in particular sleep apnea, nocturnal hypertension, hypoglycemia, and medication overuse; intracranial disorders must also be excluded. However, the presence of sleep apnea syndrome does not necessarily exclude the diagnosis of hypnic headache [4].

Primary Stabbing Headache (PSH)

PSH is characterized by transient and localized stabs of pain in the head, lasting seconds and occurring spontaneously in the absence of organic cranial disease. Stabs recur with irregular frequency, generally low, one or a few per day. No cranial autonomic symptoms occur, which aids in differentiating PSH from chronic SUNA. It may move from one area to another, in either the same or the opposite hemicranium. When stabs are strictly localized to one area, structural changes at this site and in the distribution of the affected cranial nerve must be excluded. Primary stabbing headache is more commonly experienced by people with migraine, in which case stabs tend to be localized to the site habitually affected by migraine headaches [4].

Secondary Chronic Daily Headaches

Typically, a secondary headache is diagnosed when a headache occurs de novo in close temporal relationship with another disorder able to cause headache. This remains true even when the headache has the characteristics of a primary headache and has a chronic course (migraine, tension-type headache, trigeminal autonomic cephalalgias, or another primary headache). When a preexisting primary headache becomes chronic in close temporal relation to such a causative disorder, both the primary and the secondary diagnoses should be given, provided that there is good evidence that the disorder can cause headache. This evidence of causation can be clinical (i.e., orthostatic headache in patients with low cerebrospinal fluid pressure/volume) or based on investigations (i.e., imaging in patients with brain tumors or elevated erythrocyte sedimentation rate in patients with giant-cell arteritis) [4]. Below are the most frequent known secondary chronic daily headaches.

CDH Attributed to Trauma

Persistent Headache Attributed to Traumatic Injury to the Head

This is a headache that began within 7 days of a head trauma (or within 7 days after discontinuation of medication (s) that impaired ability to sense or report headache following the injury to the head) and lasted more than 3 months. The trauma can be a direct blow to the head, whiplash injury, or craniotomy (about a quarter of patients develop persistent headache after craniotomy). Interestingly, the persistence of headache is inversely correlated with the severity of head trauma [10]. When headache following head injury becomes persistent, the possibility of another secondary headache should be considered, including medication-overuse headache.

CDH Attributed to Cranial Vascular Disorders

CDH Attributed to Giant-Cell Arteritis (GCA)

Headache may be the sole symptom of GCA, but other symptoms (i.e., polymyalgia rheumatica, jaw claudication) usually accompany it. The variability in the features of the headache attributed to GCA and in other symptoms of GCA is such that any recent persistent headache in a patient over 60 years of age should raise concern for GCA and lead to appropriate investigations [4] and treatment rapidly administered. Duration of headache and the need for corticosteroid treatment often extend for months to years. Headache of giant-cell arteritis is due to inflammation of the cranial arteries, especially branches of the external carotid artery. Recent repeated attacks of amaurosis fugax associated with headache are suggestive of GCA and should prompt urgent investigations, due to risk of severe complications, especially the major risk of blindness. The main risk after vision loss in one eye, usually irreversible, is vision loss in the other eye. Patients with GCA are also at risk of cerebral ischemic events and of dementia. Since this condition can affect arteries that are peridural, other organ systems can suffer infarctions.

Chronic Headache Attributed to Reversible Cerebral Vasoconstriction Syndrome (RCVS)

Headache caused by reversible cerebral vasoconstriction syndrome can be the sole symptom of RCVS and typically manifest with recurring thunderclap headache up to 12 weeks, often triggered by sexual activity, exertion, certain medications, Valsalva maneuvers, or emotion [4]. Recent studies indicate that, in a significant proportion of cases, patients go on to develop chronic daily headache, without the thunderclap appearance but with features that are similar to chronic migraine, chronic tension-type, or other primary headaches, including medication-overuse headache [12].

CDH Attributed to Intracranial Nonvascular Disorders

Chronic Headache Attributed to Increased Cerebrospinal Fluid Pressure

Idiopathic intracranial hypertension (IIH) or "pseudotumor cerebri" is the headache type that is caused by spontaneously increased cerebrospinal fluid (CSF) pressure, usually accompanied by other symptoms and/or clinical signs of increased intracranial pressure, especially papilledema. Idiopathic intracranial hypertension may or may not have an identifiable cause. Elevated CSF pressure can also occur as a result of cerebral venous sinus thrombosis, various medications, or other medical conditions such as renal disease or endocrinopathies. The cerebrospinal fluid opening pressure is more than 250 mm CSF, carefully measured in lateral decubitus. Although more common in obese females, IIH can also occur in nonobese males. The presence of transient visual obscurations and intracranial noises may provide clues [3]. The headache often remits after normalization of CSF pressure but may require prolonged and comprehensive chronic daily headache management based on the phenotype of the headache.

Chronic Headache Attributed to Low Cerebrospinal Fluid Pressure/Volume

Spontaneous intracranial hypotension: This headache occurs due to low cerebrospinal fluid (CSF) pressure/volume or CSF leakage, usually accompanied by neck pain/stiffness, tinnitus, changes in hearing, photophobia, and nausea. Headache that significantly worsens soon after sitting upright or standing and/or improves after lying horizontally is likely to be caused by low CSF pressure, but this cannot be relied upon as a diagnostic criterion [4]. Typically, the cerebrospinal fluid pressure is lower than 60 mm CSF and successful sealing of the CSF leak usually resolves the headache. This headache diagnosis is usually delayed and follows a chronic course. The orthostatic nature of the headache can be prominent initially but may become less obvious over time. Occasionally, orthostatic headache is never present, and patients may notice that their headaches begin and increase gradually after rising in the morning [3] or the positional component is even paradoxical. In that case it is necessary to go back and review the history and early imaging to ensure that a cause for a presumable spontaneous intracranial hypotension was not missed [13].

Chronic Headache Attributed to Intracranial Neoplasia

This type of headache is caused by an intracranial neoplasm, in the absence of a primary chronic headache disorder or making a preexistent primary disorder chronic. A pattern of a progressive headache, often worse in the morning, is usually elicited. Not uncommonly, the headache caused by intracranial tumors mimics a primary headache clinically [14].

Chronic Headache Attributed to Chiari Malformation Type I (CM1)

Headache caused by Chiari type I malformation is usually occipital or suboccipital, of short duration (less than 5 min), and provoked by cough or other Valsalva-like maneuvers. Almost all (95%) patients with CM1 report a constellation of five or more distinct symptoms. If headache is due to Chiari malformation, it remits after the successful treatment of this congenital condition [4]. Evidence of headache causation, based on specific ICHD-3 beta criteria, are required as CM1 is often asymptomatic and decompressive surgery is not indicated and has significant potential for morbidity. Cerebrospinal fluid leak, which can mimic CM1, needs to be excluded.

Chronic Headache Attributed to Noninfectious Inflammatory Disease

This type of headache occurs in the presence of a noninfectious inflammatory intracranial disease, usually with lymphocytic pleocytosis in the cerebrospinal fluid. It remits after resolution of the inflammatory disorder. Examples of conditions that can be suspected include chronic inflammatory conditions like neurosarcoidosis, lupus, Behcet's syndrome, autoimmune encephalitis, and others [4].

CDH Attributed to Long-Term Use of Medications

Chronic Headache Attributed to Long-Term Use of Non-Headache Medication

This headache type is present on more than 15 days per month and develops as an adverse event during long-term use of a medication taken for purposes other than the treatment of headache and is not necessarily reversible. Evidence of causation is required as follows: headache has developed in temporal relation to the commencement of medication intake and one or more of the following: headache has significantly worsened after an increase in dosage of the medication, or headache has significantly improved or resolved after a reduction in dosage or cessation of the medication, and the medication is recognized to cause headache [4]. Some common medications causing headache include monoamine oxidase inhibitors, calcium channel blockers, nonsteroidal anti-inflammatory agents, caffeine, ranitidine, estrogen compounds, and vasopressor agents [15].

Medication-Overuse Headache (MOH)

This is a headache occurring in 15 or more days per month, developing as a consequence of regular overuse of acute or symptomatic headache medication (on 10 or more or 15 or more days per month, depending on the overused medication) for more than 3 months. By current definition, it has to occur in a patient with a preexisting headache disorder. Among those with a previous primary headache diagnosis, most have migraine or tension-type headache (or both); only a small minority has other primary headache diagnoses such as chronic cluster headache or new daily persistent headache.

It usually, but not invariably, resolves after the overuse is stopped but may take time. In almost all cases, this necessitates diary follow-up [4]. The diagnosis of medication-overuse headache is extremely important. Approximately half of people with headache on 15 or more days per month for more than 3 months have MOH, and they constitute a large proportion of the patients presenting to headache clinics. Prevention of MOH is especially important in patients prone to frequent headaches that are likely to consume frequent medications. Medication overuse may be responsible, in part for the transformation of episodic migraine into chronic migraine and for the perpetuation of the syndrome [9]. However, medication-overuse headache is an interaction between a therapeutic agent used excessively and a susceptible patient. There is growing interest and research in this area, and this is reflected in the ongoing scholarly controversy about whether symptomatic overuse is a cause or a consequence of CDH [3].

CDH Attributed to Infections

CDH Attributed to Intracranial Infections

Chronic headache attributed to bacterial meningitis or meningoencephalitis: This is a headache that has been present for >3 months and fulfills criteria for headache attributed to bacterial meningitis or meningoencephalitis and in which bacterial meningitis or meningoencephalitis remains active or has resolved within the last 3 months [4].

Chronic headache attributed to intracranial fungal or other parasitic infection: This type of headache fulfills criteria for headache attributed to intracranial fungal or other parasitic infection, in which the intracranial fungal or other parasitic infection remains active or has resolved within the last 3 months. The headache has been present for >3 months. Examples include coccidioidomycosis, neurocysticercosis, aspergillosis, and cryptococcosis [16].

CDH Attributed to Systemic Infections

Chronic headache attributed to systemic bacterial infection. Chronic headache attributed to systemic viral infection. Chronic headache attributed to other systemic infection.

This type of headache is present for >3 months and fulfills criteria for headache attributed to bacterial, viral, or other systemic infection, in which the systemic infection remains active or has resolved within the last 3 months. Examples include Lyme disease, tuberculosis, or HIV [4].

CDH Attributed to Disorders of Homeostasis

Chronic Headache Attributed to Sleep Apnea

This is a morning headache, occurring on more than 15 days/month, usually bilateral and with a duration of less than 4 hours, caused by sleep apnea, and resolving with successful treatment of sleep apnea. A definitive diagnosis requires overnight polysomnography. Obstructive sleep apnea frequently leads to daily headaches upon awakening and should be considered in patients with a snoring history, large neck size, or obesity. Although morning headache is significantly more common in patients with sleep apnea than in the general population, headache present upon awakening is a nonspecific symptom which occurs in a variety of primary and secondary headache disorders, in sleep-related respiratory disorders other than sleep apnea (e.g., Pickwickian syndrome, chronic obstructive pulmonary disorder), and in other primary sleep disorders such as periodic leg movements of sleep [4].

Chronic Headache Attributed to Hypothyroidism

This is an uncommon type of headache, usually bilateral, non-pulsatile, and constant, in patients with hypothyroidism and remitting after normalization of thyroid hormone levels. It may follow a chronic course if not recognized and treated timely. There is a female preponderance and often a history of migraine in childhood [4, 17, 18].

CDH or Chronic Facial Pain Attributed to Disorder of the Cranium, Neck, Eyes, Ears, Nose, Sinuses, Teeth, Mouth, or Other Facial or Cervical Structures.

Chronic Headache Attributed to Disorder of Cranial Bone

This type of headache can appear in patients with chronic bone diseases like osteomyelitis, multiple myeloma, or Paget disease and may lead to diagnosis of such conditions [4].

Cervicogenic Headache

This CDH, typically unilateral, is caused by a disorder of the cervical spine and its component bony, disc, and/or soft tissue elements, usually but not invariably accompanied by neck pain. The diagnosis requires evidence of a lesion within the cervical spine or soft tissues of the neck, known to cause headache, and also evidence of causation: temporal relationship, reduced cervical range of motion, and headache made significantly worse by provocative maneuvers. The headache is abolished following diagnostic blockade of a cervical structure or its nerve supply. This needs to be distinguished in particular from migraine and tension-type headache or from the rarer TACs. Cervical spondylosis and osteochondritis may or may not be valid causes of cervicogenic headache [4]. Cervicogenic headache remains a controversial diagnosis, at the boundary between medical/surgical specialties.

Chronic Headache Attributed to Retropharyngeal Tendonitis

This is a headache caused by inflammation or calcification in the retropharyngeal soft tissues and usually brought on by stretching or compression of upper cervical prevertebral muscles and/or swallowing [4]. Upper carotid dissection (or another lesion in or around the carotid artery) should be excluded as well as disorders of other structures in the head and neck, i.e., Eagle syndrome [19].

Chronic Headache Attributed to Craniocervical Dystonia

This is a headache caused by dystonia involving neck muscles, with abnormal movements or defective posturing of the neck or head due to muscular hyperactivity. Headache location corresponds to the location of the dystonic muscle(s) [4].

Chronic Headache Attributed to Chronic or Recurring Rhinosinusitis

This type of headache is caused by a chronic infectious or inflammatory disorder of the paranasal sinuses and associated with other symptoms and/or clinical signs of the disorder. It is controversial whether chronic sinus pathology can produce persistent headache. Recent studies seem to support such causation [4]. Sphenoid sinusitis may masquerade as an intractable headache, unresponsive to analgesics and interfering with sleep, and can occur without associated nasal symptoms [9].

Chronic Headache Attributed to Temporomandibular Disorder (TMD)

This headache type is caused by a disorder involving structures in the temporomandibular region. The head pain is produced or exacerbated by active jaw movements and, when unilateral, is ipsilateral to the side of the temporomandibular disorder. It is usually most prominent in the preauricular areas of the face, masseter muscles, and/or temporal regions. A review of a large group of patients with TMD found that their headache could be attributed to this condition in only 5.1% of cases [20].

Chronic Headache Attributed to Other Disorders of the Cranium, Neck, Eyes, Ears, Nose, Sinuses, and Teeth

This is a headache and/or facial pain caused by a disorder, known to cause headache, of the cranium, neck, eyes, ears, nose, sinuses, teeth, mouth, or other facial or cervical structures not described above. Attention should be paid during the history and physical examination to exclude cervical spine, temporomandibular joint (TMJ), or dental pathology as the culprit in chronic cranial, nuchal, or facial pain [3].

CDH Headache Attributed to Psychiatric Disorders

Chronic Headache Attributed to Somatization Disorder (Currently Somatic Symptom Disorder in DSM-5)

This type of headache occurs as part of the symptomatic presentation of a somatization disorder including all of the following: at least four pain symptoms, two gastrointestinal symptoms, one sexual (other than pain), and one pseudoneurological. The patient's suffering is authentic, whether or not it is medically explained. Patients typically experience distress and a high level of functional impairment. The symptoms may or may not accompany diagnosed general medical disorders or psychiatric disorders. There may be a high level of medical care utilization, which rarely alleviates the patient's concerns [4].

Painful Cranial Neuropathies and Other Facial Pains

Classical Trigeminal Neuralgia

The classical type of trigeminal neuralgia commonly develops without apparent cause other than neurovascular compression. It is diagnosed when at least three attacks of unilateral facial pain have occurred in one or more divisions of the trigeminal nerve, with no radiation beyond the trigeminal distribution. Classical trigeminal neuralgia usually appears in the second or third divisions of that nerve. Pain has at least three of the following four characteristics: recurring in paroxysmal attacks lasting from a fraction of a second to 2 minutes; severe intensity; electric shock-like, shooting, stabbing, or sharp in quality; and precipitated by innocuous stimuli to the affected side of the face. Some attacks may be, or appear to be, spontaneous, but there must be at least three that are precipitated in this way to meet this criterion. Following a painful paroxysm, there is usually a refractory period during which pain cannot be triggered [4]. Often, there is a slight ipsilateral focal muscle twitch simultaneous with pain paroxysm—tic douloureux. The pain never crosses to the opposite side, but it may rarely occur bilaterally (especially in multiple sclerosis). Mild autonomic symptoms such as lacrimation and/or redness of the eye may occasionally be present, but they are typically absent. The duration of pain attacks can change over time and become more prolonged as well as severe, often leading to weight loss and even suicide. Evolution is unpredictable, but, between paroxysms, most patients are asymptomatic, and spontaneous remissions can occur.

Postherpetic Trigeminal Neuropathy (Trigeminal PHN)

This type of chronic headache is characterized by a unilateral head and/or facial pain persisting or recurring for at least 3 months in the distribution of one or more branches of the trigeminal nerve, with variable sensory changes, caused by herpes zoster virus. It is more prevalent in the elderly and involves the first division of the trigeminal nerve most commonly, as opposed to classical trigeminal neuralgia [4]. Postherpetic trigeminal neuropathy is associated with three different types of pain: a constant deep aching and burning pain; an intermittent, transient pain with a sharp, jabbing, or electric shock-like quality; and a sharp, radiating dysesthesia triggered by light tactile stimulation of specific trigger areas (allodynia) [21].

Chronic Occipital Neuralgia

This is a unilateral or bilateral paroxysmal, shooting, or stabbing pain in the posterior part of the scalp, in the distribution of the greater, lesser, or third occipital nerves, sometimes accompanied by diminished sensation or dysesthesia in the affected area and commonly associated with tenderness over the involved nerve(s). This must be distinguished from occipital referral of pain arising from the atlantoaxial or upper zygapophyseal joints or from tender trigger points in neck muscles or their insertions [4]. Occipital neuralgia occurs rarely and is probably overdiagnosed.

Burning Mouth Syndrome (BMS)

This represents an intraoral burning or synesthetic sensation, recurring daily for more than 2 h per day more than 3 months, without clinically evident causative lesions. The pain is usually bilateral, and its intensity fluctuates. The most common site is the tip of the tongue. Subjective dryness of the mouth, dysesthesia, and altered taste may be present. There is a high menopausal female prevalence, and some studies show comorbid psychosocial and psychiatric disorders [4, 22]. There may be multiple local or systemic causes for the BMS (like candidiasis, lichen planus, hyposalivation, medication-induced anemia, deficiencies of vitamin B12 or folic acid, Sjögren's syndrome, diabetes) and even infections, like alpha-herpes viruses [23].

Persistent Idiopathic Facial Pain (PIFP)

This headache type was previously called "atypical facial pain." It consists of persistent facial and/or oral pain, with varying presentations but recurring daily for more than 2 h per day more than 3 months, in the absence of clinical neurological deficit. Persistent idiopathic facial pain

(PIFP) may originate from a minor operation or injury to the face, maxillae, teeth, or gums but persists after healing of the initial noxious event and without any demonstrable local cause. The pain of PIFP can have sharp exacerbations and is aggravated by stress. The pain may be described as either deep or superficial. With time, it may spread to a wider area of the craniocervical region [4]. An active dental cause has to be excluded by appropriate investigations, and thorough knowledge of the trigeminal nerve anatomy is required [11].

Chronic Central Poststroke Pain (CPSP)

This type of headache is usually a unilateral facial and/or head pain, with varying presentations involving parts or all of the craniocervical region and associated with impaired sensation, occurring within 6 months and caused by a stroke. It is not explained by a lesion of the peripheral trigeminal or other cranial or cervical nerves. Symptoms may also involve the trunk and limbs of the affected side [4]. Craniocervical pain following a thalamic or lateral medullary lesion is usually part of specific sensory syndromes.

References

1. Silberstein SD, Lipton RD, Saper JR. Chronic daily headache. In: Silberstein SD, Lipton RD, Dodick DW, editors. Wolff's headache. 8th ed. New York: Raven Press; 2008. p. 315–77.
2. Tepper S, Tepper D. Diagnosis of primary chronic daily headaches. In: Tepper S, Tepper DE, editors. The Cleveland clinic manual of headache therapy. 2nd ed. Heidelberg New York Dordrecht London: Springer; 2014. p. 49.
3. Gladstone J, Eross E, Dodick D. Chronic daily headache: a rational approach to a challenging problem. Semin Neurol. 2003;23(3):265–75.
4. Headache Classification Committee of the International Headache Society (IHS). The international classification of headache disorders, 3rd edition (beta version). Cephalalgia. 2013;36(3):630–808.
5. Cowan PR, Rapoport A, Blythe J. Comprehensive clinical report [Internet]. Available from http://www.bontriage.com
6. Olesen J, Rasmussen BK. The international headache society classification of chronic daily and near-daily headaches: a critique of the criticism. Cephalalgia. 1996;16(6):407–11.
7. Lipton RB, Serrano D, Buse DC, Pavlovic JM, et al. Improving the detection of chronic migraine: development and validation of identify chronic migraine (ID-CM). Cephalalgia. 2016;36(3):203–15.
8. Dodick DW, Loder EW, Manack Adams A, Buse DC, Fanning KM, Reed ML, Lipton RB. Assessing barriers to chronic migraine consultation, diagnosis and treatment: results from the chronic migraine epidemiology and outcomes (CAMEO) study. Headache. 2016;56(5):821–34.
9. Dodick DW, Silberstein SD. Chronic migraine. In: Dodick DW, Silberstein SD, editors. Migraine. 3rd ed. New York: Oxford University Press; 2016. p. 193–242.
10. Jensen R, Olesen J. Other refractory headaches: chronic tension-type headache, new daily persistent headache, cluster headache and other trigeminal autonomic cephalalgias, and posttraumatic headache. In: Schulman EA, Levin M, Lake III AE, Loder E, editors. Refractory migraine mechanism and management. New York: Oxford University Press; 2010. p. 373–96.
11. Purdy A. Differential diagnosis and investigation of refractory headache. In: Schulman EA, Levin M, Lake III AE, Loder E, editors. Refractory migraine mechanism and management. New York: Oxford University Press; 2010. p. 69–79.
12. John S, Singha AB, Calabrese L, Uchino K, Hammad T, Tepper S, Stillman M, Mills B, Thankachan T, Hajj-Ali RA. Long-term outcomes after reversible cerebral vasoconstriction syndrome. Cephalalgia. 2016;36(4):387–94.
13. Mokri B. Low cerebrospinal headache syndromes. Neurol Clin. 2004;22(1):55–74.
14. Forsyth PA, Posner JB. Headaches in patients with brain tumors: a study of 111 patients. Neurology. 1993;43(9):1678–83.
15. Lipton RB, Saper JR, Silberstein SD. Turning treatment failure into treatment success. In: Silberstein SD, Lipton RD, Dodick DW, editors. Wolff's headache. 8th ed. New York: Raven Press; 2008. p. 793–803.
16. Baldwin K, Whiting C. Chronic meningitis: simplifying a diagnostic challenge. Curr Neurol Neurosci Rep. 2016;16(3):30. https://doi.org/10.1007/s11910-016-0630-0.
17. Lima Carvalho MF, de Medeiros JS, Valenca MM. Headache in recent onset hypothyroidism: prevalence, characteristics and outcome after treatment with levothyroxine. Cephalgia. 2016;37(10):938–46. pii: 0333102416658714. [Epub ahead of print]
18. Moreau T, Manceau E, Giroud-Baleydier F, Giroud M. Headache in hypothyroidism. Prevalence and outcome under thyroid hormone therapy. Cephalalgia. 1998;18(10):687–9.
19. Badhey A, Jategaonkar A, Angliin Kovacs AJ, Kadakia S, De Deyn PP, Ducic Y, Schantz S, Shin E. Eagle syndrome: a comprehensive review. Clin Neurol Neurosurg. 2017;159:34–8.

20. Di Paolo C, D'Urso A, Papi P, Di Sabato F, Rosella D, Pompa G, Polimeni A. Temporomandibular disorders and headache: a retrospective analysis of 1198 patients. Pain Res Manag. 2017;2017:3203027. https://doi.org/10.1155/2017/3203027. Epub 2017 Mar 21

21. Fromm GH. Facial pain with herpes zoster and postherpetic neuralgia and a comparison with trigeminal neuralgia. In: Herpes zoster and Postherpetic neuralgia. 2nd ed. Amsterdam: Elsevier; 2001. p. 151–9.

22. Jääskeläinen SK, Woda A. Burning mouth syndrome. Cephalalgia. 2017;37(7):627–47.

23. Nagel MA, Gilden D. Burning mouth syndrome associated with varicella zoster virus. BMJ Case Rep. 2016;2016:bcr2016215953. https://doi.org/10.1136/bcr-2016-215953.

Chronic Migraine: Epidemiology, Mechanisms, and Treatment

Teshamae S. Monteith

Chronic Migraine: Diagnosis and Classification

Chronic migraine is a highly disabling primary headache disorders that accounts for the greatest portion of chronic daily headache [1]. Chronic migraine differs from episodic migraine by the frequency of headache days and associated symptoms, and it has been suggested that chronic migraine represents one end of the clinical spectrum [2]. According to the International Classification of Headache Disorders-3 (ICHD-3), chronic migraine is diagnosed in individuals that have headaches that occur at least 15 days per month for more than 3 months (Table 4.1) [3, 4]. Eight of the days must have features of migraine with or without aura, which includes sensitivity to sensory stimulation, throbbing headache, and gastrointestinal symptoms (nausea). Although not a part of the official classification, non-headache symptoms including fatigue, cognitive impairment, mood disturbance, neck pain, brainstem symptoms, and other systemic symptoms may be present and can be equally disabling. The premonitory and postdrome phase of a migraine attacks occurs before and after headache, respectively; these phases are often lost or less distinct in individuals with chronic migraine. Alternative

criteria in the appendix section of the ICHD-3 include chronic migraine with pain-free periods versus chronic migraine with continuous pain. Overall, the classification system can be both useful for both clinical and research purposes; however, there are limitations and a continued need for a biologically driven approach to identify clinically relevant heterogeneity in chronic migraine.

Chronic migraine is no longer considered a complication of migraine and is recognized in individuals that have had at least five attacks fulfilling criteria for migraine with/or without aura. The diagnosis allows for the patient perception of migraine at the onset if relieved by migraine-specific abortive treatments, such as triptans and ergotamine derivatives, so that treatment does not limit the diagnosis. Patient perception has been included because associated features vary during the day and it is difficult to keep a patient medication-free to determine the natural history of an attack. Medication overuse of acute analgesics often occurs with chronic migraine. In the previous ICHD-2R classification system, medication overuse headache had to be excluded before the diagnosis of chronic migraine could be made [5]. According to revised ICHD-3, the presence of medication overuse headache no longer excludes a diagnosis of chronic migraine; both should be coded together when present. Medication overuse headache will be discussed elsewhere in this book (Chap. 14).

In clinical practice, chronic migraine is often underdiagnosed and undertreated. There are several reasons why this may be the case. Patients

T. S. Monteith
Department of Neurology, Miller School of Medicine, University of Miami, Miami, FL, USA
e-mail: tmonteith@med.miami.edu

© Springer International Publishing AG, part of Springer Nature 2019
M. W. Green et al. (eds.), *Chronic Headache*, https://doi.org/10.1007/978-3-319-91491-6_4

Table 4.1 Diagnostic criteria for transformed migraine and chronic migraine

ICHD-3 episodic migraine	Silberstein-Lipton TM	ICHD-2R chronic migraine	ICHD-3 chronic migraine

A. At least five attacks fulfilling criteria B–D
B. Headache attacks lasting 4–72 h (untreated or unsuccessfully treated)
C. Headache has at least two of the following four characteristics:
  1. Unilateral location
  2. Pulsating quality
  3. Moderate or severe pain intensity
  4. Aggravation by or causing avoidance of routine physical activity (e.g., walking or climbing stairs)
D. During headache at least one of the following:
  1. Nausea and/or vomiting
  2. Photophobia and phonophobia
E. Not better accounted for by another ICHD-3 diagnosis
	Daily or almost daily (>15 days a month) head pain for >1 month
	Average headache duration of >4 h (if untreated)
	At least one of the following:
	  History of episodic migraine meeting any IHS criterion 1.1–1.6
	  History of increasing headache frequency with decreasing severity of migrainous features over at least 3 months
	Headache at some time meets IHS criteria for migraine 1.1–1.6 other than duration
	Does not meet criteria for new daily persistent headache (4.7) or hemicrania continua (4.8)
		Headache on ≥15 days/month for 3 months
		Occurring in a patient who has had at least five attacks fulfilling criteria for 1.1 migraine without aura
		On ≥8 days per month, for at least 3 months, headache fulfills criteria for migraine C1 and/or C2 below, that is, has fulfilled criteria for pain and associated symptoms of migraine without aura
		Has at least two of a–d:
		(a) Unilateral location
		(b) Pulsating quality
		(c) Moderate or severe pain intensity
		(d) Aggravated by or causing avoidance of routine physical activity and at least one of a or b
		  (a) Nausea and/or vomiting
		  (b) Photophobia and phonophobia
		Treated or relieved with triptans or ergotamine before the expected development of C1 above
		No medication overuse and not attributable to other causative disorder
			Headache on ≥15 days per month for at least 3 months
			Occurring in a patient who has had at least five attacks fulfilling criteria for 1.1 migraine without aura and/or 1.2 *migraine with aura*
			On ≥8 days per month for at least 3 months 1 or more of the following criteria were fulfilled
			Criteria C and D for 1.1 *migraine without aura*
			Criteria B and C for 1.2 *migraine with aura*
			Headache considered by patient to be onset migraine and relieved by a triptan or an ergotamine derivative
			Not better accounted for by another ICHD-3 diagnosis

The diagnostic criteria for chronic migraine have evolved over time and results in variability in estimated prevalence globally. The chart is adapted from Silberstein et al. Headache 2014 [4]. Episodic migraine refers to migraine occurring <15 days per month and can be further divided into low-frequency migraine (1–4 days per month) and high-frequency migraine (10–14 days per month)

sometimes report only the most severe headaches, while minimizing relatively mild to moderate headache days [6]. The diagnosis may also be a challenge to make because migraine-associated symptoms may be reduced over time or be so mild that they are not diagnosed as having migraine. The Lipton-Silberstein classification system defines transformed migraine when individuals have headache 15 or more headache days per month (not necessarily migraine), with a current or past history of migraine [7]. Transformed migraine may be diagnosed in patients that would otherwise be classified as chronic tension-type headache and migraine [4]. Transformed migraine is not recognized in the ICHD-3 classification; however, some

data support the observation that non-migraine headache may increase in frequency as the illness progresses so that transformed migraine may be a transitional stage of chronification [8].

Currently, there is no universally accepted objective test for the diagnosis of chronic migraine. The best accepted methods for the diagnosis of chronic migraine, in addition to self-reported history, are migraine diaries, which are often associated with poor compliance, missing data, and recall bias. As chronic migraine is underdiagnosed, several attempts have been made to improve the detection. Identify Chronic Migraine (ID-CM) is a simple self-administered tool that is both sensitive and specific and facilitates the accurate diagnosis of most people with chronic migraine [9]. Automated migraine classification with machine learning techniques have also been developed for use in patients undergoing magnetic resonance imaging with diffusion tensor imaging [10]. Early results found that pain, analgesics, and left uncinate nuclei, an area that connects pain with emotions, were most useful for classification. According to a meta-analysis of CSF and blood samples of chronic migraine, the most robust findings for biochemical markers include increased glutamate, calcitonin gene-related peptide (CGRP), nerve growth factor, and decreased beta-endorphin [11]. Pituitary adenylate cyclase-activating polypeptide (PACAP) appears to play a role in nociception and migraine, although an early study showed no change in interictal PACAP levels in the peripheral blood of women with chronic migraine [12]. Widely accepted and systematic detection methods with high rates of accuracy are lacking.

Epidemiology and Impact

Chronic migraine is a debilitating primary headache disorder affecting 1.4–2.2% [1] of the population and is associated with a higher headache impact when compared to episodic migraine [1, 13]. The prevalence of chronic migraine is 2.5–6.5 greater in women [1]. In comparison to episodic migraine, individuals with chronic migraine have statistically lower household incomes, have a higher likelihood of being occupationally disabled, and are less likely to be employed full time [14]. According to the International Burden of Migraine Study, chronic migraine has three times the mean total annual cost of headache compared to episodic migraine [15], significantly greater direct medical costs and indirect costs. Pharmaceutical utilization made up the largest portion of direct medical costs in both groups. Family burdens were also greater with increased headache frequency [16]. Patients with chronic migraine also have higher rates of anxiety, depression, respiratory illness, higher rates of allergies, cardiovascular disorder and heart disease, obesity, chronic pain, and ulcers [14]. These common comorbidities in chronic migraine may contribute

to the overall functional impairment. In addition, longitudinal population studies have identified other risk factors for chronic daily headache such as head and neck injury [17], high caffeine intake [18], habitual snoring [19], insomnia [20], stressful life events [21], caucasians, female sex, less education, and previously married (divorced, separated, widowed) [22].

The rate of new onset chronic migraine is 2.5% in persons with episodic migraine after 1 year according to the American Migraine Prevalence and Prevention Study (AAMPS) [23]. The clinical progression to chronic migraine generally occurs gradually with an increase in attack frequency over time; in other cases, chronic migraine may occur suddenly. Moreover, there is a significant variability in the frequency of headache depending on the frequency of sampling in epidemiological studies. An analysis from the Chronic Migraine Epidemiology and Outcomes (CaMEO) Study, a longitudinal survey of US adults with episodic and chronic migraine, illustrated the natural fluctuations over the course of 1 year between episodic migraine and chronic migraine during 3-month intervals [24]. The investigators found that among 5465 respondents with episodic migraine, 92.4% had episodic migraine in all periods of sampling or waves of data, while 7.6% had chronic migraine in at least one wave. There were 526 respondents with chronic migraine at baseline of which 26% had chronic migraine at every point and 73.4% had episodic migraine at least once. The studies suggest that there are frequent transitions between episodic migraine and chronic migraine in persons with migraine at 3 months intervals during a 12-month period. More studies are needed to understand the transitions between episodic migraine and chronic migraine and to better identify individuals in the pre-chronic migraine state who may be at a greater risk for personal, occupational, and social loss due to migraine progression.

Predictors of progression have important clinical significance (Fig. 4.1). In addition, there are a number of migraine-specific and treatment-related risk factors. In the American Migraine Prevalence and Prevention Study of 5681 eligible study respondents, the Migraine Treatment Optimization Questionnaire (mTOQ-4) was used to determine

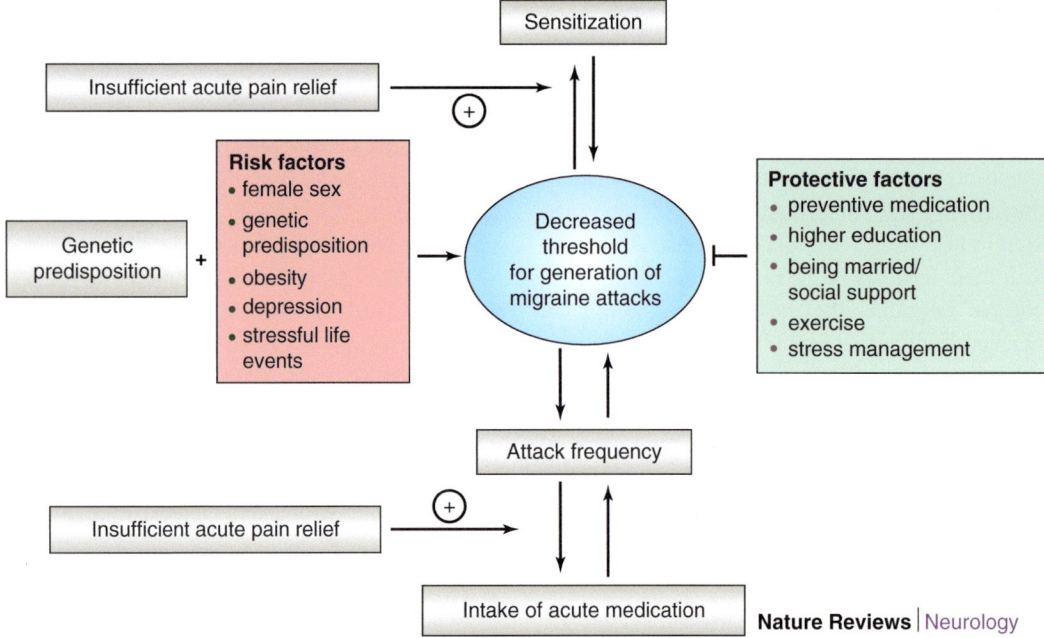

Fig. 4.1 Multiple factors contribute to migraine chronification. (May A, Schulte LH. Chronic migraine: Risk factors, mechanisms and treatment. Nat Rev Neurol 2016;12:455–64. Reprinted with permission from Springer Nature)

treatment responses and a logistic regression model was used to examine transition from episodic migraine to chronic migraine. The study found that ineffective acute treatment of episodic migraine was associated with new onset chronic migraine over the course of 1 year [25]. When compared to the maximum treatment efficacy group, the very poor treatment efficacy group had more than a two-fold-increased risk of chronic migraine. Medication overuse of acute analgesics is a commonly recognized risk factor for chronic migraine and migraine progression. The risk of migraine progression is associated with the use of butalbital-containing compounds (>5 days per month) and opiate drugs (>8 days per month) as compared to acetaminophen used as a reference [23]. A baseline high attack frequency is also associated with migraine progression as well as frequent and persistent nausea [26].

Predictors of remission and progression have been explored in epidemiological samples of chronic migraine. In a study of 383 respondents over a 2-year period, 34% had persistent chronic migraine and 26% had remittance of their chronic migraine state [27]. Predictors of remission include the baseline headache frequency and absence of allodynia; remission rates are associated with decreases in headache-related disability

in addition to less headache days. After a multivariate analysis, predictors of remission included headache frequency (15–19 vs. 25–31, headache days/month; odds ratio [OR] 0.29; 95% confidence interval [CI] 0.11–0.75) and absence of allodynia (OR 0.45; 95% CI 0.23–0.89). As expected, those with persistent chronic migraine had increased disability, and those with remitted chronic migraine had reduced disability.

Pathophysiology

Chronic migraine is thought to involve multiple levels of the central nervous system and include biochemical, physiological, functional, and structural alterations. In a meta-analysis of 375,000 individuals with migraine, 38 genetic loci were found for migraine [28]. The GWAS (genome wide association study) has some limitations but implicates both neuronal and vascular cells, indicative of a neurovascular disorder. They also point to supporting glia, pain signaling pathways and multiple influences that may lead to a progressive, maladaptive state. The genetic underpinnings of chronic migraine are unknown but are likely polygenic similar to

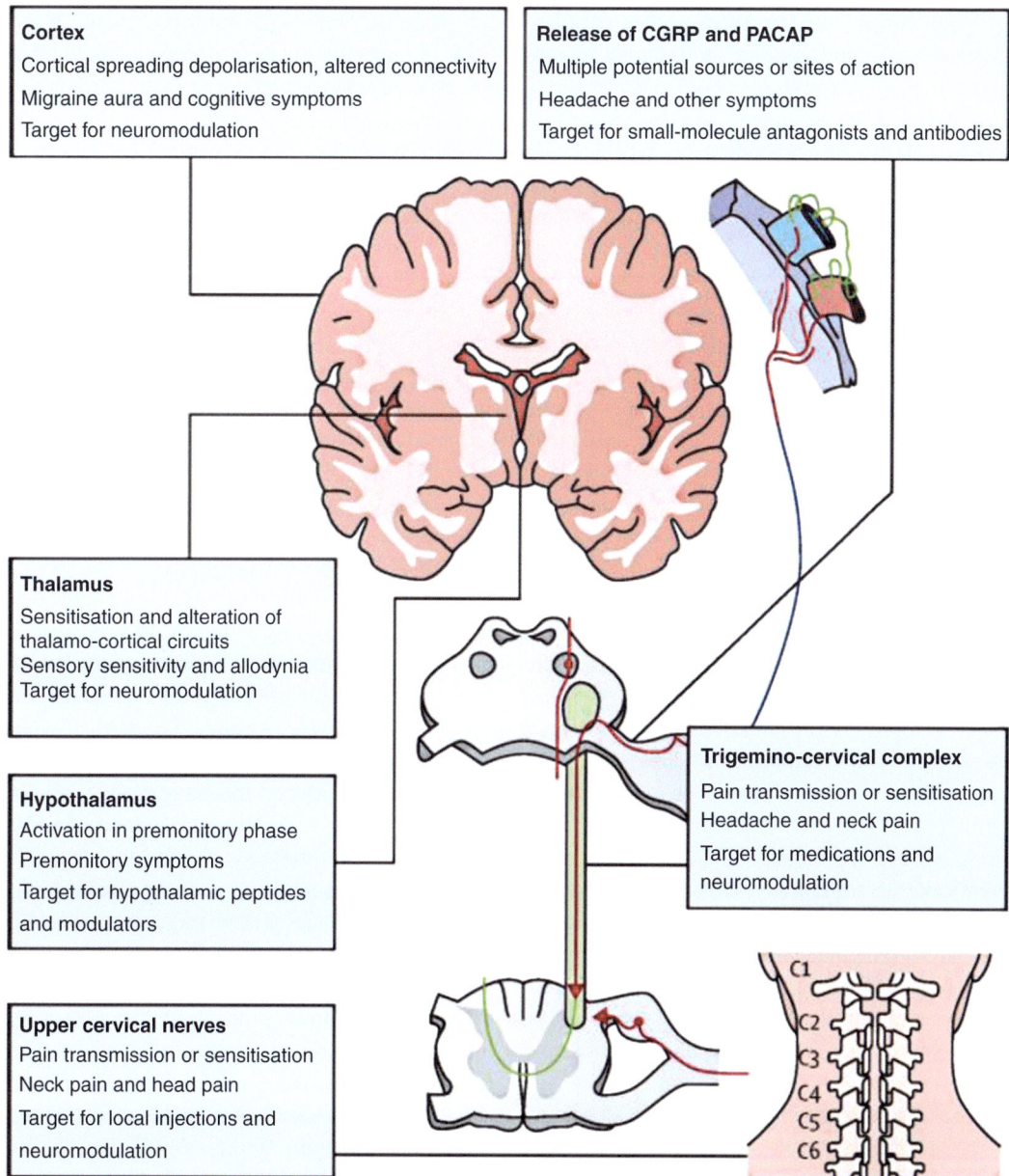

Cortex

Cortical spreading depolarisation, altered connectivity

Migraine aura and cognitive symptoms

Target for neuromodulation

Release of CGRP and PACAP

Multiple potential sources or sites of action

Headache and other symptoms

Target for small-molecule antagonists and antibodies

Thalamus

Sensitisation and alteration of thalamo-cortical circuits
Sensory sensitivity and allodynia
Target for neuromodulation

Hypothalamus

Activation in premonitory phase

Premonitory symptoms

Target for hypothalamic peptides and modulators

Upper cervical nerves

Pain transmission or sensitisation

Neck pain and head pain

Target for local injections and neuromodulation

Trigemino-cervical complex

Pain transmission or sensitisation
Headache and neck pain

Target for medications and neuromodulation

Fig. 4.2 The diagram illustrates the multiple levels of the peripheral and central nervous system involvement in the pathophysiology of chronic migraine. There are a number of targets for medications, antibodies, small molecule antagonists, peptides and modulators, neuromodulation devices, and injection therapies as treatment for migraine. Emerging evidence supports the potential for targeted treatments in chronic migraine; however, more investigations are needed. (Charles A. The pathophysiology of migraine: implications for clinical management. Lancet. 2018;17(2):174–82. Reprinted with permission from Elsevier)

episodic migraine. Significant progress has been made for the past few decades in the understanding of the peripheral and central pathways, important neuropeptides, neurotransmitters, and receptors involved in migraine pathophysiology, although with somewhat lesser knowledge of chronic migraine. There has been much debate as to the level in which peripheral trigeminal nociceptive activation is involved in migraine attacks. An extracranial hypothesis that includes an inflammatory profile has been suggested in a small series of chronic migraine patients [29], although chronic tenderness of pericranial muscles may be a consequence of frequent attacks as well. It is plausible that both the peripheral and central systems are involved (Fig. 4.2) One-quarter of patients experience migraine with aura, transient neurological disturbances in the visual, sensory, motor, and language systems. The electrophysiological correlate for migraine aura is cortical spreading depression (2-6 mm/min), a slowly propagating wave of neuronal and glial depression consisting of electrophysiological hyperactivity followed by cortical inhibition [30]. Cortical spreading depression can activate trigeminal nociception and trigger headache mechanisms, as supported by animal studies [31]. Cortical spreading depression may also activate or disinhibit central trigeminal sensory neurons, supported by preclinical studies [32]. As most migraine attacks do not begin with aura and migraine headache may occur during the aura phase, aura has been postulated as a brain state and other mechanisms of attack initiation have been proposed [33]. Alternatively, lowered thresholds of activation due to enhanced cyclical brainstem activity may also contribute to chronic migraine [34]. The hallmarks of chronic migraine are repetitive activation and sensitization of the trigeminovascular system, which includes the sensory peripheral projections to the pain-producing dura mater and central projections to the trigeminal nucleus caudalis in the brainstem. Central projections are then sent to the trigeminothalamic tract, to the thalamus, and the cortex.

The distinct pathological drivers associated with chronic migraine are poorly understood, although there appear to be significant brain changes [2]. For example, an imaging study suggested that the ICHD-3 diagnosis of chronic migraine as compared to episodic migraine could be adequately classified based on regional changes in cortical thickness, surface area, and volumes [35]. In another magnetic resonance imaging study with voxel-based morphometry, there were significant gray matter reductions in the left and right anterior cingulate, left amygdala, left and right insular lobe, left parietal operculum, left parietal operculum, and left, middle,

left inferior, and right inferior frontal gyrus [36]. Significant positive correlations between the attack frequency and gray matter reductions have been shown in the anterior cingulate cortex. Moreover, another imaging study of non-heme iron deposition in the periaqueductal gray, an area of descending antinociceptive neuronal network, found statistically significant differences in episodic migraine and chronic daily headache as compared to controls and positive correlations with the duration of illness. The investigators hypothesized that iron homeostasis in the periaqueductal gray matter is persistent and progressively impaired due to iron-catalyzed free radical injury from repeated migraine attacks [37]. Taken together, the findings suggest that repeated migraine attacks might be associated with changes in brain structure.

Historically, both cortical and brainstem regions have been implicated in the pathophysiology of migraine [38]. Patients with chronic migraine have enhanced cortical excitability as compared to episodic migraine. The cortical excitability is thought to be intrinsic or due to reduced intracortical inhibitory mechanisms [2, 38]. In one study using transcranial magnetic stimulation indexes of cortical excitability, the magnetic suppression of perceptual accuracy was significantly reduced in 25 chronic migraine patients as compared to episodic subjects and controls [39]. In a subset of the patients with chronic migraine, PET imaging showed increased metabolism in the pons and right temporal cortex; the medial frontal, parietal, and somatosensory cortices and the bilateral caudate nuclei had decreased metabolism. Imaging studies with PET have also supported the role of the pons. In another study of chronic migraine with suboccipital stimulators, activation in the dorsal pons was similar to that in episodic migraine; however, persistent activation after stimulation suggests the structure may play a key role in the pathophysiology of chronic migraine [40]. Taken together, the activation and inhibitory patterns of the brainstem, the pons in particular, suggest that cortical excitability is "raised" and may result in a higher susceptibility to migraine triggers [41]. Another investigation to better understand light aversion was performed in 18 episodic migraineurs, 17 chronic migraineurs, and 19 healthy controls. The investigators used high resolution brainstem imaging to determine the effects of visual stimulation on activation of the spinal trigeminal nucleus [42]. The study showed that individuals with chronic migraine had enhanced activation within the spinal trigeminal nucleus as compared to healthy controls. Activation was also greater in the spinal trigeminal nucleus when comparing migraine with headaches during scanning with migraine without headaches. In addition, there was enhanced activity of the right superior colliculus in chronic migraine as compared to healthy controls. The study provides evidence for visual-nociceptive integration on the brainstem level in chronic migraine and ultimately illustrates sensory processing dysfunction.

Migraine chronification is also associated with dysfunctional thalamocortical pathways; specifically, electrophysiological studies have suggested that there is an increase in the strength of connections between the thalamus and the cortex in chronic migraine as compared to episodic migraine between attacks [43]. In a MR spectroscopy investigation of the bilateral medial walls of the brain in individuals with chronic migraine, the investigators assessed the metabolite alternations as compared to matched episodic migraine and headache-free controls; the thalamus, occipital lobe, and anterior cingulate cortex were analyzed as region of interests to determine if N-acetyl-aspartate, a marker of neuronal integrity, was reduced [44]. Reduced N-acetyl-aspartate metabolism and altered interregional N-acetyl-aspartate correlations were found, thus supporting the role of thalamocortical dysfunction in migraine chronification.

Recent studies suggest a key role for the hypothalamus in both migraine and chronic migraine. In a PET imaging study of nitroglycerin-triggered acute migraine attacks, brain activation patterns were elucidated during the premonitory phase; the hypothalamus in particular is associated with many of the premonitory symptoms and was activated early before migraine pain began [45]. Interestingly, a functional MRI investigation using painful ammonia stimulation in 17 chronic migraineurs, 18 episodic migraineurs, and 19 healthy controls suggested that the hypothalamus might also be the mediator of chronic migraine [46]. Moreover, the activation patterns suggested that the anterior hypothalamus might play a role in attack generation and migraine chronification as opposed to the posterior aspect, which appears to be important for the acute pain phase. Many questions remain such as mechanisms of migraine initiation, propagation, and termination, which could then lead to a better understanding of chronic migraine mechanisms.

Resting-state FMRI is a type of functional brain imaging that can be used to assess regional interactions that occur when an individual is not performing a specific task. With this technique, significant differences in functional connections with affective pain regions were demonstrated in chronic migraine as compared to controls. In addition, there were significant correlations between the number of years with chronic migraine and functional connectivity strength between the anterior insula with the periaqueductal gray and the anterior insula with the medial dorsal thalamus [47].

Central sensitization is a pivotal process that occurs in chronic migraine. When central sensitization occurs, the nervous system goes through a process of windup resulting in a persistent state of high reactivity. Central sensitization is a maladaptive state mediated by sensitization of the central trigeminovascular neurons in the nucleus caudalis, spinal cord, and posterior thalamic nuclei [48]. Clinically, central sensitization often manifests as hypersensitivity to non-painful stimuli known as "allodynia in addition to persistent headache. Dysfunctional pain modulation, either due to descending pain facilitation of nociception or impairments in descending inhibitory pathways, contributes to central sensitization. Cutaneous allodynia has been investigated in an intrinsic resting-state FMRI study of chronic migraine, which showed modulation of brain networks in women [49]. In the study, the frequency of moderate and severe headaches was associated with decreased connectivity in the salience network, while cutaneous allodynia was associated with an increased connectivity with the central executive network. The presence of cutaneous allodynia correlates with migraine severity, migraine-associated symptoms, and other migraine features such as aura [50].

Management and Treatment

A number of barriers to chronic migraine care exist. There are hurdles in obtaining a consultation, diagnosis, and treatment, resulting in a large unmet need [16]. The primary goals of care for chronic migraine are to reduce headache frequency, relieve pain, restore function, and prevent progression. All patients with chronic migraine require acute and preventive treatments. Medication overuse when present should be addressed for optimal outcomes. A through history and physical examination is necessary to rule out secondary causes of chronic headaches, which may resemble chronic migraine. Systemic symptoms such as fever and weight loss or secondary risk factors such as systemic cancer and HIV disease are important considerations. Neurological symptoms or signs, sudden onset of headache, older age (>50), new onset, or change in clinical features are indications for further evaluations [51]. Patients with chronic migraine should have an extensive evaluation of common triggers: change in routine, stress, stress letdown, changes in sleep patterns, hormonal changes, environmental changes (weather change, humidity, loud noises, exposure to bright/flickering lights, computer screens, foods, dehydration and skipped meals.

There are a number of comorbidities that should be assessed in individuals with chronic migraine. Depression is a risk factor for the transformation of episodic migraine to chronic migraine [52]. The greater the severity of depression, the greater the risk of chronic migraine. Anxiety and depression are also strongly associated with both chronic migraine and migraine progression. Non-cephalic pain is a risk factor for new onset chronic migraine and chronic migraine progression [53]. Neck pain in particular is a common symptom associated with migraine and when related to neck pathology may contribute to the activation of the trigeminocervical complex. Opiates used to treat non-cephalic pain may lead to high rates of morbidity, mortality, misuse, and potentially medication overuse headache in patients with chronic migraine. Poor sleep quality may contribute to high frequencies of migraine, and migraine may aggravate sleep [14]. Obesity is a risk factor for transformed migraine but can also be a consequence of prophylactic treatment and inactivity due to movement sensitivity experienced by migraineurs [54–56]. In one study of women with migraine (4–20 days per month) that were overweight or obese, behavioral weight loss intervention yielded sustained reductions in migraine headaches similar to migraine education. Overall, the benefits of multidisciplinary interventions that target comorbidities for reduction in migraine days require further exploration in patients with chronic migraine.

The careful selection of migraine patients for preventive treatments may reduce the likelihood of progression from episodic migraine to chronic migraine [57]. There are five US FDA-approved preventive treatments for episodic migraine, which include two anticonvulsants (topiramate and valproate) and three antihypertensive beta-blockers (metoprolol, propranolol, timolol). According to expert consensus, oral preventive treatments for episodic migraine such as antihypertensive (beta-blockers, angiotensin receptor blockers, angiotensin-converting enzyme inhibitors), antidepressants (tricyclic antidepressants, serotonin-norepinephrine reuptake inhibitors), and anticonvulsants may be also helpful for chronic migraine; however, the evidence is lacking except for topiramate [58]. OnabotulinumtoxinA injection therapy is FDA approved for preventive treatment of chronic migraine but not episodic migraine. Smaller randomized control studies of chronic daily headache (or high-frequency headache) include amitriptyline [59], sodium valproate [60], gabapentin [61], and tizanidine [62, 63]. Open-label studies provide weaker evidence for memantine [64], pregabalin [65], milnacipran [66], atenolol, and zonisamide [67]. Adherence is problematic as persistent use of oral prophylactic medications among chronic migraine patients is low at 6 months and declines even further by 12 months [68].

Acute treatment is based on studies for acute migraine attacks in episodic migraine. According the American Headache Society evidence assessment, triptans are migraine-specific treatments considered effective (level A) [69]. Dihydroergotamine and ergotamine, some nonsteroidal anti-inflammatory agents, and neuroleptics may also help acute migraine days of chronic migraine. Two-hour pain-free rates are lower in chronic migraine as compared to episodic migraine. Cutaneous allodynia, major depression, and the use of nonsteroidal anti-inflammatory drugs are associated with poor treatment responses [70]. In contrast, acute medication optimization is associated with use of triptans and preventive medications. Newer agents in the class of CGRP antagonists, ubrogepant and rimegepant [71], and the 5-HT (1F) receptor agonist lasmiditan [72] are non-vasoconstrictive drugs under clinical development. Ultimately, there is a great need for well-designed studies to test the efficacy and safety of novel therapeutics for chronic migraine.

Established and Emerging Pharmacological Treatments

Topiramate

Topiramate is an anticonvulsant FDA approved for the treatment of migraine (Table 4.2). Topiramate has a broad mechanism of action including enhancing inhibitory effects and minimizing excitatory affects that result in its antimigraine action. Topiramate regulates cell membrane ion channels (potassium, calcium, sodium), modulates neurotransmitter release (glutamate, gamma-aminobutyric acid), and inhibits some carbonic anhydrase isozymes [73]. Electrophysiological studies indicate that topiramate has modulatory effects within the trigeminovascular and trigeminothalamic pathway and mechanisms involved in cortical spreading depression [74, 75]. Studies also indicate that the inotropic glutamate receptor, specifically the kainate receptor, is a potential target. Topiramate also modulates thalamocortical networks in humans [76].

The efficacy and safety of topiramate in the treatment of chronic migraine is supported by two large multicenter randomized double-blind, placebo-controlled clinical trials. In the TOP-CHROME study, efficacy and safety were evaluated at doses ranging between 50 and 200 mg/day (average dose 100 mg/day) [77]. Topiramate significantly reduced the mean number of monthly migraine days ($\pm$SD) by 3.5 ± 6.3, compared with placebo (-0.2 ± 4.7, $P < 0.05$). In the Topiramate Chronic Migraine Study, the active treatment arm (mean maintenance dose 86 mg/day) resulted in a statistically significant mean reduction of migraine/migrainous headache days (topiramate -6.4 vs. placebo -4.7, $P = 0.010$) and migraine headache days relative to baseline (topiramate -5.6 vs. placebo -4.1, $P = 0.032$) [78]. Topiramate was also effective in the treatment of patients with chronic migraine with and without acute medication overuse, suggesting detoxification prior to initiating prophylactic therapy may not be required for all patients [79]. In the INTREPID study, a multicenter, randomized, double-blind study comparing topiramate to placebo for the prevention of migraine progression, topiramate failed to prevent new onset chronic daily migraine at month 6 which may have been due to unexpectedly low transition rates in the placebo arm and short observation period [80]. However, topiramate reduced both headache and migraine headache days [81]. The efficacy of propranolol added to topiramate in chronic migraine was also assessed in subjects inadequately controlled with topiramate [82]. The study provided class II evidence that propranolol added to topiramate did not result in moderate to severe headache rate reduction at 6 months.

Paresthesias are a common side effect in both chronic migraine clinical trials. In clinical practice, cognitive side effects are a common cause of discontinuation. Extended-release formulations may have significantly less cognitive side effects due to stable steady-state plasma concentrations. This is supported by verbal fluency studies that showed less impairment with topiramate extended release as compared to the immediate release in healthy volunteers [83]. Extended release may improve compliance without significant consequences in plasma concentrations due to dosing irregularities [84]. In addition, topiramate is

Table 4.2 Pharmaceutical preventive treatment for chronic migraine

Name	Class	Route of administration	Clinical phase	Primary endpoints	Safety profiles
Topiramate	Anticonvulsant	Oral	Phase 3 (TOP-CHROME, Topiramate Chronic Migraine Study)	Significantly reduced the mean number of monthly migraine days/migrainous days	Paresthesia, nausea, dizziness, dyspepsia, fatigue, anorexia, cognitive impairment, renal stones
OnabotulinumtoxinA	Neurotoxin	Intramuscular	Phase 3 (PREEMPT 1)	No significant between-group difference for onabotulinumtoxinA versus placebo was observed for headache episodes	Neck pain, headache, weakness, ptosis, injection site pain
			Phase 3 (PREEMPT 2)	OnabotulinumtoxinA was statistically significantly superior to placebo for frequency of headache days	
Fremanezumab	Monoclonal antibodies to CGRP	Subcutaneous, intravenous	Phase 3 randomized controlled studies	The least squares mean (±SE) reduction in the average number of headache days per month with quarterly and monthly dosing	No serious adverse events related to the study drug; injection site reactions were common
Erenumab	Monoclonal antibodies to CGRP receptor	Subcutaneous	FDA approved	Reduced monthly migraine days	No serious adverse events related to the study drug; injection site reactions were common
Galcanezumab	Monoclonal antibodies to CGRP	Subcutaneous	Phase 3, REGAIN	Mean change from baseline in monthly migraine headache days over the 3-month period	No serious adverse events related to the study drug; injection site reactions were common
Eptinezumab	Monoclonal antibodies to CGRP	Intravenous	Phase 3 PROMISE 2	Reduction of monthly migraine days	No serious adverse events related to the study drug; injection site reactions were common

considered weight neutral, but a subset of patients treated may experience weight loss. It acts as a carbonic anhydrase inhibitor, which may lead to the development of renal stones. Post-marketing evidence has shown an increase risk of oral clefts with first trimester fetal exposure (Category D). In addition, long-term studies of topiramate are needed to assess osteoporosis-fracture risk [85].

OnabotulinumtoxinA

Botulinum toxin is a protein produced by the bacteria *Clostridium botulinum* and exists in seven antigenically and serologically distinct forms named as A–G [86]. OnabotulinumtoxininA delivered to extracranial dermatomes is the first FDA-approved treatment for chronic migraine. In addition to its well-described inhibition of acetylcholine from cholinergic nerve endings at the skeletal neuromuscular junction, the onabotulinumtoxinA mode of action is initiated by the cleavage of proteins required for trigeminal nerve activation and signaling. The toxin binds to afferent nerve terminals by connecting with high affinity sites. The neuron confines the toxin into a vesicle once bound to the nerve terminal. The vesicle moves into the cell and once activated exits into the cytoplasm and cleaves soluble *N*-ethylmaleimide-sensitive factor attachment protein receptor (SNARE) proteins. SNARE proteins mediate vesicle release of neurotransmitters but are also involved in the transport of channels and receptors. The cleavage of SNARE proteins prevents the cell from releasing vesicles of substance P, bradykinin, CGRP, and glutamate [87]. In a recent study by Burstein et al., onabotulinumtoxinA selectively inhibited peripheral C mechanonociceptors in the trigeminovascular neurons [88]. OnabotulinumtoxinA injections into the C-meningeal nociceptors in the dura inhibited responses to mechanical stimulation and reversed and prevented the development of mechanical hypersensitivity. The experiments showed that onabotulinumtoxinA prevents the fusion of high threshold mechanosensitive ion channels to the nerve terminal membrane, thus interfering with the expression of the ion channel linked to mechanical pain.

Antinociceptive central effects of onabotulinumtoxinA likely occur through axonal transport. OnabotulinumtoxinA can be taken up peripherally and undergoes transcytosis to cleave SNARE proteins at the trigeminal ganglion and the trigeminal nucleus caudalis preventing downstream events. Early investigations suggest the antinociceptive effects may therefore involve different sites of the trigeminal system and interaction with the central endogenous opioid system [89].

OnabotulinumtoxinA injected to 31 sites in the procerus, corrugator, frontalis, temporalis, occipitalis, and posterior cervical injections including the trapezius is safe and efficacious for the treatment of chronic migraine. The FDA approval was based on two-phase III clinical trials over a 24-week randomized, double-blind phase followed by a 32-week open-label phase. In PREEMPT 1, there were no between-group differences for the primary endpoint of mean change from baseline in headache episode frequency at week 24 [90]. Both migraine and headache days were significant secondary endpoints. For the PREEMPT 2 trial, the primary endpoint was the mean change in headache days per 28 days from baseline to weeks 21–24 posttreatment [91]. OnabotulinumtoxinA was statistically significantly superior to placebo for the primary endpoint, frequency of headache days per 28 days relative to baseline (-9.0 botulinum toxin A/-6.7 placebo, $P < 0.001$). OnabotulinumtoxinA was significantly favored in all secondary endpoint comparisons including change from baseline in the frequency of migraine days, frequency of moderate/severe headache days, cumulative total headache hours on headache days, frequency of headache episodes, in total HIT-6 scores, frequency of acute headache pain medication intakes, and frequency of triptan intake. In pooled studies of PREEMPT 1 and PREEMPT 2 (Fig. 4.3), 1384 qualified adults with chronic migraine were randomized to onabotulinumtoxinA (155–195 U) or placebo injections every 12 weeks [92]. The analyses demonstrated a large mean decrease from baseline in frequency of headache days, with statistically significant between-group differences favoring onabotulinumtoxinA over

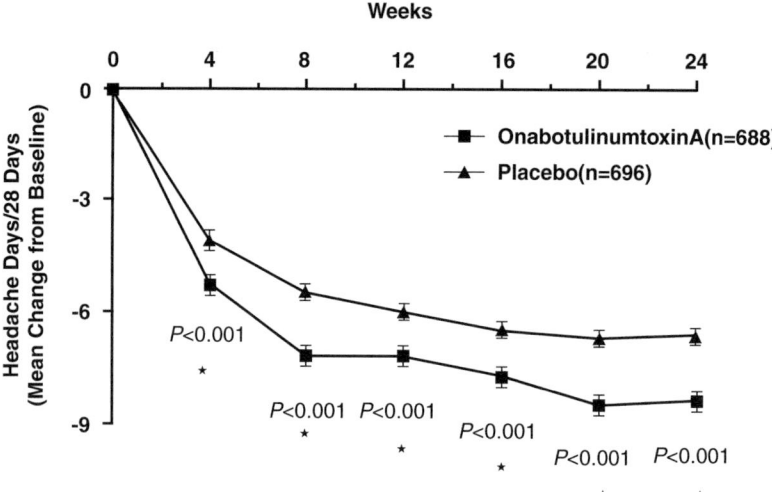

Fig. 4.3 OnabotulinumtoxinA for the treatment of chronic migraine: pooled results from the double-blind, randomized, placebo-controlled PREEMPT studies. The pooled PREEMPT results demonstrate a large mean decrease from baseline headache days of 19.9 ± 0.1 onabotulinumtoxinA group versus 19.8 ± 0.1 placebo group, $P = 0.498$. The analyses show statistically significant between-group differences favoring onabotulinumtoxinA over placebo at week 24 (-8.4 vs. -6.6) $P < 0.001$) and at all time points expressed as mean ± standard error. All secondary endpoints were met except frequency of acute headache pain medication intakes. Adverse events were mild to moderate and few discontinued due to adverse events. (Dodick DW, et al. [92]. Reprinted with permission from John Wiley and Sons)

placebo at week 24 (-8.4 vs. -6.6; $P < 0.001$) and at all other time points. The study met all secondary endpoints including mean change from baseline to week 24 in frequency of migraine/probable migraine days, frequency of moderate/severe headache days, total cumulative hours of headache on headache days, frequency of headache episodes, frequency of migraine/probable migraine episodes, and the proportion of patients with severe (≥ 60) Headache Impact Test-6 score at week 24, except frequency of acute headache pain medication intakes. In an open-label prospective study comparing baseline to week 24, Generalized Anxiety Disorder questionnaires and Beck Depression Inventory II tests showed significant improvement in anxiety and depression symptoms posttreatment [93]. Although the PREEMPT trials did not show a superior benefit of injections with 195 U as compared to 155 U, an open-label prospective study showed superior efficacy of 195 U as compared to 155 U over 2 years in chronic migraine with medication overuse headache. Treatment-related adverse events were transient and mild to moderate [94]. Additional clinical trials are needed to inform the

optimal dosing, injection frequency and sites for potentially improved outcomes.

The safety profile of onabotulinumtoxinA has been extensively reviewed for the treatment of chronic migraine and other indications. Adverse events were generally considered mild or moderate, no unexpected treatment-related adverse events were identified, and discontinuation rates were low. The most common treatment-related side effects were neck pain, muscular weakness, eyelid ptosis, musculoskeletal pain, injection site pain, headache, myalgia, and musculoskeletal stiffness. Long-term treatment benefits and safety were reported in a cohort of chronic migraine and medication overuse headache patients over a course of 3 years of therapy [95]; no serious adverse events were reported. Optimal outcomes may be achieved with a greater consideration for the functional anatomy including the peripheral nerves and muscles targeted during the PREEMPT clinical program (Figs. 4.4 and 4.5).

A number of investigations have tried to determine predictors or markers of onabotulinumtoxinA response. One study found that

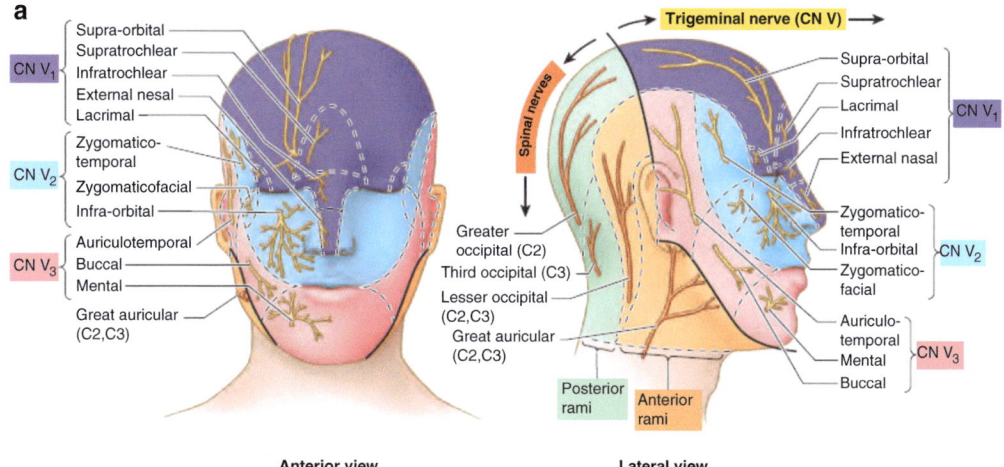

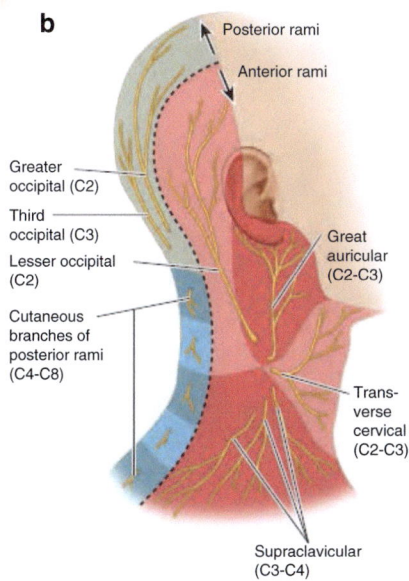

Fig. 4.4 Important functional anatomy behind the PREEMPT injections paradigm includes the distribution of peripheral nerves: (**a**) anterior and lateral view of the tri-geminal (CN V) and occipital (C2, C3) sensory nerves and (**b**) cervical sensory nerves (C2, C3). (Moore KL, et al. [96]. Reprinted with permission from Wolters Kluwer Health)

pretreatment vasoactive intestinal peptide and CGRP levels were predictors of response to onabotulinumtoxinA and interictal plasma levels of CGRP can be lowered with onabotulinumtoxinA [68, 97]. Another study of chronic migraine patients found structural and functional brain changes in onabotulinumtoxinA responders versus nonresponders [98]. The responders showed significant cortical thickening in the right primary somatosensory cortex, anterior insula, and left superior temporal gyrus

(STG) and pars opercularis compared to nonresponders. Disease duration was negatively correlated with cortical thickness in frontoparietal and temporo-occipital regions in the responders only. The investigators were also able to distinguish between responders and nonresponders based on seed based resting-state functional connectivity analysis. The authors concluded that elucidating tools to detect central nervous system changes might lead to markers for disease de-chronification.

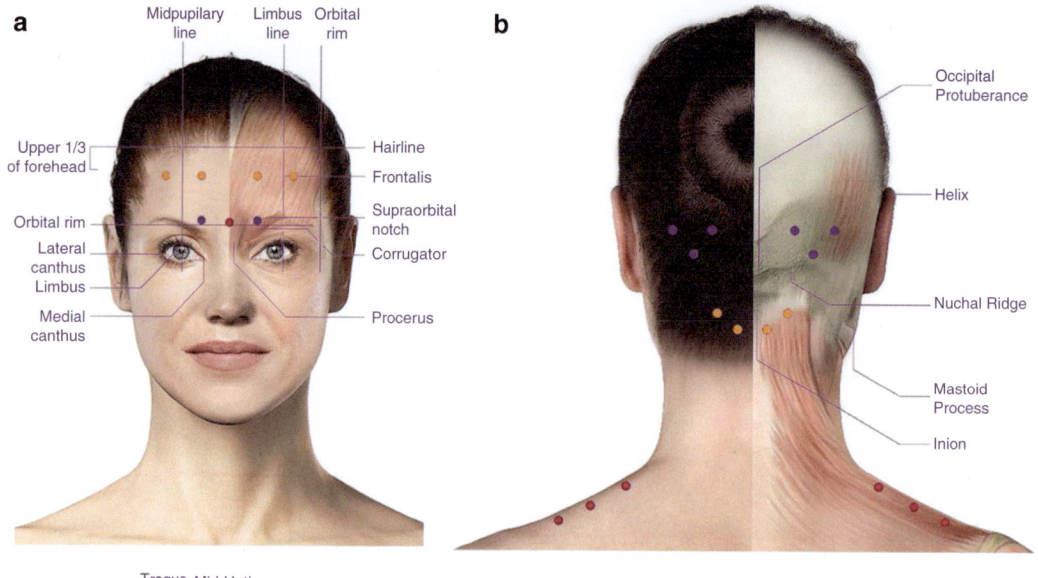

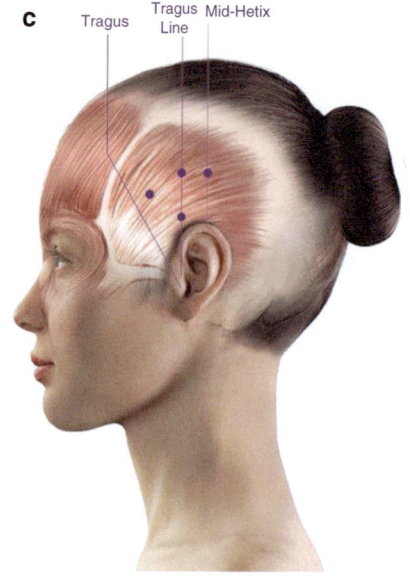

Fig. 4.5 The fixed-site, fixed-dose PREEMPT injection site locations of the pivotal trials: (**a**) corrugator, as depicted by purple dots; procerus, as depicted by the red dot; frontalis, as depicted by orange dots, (**b**) occipitalis area, as depicted by purple dots; cervical paraspinal area, as depicted by orange dots; trapezius, as depicted by red dots, and (**c**) temporalis, as depicted by purple dots. (Blumenfeld AM, et al. [99]. Reprinted with permission from John Wiley and Sons)

Monoclonal Antibodies to the Calcitonin Gene-Related Peptide or Its Receptor

A number of preclinical and clinical studies overwhelmingly support a role of calcitonin gene-related peptide (CGRP) in the pathophysiology of both migraine and chronic migraine [100].

CGRP is a 37-amino acid neuropeptide formed from alternative splicing of the calcitonin/CGRP gene located on chromosome [100]. CGRP is found in nociceptive tissue and is a strong cerebral vasodilator. CGRP is uniquely increased in the extracerebral circulation during the headache phase of migraine [101], but not neuropeptides such as substance P, VIP, and NPY. CGRP

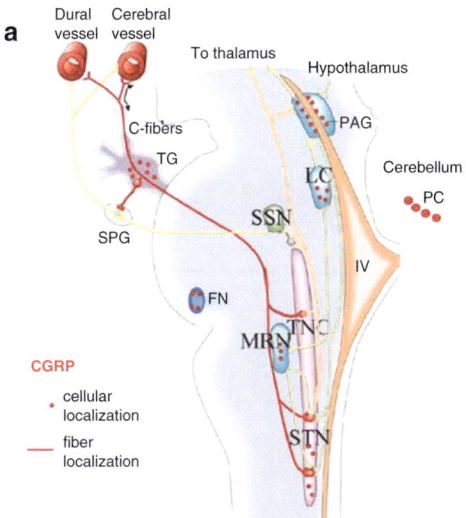

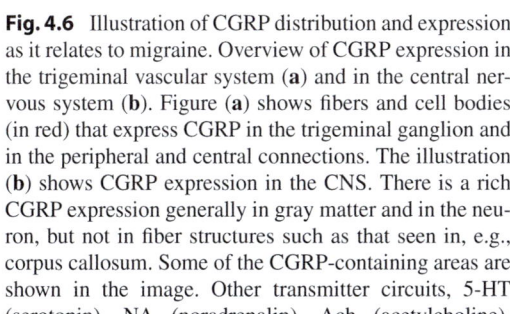

Fig. 4.6 Illustration of CGRP distribution and expression as it relates to migraine. Overview of CGRP expression in the trigeminal vascular system (**a**) and in the central nervous system (**b**). Figure (**a**) shows fibers and cell bodies (in red) that express CGRP in the trigeminal ganglion and in the peripheral and central connections. The illustration (**b**) shows CGRP expression in the CNS. There is a rich CGRP expression generally in gray matter and in the neuron, but not in fiber structures such as that seen in, e.g., corpus callosum. Some of the CGRP-containing areas are shown in the image. Other transmitter circuits, 5-HT (serotonin), NA (noradrenalin), Ach (acetylcholine), dopamine, and GABA (gamma-aminobutyric acid), are also included in the image, visualizing the complexity of transmitter interactions. *TG* trigeminal ganglion, *SPG* sphenopalatine ganglion, *PAG* periaqueductal gray, *PC* Purkinje cells, *LC* locus coeruleus, *SSN* superior salivatory nucleus, *IV* 4th ventricle, *FN* facial nucleus, *TNC* trigeminal nucleus caudalis, *MRN* raphe magnus nucleus, *STN* spinal trigeminal nucleus, *Me5* mesencephalic trigeminal nucleus, *Med* medial cerebellar nucleus, *Pn* pontine nucleus, *IO* inferior olive. (Edvinsson L, Warfvinge K [102]. Reprinted with permission from Sage Publications)

and its receptor components, RAMP1 and CLR, are found abundantly in the trigeminovascular system (Fig. 4.6) and are released in the peripheral endings in the meninges and in the central endings in the medullary and upper cervical dorsal horn [103]. Taken together, the role of CGRP in migraine is evidenced by its release during acute migraine attacks [104] and normalization by triptans [105] and small molecule CGRP receptor antagonists [106], as well as persistent CGRP elevation in chronic migraine as mentioned previously. CGRP function-blocking monoclonal antibodies represent the first mechanism-based preventive treatment for both migraine and chronic migraine. To date, there are four monoclonal antibodies to the CGRP peptide or receptor with phase II/III evidence to support efficacy and safety for the treatment of both episodic and chronic migraine (Fig. 4.7). Additional efforts to target the PACAP pathway for potential preventive treatment of chronic migraine are underway.

Erenumab is a monoclonal antibody that targets the CGRP receptor. A phase 2 randomized double-blind, placebo-controlled study of erenumab showed that erenumab 70 mg and 140 mg reduced monthly migraine days versus placebo (both doses −6.6 days vs. placebo −4.2 days; difference −2.5, 95% CI −3.5 to −1.4, $P < 0.0001$) from weeks 9 to 12 [107]. The study drug also met several secondary endpoints including achievement of at least 50% reduction from baseline in monthly migraine days (i.e., 50% responder rate), change from baseline in days on which acute migraine-specific drugs were used, and change from baseline in cumulative headache hours. Erenumab was the first monoclonal antibody to the CGRP receptor that was FDA approved for the preventive treatment of migraine.

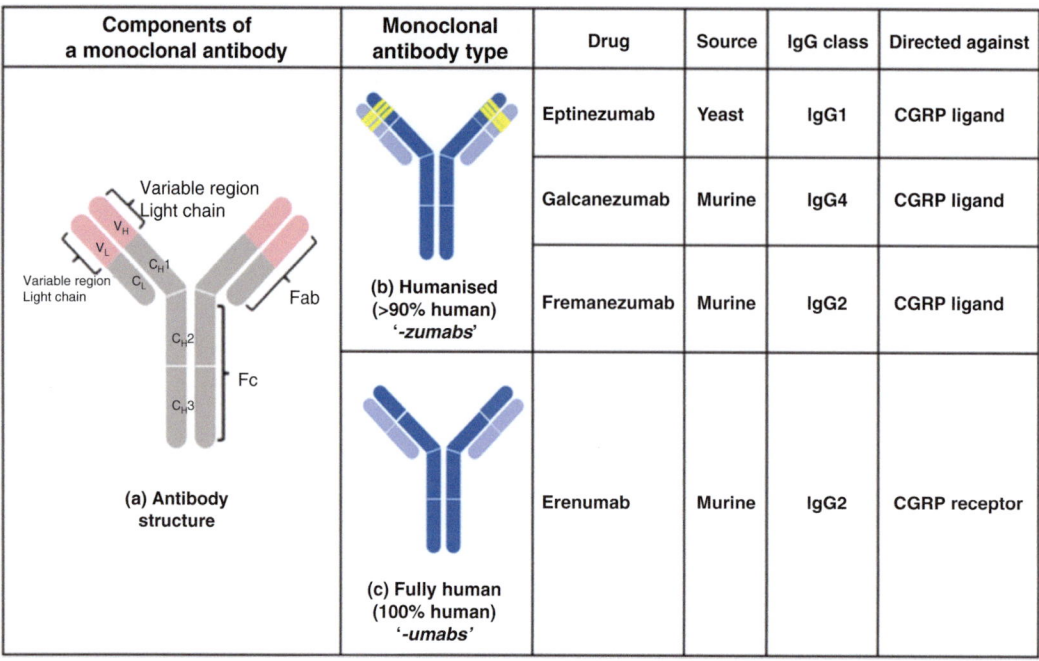

Components of a monoclonal antibody	Monoclonal antibody type	Drug	Source	IgG class	Directed against
		Eptinezumab	Yeast	IgG1	CGRP ligand
		Galcanezumab	Murine	IgG4	CGRP ligand
	(b) Humanised (>90% human) '-zumabs'	Fremanezumab	Murine	IgG2	CGRP ligand
(a) Antibody structure		Erenumab	Murine	IgG2	CGRP receptor
	(c) Fully human (100% human) '-umabs'				

Fig. 4.7 Overview of structure of antibody and monoclonal antibodies: novel mechanisms targeting the CGRP pathway. Eptinezumab, galcanezumab, and fremanezumab humanized and are directed against the CGRP ligand; erenumab is fully human and directed against the CGRP receptor. The potential therapeutic significance of these differences is currently unknown. (Ong JJY, et al. [108]. Reprinted with permission from Springer)

In another phase 3 study of fremanezumab for chronic migraine, subjects were randomized to quarterly, monthly, and placebo injections [109]. The least squares mean (±SE) reduction in the average number of headache days per month was 4.3 ± 0.3 with fremanezumab quarterly, 4.6 ± 0.3 with fremanezumab monthly, and 2.5 ± 0.3 with placebo ($P < 0.001$) for both comparisons with placebo. For secondary endpoints, the number of migraine days, headache-related disability, 50% responder rates, and days with acute medication use were significantly reduced with quarterly and monthly dosing. The study confirmed the long-lasting benefits of subcutaneous injections, which may be beneficial for improving drug compliance.

In the phase 3, randomized, double-blind, placebo-controlled trial (REGAIN), two doses of galcanezumab administered subcutaneously (120 or 240 mg once monthly, following a 240 mg starting dose) were compared with placebo for the treatment of chronic migraine [110]. The primary endpoint, the overall mean change in the number of monthly migraine headache days from months 1

to 3, was met. The least squares mean change from baseline (SE) was 4.8 days for the 120 mg dose and 4.6 days for the 240 mg dose as compared to a reduction of 2.7 days for placebo ($P < 0.001$). Secondary endpoints met included statistically significant improvement compared to placebo response rates and measures of daily activities.

Eptinezumab is a CGRP receptor antibody that is 100% bioavailable. In a randomized, placebo-controlled Phase 3 study (PROMISE 2) of eptinezumab with quarterly infusions, there was a significant reduction in monthly migraine days from 8.2 days at baseline compared to 5.6 for placebo, $P < 0.001$ [111]. Key secondary endpoints that were met included significant rapid day one prevention and significantly greater responder rates that were sustained for month 1 through 3 (50%, 75%, and 100%). Collectively, the observed safety profiles across the four monoclonal antibodies were similar to placebo-treated subjects. There were no severe adverse effects attributed to the study drug.

CGRP human or humanized monoclonal antibodies are large molecules with a site of action that is likely in the periphery, outside the blood-brain barrier. Fremanezumab, a humanized monoclonal antibody, was used to test the selective inhibitory effect on the activity of second-order trigeminovascular dorsal horn neurons that receive peripheral input from the cranial dura [112]. The investigators found selective central inhibition of high threshold but not wide dynamic range class of dorsal horn neurons [113]. Additional studies on the evoked activity of mechanosensitive primary afferent neurons in the trigeminal ganglion show that thinly myelinated Aδ meningeal nociceptors are possibly the peripheral site of action of fremanezumab for headache prevention [112]. Other animal studies have shown existing CGRP receptor-binding sites and expression of the receptor in the trigeminal ganglion, outside the blood-brain barrier [114]. Taken together, the investigators postulate that the selectivity may explain differences in responder rates of CGRP monoclonal antibodies, but confirmatory studies are needed. Additional studies will need to determine if there a difference between antibodies to CGRP versus its receptor. Further quantification of neutralizing anti-drug antibodies and the potential impact on efficacy is yet to be determined. The biological differences of those that had a 100% response to the treatment, the so-called super responders, should also be elucidated. In addition, the efficacy of CGRP monoclonal antibodies for the treatment of medication overuse headache, refractory cases of chronic migraine, and special populations (i.e., vascular disease) should be determined.

Nonpharmacological Treatments and Other Interventions

Acupuncture

Acupuncture is a Chinese technique that uses thin needles inserted in the skin at specified acupuncture points to restore Qi, vital energy, and treat a variety of conditions. In a Cochrane review of migraine, the authors found adding acupuncture to symptomatic treatment of attacks reduces the frequency of headaches, and the benefits may be similar to prophylactic drugs [115]. A small effect

over sham was found. Few sham-controlled studies exist for chronic migraine prevention. A randomized controlled trial of acupuncture versus topiramate in 66 consecutive patients with chronic migraine over a 12-week period was conducted [116]. In the acupuncture group, the median change in the mean number of moderate/severe headache days during 4 weeks for patients with higher baseline headache days (>20 days) was significantly greater than that for lower baseline headache days (≤20 days) (median ± interquartile range: -12 ± 2 vs. -10 ± 1 days, $P = 0.01$) in the acupuncture group. Patients with throbbing symptoms had a better prognosis and higher scores in general. Their expectations predicted responses to both groups. Long-term studies are needed to determine sustained benefits of acupuncture.

Behavioral Therapy

Cognitive behavioral therapy, mindfulness, relaxation therapy, and biofeedback are commonly used non-pharmaceutical interventions for the treatment of migraine. For some individuals, access to behavioral therapies is a major limitation. However, internet-based treatment programs utilizing relaxation, biofeedback, and stress management have proved to be effective for chronic headaches and have the potential to reach a larger number of patients with less cost [117].

Several clinical trials have tested cognitive behavioral therapy for chronic migraine. Cognitive behavioral therapy is a common form of psychotherapy to assist with the management of emotional and physical symptoms, coping, and maladaptive thinking and behaviors that may be associated with chronic pain. A randomized placebo-controlled trial of 135 pediatric patients with chronic migraine compared amitriptyline with cognitive behavioral therapy versus amitriptyline and headache education [118]. The primary endpoint was headache days. In children and adolescents with chronic migraine, amitriptyline with cognitive behavioral therapy had a greater reduction in headache days and migraine-related disability compared to the use of amitriptyline with headache education. At baseline, there were a mean (SD) of 21 (5) days with headache per 28 days. At the 20-week endpoint, days with headache were reduced by 11.5 for the cognitive behavioral therapy plus amitriptyline group versus 6.8 for the headache education plus amitriptyline group (difference, 4.7 [95% CI, 1.7–7.7] days; $P = 0.002$). The secondary endpoint, the mean (SD) PedMIDAS, was 68 (32) points. The PedMIDAS decreased by 52.7 points for the CBT group versus 38.6 points for the headache education group (difference, 14.1 [95% CI, 3.3–24.9] points; $P = 0.01$). The findings support the efficacy of cognitive behavioral therapy in treatment of pediatric populations with chronic migraine.

Behavioral therapy may also be effective for the treatment of comorbidities associated with chronic migraine. Behavioral therapies may be of particular benefit, as stress is associated with poor outcomes to acute treatment in chronic migraine [119]. These interventions may address pain catastrophizing and treat psychiatric disease, both strongly associated with chronic migraine, migraine-related disability, and impact [120, 121]. In addition, behavioral therapies are widely accepted approaches to treatment of insomnia. In a study of behavioral insomnia treatment for chronic migraine with comorbid insomnia, outcomes were compared in patients that received 30-min biweekly sessions of cognitive behavioral therapy for insomnia versus training in the daily practice of skills pertaining to keeping a consistent food/liquid intake, range of motion exercises, and acupressure as a control [122]. Both groups received reduction in headache frequency, but only the cognitive behavioral treatment interventional group had significantly larger increases in total sleep time and sleep efficiency.

Chronic migraine with medication overuse is associated with high rates of relapse after withdrawal treatment [123], yet few studies have tested behavioral interventions. In a study comparing pharmacological prophylaxis to mindfulness-based training for the treatment of chronic migraine after withdrawal from medication overuse, headache frequency and medication use was similar after 1-year follow-up [124]. Another pilot study showed benefits of biofeedback added to traditional pharmacotherapy for reducing headache frequency and acute medication use [125]. Although initial studies are

promising, further research is needed in larger populations to investigate behavioral interventions in addition to pharmacotherapies and withdrawal protocols.

Peripheral Neurostimulation for Chronic Migraine

Peripheral neurostimulation has been used to treat refractory chronic migraine for years. To date, there are three FDA-approved devices for the acute and preventive treatment of migraine and no specific approvals for chronic migraine. Single-pulse transcranial magnetic stimulation (TMS) is approved for the acute treatment of migraine with aura and for migraine prevention. The efficacy of TMS on chronic migraine was reviewed in a meta-analysis of randomized, double-blind, sham-controlled trials [126]. According to the results, TMS for the treatment of chronic migraine was not significant (OR 2.93; 95% CI 0.71–12.15; $P = 0.14$). A small sample size may have accounted for the results. Further studies are needed as a preliminary randomized investigation using high-frequency deep TMS showed a reduction in the frequency and intensity of migraine attack, drug overuse, and depressive symptoms [127]. Supraorbital transcutaneous stimulation with the Cefaly device is also FDA approved for the acute and preventive treatment of migraine but not for chronic migraine. In a small open-label study of 23 consecutive chronic migraine patients designed to determine the efficacy of supraorbital transcutaneous stimulation with the Cefaly device, 35% of the patients enrolled had 50% reduction in monthly migraine days and 50% reduction in monthly medication use over 4 months [128]. In addition, there was greater than 50% reduction in acute medication consumption in over half the patients.

The gammaCore device is FDA approved as a noninvasive vagus nerve stimulation device for the acute treatment of cluster headache and has been approved for migraine as well [129]. Potential antimigraine mechanisms are supported by animal models that show vagus nerve stimulation suppresses acute activation of the trigeminocervical neurons [130], cortical spreading depression [131], and treat trigeminal allodynia [132]. The evidence for migraine attack treatment is based on pain-free rates of moderate to severe attacks in the PRESTO study [133], a randomized, sham-controlled study showing efficacy, tolerability, and safety with no serious or adverse events. The evidence for noninvasive vagus nerve stimulation for the treatment of chronic migraine is limited by trial design. Another small study using trans-cutaneous stimulation of the auricular branch of the vagal nerve (t-VNS) showed efficacy and safety [134]. The results of the EVENT study, a multicenter, prospective double-blind, sham-controlled pilot study of noninvasive vagus nerve stimulation for chronic migraine, suggest that persistent use may reduce the number of head-ache days over time [135].

A protocol with 12 transcranial direct current stimulation sessions was investigated in a ran-domized, sham-controlled trial in subjects with chronic migraine [136]. Intragroup comparisons exhibited greater reduction in headache impact and pain intensity and a higher quality of life after treatment with anodal stimulation of the left primary motor and dorsolateral prefrontal cortex but not in the sham group. Larger studies are needed to establish efficacy and determine the optimal site of cortical stimulation.

The effectiveness of occipital nerve stimu-lation has been tested in multiple-randomized placebo-controlled trials; a meta-analysis showed a modest effect size for chronic migraine. Fre-quent complications included lead migration, infection, and need for surgical revision [137]. A small series of patients with a combination of occipital nerve and supraorbital nerve stimula-tion has shown positive benefits [138]; however, large randomized controlled studies are needed to confirm these findings given the potential for surgical complications.

Peripheral Nerve Blockade

Peripheral nerve blockade is generally cost-effective and safe. Occipital nerve blockade for the treatment of chronic migraine has shown mixed results for short-term prophylaxis. In a mixed cohort consisting of episodic and chronic migraine, occipital nerve blockade was no better than placebo [139]. In another study of chronic migraine, greater occipital blockade was random-ized in a double-blind and placebo-controlled study using bupivacaine versus placebo [140]. After weekly injections for 4 weeks, there was a significant reduction in duration of headache hours and the VAS score. Another study using a bilateral greater occipital nerve block with bupi-vacaine 0.5% or sham with normal saline showed superiority in reducing moderate or severe head-ache days for the week following the injection [141]. After the greater occipital nerve block, there was an increase in pressure pain thresholds in the trigeminal area supporting an effect on the central sensitization at the trigeminal nucleus caudalis. Nerve blocks may be particularly use-ful for certain populations, such as in pregnancy.

The sphenopalatine ganglion is a target of interest for the treatment of migraine as studies have suggested a link between parasympathetic ganglia and the sensory trigeminal system. Para-sympathetic activity may contribute to migraine by activation or sensitization of the intracranial nociceptors and the sphenopalatine ganglion, the largest extracranial parasympathetic ganglion of the head [142]. Furthermore, immunohistochem-ical studies have shown CGRP receptor compo-nents and CGRP-immunoreactive fibers were found in the sphenopalatine ganglion [143]. In one randomized placebo-controlled trial, repeti-tive transnasal sphenopalatine ganglion blockade was found to be effective for the acute treatment of chronic migraine [144]. Long-term efficacy was also established with blockade twice per week for 6 weeks [145]. Taken together, peripheral nerve blocks appear promising; however, large, multicenter, randomized, placebo-controlled tri-als are needed for wider acceptance in the treat-ment of chronic migraine.

Refractory Chronic Migraine and Clinical Trial Considerations

Tertiary headache centers are referral cen-ters, often treating refractory cases of chronic migraine. The term refractory chronic migraine is not recognized as a part of the IHCD-3 but has important clinical and research implications.

A proposed definition of refractory chronic migraine was published by the Refractory Headache Special Interest Section of the American Headache Society [146]. The definition requires significant impairment of quality of life despite trigger management and adequate trials of acute and preventive medications. Patients should have a poor response to two of four drug classes including beta-blockers, anticonvulsants, tricyclics, and calcium channel blockers when tried for at least 2 months. The criteria also require a lack of response to triptans and dihydroergotamine (DHE) intranasal or injectable formulation and either nonsteroidal anti-inflammatory drugs (NSAIDs) or combination analgesic. Modifiers for medication overuse and disability were also proposed. The European Headache Federation Expert Group of refractory chronic migraine characterizes refractory chronic migraine patients by their enormous disability, high risks of serious adverse events, and potential exposures to uncontrolled applications on therapeutics not yet validated [147]. In contrast to the American Headache Society criteria, medication overuse is not included, and adequate treatment of psychiatric or other comorbidities is proposed. For the American Headache Society criteria, failure to respond to onabotulinumtoxinA is not included as it was not yet approved for chronic migraine at the time of publication. Further studies will be needed to evaluate the definitions of refractoriness for prognosis, resource utilization, and treatment stratification.

In cases of disability, excessive emergency room visits, and multiple complex comorbidities, referrals to specialized headache centers may be helpful to prevent complications and progression [148]. Tertiary headache centers provide access to inpatient care, infusions, and coordination of care to optimize management. In the outpatient setting, the use of telemedicine, electronic diaries, and migraine trigger apps may facilitate communication and enhance care for refractory patients. Common inpatient treatment protocols for chronic migraine refractory to outpatient approaches include intravenous dihydroergotamine, lidocaine, and ketamine [149–151]. Both comprehensive inpatient management and integrated headache care networks have been established; however; further, research is needed to assess sustained benefits and predictors of outcome [152].

Clinical trials should be designed to include clinical meaningful endpoints that may be useful in guiding treatment considerations for refractory cases. In addition to headache days with moderate to severe intensity, frequency of migraine episodes and migraine days as suggested by the Task Force of the International Headache Society Clinical Trials Subcommittee [153], responder rates, quality of life measures, disability assessments, acute medication usage, discontinuation rates, safety, and tolerability profiles are meaningful considerations [154]. Attempts should be made to recruit real-world patients who have not responded to multiple preventive medications, have experienced continuous headache [155], and have significant comorbidities to obtain real-world insights. Over the past several decades, there has been progress in novel therapeutics for chronic migraine. Treatment options should be both efficacious and cost-effective, with lost productivity taken into consideration for the development of health policies. Taken together, partnerships with academia, industry, patient groups, and federal agencies are needed to further progress, improve care, and reduce disability associated with chronic migraine.

References

1. Natoli JL, Manack A, Dean B, et al. Global prevalence of chronic migraine: a systematic review. Cephalalgia. 2010;30(5):599–609.
2. Aurora SK. Spectrum of illness: understanding biological patterns and relationships in chronic migraine. Neurology. 2009;72(5 Suppl):S8–13.
3. Headache Classification Committee of the International Headache Society (IHS). The international classification of headache disorders, 3rd edition. Cephalalgia. 2018;38(1):1–211.
4. Silberstein SD, Lipton RB, Dodick DW. Operational diagnostic criteria for chronic migraine: expert opinion. Headache. 2014;54(7):1258–66.
5. Headache Classification Subcommittee of the International Headache Society. The international classification of headache disorders: 2nd edition. Cephalalgia. 2004;24(Suppl 1):9–160.

6. Bigal ME, Sheftell FD, Tepper SJ, Rapoport AM, Lipton RB. Migraine days decline with duration of illness in adolescents with transformed migraine. Cephalalgia. 2005;25(7):482–7.

7. Silberstein SD, Lipton RB, Sliwinski M. Classification of daily and near-daily headaches: field trial of revised IHS criteria. Neurology. 1996;47(4): 871–5.

8. Bigal ME, Rapoport AM, Sheftell FD, Tepper SJ, Lipton RB. Chronic migraine is an earlier stage of transformed migraine in adults. Neurology. 2005;65(10):1556–61.

9. Lipton RB, Serrano D, Buse DC, et al. Improving the detection of chronic migraine: development and validation of identify chronic migraine (ID-CM). Cephalalgia. 2016;36(3):203–15.

10. Garcia-Chimeno Y, Garcia-Zapirain B, Gomez-Beldarrain M, Fernandez-Ruanova B, Garcia-Monco JC. Automatic migraine classification via feature selection committee and machine learning techniques over imaging and questionnaire data. BMC Med Inform Decis Mak. 2017;17(1):38.

11. van Dongen RM, Zielman R, Noga M, et al. Migraine biomarkers in cerebrospinal fluid: a systematic review and meta-analysis. Cephalalgia. 2017;37(1):49–63.

12. Cernuda-Morollon E, et al. No change in interictal PACAP levels in peripheral blood in women with chronic migraine. Headache. 2016;56(9):1448–54.

13. Buse D, Manack A, Serrano D, et al. Headache impact of chronic and episodic migraine: results from the American Migraine Prevalence and Prevention study. Headache. 2012;52(1):3–17.

14. Buse DC, Manack A, Serrano D, Turkel C, Lipton RB. Sociodemographic and comorbidity profiles of chronic migraine and episodic migraine sufferers. J Neurol Neurosurg Psychiatry. 2010;81(4):428–32.

15. Messali A, Sanderson JC, Blumenfeld AM, et al. Direct and indirect costs of chronic and episodic migraine in the United States: a web-based survey. Headache. 2016;56(2):306–22.

16. Dodick DW, Loder EW, Manack Adams A, et al. Assessing barriers to chronic migraine consultation, diagnosis, and treatment: results from the Chronic Migraine Epidemiology and Outcomes (CaMEO) study. Headache. 2016;56:821.

17. Couch JR, Lipton RB, Stewart WF, Scher AI. Head or neck injury increases the risk of chronic daily headache: a population-based study. Neurology. 2007;69(11):1169–77.

18. Scher AI, Stewart WF, Lipton RB. Caffeine as a risk factor for chronic daily headache: a population-based study. Neurology. 2004;63(11):2022–7.

19. Scher AI, Lipton RB, Stewart WF. Habitual snoring as a risk factor for chronic daily headache. Neurology. 2003;60(8):1366–8.

20. Odegård SS, Sand T, Engstrøm M, Stovner LJ, Zwart JA, Hagen K. The long-term effect of insomnia on primary headaches: a prospective population-based cohort study (HUNT-2 and HUNT-3). Headache. 2011;51(4):570–80.

21. Scher AI, Stewart WF, Buse D, Krantz DS, Lipton RB. Major life changes before and after the onset of chronic daily headache: a population-based study. Cephalalgia. 2008;28(8):868–76.

22. Scher AI, Stewart WF, Ricci JA, Lipton RB. Factors associated with the onset and remission of chronic daily headache in a population-based study. Pain. 2003;106(1–2):81–9.

23. Bigal ME, Serrano D, Buse D, Scher A, Stewart WF, Lipton RB. Acute migraine medications and evolution from episodic to chronic migraine: a longitudinal population-based study. Headache. 2008;48(8):1157–68.

24. Serrano D, Lipton RB, Scher AI, et al. Fluctuations in episodic and chronic migraine status over the course of 1 year: implications for diagnosis, treatment and clinical trial design. J Headache Pain. 2017;18(1):101.

25. Lipton RB, Fanning KM, Serrano D, Reed ML, Cady R, Buse DC. Ineffective acute treatment of episodic migraine is associated with new-onset chronic migraine. Neurology. 2015;84(7):688–95.

26. Reed ML, Fanning KM, Serrano D, Buse DC, Lipton RB. Persistent frequent nausea is associated with progression to chronic migraine: AMPP study results. Headache. 2015;55(1):76–87.

27. Manack A, Buse DC, Serrano D, Turkel CC, Lipton RB. Rates, predictors, and consequences of remission from chronic migraine to episodic migraine. Neurology. 2011;76(8):711–8.

28. Gormley P, Anttila V, Winsvold BS, et al. Meta-analysis of 375,000 individuals identifies 38 susceptibility loci for migraine. Nat Genet. 2016;48:856–66.

29. Perry CJ, Blake P, Buettner C, Papavassiliou E, Schain AJ, Bhasin MK, Burstein R. Upregulation of inflammatory gene transcripts in periosteum of chronic migraineurs: implications for extracranial origin of headache. Ann Neurol. 2016;79(6):1000–13.

30. Leao AAP. Spreading depression of activity in thecerebral cortex. J Neurophysiol. 1944;7:359–90.

31. Zhang X, Levy D, Noseda R, Kainz V, Jakubowski M, Burstein R. Activation of meningeal nociceptors by cortical spreading depression:Implications for migraine with aura. J Neurosci. 2010;30(26):8807–14.

32. Zhang X, Levy D, Kainz V, Noseda R, Jakubowski M, Burstein R. Activation of central trigeminovascular neurons by cortical spreading depression. Ann Neurol. 2011;69:855-865.

33. Hansen JM, Lipton RB, Dodick DW, et al.Migraine headache is present in the aura phase:A prospective study. Neurology.2012;79:2044-2049.

34. Dodick DW. A Phase-by-Phase Review of Migraine Pathophysiology.Headache. 2018;58Suppl 1:4-16.

35. Schwedt TJ, Chong CD, Wu T, Gaw N, Fu Y, Li J. Accurate classification of chronic migraine via brain magnetic resonance imaging. Headache. 2015;55(6):762–77.

36. Valfre W, Rainero I, Bergui M, Pinessi L. Voxel-based morphometry reveals gray matter abnormalities in migraine. Headache. 2008;48(1):109–17.

37. Welch KMA, Nagesh V, Aurora SK, Gelman N. Periaqueductal gray matter dysfunction in migraine: cause or the burden of illness? Headache. 2001;41(7):629–37.

38. Aurora SK. Is chronic migraine one end of a spectrum of migraine or a separate entity? Cephalalgia. 2009;29(6):597–605.

39. Aurora SK, Barrodale PM, Tipton RL, Khodavirdi A. Brainstem dysfunction in chronic migraine as evidenced by neurophysiological and positron emission tomography studies. Headache. 2007;47(7):996–1003; discussion 1004–1007.

40. Matharu MS, Bartsch T, Ward N, Frackowiak RS, Weiner R, Goadsby PJ. Central neuromodulation in chronic migraine patients with suboccipital stimulators: a PET study. Brain. 2004;127(Pt 1):220–30.

41. Mathew NT. Pathophysiology of chronic migraine and mode of action of preventive medications. Headache. 2011;51(Suppl 2):84–92.

42. Schulte et al. Visual stimulation leads to activation of the nociceptive trigeminal nucleus in chronic migraine. Neurology.2018;90(22).

43. Coppola G, Iacovelli E, Bracaglia M, Serrao M, Di Lorenzo C, Pierelli F. Electrophysiological correlates of episodic migraine chronification: evidence for thalamic involvement. J Headache Pain. 2013;14:76.

44. Niddam DM, Lai KL, Tsai SY, et al. Neurochemical changes in the medial wall of the brain in chronic migraine. Brain. 2017;141(2):377–90.

45. Maniyar FH, Sprenger T, Monteith T, Schankin C, Goadsby PJ. Brain activations in the premonitory phase of nitroglycerin-triggered migraine attacks. Brain. 2014;137(Pt 1):232–41.

46. Schulte LH, Allers A, May A. Hypothalamus as a mediator of chronic migraine: evidence from high-resolution fMRI. Neurology. 2017;88(21):2011–6.

47. Schwedt TJ, Schlaggar BL, Mar S, et al. Atypical resting-state functional connectivity of affective pain regions in chronic migraine. Headache. 2013;53(5):737–51.

48. Bernstein C, Burstein R. Sensitization of the trigeminovascular pathway: perspective and implications to migraine pathophysiology. J Clin Neurol. 2012;8(2):89–99.

49. Androulakis XM, Krebs K, Peterlin BL, et al. Modulation of intrinsic resting-state fMRI networks in women with chronic migraine. Neurology. 2017;89(2):163–9.

50. Young WB. Allodynia as a complication of migraine: background and management. Curr Treat Options Neurol. 2009;11(1):3–9.

51. Dodick DW. Adv Stud Med. 2003;3(6C):S550-S555.

52. Ashina S, Serrano D, Lipton RB, et al. Depression and risk of transformation of episodic to chronic migraine. J Headache Pain. 2012;13(8):615–24.

53. Scher AI, Buse DC, Fanning KM, Kelly AM, Franznick DA, Adams AM, Lipton RB. Comorbid pain and migraine chronicity: The Chronic Migraine Epidemiology and Outcomes Study. Neurology. 2017;89(5):461–8.

54. Farris SG, Thomas JG, Abrantes AM, et al. Pain worsening with physical activity during migraine attacks in women with overweight/obesity: a prospective evaluation of frequency, consistency, and correlates. Cephalalgia. 2017:333102417747231.

55. Bigal ME, Lipton RB. Obesity is a risk factor for transformed migraine but not chronic tension-type headache. Neurology. 2006;67(2):252–7.

56. Bond DS, Thomas JG, Lipton RB, et al. Behavioral weight loss intervention for migraine: a randomized controlled trial. Obesity (Silver Spring). 2018;26(1):81–7.

57. Midgette LA, Scher AI. The epidemiology of chronic daily headache. Curr Pain Headache Rep. 2009;13(1):59–63.

58. Loder E, Burch R, Rizzoli P. The 2012 AHS/AAN guidelines for prevention of episodic migraine: a summary and comparison with other recent clinical practice guidelines. Headache. 2012;52(6):930–45.

59. Couch JR. Amitriptyline in the prophylactic treatment of migraine and chronic daily headache. Headache. 2011;51(1):33–51.

60. Yurekli VA, Akhan G, Kutluhan S, Uzar E, Koyuncuoglu HR, Gultekin F. The effect of sodium valproate on chronic daily headache and its subgroups. J Headache Pain. 2008;9(1):37–41.

61. Spira PJ, Beran RG. Gabapentin in the prophylaxis of chronic daily headache: a randomized, placebo-controlled study. Neurology. 2003;61(12):1753–9.

62. Saper JR, Lake AE III, Cantrell DT, Winner PK, White JR. Chronic daily headache prophylaxis with tizanidine: a double-blind, placebo-controlled, multicenter outcome study. Headache. 2002;42(6):470–82.

63. May A, Schulte LH. Chronic migraine: risk factors, mechanisms and treatment. Nat Rev Neurol. 2016;12(8):455–64.

64. Charles A, Flippen C, Romero Reyes M, Brennan KC. Memantine for prevention of migraine: a retrospective study of 60 cases. J Headache Pain. 2007;8(4):248–50.

65. Calandre EP, Garcia-Leiva JM, Rico-Villademoros F, Vilchez JS, Rodriguez-Lopez CM. Pregabalin in the treatment of chronic migraine: an open-label study. Clin Neuropharmacol. 2010;33(1):35–9.

66. Engel ER, Kudrow D, Rapoport AM. A prospective, open-label study of milnacipran in the prevention of headache in patients with episodic or chronic migraine. Neurol Sci. 2014;35(3):429–35.

67. Pascual-Gomez J, Alana-Garcia M, Oterino A, Leira R, Lainez-Andres JM. Preventive treatment of chronic migraine with zonisamide: a study in patients who are refractory or intolerant to topiramate. Rev Neurol. 2008;47(9):449–51.

68. Cernuda-Morollon E, Ramon C, Martinez-Camblor P, Serrano-Pertierra E, Larrosa D, Pascual J. OnabotulinumtoxinA decreases interictal CGRP plasma levels in patients with chronic migraine. Pain. 2015;156(5):820–4.

69. Marmura MJ, Silberstein SD, Schwedt TJ. The acute treatment of migraine in adults: the American Headache Society evidence assessment of migraine pharmacotherapies. Headache. 2015;55(1):3–20.

70. Serrano D, Buse DC, Manack Adams A, Reed ML, Lipton RB. Acute treatment optimization in episodic and chronic migraine: results of the American

Migraine Prevalence and Prevention (AMPP) Study. Headache. 2015;55(4):502–18.

71. Holland PR, Goadsby PJ. Targeted CGRP small molecule antagonists for acute migraine therapy. Neurotherapeutics. 2018;15(2):304–12. https://doi.org/10.1007/s13311-018-0617-4. Review. PMID: 29556965

72. Färkkilä M, et al. Efficacy and tolerability of lasmiditan, an oral 5-HT(1F) receptor agonist, for the acute treatment of migraine: a phase 2 randomised, placebo-controlled, parallel-group, dose-ranging study. Lancet Neurol. 2012;11(5):405–13. https://doi.org/10.1016/S1474-4422(12)70047-9.

73. Aurora SK, Brin MF. Chronic migraine: an update on physiology, imaging, and the mechanism of action of two available pharmacologic therapies. Headache. 2017;57(1):109–25.

74. Hoffmann J, Akerman S, Goadsby PJ. Efficacy and mechanism of anticonvulsant drugs in migraine. Expert Rev Clin Pharmacol. 2014;7(2):191–201.

75. Andreou AP, Goadsby PJ. Topiramate in the treatment of migraine: a kainate (glutamate) receptor antagonist within the trigeminothalamic pathway. Cephalalgia. 2011;31(13):1343–58.

76. Hebestreit JM, May A. Topiramate modulates trigeminal pain processing in thalamo-cortical networks in humans after single dose administration. PLoS One. 2017;12(10):e0184406.

77. Diener HC, Bussone G, Van Oene JC, Lahaye M, Schwalen S, Goadsby PJ. Topiramate reduces headache days in chronic migraine: a randomized, double-blind, placebo-controlled study. Cephalalgia. 2007;27(7):814–23.

78. Silberstein SD, Lipton RB, Dodick DW, et al. Efficacy and safety of topiramate for the treatment of chronic migraine: a randomized, double-blind, placebo-controlled trial. Headache. 2007;47(2):170–80.

79. Diener HC, Dodick DW, Goadsby PJ, et al. Utility of topiramate for the treatment of patients with chronic migraine in the presence or absence of acute medication overuse. Cephalalgia. 2009;29(10):1021–7.

80. Silberstein SD. Topiramate in migraine prevention: a 2016 perspective. Headache. 2017;57(1):165–78.

81. Lipton RB, Silberstein S, Dodick D, et al. Topiramate intervention to prevent transformation of episodic migraine: the topiramate INTREPID study. Cephalalgia. 2011;31(1):18–30.

82. Silberstein SD, Dodick DW, Lindblad AS, et al. Randomized, placebo-controlled trial of propranolol added to topiramate in chronic migraine. Neurology. 2012;78(13):976–84.

83. Johnson J, Brittain S, Schwabe S. Cognitive effects of extended-release once-daily SPN-538 (Trokendi XR™) vs bid immediate-release topiramate (TPM-IR, Topamax®) in healthy volunteers. Neurology. 2014;82(10 Suppl):S43.002.

84. Brittain ST, Wheless JW. Pharmacokinetic simulations of topiramate plasma concentrations following dosing irregularities with extended-release vs. immediate-release formulations. Epilepsy Behav. 2015;52(Pt A):31–6.

85. Shen C, Chen F, Zhang Y, Guo Y, Ding M. Association between use of antiepileptic drugs and fracture risk: a systematic review and meta-analysis. Bone. 2014;64:246–53.

86. Lovati C, Giani L. Action mechanisms of Onabotulinum toxin-A: hints for selection of eligible patients. Neurol Sci. 2017;38(Suppl 1):131–40.

87. Schaefer SM, Gottschalk CH, Jabbari B. Treatment of chronic migraine with focus on botulinum neurotoxins. Toxins. 2015;7(7):2615–28.

88. Burstein R, Zhang X, Levy D, Aoki KR, Brin MF. Selective inhibition of meningeal nociceptors by botulinum neurotoxin type A: therapeutic implications for migraine and other pains. Cephalalgia. 2014;34(11):853–69.

89. Drinovac Vlah V, Filipovic B, Bach-Rojecky L, Lackovic Z. Role of central versus peripheral opioid system in antinociceptive and anti-inflammatory effect of botulinum toxin type A in trigeminal region. Eur J pain 2,2,3 (583–591), 2017.

90. Aurora SK, Dodick DW, Turkel CC, et al. OnabotulinumtoxinA for treatment of chronic migraine: results from the double-blind, randomized, placebo-controlled phase of the PREEMPT 1 trial. Cephalalgia. 2010;30(7):793–803.

91. Diener HC, Dodick DW, Aurora SK, et al. OnabotulinumtoxinA for treatment of chronic migraine: results from the double-blind, randomized, placebo-controlled phase of the PREEMPT 2 trial. Cephalalgia. 2010;30(7):804–14.

92. Dodick DW, Turkel CC, DeGryse RE, et al. OnabotulinumtoxinA for treatment of chronic migraine: pooled results from the double-blind, randomized, placebo-controlled phases of the PREEMPT clinical program. Headache. 2010;50(6):921–36.

93. Boudreau GP, Grosberg BM, McAllister PJ, Lipton RB, Buse DC. Prophylactic onabotulinumtoxinA in patients with chronic migraine and comorbid depression: an open-label, multicenter, pilot study of efficacy, safety and effect on headache-related disability, depression, and anxiety. Int J Gen Med. 2015;8: 79–86.

94. Negro A, Curto M, Lionetto L, Martelletti P. A two years open-label prospective study of OnabotulinumtoxinA 195 U in medication overuse headache: a real-world experience. J Headache Pain. 2015;17(1):1.

95. Guerzoni S, Pellesi L, Baraldi C, et al. Long-term treatment benefits and prolonged efficacy of onabotulinumtoxinA in patients affected by chronic migraine and medication overuse headache over 3 years of therapy. Front Neurol. 2017;8:586.

96. Moore KL, Dalley AF, Agur AMR. Clinically oriented anatomy. 7th ed. Philadelphia, PA: Lippincott Williams & Wilkins; 2013.

97. Cady R, Turner I, Dexter K, Beach ME, Durham P. An exploratory study of salivary calcitonin gene-related peptide levels relative to acute interventions and preventative treatment with onabotulinumtoxinA in chronic migraine. Headache. 2014;54(2):269–77.

98. Hubbard CS, Becerra L, Smith JH, et al. Brain changes in responders vs. non-responders in chronic migraine: markers of disease reversal. Front Hum Neurosci. 2016;10:497.

99. Blumenfeld AM, Silberstein SD, Dodick DW, Aurora SK, Brin MF, Binder WJ. Insights into the functional anatomy behind the PREEMPT injection paradigm: guidance on achieving optimal outcomes. Headache. 2017;57:766–77.

100. Edvinsson L. The journey to establish CGRP as a migraine target: a retrospective view. Headache. 2015;55(9):1249–55.

101. Goadsby PJ, Edvinsson L, Ekman R. Vasoactive peptide release in the extracerebral circulation of humans during migraine headache. Ann Neurol. 1990;28:183–7.

102. Edvinsson L, Warfvinge K. Recognizing the role of CGRP and CGRP receptors in migraine and its treatment. Cephalalgia. 2017;333102417736900.

103. Storer RJ, Akerman S, Goadsby PJ. Calcitonin gene-related peptide (CGRP) modulates nociceptive trigeminovascular transmission in the cat. Br J Pharmacol. 2004;142(7):1171–81.

104. Goadsby PJ, Edvinsson L, Ekman R. Release of vasoactive peptides in the extracerebral circulation of humans and the cat during activation of the trigeminovascular system. Ann Neurol. 1988;23(2):193–6.

105. Vanmolkot F, Van der Schueren B, de Hoon J. Sumatriptan causes parallel decrease in plasma CGRP concentration and migraine headache during nitroglycerin-induced migraine attack. Cephalalgia. 2006;26(8):1037–8; author reply 1038–9.

106. Olesen J, Diener HC, Husstedt IW, Goadsby PJ, BIBN 4096 BS Clinical Proof of Concept Study Group, et al. Calcitonin gene-related peptide receptor antagonist BIBN 4096 BS for the acute treatment of migraine. N Engl J Med. 2004;350(11):1104–10.

107. Ong JJY, Wei DY, Goadsby PJ. Recent advances in pharmacotherapy for migraine prevention: from pathophysiology to new drugs. Drugs. 2018;78:411. https://doi.org/10.1007/s40265-018-0865-y.

108. Tepper S, Ashina M, Reuter U, et al. Safety and efficacy of erenumab for preventive treatment of chronic migraine: a randomised, double-blind, placebo-controlled phase 2 trial. Lancet Neurol. 2017;16(6):425–34.

109. Silberstein SD, Dodick DW, Bigal ME, Yeung PP, et al. Fremanezumab for the preventive treatment of chronic migraine. N Engl J Med. 2017;377(22):2113–22.

110. Detke H, Wang S, Skljarevski V, Ahl J, Millen B, Aurora S, Yang JY. A phase 3 placebo-controlled study of galcanezumab in patients with chronic migraine: results from the 3-month double-blind treatment phase of the REGAIN study. American Headache Society, 2017. Poster sponsored by Eli Lilly and Company and/or one of its subsidiaries.

111. Lipton, R. et al. A Phase 3, Randomized, Double-blind, Placebo-Controlled Study to Evaluate the Efficacy and Safety of Eptinezumab for the Preventive Treatment of Chronic Migraine: Results of the PROMISE-2 (PReventionOf Migraine via Intravenous eptinezumab Safety and Efficacy–2) Trial. Plenary Presentation. American Academy of Neurology Conference, 2018

112. Melo-Carrillo A, Strassman AM, Nir RR, et al. Fremanezumab-A humanized monoclonal anti-CGRP antibody-inhibits thinly myelinated (Adelta) but not unmyelinated (C) meningeal nociceptors. J Neurosci. 2017;37(44):10587–96.

113. Melo-Carrillo A, Noseda R, Nir RR, et al. Selective inhibition of trigeminovascular neurons by fremanezumab: a humanized monoclonal anti-CGRP antibody. J Neurosci. 2017;37(30):7149–63.

114. Eftekhari S, Salvatore CA, Johansson S, Chen TB, Zeng Z, Edvinsson L. Localization of CGRP, CGRP receptor, PACAP and glutamate in trigeminal ganglion. Relation to the blood-brain barrier. Brain Res. 2015;1600:93–109.

115. Linde K, Allais G, Brinkhaus B, et al. Acupuncture for the prevention of episodic migraine. Cochrane Database Syst Rev. 2016(6):CD001218.

116. Yang CP, Chang MH, Li TC, Hsieh CL, Hwang KL, Chang HH. Predicting prognostic factors in a randomized controlled trial of acupuncture versus topiramate treatment in patients with chronic migraine. Clin J Pain. 2013;29(11):982–7.

117. Devineni T, Blanchard EB. A randomized controlled trial of an internet-based treatment for chronic headache. Behav Res Ther. 2005;43(3):277–92.

118. Powers SW, Kashikar-Zuck SM, Allen JR, et al. Cognitive behavioral therapy plus amitriptyline for chronic migraine in children and adolescents: a randomized clinical trial. JAMA. 2013;310(24):2622–30.

119. Cha MJ, Kim BK, Moon HS, Ahn JY, et al. Stress is associated with poor outcome of acute treatment for chronic migraine: a multicenter study. Pain Med. 2017. https://doi.org/10.1093/pm/pnx269.

120. Buse DC, Silberstein SD, Manack AN, Papapetropoulos S, Lipton RB. Psychiatric comorbidities of episodic and chronic migraine. J Neurol. 2013;260(8):1960–9.

121. Seng EK, Buse DC, Klepper JE, J Mayson S, et al. Psychological factors associated with chronic migraine and severe migraine-related disability: an observational study in a tertiary headache center. Headache. 2017;57(4):593–604.

122. Smitherman TA, Walters AB, Davis RE, et al. Randomized controlled pilot trial of behavioral insomnia treatment for chronic migraine with comorbid insomnia. Headache. 2016;56(2):276–91.

123. Raggi A, Giovannetti AM, Leonardi M, et al. Predictors of 12-months relapse after withdrawal treatment in hospitalized patients with chronic migraine associated with medication overuse: a longitudinal observational study. Headache. 2017;57(1):60–70.

124. Grazzi L, Sansone E, Raggi A, D'Amico D, et al. Mindfulness and pharmacological prophylaxis after

withdrawal from medication overuse in patients with chronic migraine: an effectiveness trial with a one-year follow-up. J Headache Pain. 2017;18(1):15.

125. Rausa M, Palomba D, Cevoli S, et al. Biofeedback in the prophylactic treatment of medication overuse headache: a pilot randomized controlled trial. J Headache Pain. 2016;17(1):87.

126. Lan L, Zhang X, Li X, Rong X, Peng Y. The efficacy of transcranial magnetic stimulation on migraine: a meta-analysis of randomized controlled trails. J Headache Pain. 2017;18(1):86.

127. Rapinesi C, Del Casale A, Scatena P, et al. Add-on deep transcranial magnetic stimulation (dTMS) for the treatment of chronic migraine: a preliminary study. Neurosci Lett. 2016;623:7–12.

128. Di Fiore P, Bussone G, Galli A, et al. Transcutaneous supraorbital neurostimulation for the prevention of chronic migraine: a prospective, open-label preliminary trial. Neurol Sci. 2017;38(Suppl 1):201–6.

129. Goadsby P, Grosberg BM, Mauskop A, Cady R, Simmons KA. Effect of noninvasive vagus nerve stimulation on acute migraine: an open-label pilot study. Cephalalgia. 2014;34(12):986–93.

130. Akerman S, Simon B, Romero-Reyes M. Vagus nerve stimulation suppresses acute noxious activation of trigeminocervical neurons in animal models of primary headache. Neurobiol Dis. 2017;102:96–104.

131. Chen SP, Ay I, de Morais AL, Qin T, et al. Vagus nerve stimulation inhibits cortical spreading depression. Pain. 2016;157(4):797–805.

132. Oshinsky ML, Murphy AL, Hekierski H Jr, Cooper M, Simon BJ. Noninvasive vagus nerve stimulation as treatment for trigeminal allodynia. Pain. 2014;155(5):1037–42.

133. Tassorelli C. Noninvasive vagus nerve stimulation as acute therapy for migraine: The randomized PRESTO study. Neurology.2018 Jun 15.pii: 10.1212 WNL.0000000000005857. doi: 10.1212/WNL.0000000000005857. [Epub ahead of print]

134. Straube A, Ellrich J, Eren O, Blum B, Ruscheweyh R. Treatment of chronic migraine with transcutaneous stimulation of the auricular branch of the vagal nerve (auricular t-VNS): a randomized, monocentric clinical trial. J Headache Pain. 2015;16:543.

135. Silberstein SD, Calhoun AH, Lipton RB, et al. Chronic migraine headache prevention with noninvasive vagus nerve stimulation: the EVENT study. Neurology. 2016;87(5):529–38.

136. Andrade SM, de Brito Aranha REL, de Oliveira EA, et al. Transcranial direct current stimulation over the primary motor vs prefrontal cortex in refractory chronic migraine: a pilot randomized controlled trial. J Neurol Sci. 2017;378:225–32.

137. Chen YF, Bramley G, Unwin G, Hanu-Cernat D, Dretzke J, Moore D, Bayliss S, Cummins C, Lilford R. Occipital nerve stimulation for chronic migraine--a systematic review and meta-analysis. PLoS One. 2015;10(3):e0116786.

138. Reed KL, Black SB, Banta CJ II, Will KR. Combined occipital and supraorbital neurostimulation for the treatment of chronic migraine headaches: initial experience. Cephalalgia. 2010;30(3):260–71.

139. Dilli E, Halker R, Vargas B, et al. Occipital nerve block for the short-term preventive treatment of migraine: a randomized, double-blinded, placebo-controlled study. Cephalalgia. 2015;35(11):959–68.

140. Inan LE, Inan N, Karadas O, et al. Greater occipital nerve blockade for the treatment of chronic migraine: a randomized, multicenter, double-blind, and placebo-controlled study. Acta Neurol Scand. 2015;132(4):270–7.

141. Cuadrado ML, Aledo-Serrano A, Navarro P, et al. Short-term effects of greater occipital nerve blocks in chronic migraine: a double-blind, randomised, placebo-controlled clinical trial. Cephalalgia. 2017;37(9):864–72.

142. Yarnitsky D, Goor-Aryeh I, Bajwa ZH, Ransil BI, Cutrer FM, Sottile A, Burstein R. 2003 Wolff Award: Possible parasympathetic contributions to peripheral and central sensitization during migraine. Headache. 2003;43(7):704–14.

143. Csati A, Tajti J, Tuka B, Edvinsson L, Warfvinge K. Calcitonin gene-related peptide and its receptor components in the human sphenopalatine ganglion -- interaction with the sensory system. Brain Res. 2012;1435:29–39.

144. Cady R, Saper J, Dexter K, Manley HR. A double-blind, placebo-controlled study of repetitive transnasal sphenopalatine ganglion blockade with tx360((R)) as acute treatment for chronic migraine. Headache. 2015;55(1):101–16.

145. Cady RK, Saper J, Dexter K, Cady RJ, Manley HR. Long-term efficacy of a double-blind, placebo-controlled, randomized study for repetitive sphenopalatine blockade with bupivacaine vs. saline with the Tx360 device for treatment of chronic migraine. Headache. 2015;55(4):529–42.

146. Schulman EA, Peterlin BL, Lake AE III, et al. Defining refractory migraine: results of the RHSIS Survey of American Headache Society members. Headache. 2009;49(4):509–18.

147. Martelletti P, Katsarava Z, Lampl C, et al. Refractory chronic migraine: a consensus statement on clinical definition from the European Headache Federation. J Headache Pain. 2014;15:47.

148. Lee HJ, Choi KS, Won SY, et al. Topographic relationship between the supratrochlear nerve and corrugator supercilii muscle--can this anatomical knowledge improve the response to botulinum toxin injections in chronic migraine? Toxins. 2015;7(7):2629–38.

149. Nagy AJ, Gandhi S, Bhola R, Goadsby PJ. Intravenous dihydroergotamine for inpatient management of refractory primary headaches. Neurology. 2011;77(20):1827–32.

150. Rosen N, Marmura M, Abbas M, Silberstein S. Intravenous lidocaine in the treatment of refractory

headache: a retrospective case series. Headache. 2009;49(2):286–91.

151. Pomeroy JL, Marmura MJ, Nahas SJ, Viscusi ER. Ketamine infusions for treatment refractory headache. Headache. 2017;57(2):276–82.

152. Lake AE III, Saper JR, Hamel RL. Comprehensive inpatient treatment of refractory chronic daily headache. Headache. 2009;49(4):555–62.

153. Silberstein S, Tfelt-Hansen P, Dodick DW, Limmroth V, Lipton RB, Pascual J, Wang SJ, for the Task Force of the International Headache Society Clinical Trials Subcommittee. Guidelines for controlled trials of prophylactic treatment of chronic migraine in adults. Cephalalgia. 2008;28:484–95.

154. Dodick DW, Turkel CC, DeGryse RE, et al. Assessing clinically meaningful treatment effects in controlled trials: chronic migraine as an example. J pain. 2015;16(2):164–75.

155. Trimboli M, Al-Kaisy A, Andreou A, Murphy M, Lamru G. Non-invasive vagus nerve stimulation for the management of refractory primary chronic headaches: a real-world experience. Cephalalgia. 2017;2017:1–10.

Yogi's Headache: Chronic Tension-Type Headache

Duren Michel Ready, Weiwei Dai,
Linda Kirby Keyser, and Cristina Cabret-Aymat

If baseball great Yogi Berra were to comment on tension-type headache, he might say, "That headache is so common, you'd never see it." Tension-type headache (TTH) is the second most common condition worldwide, surpassed only by dental carries in incidence. It occurs so commonly that its incidence is considered a normal part of life [1].

TTH has become known as a "featureless" headache and defined by what it is not [2]. It has been called "muscular contraction", "psychogenic", "psychomyogenic", "stress", and "nonmigrainous" headache. The pain related to TTH typically lacks localization (mostly diffuse and bilateral), mild to moderate in severity, and not pulsatile or worsened by activity. There is an absence of neurological and autonomic features such as aura, lacrimation, nasal congestion, and rhinorrhea). The pain is described as an ache or an external pressure-type (vise-like) sensation [3]. There is often accompanying pericranial muscle tenderness to palpation [4]. The challenge with identifying TTH by "what it is not" begs the question, what is it? We are left then with the fundamental answer, "It hurts."

The heterogeneous characteristics led the first International Headache Society Classification Committee to choose the term "tension-type" in order to represent an uncertain etiology while acknowledging that physical and psychological "tension" somehow plays a role [5]. As TTH's pathogenesis has remained unclear, the terminology has remained in the subsequent editions of the International Classification of Headache Disorders (ICHD) (now in its third edition). It was hoped that codifying TTH's varied or uncertain etiology could facilitate future research [2].

Infrequent Episodic Tension-Type Headache
Description: Infrequent episodes of headache, typically bilateral, pressing, or tightening in quality and of mild to moderate intensity, lasting minutes to days. The pain does not worsen with routine physical activity and is not associated with nausea, but photophobia or phonophobia may be present.

D. M. Ready (✉) · L. K. Keyser · C. Cabret-Aymat
Central Texas Headache Fellowship, Headache Medicine, Baylor Scott and White, Temple, TX, USA
e-mail: duren.ready@bswhealth.org

W. Dai
Neurology, Presbyterian Hospital,
Rio Rancho, NM, USA

Diagnostic Criteria

A. At least ten episodes of headache occurring on <1 day per month on average (<12 days per year) and fulfilling criteria B–D
B. Lasting from 30 min to 7 days
C. At least two of the following four characteristics:
  1. Bilateral location
  2. Pressing or tightening (nonpulsating) quality
  3. Mild or moderate intensity
  4. Not aggravated by routine physical activity such as walking or climbing stairs
D. Both of the following:
  1. No nausea or vomiting
  2. No more than one of photophobia or phonophobia
E. Not better accounted for by another ICHD-3 diagnosis

Frequent Episodic Tension-Type Headache
Description: Frequent episodes of headache, typically bilateral, pressing or tightening in quality and of mild to moderate intensity, lasting minutes to days. The pain does not worsen with routine physical activity and is not associated with nausea, but photophobia or phonophobia may be present.

Diagnostic Criteria

A. At least ten episodes of headache occurring on 1–14 days per month on average for >3 months (≥12 and <180 days per year) and fulfilling criteria B–D
B. Lasting from 30 min to 7 days
C. At least two of the following four characteristics:
  1. Bilateral location
  2. Pressing or tightening (nonpulsating) quality
  3. Mild or moderate intensity

4. Not aggravated by routine physical activity such as walking or climbing stairs
D. Both of the following:
  1. No nausea or vomiting
  2. No more than one of photophobia or phonophobia
E. Not better accounted for by another ICHD-3 diagnosis

Unfortunately, the absence of clear diagnostic criteria in the ICHD 2 allowed individuals with TTH to be diagnosed as having mild migraine, as there is a significant overlap between these two conditions. Many migraine characteristics may be seen in TTH: worsened by physical activity (27.7%), pulsating quality (17.5%), anorexia (18.2%), photophobia (10.6%), unilateral headache (10%), or nausea (4.2%) [6]. The comorbidity of migraine and TTH is even more common in children with 58.4% of children with migraine also having TTH and 68.1% of children with TTH also having migraine [7] (Table 5.1).

The lifetime incidence of tension-type headache is estimated to be between 30 and 78% [8]. The annual US prevalence for chronic tension-type headache (CTTH) is estimated to be 2.2% [9]. The worldwide prevalence has been consistently estimated to be between 2 and 3% [10]. There is a slight female predominance in episodic tension-type headache (ETTH) about 5:4. Typically, TTH develops prior to age 30 with

Table 5.1 Clinical features of tension-type headache (TTH) vs. migraine

Clinical features of TTH	Clinical features of migraine
Bilateral pain	Unilateral pain (chronic migraine can be bilateral)
Pressing, burning pain	Pulsatile pain
Mild to moderate pain	Moderate to intense pain
Not aggravated by physical activity	Aggravated by physical activity
Nausea and vomiting generally absent	Nausea and vomiting usually present
Only photophobia or phonophobia	Usual photophobia ± phonophobia

peak prevalence between 40 and 49 and subsequent decrease with age in both sexes [9].

As the incidence of TTH is much greater than migraine, it has a greater societal burden. Rasmussen et al. reported that 5% of the working population (age 25–64) missed 4 days/year due to headache, 2% missed 20 days/year from headache, and 59% of people with TTH felt that it interfered with their activities [11]. A Danish study found that lost workdays from TTH was three times higher than migraine [12]. These lost workdays accounted for approximately 10% of *all* lost workdays.

Beyond the societal costs, the individual experience and resulting disability is also great. These costs produce suffering through impaired personal functioning, lost wages, and overall reduced quality of life. Unfortunately, these costs are difficult to quantify which may lead to minimizing TTH impact. Tension-type headache frequency (instead of severity) appears to produce the greatest impact on disability and quality of life [3].

When TTH chronifies into chronic tension-type headache (CTTH), it is associated with an even greater societal cost. Considering its significant incidence and cost, it is difficult to understand why it is neglected, and this neglect has left us with few effective interventions [13].

Chronic Tension-Type Headache

Description: A disorder evolving from frequent episodic tension-type headache, with daily or very frequent episodes of headache, typically bilateral, pressing or tightening in quality and of mild to moderate intensity, lasting hours to days, or unremitting. The pain does not worsen with routine physical activity but may be associated with mild nausea, photophobia, or phonophobia.

Diagnostic Criteria

A. Headache occurring on ≥15 days per month on average for >3 months (≥180 days per year), fulfilling criteria B–D
B. Lasting hours to days, or unremitting

C. At least two of the following four characteristics:
   1. Bilateral location
   2. Pressing or tightening (non-pulsating) quality
   3. Mild or moderate intensity
   4. Not aggravated by routine physical activity such as walking or climbing stairs
D. Both of the following:
   1. No more than one of photophobia, phonophobia, or mild nausea
   2. Neither moderate or severe nausea nor vomiting
E. Not better accounted for by another ICHD-3 diagnosis

Tension-Type Headache as a Spectrum

…nothing is more helpful to a clear understanding, prompt recognition, and sound memory than a well ordered arrangement into classes, primary and subordinate…(Yet) Nature, as the saying goes, makes no jumps and passes from extreme to extreme only through a mean. She always produces a species intermediate between higher and lower types, species of doubtful classification linking one type with another and having something in common with both…
John Ray, who invented the concept of species (1682)

An overwhelming number of migraineurs have comorbid TTH, especially those with chronic migraine. This concurrence is what gave rise to the convergence hypothesis [14]. The low-grade background headache that is observed in medication-overuse induced chronic migraine is phenotypically similar to TTH [15]. CTTH also shares many clinical features with fibromyalgia, and they are often comorbid [16]. Additionally, migraine, fibromyalgia, and TTH are more common in women, may in some have a genetic basis, many similar triggers, and are comorbid with depression and anxiety [17]. A recently proposed pain model for CTTH postulated a referred pain from trigger points in the craniocervical muscles and mediated via the spinal cord and the trigeminal nucleus caudalis.

Pain is ultimately an individual perceptual experience. Don Price identified the components of the peripheral pain experience as sensory discriminative (signal) and affective motivational (suffering). These distinct components, once integrated in the cerebral cortex, become the pain experience. The sensory discriminative pathway commences when stimuli transmitted from the peripheral nervous system are transmitted to second-order neurons in the dorsal horn of the spinal cord and then ascends through the spinothalamic track to the thalamus and ultimately to the contralateral sensory cortex. This signal is transmitted along heavily myelinated nerve fibers allowing for precise recognition of the quality, quantity, and location of the signal.

The affective motivational pathway branches off the spinothalamic tract to form the parabrachial track and is then bilaterally distributed throughout the cortex to the limbic system (amygdala, insula, hippocampus, caudate, anterior cingulate gyrus, prefrontal cortex, and the supraorbital cortex).

This pathway is responsible for the subjective experience associated with the signal. Limbically augmented pain (pain greater than the sum of its parts) suggests that pain and mood share many common pathways. The shared common pathways help us understand how unmanaged stress, past traumas, or depression amplify suffering beyond the sum product of stress.

Tension-Type Headache Pathophysiology and Clinical Findings

Historically it was believed that TTH was the result of muscle contraction and head and neck muscle ischemia [18]. Subsequent electromyographic (EMG) studies refuted this etiology [19]. Furthermore, studies have demonstrated normal muscle lactate levels in CTTH, thereby making increased muscle contraction an unlikely etiology for TTH [20].

Fundamentals

In TTH, there is increased nociceptive input into the central nervous system. Injection of algogenic solution produces increased nociception to pressure, thermal, and electrical stimulation. This increased sensitivity is seen in cephalic and extracephalic musculature [18]. Subsequently, amplified nociceptive input from pericranial and cervical muscles provokes changes in second-order neurons in the spinal cord dorsal horn and the spinal trigeminal nucleus. Over time, these second-order neurons undergo plastic changes increasing sensitivity to stimulation. The end result is central sensitization. A likely product of the central sensitization is increased muscle contraction that is seen in CTTH [21]. The increased baseline muscle tone appears to be a consequence rather than a cause of the increased pain. The central sensitization has been confirmed in CTTH by examining the nociceptive flexion reflex R3 component [22], suprathreshold (single or repetitive) electrical thresholds [23], and cortical potential evoked by supraorbital laser heat stimulation [24]. In a properly functioning system the hyperexcitability of the interneurons would be inhibited by input from the periaqueductal gray. The absence of effective descending pain modulation confirms the involvement of central mechanism in CTTH [3].

Differences Between ETTH and CTTH

In ETTH, the pericranial myofascial mechanisms are likely significant. However, in CTTH alterations in central pain processing are generally accepted as causative [15]. High density EEG brain mapping has demonstrated abnormal processing of sensory evoked potentials in CTTH and descending modulation of nociceptive input [25]. A causative central mechanism is supported by evidence of specific disruption of the trigeminal pathway via suppression of the R2 component of the blink reflex. However, this mechanism was only observed in CTTH [26].

Chemical

Multiple algogenic chemical mediators (glutamate, bradykinin, prostaglandin E2, glucose or pyruvate) have been identified in tender muscle tissue in CTTH [27]. These substances may be released at trigger points locally and in distal pain-free tissues [28]. Algogenic substance release decreases nociceptive threshold, generating a cycle of peripheral sensitization in TTH [29]. In addition, calcitonin gene-related peptide (CGRP), a potent migraine provocateur, has been demonstrated in people with "pulsatile" CTTH [30].

Pericranial Tenderness

Pericranial muscle tenderness is a common finding in TTH. The increased tenderness to palpation is present in adults with both frequent ETTH and CTTH. However, in children, it seems to be only present in CTTH [31–33]. When present, pericranial tenderness correlates with headache frequency and intensity. Typically the muscle tenderness is diffused, perceived as a spasm, or associated with a "trigger point" in a tight muscle. Pericranial tenderness can be present even on headache-free days. Given the consistent finding of pericranial tenderness, it is considered to be a precipitant and not a product of TTH [3].

Pericranial tenderness initiates a feedback loop that can, over time, induce central sensitization in the cortex by increasing attention to and emotional response to pain [34]. It has recently been demonstrated that the central sensitization associated with this phenomenon can be accelerated by inadequate sleep [35].

Pain Pressure Point

The scalp, neck, and jaw muscle and tendon tenderness is observed during and between attacks. There appears to be some correlation between the observed muscle tenderness and TTH severity and frequency [36, 37]. This tenderness is the best documented finding in ETTH and CTTH [1]. Pressure pain thresholds (PPT—the lowest pressure stimulus that is perceived as painful) and pressure pain tolerance thresholds (PPTol—the maximum pressure stimulus that is tolerated) in cephalic and extracephalic regions are lower in CTTH when compared to controls [38, 39]. Increased pressure pain detection has also been identified in infrequent TTH [40, 41]. Interestingly, the increased pressure pain sensitivity is not evenly distributed. In the temporalis, the anterior aspect is the most sensitive [42].

Myofascial Trigger Points

Trigger points are a palpable hard nodule in a "taunt band" of skeletal muscle. "Active" trigger points are painful spontaneously, and "latent" trigger points are painful when palpated. Active trigger points are associated with higher bradykinin levels and other chemical mediators [28]. They are also associated with local and referred pain [28, 43]. When active trigger points are present in TTH, patients have greater headache intensity, frequency, and duration [44]. In CTTH there are more active trigger points than controls, which suggest that they are involved in TTH pathophysiology [45].

Multiple clinical trials have demonstrated the significance of active trigger points in CTTH [46]. Trigger points have been identified in the suboccipital [47], upper trapezius [48], superior oblique [49], sternocleidomastoid [50], temporalis [51], and lateral rectus [52] muscles. These widespread trigger points support the Fernandez-de-las-Peñas et al. model involving peripheral nociceptor sensitization through active trigger points and then central sensitization via the continued afferent discharge to the trigeminal nucleus caudalis. In this model the muscle tenderness is the product, and the trigger point referred pain becomes one of the significant causes of CTTH [53]. Trigger point activity should not obscure the need to address other factors associated with TTH and its progression such as forward head posture [54], muscle atrophy [55], altered muscle pattern recruitment [56], or psychological factor [57]. These additional peripheral factors add to the central sensitizing process.

Neuroplastic Changes and Central Sensitization

Central nervous system hyperexcitability and reduced inhibitory pain mechanisms are involved in TTH nociception [58]. CTTH patients report hypersensitivity to stimulus in cephalic and extra-cephalic non-symptomatic locations, demonstrating increased synaptic nociceptive transmission within the central nervous system [59]. Lowered pressure pain threshold has been demonstrated in the trapezius, frontalis, and temporalis muscles in TTH and CTTH [60].

Pressure pain thresholds for infrequent TTH are normal. However, in frequent TTH and CTTH, they are decreased [3]. This lowered threshold is consistent with what is observed in other central pain conditions [61]. Fibromyalgia (FMS), a classical central pain disorder, is highly comorbid with CTTH. In ETTH, FMS is estimated to be present in 35% of patients. Once it progresses to CTTH, the incidence climbs as high as 44% [62, 63].

This central neuronal sensitization appears to be important in CTTH pathogenesis [59]. Neuroplastic changes, such as the nociceptive flexion reflex R3 component [22] and evoked cortical potential via supraorbital laser heat stimulation, have been reported [24]. However, the most significant change is pericranial muscle tenderness to palpation. In adults, this is the most typical finding [64]. This tenderness is not limited to the pericranial musculature but is also observed in the neck and shoulders.

Clinical Signs of Central Sensitization [4]

1. Generalized pericranial muscle and nerve tenderness
2. Widespread pressure and electrical pain sensitivity
3. Comorbid with fibromyalgia syndrome
4. Presence of non-restorative sleep
5. Comorbid with anxiety, depression, mood disorders, coping mechanisms

---

A 12-year longitudinal study found that patients who developed CTTH had normal tenderness scores and pain pressure threshold prior to the onset of TTH symptoms. These findings suggest that sensitization is a consequence and not a trigger of CTTH [65]. The persistent trigger point activation induces negative neuroplastic changes in second-order neurons in the dorsal horn and spinal trigeminal nucleus producing increased pericranial and cervical muscle tenderness [66]. Diminished descending nociceptive inhibition at the dorsal horn is supported by the finding that in CTTH there are deficiencies in diffuse noxious inhibitory pain control (DINC) mechanisms [67–69].

MRI of the brain in CTTH patients reveals significantly reduced gray matter density in the pain matrix (cingulate, insular, orbitofrontal cortex, right posterior temporal lobe, bilateral parahippocampus, dorsal rostral and ventral pons, and right cerebellum) [70]. However, the reduction in gray matter may suggest neuronal damage, but that is not always the case [71]. The gray matter density reduction is positively correlated with headache burden over time. These findings are similar to other chronic central pain disorders and suggest that it is a consequence of the continued pain state [72].

Stress and Genetics

While stress is generally accepted to be one of the most significant TTH triggers, its causative pathway is unclear [68]. Stress, whether psychological or environmental, seems to have a greater impact than genetics [15]. Stressors (and the failure to recover from stressors) are additive TTH risk factors [15]. These stressors may include hunger, thirst, lack of restorative sleep, and homeostasis disruptions. Patients may often report a TTH on a "bad" day. This effect may be by a direct mechanism or by worsening comorbidity, such as depression, anxiety, or insomnia [3].

While no specific genetic locus has been identified in CTTH, epidemiological studies have found that first-degree relatives of CTTH patients have a 3.1-fold increase in the odds of having CTTH [73, 74]. This would suggest that developing CTTH is a product of genetic and environmental factors [75]. However, it would appear that stress-producing environmental factors exert a greater influence than genetics [76]. Stress increases attention and vigilance to pain which amplifies the pain experience. When compared to controls, TTH sufferers demonstrate greater stress-induced pain sensitivity. This in turn triggers a "stress" headache [77]. Additionally, stress enhances myofascial tissue activation and sensitization peripherally and decreases nociceptive thresholds centrally [68].

Tension-Type Headache Clinical Issues

Population-based studies have shown that increased pain sensitivity increases the prevalence and frequency of tension-type headache [78]. The nonspecific and widespread sensitivity in TTH suggests central nervous system impairment by increased excitability in dorsal horn and supraspinal neurons [4]. The increased sensitivity is observed ictally and interictally [79].

Cervical range of motion is also impaired in TTH with a more pronounced forward head posture while sitting and standing [54]. These findings seem to correlate with headache frequency and duration and the cervical range of motion impairment directly linked to the degree of forward head posture.

Tension-Type Headache Clinical and Physical Findings

The experience of muscle pain occurs when muscle nociceptors are excited. These free nerve endings respond to mechanical (thermal/chemical) stimulation and endogenous algogenic neurotransmitters (bradykinin/serotonin/prostaglandin E2) [29]. The marked heterogeneity of TTH pathophysiological and significant environmental contributions suggests multiple pathways that may be contributing in tandem or isolation [80].

Secondary Headache

Since many TTH features are nonspecific, it should only be diagnosed after any secondary headache disorder has been excluded [81]. Headaches associated to giant cell arteritis may resemble TTH but typically presents with severe unilateral pain and jaw claudication [3]. A nonspecific headache may be the product of a homeostatic disorder such as anemia, hypothyroidism, hepatic, or renal disease. A systemic infection (bacterial or viral) may also have headache as a symptom. Because of the symptom overlay between primary and secondary headache symptoms, it is essential to elicit the temporal pattern of the headache [15].

Cervicogenic

It is not uncommon for cervicogenic headaches to present with TTH characteristics. The pathology may involve the discs, osseous structures, or structural alignment [15]. Common clinical features such as side-locked pain, pain worsened by moving the head, pain that is provoked by pressing the fingers into the neck muscles, and pain that radiates from the back to the front can be seen in both TTH and many secondary headaches [82].

Comorbidities

Insomnia is one of the most common comorbidities seen in TTH. Continued sleep deprivation appears to lower pain thresholds [83]. One prospective trial demonstrated that insomniacs were more likely to develop TTH over a decade [84]. Polysomnographic studies in TTH detected notably greater rates of insomnia, daytime tiredness, anxiety, and reduced subjective sleep quality compared with controls. Remarkably, TTH patients had no sleep-time differences or additional slow-wave sleep (a marker of increased sleep quality). These findings suggest that TTH patients may have greater sleep requirements [35]. Addressing this comorbidity is essential as disturbed sleep has been shown to be a poor prognostic factor in TTH [85].

Temporomandibular disorder (TMD) may be a secondary cause of headache and can resemble TTH. Temporomandibular joint (TMJ) pain usually originates from the joint or the muscles of mastication. This disorder is common in TTH and migraine [86]. The relationship between TMD and these primary headaches appears bidirectional with each condition worsening the other [87]. Similar to CTTH, TMD has also been associated with cutaneous allodynia (a marker for central sensitization) suggesting a pathophysiological mechanism for the bidirectional influence [88].

Mood/Behavioral

As seen in other chronic pain conditions, mood disorders are common in CTTH [89]. One meta-analysis reported that children and adolescents with TTH had more psychopathological symptoms similar to what is seen in migraine [90]. It is estimated that the chance of developing a secondary depression is 25% in CTTH. CTTH patients additionally exhibit higher anxiety rates [91]. In combination, depression and anxiety may accelerate headache frequency by lowering pain threshold [92]. There are also higher rates of catastrophizing and avoidance in CTTH [18].

ETT/CTTH Treatment

Treatment for TTH involves pharmacological, behavioral, physical, and procedural therapies. It is further subdivided into acute and preventive therapy [15]. Interventions seem to be effective in ETTH and may prevent progression to CTTH [4] where their effectiveness may be limited [89]. Unfortunately, research has not demonstrated a robust response [93]. As in migraine, as TTH becomes chronic, it becomes more difficult to treat [89].

The European Federation of Neurological Sciences (now the European Academy of Neurology) published TTH treatment guidelines in 2010 [94]. These guidelines recommended the use of nonpharmacological interventions despite the weakness (or in some cases the absence) of robust scientific evidence. Acute ETTH treatment recommendations included simple analgesics and NSAIDs followed by caffeinated combination analgesics. The guidelines argue against the acute use of triptans, muscle relaxants, and opioids. The typical admonition about avoiding medication-overuse headache was also included. Amitriptyline, followed by mirtazapine, and venlafaxine were recommended for TTH prophylaxis. The guidelines pointed out that the efficacy of prophylactic medication is limited and frequently causes problematic adverse effects.

A likely explanation for promoting nonpharmacological intervention (in spite of their weak evidence) is that many of these treatments promote positive lifestyle changes that enhance resilience. This may block the most common trigger of TTH "stress."

Acute Treatment

Consistent with the EFNS guidelines, clinical practice demonstrates that NSAIDs are first-line therapy for TTH [95]. Ibuprofen (between 400 and 800 mg) is a reasonable first choice for acute ETTH [4]. One trial demonstrated the benefit of a COX-2 inhibitor, lumiracoxib (200–400 mg), for ETTH [96] (Table 5.2).

Triptans have been demonstrated to effectively treat acute TTH in individuals with comorbid migraine [97]. However, medication cost will likely limit triptan usage in TTH.

Prophylactic

Tricyclic antidepressants, especially amitriptyline, are the first-line therapeutic agents for TTH (both ETTH and CTTH) [2]. Most studies initiate amitriptyline between 10 and 25 mg titrating upward to 75 mg in CTTH [15]. Clomipramine may be superior to amitriptyline, but adverse

Table 5.2 Recommended drugs for acute treatment of tension-type therapy

Substance	Dose (mg)	Level	Comment
Ibuprofen	200–800	A	Gastrointestinal side effects, risk of bleeding
Ketoprofen	25	A	Side effects as for ibuprofen
Aspirin	500–1000	A	Side effects as for ibuprofen
Naproxen	375–550	A	Side effects as for ibuprofen
Diclofenac	12.5–100	A	Side effects as for ibuprofen, only doses of 12.5–25 mg tested in TTH
Paracetamol	1000 (oral)	A	Less risk of gastrointestinal side effects compared with NSAIDs
Caffeine comb.	65–200	B	See below[a]

[a]The level of recommendation considers side effects and consistency of the studies. There is sparse evidence for optimal doses. The most effective dose of a drug well tolerated by a patient should be chosen; NSAID, nonsteroidal anti-inflammatory drugs; TTH, tension-type headache; a combination with caffeine 65–200 mg increases the efficacy of ibuprofen and APAP but possibly also the risk for developing medication-overuse headache. Level of recommendation of combination drugs containing caffeine is therefore B

events often limit its use. Nortriptyline typically has a better side effect profile to amitriptyline, and it may be a reasonable alternative for those who have difficulty tolerating amitriptyline. Doxepin (especially if there is comorbid insomnia) is a reasonable second-line TCA choice [80]. Protriptyline has been shown to be beneficial in CTTH [3], but side effects may limit its utility.

Mirtazapine (an antidepressant that acts at alpha -2 and histamine -1 receptors increasing serotonin and norepinephrine) has demonstrated efficacy at 30 mg daily dosing even in amitriptyline nonresponders [98]. Unfortunately this dosage produces fatigue and weight gain and lower doses were not effective.

Venlafaxine was shown to benefit ETT patients with comorbid depression, but not in CTTH [99]. Another SNRI, duloxetine at 60 mg/day, demonstrated significant headache improvement in an open-label trial in chronic migraine and CTTH patients with major depression [100].

Typically, muscle relaxants have limited utility in TTH. Tizanidine, a centrally acting anti-spasticity agent, demonstrated some benefit with doses between 6 and 18 mg/day. Additional benefit was seen for tizanidine 4 mg combined with amitriptyline 20 mg in CTTH over amitriptyline alone [101].

Topiramate in a prospective open-label trial produced a 50% improvement in CTTH severity and frequency [102]. Other membrane-stabilizing medications have no evidence supporting their use [3] (Table 5.3).

Table 5.3 Recommended drugs for prevention of tension-type headaches

Substance	Daily dose (mg)	Level of recommendation
Drug of first choice		
Amitriptyline	30–75	A
Drugs of second choice		
Mirtazapine	30	B
Venlafaxine	150	B
Drugs of third choice		
Clomipramine	75–150	B
Maprotiline	75	B
Mianserin	30–60	B

The level of recommendation considers side effects and number and quality of the studies

Procedural Interventions

Trials of botulinum toxin A for TTH have yielded contradictory results. One trial showed benefit for headache duration and patient assessment scores while failing to demonstrate any improvement in headache-free days [103]. A latter trial showed significant improvement for headache days, intensity, and related disability [104]. Unfortunately, these benefits have not been confirmed in placebo-controlled double blinded trials [105].

Pericranial trigger point injections with lidocaine in patients with frequent TTH were shown to reduce headache frequency and severity [106]. Fernández-de-las-Peñas, et al. developed a preliminary clinical prediction rule to identify CTTH patients who might benefit from short-term success with a muscle trigger point therapy. The clinical rule has four variables: headache duration <8.5 h/day, headache frequency <5.5 days/week, bodily pain <47, and vitality <47.5.[1] One-month improvement was associated with two variables: headache frequency <5.5 days/week and bodily pain <47 [107].

Acupuncture trials and systematic reviews have also yielded conflicting results. One review demonstrated superiority over sham acupuncture at both early and late follow-up [108]. The combined results also demonstrated superiority over pharmacological intervention in headache frequency and intensity, functioning, and response. In contrast, a more recent meta-analysis concluded that acupuncture (when compared to sham acupuncture) had limited efficacy for reducing TTH frequency [109].

Behavioral Therapy

Cognitive behavioral therapy (CBT) and relaxation therapies have been shown to have a robust synergistic effect in lowering severity CTTH when combined with amitriptyline [110] (Table 5.4). Younger patients tend to be more responsive to behavioral therapies [95].

Table 5.4 Non-pharmacological treatments for tension of tension-type headache

Treatment	Level of recommendation
EMG biofeedback	A
Cognitive-behavioral therapy	C
Relaxation training	C
Physical therapy	C
Acupuncture	C

The level of recommendation considers number and quality of the studies

A level A rating (effective) required at least one convincing class I study or two consistent convincing class II studies. A level B rating (probably effective) required at least one convincing class II study or overwhelming class III evidence. A level C rating (possibly effective) required at least two convincing class III studies

Data from the guidelines from the European Federation of Neurological Societies [94]

[1] As measured on the Medical Outcomes Study SF-36

Electromyography biofeedback that allows patients to learn control over pericranial muscle tension has demonstrated effectiveness for TTH [111]. This meta-analysis reported a significant medium to large benefit that was stable over 15 months. The greatest improvement was seen in headache frequency.

Exercise and physical therapy have demonstrated benefit in TTH. Some recent trials have demonstrated benefit for physical therapy in CTTH for headache frequency, duration, and intensity [112–114].

Conclusion

Tension-type headache remains an underdiagnosed and undertreated entity with poorly understood pathophysiology. However, the burden of tension-type headache, both individually and for society is significant and the inescapable association with stress suggests that TTH may be a marker for a variety of social and personal circumstances requiring our attention. Sufferers deserve attention and care. These headaches may just simply be telling us that we need to be taking better care of ourselves.

References

1. Bezov D, Ashina S, Jensen R, Bendtsen L. Pain perception studies in tension-type headache. Headache. 2011;51(2):262–71.
2. Fernández-de-las-Peñas C, Schoenen J. Chronic tension-type headache: what is new? Curr Opin Neurol. 2009;22(3):254–61.
3. Kaniecki R, Diamond S, Cady RK, Diamond ML, Martin VT. Headache and migraine biology and management. New York: Academic; 2015.
4. de Tommaso M, Fernández-de-Las-Penas C. Tennsion type headache. Curr Rheumatol Rev. 2016;12(2):127–39.
5. Headache Classification Committee of the International Headache Society. Classification and diagnostic criteria for headache disorders, cranial neuralgias and facial pain. Cephalalgia. 1998;8(Suppl 7):1–96.
6. Rasmussen BK, Jensen R, Olesen J. A population-based analysis of the criteria of the International Headache Society. Cephalalgia. 1991;11:129–34.
7. Turkdogan D, Cagirici S, Soylemez D, et al. Characteristics and overlapping features of migraine and tension-type headache. Headache. 2006;46:461–8.

8. Bendtsen L, Jensen R. Tension-type headache: the most common, but also the most neglected, headache disorder. Curr Opin Neurol. 2006;19:305–9.

9. Schwartz BS, Stewart WF, Simon D, Lipton R. Epidemiology of tension-type headache. JAMA. 1998;279:381–3.

10. Stovner L, Hagen K, Jensen R, et al. The global burden of headache: a documentation of headache prevalence and disability worldwide. Cephalalgia. 2007;27(3):193–210.

11. Rasmussen BK, Jensen R, Olesen J. Epidemiology of tension-type headache in a general population. In: Olesen J, Schoenen J, editors. Tension-type headache: classification, mechanisms, and treatment. New York: Raven Press; 1993. p. 9–13.

12. Rasmussen B, Jensen R, Olesen J. Impact of headache on sickness absence and utilization of medical services: a Danish population study. J Epidemiol Community Health. 1992;46:443–6.

13. Fernández-de-Las-Peñas C. What do we know about chronic tension-type headache? Discov Med. 2009;8(43):232–6.

14. Cady RK. The convergence hypothesis. Headache. 2007;47:S44–51.

15. Kaniecki RG. Tension-type headache. Continuum (Minneap Minn). 2012;18(4):823–34.

16. Kanaan RA, Lepine JP, Wessely SC. The association or otherwise of the functional somatic syndromes. Psychosom Med. 2007;69:855–9.

17. Marcus DA, Bernstein C, Rudy TE. Fibromyalgia and headache: an epidemiological study supporting migraine as part of the fibromyalgia syndrome. Clin Rheumatol. 2005;24:595–601.

18. Bendtsen L, Jensen R. Tension-type headaches. Neurol Clin. 2009;27:525–35.

19. Jensen R. Pathophysiological mechanisms of tension-type headache: a review of epidemiological and experimental studies. Cephalalgia. 1999;19:602–21.

20. Ashina M, Stallknecht B, Bendtsen L, et al. In vivo evidence of altered skeletal muscle blood flow in chronic tension-type headache. Brain. 2002;125:320–6.

21. Jensen R, Fuglsang-Frederiksen A, Olesen J. Quantitative surface EMG of pericranial muscles in headache: a population study. Electroencephalogr Clin Neurophysiol. 1994;93:355–44.

22. Filatova E, Latysheva N, Kurenkov A. Evidence of persistent central sensitization in chronic headaches: a multimethod study. J Headache Pain. 2008;9:295–300.

23. Ashina S, Bendtsen L, Ashina M, et al. Generalized hyperalgesia in patients with chronic tension type headache. Cephalalgia. 2006;26:940–8.

24. de Tommaso M, Libro G, Guido M, Sciruicchio V, Losito L, Puca F. Heat pain thresholds and cerebral event-related potentials following painful CO$_2$ laser stimulation in chronic tension-type headache. Pain. 2003;104:111–9.

25. Buchgreitz L, Egsgaard LL, Jensen R, Arendt-Nielsen L, Bendtsen L. Abnormal pain processing in chronic tension-type headache: a high-density EEG brain mapping study. Brain. 2008;131:3232–8.

26. Sohn J, Choi H, Kim C. Differences between episodic and chronic tension-type headache in nociceptive-specific trigeminal pathways. Cephalalgia. 2013;33:330–9.

27. Ashina M, Stallknecht B, Bendtsen L, et al. Tender points are not sites of ongoing inflammation: in vivo evidence in patients with chronic tension-type headache. Cephalalgia. 2003;23:109–16.

28. Shah JP, Danoff JV, Desai MJ, et al. Bio-chemicals associated with pain and inflammations are elevated in sites near to and remote from active myofascial trigger points. Arch Phys Med Rehabil. 2008;89:16–23.

29. Arendt-Nielsen L. Headache: muscle tension, trigger points and referred pain. Int J Clin Pract Suppl. 2015;(182):8–12.

30. Ashina M, Bendtsen L, Jensen R, et al. Plasma levels of calcitonin gene-related peptide in chronic tension-type headache. Neurology. 2000;55:1335–40.

31. Metsahonkala L, Anttila P, Laimi K, et al. Extracephalic tenderness and pressure pain threshold in children with headache. Eur J Pain. 2006;10:581–5.

32. Anttila P, Metsähonkala L, Mikkelsson M, et al. Muscle tenderness in pericranial and neck-shoulder region in children with headache: a controlled study. Cephalalgia. 2002;22:340–4.

33. Soee AB, Skov L, Kreiner S, Tornoe B, Thomsen LL. Pain sensitivity and peri-cranial tenderness in children with tension-type headache: a controlled study. J Pain Res. 2013;6:425–34.

34. de Tommaso M, Shevel E, Pecoraro C, et al. Topographic analysis of laser evoked potentials in chronic tension-type headache: correlations with clinical features. Int J Psychophysiol. 2006;62:38–45.

35. Engstrøm M, Hagen K, Bjørk M, Stovner LJ, Stjern M, Sand T. Sleep quality, arousal and pain thresholds in tension-type headache: a blinded controlled polysomnographic study. Cephalalgia. 2014;34:455–63.

36. Drummond P. Scalp tenderness and sensitivity to pain in migraine and tension headache. Headache. 1987;27:45–50.

37. Lipchik GL, Holroyd KA, O'Donnell FJ, et al. Exteroceptive suppression periods and pericranial muscle tenderness in chronic tension-type head-ache: effects of psychopathology, chronicity and disability. Cephalalgia. 2000;20:638–46.

38. Schoenen J, Bottin D, Hardy F, Gerard P. Cephalic and extra-cephalic pressure pain thresholds in chronic tension type headache. Pain. 1991;47:145–9.

39. Sandrini G, Antonaci F, Pucci E, Bono G, Nappi G. Comparative study with EMG, pressure algometry and manual palpation in tension-type headache and migraine. Cephalalgia. 1994;14:451–7.

40. Schmidt-Hansen PT, Svensson P, Bendtsen L, Graven-Nielsen T, Bach FW. Increased muscle pain sensitivity in patients with tension-type headache. Pain. 2007;129:113–21.

41. Mørk H, Ashina M, Bendtsen L, Olesen J, Jensen R. Induction of prolonged tenderness in patients with tension-type headache by means of a new

experimental model of myofascial pain. Eur J Neurol. 2003;10:249–56.

42. Fernández-de-las-Penas C, Ge HY, Cuadrado ML, et al. Bilateral pressure pain sensitivity mapping of the temporalis muscle in chronic tension type headache. Headache. 2008;48:1067–75.

43. Simons DG, Travell J, Simons LS. Myofascial pain and dysfunction: the trigger point manual, vol. 1. 2nd ed. Baltimore, MD: Williams & Wilkins; 1999.

44. Fernandez-de-las-Penas C, Cuadrado ML, Arendt-Nielsen L, Simons DG, Pareja JA. Myofascial trigger points and sensitization: an updated pain model for tension-type headache. Cephalalgia. 2007;27:383–93.

45. Marcus DA, Scharff L, Mercer S, Turk DC. Musculoskeletal abnormalities in chronic headache: a controlled comparison of headache diagnostic groups. Headache. 1999;39:21–7.

46. Fernández-de-las-Penas C, Simons DG, Gerwin RD, et al. Muscle trigger points in tension type headache. In: Fernández-de-las-Penas C, Arendt-Nielsen L, Gerwin RD, editors. Tension type and cervicogenic headache: pathophysiology, diagnosis and treatment. Baltimore: Jones & Bartlett; 2009. p. 61–76.

47. Fernández-de-las-Penas C, Alonso-Blanco C, Cuadrado ML, et al. Trigger points in the suboccipital muscles and forward head posture in tension type headache. Headache. 2006;46:454–60.

48. Fernández-de-las-Penas C, Ge H, Arendt-Nielsen L, et al. Referred pain from trapezius muscle trigger point shares similar characteristics with chronic tension type headache. Eur J Pain. 2007;11:475–82.

49. Fernández-de-las-Penas C, Cuadrado ML, Gerwin RD, Pareja JA. Referred pain from the trochlear region in tension-type headache: a myofascial trigger point from the superior oblique muscle. Headache. 2005;45:731–7.

50. Fernández-de-las-Penas C, Alonso-Blanco C, Cuadrado ML, et al. Myofascial trigger points and their relationship with headache clinical parameters in chronic tension type headache. Headache. 2006;46:1264–72.

51. Fernández-de-las-Penas C, Ge H, Arendt-Nielsen L, et al. The local and referred pain from myofascial trigger points in the temporalis muscle contributes to pain profile in chronic tension-type headache. Clin J Pain. 2007;23:786–92.

52. Fernández-de-las-Penas C, Cuadrado ML, Gerwin RD, Pareja JA. Referred pain from the lateral rectus muscle in subjects with chronic tension type headache. Pain Med. 2009;10:43–8.

53. Fernández-de-las-Peñas C, Arendt-Nielsen L, Simons DG, Cuadrado ML, Pareja JA. Sensitization in tension type headache: a pain model. In: Fernández-de-las-Peñas C, Arendt-Nielsen L, Gerwin RD, editors. Tension type and cervicogenic headache: pathophysiology, diagnosis and treatment. Baltimore, MD: Jones & Bartlett; 2009. p. 97–106.

54. Fernández-de-las-Penas C, Alonso-Blanco C, Cuadrado ML, Pareja JA. Forward head posture and neck mobility in chronic tension type headache: a

blinded, controlled study. Cephalalgia. 2006;26:314–9.

55. Fernández-de-las-Penas C, Bueno A, Ferrando J, et al. Magnetic resonance imaging of the morphometry of cervical extensor muscles in chronic tension type headache. Cephalalgia. 2007;27:355–62.

56. Fernández-de-las-Penas C, Falla D, Arendt-Nielsen L, Farina D. Cervical muscle co-activation in isometric contractions is enhanced in chronic tension type headache. Cephalalgia. 2008;28:744–51.

57. Penacoba-Puente C, Fernández-de-las-Penas C, González-Gutiérrez JL, et al. Mediating or moderating effect of anxiety and depression in headache clinical parameters and quality of life in chronic tension type headache. Eur J Pain. 2008;12:886–94.

58. Bendtsen L, Schoenen J. Synthesis of tension type headache mechanisms. In: Olesen J, Goasdby P, Ramdan NM, Tfelt-Hansen P, Welch KMA, editors. The headaches. 3rd ed. Philadelphia: Lippincott Williams & Wilkins; 2006.

59. Bendtsen L. Central sensitization in tension-type headache: possible pathophysiological mechanisms. Cephalalgia. 2000;20:486–508.

60. Abboud J, Marchand A, Sorra K, Descarreaux M. Musculoskeletal physical outcome measures in individuals with tension-type headache: a scoping review. Cephalalgia. 2013;33:1319–36.

61. Carli G, Suman AL, Biasi G, Marcolongo R. Reactivity to superficial and deep stimuli in patients with chronic musculoskeletal pain. Pain. 2002;100:259–69.

62. de Tommaso M, Sardaro M, Serpino C, et al. Fibromyalgia comorbidity in primary headaches. Cephalalgia. 2009;29:453–64.

63. de Tommaso M, Federici A, Serpino C, et al. Clinical features of headache patients with fibromyalgia comorbidity. J Headache Pain. 2011;12:629–38.

64. Langemark M, Olesen J. Pericranial tenderness in tension headache. A blind controlled study. Cephalalgia. 1987;7:249–55.

65. Buchgreitz L, Lyngberg AC, Bendtsen L, Jensen R. Increased pain sensitivity is not a risk factor but a consequence of frequent headache: a population-based follow-up study. Pain. 2008;137:623–30.

66. Bendtsen L, Fernandez-de-la-Penas C. The role of muscles in tension-type headache. Curr Pain Headache Rep. 2011;15(6):451–8.

67. Fernandez-de-la-Penas C, Cuadrado M, Pareja J. Myofascial trigger points, neck mobility, and forward head posture in episodic tension-type headache. Headache. 2007;47:662–72.

68. Cathcart S, Winefield A, Lushington K, Rolan P. Stress and tension-type headache mechanisms. Cephalalgia. 2010;30:1250–67.

69. Jensen R, Bendtsen L, Olesen J. Muscular factors are of importance in tension-type headache. Headache. 1998;38:10–7.

70. Schmidt-Wilcke T, Leinisch E, Straube A, et al. Gray matter decrease in patients with chronic tension-type headache. Neurology. 2005;65:1483–6.

71. May A. Chronic pain may change the structure of the brain. Pain. 2008;137:7–15.

72. Apkarian AV, Baliki MN, Geha PY. Towards a theory of chronic pain. Prog Neurobiol. 2009;87:81–97.

73. Ostergaard S, Russell MB, Bendtsen L, Olesen J. Comparison of first degree relatives and spouses of people with chronic tension headache. Br Med J. 1997;14:1092–3.

74. Russell MB, Iselius L, Østergaard S, Olesen J. Inheritance of chronic tension-type headache investigated by complex segregation analysis. Hum Genet. 1998;102:138–40.

75. Friederichs H, Olesen J, Russell M. Familial occurrence of chronic tension headache. Ugeskr Laeger. 1999;161:576–8.

76. Ulrich V, Gervil M, Olesen J. The relative influence of environment and genes in episodic tension-type headache. Neurology. 2004;62:2065–9.

77. Cathcart S, Petkov J, Pritchard D. Effects of induced stress on experimental pain sensitivity in chronic tension-type headache sufferers. Eur J Neurol. 2008;15:552–8.

78. Buchgreitz L, Lyngberg A, Bendtsen L, Jensen R. Increased prevalence of tension-type headache over a 12-year period is related to increased pain sensitivity: a population study. Cephalalgia. 2007;27:145–52.

79. Lindelof K, Ellrich J, Jensen R, Bendtsen L. Central pain processing in chronic tension-type headache. Clin Neurophysiol. 2009;120:1364–70.

80. Fumal A, Schoenen J. Tension-type headache: current research and clinical management. Lancet Neurol. 2008;7:70–83.

81. Sacco S, Ricci S, Carolci A. Tension-type headache and systemic medical disorders. Curr Pain Headache Rep. 2011;15:438–43.

82. Headache Classification Committee of the International Headache Society (IHS). The international classification of headache disorders, 3rd edition (beta version). Cephalalgia. 2013;33:629–808.

83. Roehrs T, Hydae M, Blaisdell B, Greenwald M, Roth T. Sleep loss and REM sleep loss are hyperalgesic. Sleep. 2006;29:144–51.

84. Odegard S, Sand T, Engstrom M, Stovner L, Zwart J, Hagen K. The long-term effect of insomnia on primary headaches: a prospective, population-based cohort study (HUNT-2 and HUNT-3). Headache. 2011;51:570–80.

85. Lyngberg A, Rasmussen B, Jorgensen T, Jensen R. Incidence of primary headache: a Danish epidemiologic follow-up study. Am J Epidemiol. 2005;161:1066–73.

86. Bellegaard V, Thede-Schmidt-Hansen P, Svensson P, Jensen R. Are headache and temporomandibular disorders related? A blinded study. Cephalagia. 2008;28:832–41.

87. Glaros A, Urban D, Locke J. Headache and temporomandibular disorders: evidence for diagnostic and behavioral overlap. Cephalalgia. 2007;27:542–9.

88. Fernandez-de-las-Penas C, Galan-del-Rio F, Fernandez-Carnero J, Pesquera J, Arendt-Nielsen L, Svensson P. Bilateral widespread mechanical pain sensitivity in women with myofascial temporomandibular joint disorder: evidence of impairment of central nociceptive processing. J Pain. 2009;10:1170–8.

89. Ailani J. Chronic tension-type headache. Curr Pain Headache Rep. 2009;13(6):479–83.

90. Balottin U, Fusar Poli P, Termine C, Molteni S, Galli F. Psychopathological symptoms in child and adolescent migraine and tension-type headache: a meta-analysis. Cephalalgia. 2012;33:112–22.

91. Solomon G. Chronic tension-type headache: advice for the viselike-headache patient. Cleve Clin J Med. 2002;69:167–72.

92. Janke EA, Holryod KA, Romanek K. Depression increases onset of tension-type headache following laboratory stress. Pain. 2004;111:230–8.

93. Verhagen AP, de Vet HC, Willemsen S, Stijnen T. A meta-regression analysis shows no impact of design characteristics on outcome in trials on tension type headaches. J Clin Epidemiol. 2008;61:813–8.

94. Bendtsen L, Evers S, Linde M, Mitsikostas DD, Sandrini G, Schoenen J, EFNS. EFNS guideline on the treatment of tension-type headache - report of an EFNS task force. Eur J Neurol. 2010;17:1318–25.

95. Semenov IA. Tension-type headaches. Dis Mon. 2015;61(6):233–5.

96. Packman E, Packman B, Thurston H, Tseng L. Lumiracoxib is effective in the treatment of episodic tension-type headache. Headache. 2005;45:1163–70.

97. Cady R, Gutterman D, Salers JA, Beach ME. Responsiveness of non-IHS migraine and tension-type headache to sumatriptan. Cephalalgia. 1997;17:588–90.

98. Bendtsen L, Jensen R. Mirtazapine is effective in the prophylactic treatment of chronic tension-type headache. Neurology. 2004;62:1706–11.

99. Zissis NP, Harmoussi S, Vlaikidis N, et al. A randomized, double-blind, placebo-controlled study of venlafaxine XR in out-patients with tension type headache. Cephalalgia. 2007;27:315–24.

100. Volpe FM. An 8-week open-label trial of duloxetine for comorbid major depressive disorder and chronic headache. J Clin Psychiatry. 2008;69:1449–54.

101. Bettucci D, Testa L, Calzoni S, et al. Combination of tizanidine and amitriptyline in the prophylaxis of chronic tension type headache: evaluation of efficacy and impact on quality of life. J Headache Pain. 2006;7:34–6.

102. Lampl C, Marecek S, May A, Bendtsen L. A prospective, open-label, long-term study of the efficacy and tolerability of topiramate in the prophylaxis of chronic tension-type headache. Cephalalgia. 2006;26:1203–8.

103. Straube A, Empl M, Ceballos-Baumann A, et al. Peri-cranial injection of botulinum toxin type A

(Dysport) for tension type headache: a multicentre, double-blind, randomized, placebo-controlled study. Eur J Neurol. 2008;15:205–13.

104. Hamdy S, Samir H, El-Sayed M, et al. Botulinum toxin: could it be an effective treatment for chronic tension-type headache? J Headache Pain. 2009;10:27–34.

105. Silberstein SD, Gobel H, Jensen R, et al. Botulinum toxin type A in the prophylactic treatment of chronic tension type headache: a multicentre, double-blind, randomized, placebo-controlled, parallel-group study. Cephalalgia. 2006;26:790–800.

106. Karadas O, Gul H, Inan L. Lidocaine injection of pericranial myofascial trigger points in the treatment of frequent episodic tension-type headache. J Headache Pain. 2013;14:44.

107. Fernández-de-las-Peñas C, Cleland J, Cuadrado M, Pareja J. Predictor variables for identifying patients with chronic tension-type headache who are likely to achieve short-term success with muscle trigger point therapy. Cephalalgia. 2008;28:264–75.

108. Sun Y, Gan T. Acupuncture for the management of chronic headache: a systematic review. Anesth Analg. 2008;107:2038–47.

109. Davis MA, Kononowech RW, Rolin SA, Spierings EL. Acupuncture for tension-type headache: a meta-analysis of randomized, controlled trials. J Pain. 2008;9:667–77.

110. Holroyd KA, O'Donnell FJ, Stensland M, Lipchik GL, Cordingley GE, Carlson BW. Management of chronic tension-type headache with tricyclic antidepressant medication, stress management therapy, and their combination. J Am Med Assoc. 2001;285(17):2208–15.

111. Nestoriuc Y, Rief W, Martin A. Meta-analysis of bio-feedback for tension-type headache: efficacy, specificity, and treatment moderators. J Consult Clin Psychol. 2008;76:379–96.

112. Torelli P, Jensen R, Olesen J. Physiotherapy for tension-type headache: a controlled study. Cephalalgia. 2004;24:29–36.

113. Van Ettekoven H, Lucas C. Efficacy of physiotherapy including a cranio-cervical training programme for tension-type headache: a randomized clinical trial. Cephalalgia. 2006;26:983–91.

114. Soderberg E, Carlsson J, Stener-Victorin E. Chronic tension-type headache treated with acupuncture, physical training and relaxation training: between group differences. Cephalalgia. 2006;26:1320–9.

Chronic Cluster Headaches

Soma Sahai-Srivastava

Chronic cluster headaches are a rare cause of chronic headaches. They are the most prominent and common type of trigeminal autonomic cephalalgias (TAC) and were described in 1941 by Horton, who also first used oxygen therapy to abort an acute cluster attack [1]. In 1952, Kunkle first used the term "cluster" to describe these headaches [2]. There are many synonyms for cluster headache, including "suicide headache" due to rare reports of suicidal behavior within this patient population.

Synonyms for Cluster Headache
Ciliary neuralgia
  Erythromelalgia of the head
  Erythroprosopalgia of Bing
  Horton's neuralgia or headache
  Harris-Horton disease
  Hemicrania angioparalytica
  Histaminic cephalalgia
  Hemicrania neuralgiformis
  Migrainous neuralgia (of Harris)
  Petrosal neuralgia (of Gardner)
  Sluder's neuralgia
  Sphenopalatine neuralgia
  Vidian neuralgia

S. Sahai-Srivastava
Clinical Professor of Neurology, Keck school of Medicine, Los Angeles, CA, USA
e-mail: sahai@usc.edu

The first vivid description of cluster headache dates to 1745, by Gerhard van Swieten, published in Latin. It serves as a stark reminder of the scourge of this rare primary headache [3]: "A healthy, robust man of middle age was, each day, at the same hour troubled by pain above the orbit of the left eye, where the nerve leaves through the bony frontal opening; after a short time the left eye began to redden and tears to flow; then he felt as if his eye was protruding from its orbit with so much pain that he became mad. After a few hours all this evil ceased and nothing in the eye appeared at all changed."

An earlier description, in *Observationes Medicae*, published in1641, Nicolaas Tulp, a well-known physician from Amsterdam, mentioned two different types of "recurring headache": migraine and a second entity which resembles cluster headache [4]. In recent years, patient advocacy organizations have raised the general awareness of this entity [5]. This has contributed to new discoveries in neuroimaging, medication therapies, and neurostimulation, which have created a better understanding of the pathophysiology and created new treatment options.

Epidemiology

Fishera reported a lifetime prevalence of cluster headaches at 124 per 100,000 and a 1-year prevalence of 53 per 100,000, with an overall male-to-female sex ratio of 4.3:6.0 [6]. Approximately

© Springer International Publishing AG, part of Springer Nature 2019
M. W. Green et al. (eds.), *Chronic Headache*, https://doi.org/10.1007/978-3-319-91491-6_6

10–20% of patients with episodic cluster develop the chronic form, which is defined as a remission period of more than a month [7]. In the general population, more recent studies suggest that prevalence of cluster headache is nearer to 1/1000 to 1/2000. However, in several European countries, extensive epidemiological studies indicate a more variable prevalence: 119 per 100,000 in Germany [8], 326 per 100,000 in Norway [9], and 279 per 100,000 in Italy [10]. These studies suggest cluster incidence is likely to be dependent upon the awareness and training specialists who see these patients. Cluster headache is a hidden underdiagnosed condition, and there may be a delay of over 5 years in accurate diagnosis and treatment [11]. Cluster headache in women is often misdiagnosed as migraine and can present with an overlap of symptoms between the two entities. Women are more likely to be diagnosed after 10 years of symptom onset than males, and significantly fewer women than men are diagnosed correctly at an initial physician visit [12].

Clinical Features

Diagnostic criteria for both episodic and chronic cluster headaches have been established [13]. The beta version of ICHD-3 has eliminated the term "primary" and "secondary" previously used to distinguish between chronic cluster headaches that arise de novo or evolve from the episodic version. Cluster headaches are considered chronic when attacks fulfilling the criteria for cluster headaches occur without remission or with remission periods lasting less than 1 month, for at least 1 year. The European Headache Federation has established a consensus statement on *refractory chronic cluster headache*, with the purpose of identifying patients who may be eligible for invasive treatments such as neurostimulators. Chronic cluster headache, with at least three severe attacks per week despite at least three consecutive trials of adequate preventive treatments, is considered refractory [14].

Cluster Headache Has Two Forms
1. Episodic: Occurs in periods lasting 7 days to 1 year separated by pain-free periods lasting 1 month.
2. Chronic: Attacks occur for more than 1 year without remission or with remission lasting less than 1 month.

Diagnostic Criteria for Cluster Headache
A. At least five attacks fulfilling criteria B–D.
B. Severe or very severe unilateral orbital, supraorbital, and/or temporal pain lasting 15–180 min (when unilateral).
C. Either or both of the following:
  1. At least one of the following symptoms or signs, ipsilateral to the headache:
    a. Conjunctival injection and/or lacrimation
    b. Nasal congestion and/or rhinorrhea
    c. Eyelid edema
    d. Forehead and facial sweating
    e. Forehead and facial flushing
    f. Sensation of fullness in the ear
    g. Miosis and/or ptosis
  2. A sense of restlessness or agitation
D. Attacks have a frequency between one every other day and eight per day for more than half of the time when the disorder is active.
E. Not better accounted for by another ICHD-3 diagnosis.

Age of onset of cluster headaches is usually 20–40 years. The male-to-female ratio is higher in chronic cluster headache (15.0) compared to episodic cluster headache (3.8). Some authors however, report that chronic cluster headaches are slightly more common in women than in men [15]. Cluster headaches are strictly unilateral, side-locked, orbital, supraorbital, or periorbital headaches that are accompanied by at least one of seven autonomic features ipsilaterally or are accompanied by a sense of restlessness and/or agitation. The maximum duration of these attacks, according to the ICHD-3 beta version criteria, is 3 h. Taga et al. reviewed migraine-like features in a large cohort of 569 cluster patients and found migrainosus features in 46% of patients [16]. After adjusting for confounding factors, they noted a more frequent association with females, a relatively younger age of onset, longer attack duration, and accompanied by more frequent sweating (OR 1.63, CI 1.02–2.21), miosis, and osmophobia. Another study with 155 cluster patients reported that 24.5% experienced at least one migrainous feature during every cluster headache attack. Nausea and vomiting were the most frequently reported of the migrainous features [17]. The clinical presentation in cluster headache patients with and without migrainous features was not significantly different, with the exception of aggravation of pain by effort (20.6% vs. 4.1%) and facial sweating (13.2% vs. 0.85%) which were more frequent in cluster patients with migrainous features [16].

Because cluster aura is seldomly discussed among clinicians, and there is little awareness even among patients, patients with cluster aura may be misdiagnosed as suffering with migraine with aura. Silberstein reported 6 cluster patients out of a series of 101 with an associated aura, 5 visual and 1 olfactory [18]. Chronic cluster patients often describe a "shadow or aura" around the eye affected by cluster attacks, described as a sensation of pressure or discomfort. Some cluster patients describe a sense of an impending event that can precede an attack and which in many cases persists between attacks. This description is provided from the author's own unpublished observation of a series of chronic cluster patients and has not been previously described. A hemiplegic variant of cluster has been recently described by Siow et al. in a series of four patients, one of them with an autosomal dominant inheritance [19]. A recently published "Leiden University Cluster headache neuro-Analysis" (LUCA) study reported that 36% of cluster patients had allodynia during attacks [20]. Female gender, younger age at onset, lifetime depression, comorbid migraine, and having recent attacks were independent risk factors for allodynia in this study. The authors suggest that central sensitization, as in migraine, is frequently seen in cluster headache.

Due to the challenges in diagnosing cluster headaches, a two-question cluster headache screening tool has been validated with the following questions: (1) attack duration <180 min and (2) the presence of conjunctival injection and/or lacrimation during attack [21]. This two-question tool had a sensitivity of 81.1% and a specificity of 100%.

The chronobiology of chronic cluster headaches is not as predictable as that of the episodic type, and there are reports of both nighttime and daytime attacks among the chronic patients [22–24]. Spring and fall are well-known cluster periods [25], though for chronic cluster patients, this seasonal rhythmicity may either completely disappear or become modified [26]. Limited scientific evidence indicates that in one-third of cases cluster remission occurs regardless of age and that features of cluster headache become less prominent over time [27]. Cluster attacks can be provoked by alcohol, histamine, and nitroglycerine.

Cluster headache profoundly affects every aspect of life from work to activities of daily living, and patients report worse working memory, disturbance of mood, and poorer quality of life compared to healthy controls. Self-reported anxiety is higher in those with chronic cluster than for episodic patients, with 75% of the former compared with 38% of the latter groups on a measure of anxiety [28]. Jensen reports that 82% of cluster headache patients from a tertiary center had decreased work ability during a cluster period and half of the patients considered it profound [29].

Differential Diagnosis

The main differential diagnoses of chronic cluster headache include chronic migraine and other TACs such as chronic paroxysmal hemicranias (CPH) and hemicrania continua.

Differential Diagnosis of Chronic Cluster Headache

Primary Headaches
   Chronic migraine
   Trigeminal autonomic cephalalgias

Chronic paroxysmal hemicrania
Hemicrania continua
Chronic SUNCT
Chronic SUNA

   Trigeminal neuralgia
   Persistent idiopathic facial pain
   Rebound analgesic headaches
   Secondary Headaches
   Vascular-vertebral artery dissection or aneurysm

Aneurysm of anterior communicating artery
Carotid aneurysm
Occipital lobe AVM
AVM middle cerebral territory
Giant cell arteritis

   Lower brainstem or upper spinal cord

Meningioma
Brainstem or upper cord infarction

   Intracranial lesions

Pituitary adenoma (prolactinoma)
Sphenoid wing meningioma

   Facial trauma
   Orbital/sinus
   Tolosa-Hunt syndrome

Chronic migraine can be difficult to distinguish from chronic cluster, especially in women, due to the presence of nausea and photophobia. Moreover, previous reports have shown that 27% of patients with migraine have at least one unilateral autonomic symptom, and this may explain the excess of cluster diagnosis in the first step of

these studies [30]. Other authors suggest that the prevalence of cluster in general population could be underestimated, particularly when patients have less painful attacks, shorter bouts, and attacks without autonomic symptoms [31] or have migraine symptoms (photophobia, phonophobia, nausea) associated with their cluster attacks [32]. All patients with side-locked, short-lasting, unilateral headache and autonomic features should receive an adequate trial of oxygen therapy during their headache, as this is a very simple and effective means of identifying clusters, which are the only headaches that respond to such treatment. It is helpful to have oxygen available in a headache clinic for a trial in such patients, such that it could be administered in an urgent care setting.

According to the ICHD-3 beta version criteria, CPH attacks last 2–310 min and do not include the criteria "sensation of restlessness or agitation."

Chronic Paroxysmal Hemicrania Has Two Forms
1. Episodic: Occurs in periods lasting 7 days to 1 year separated by pain-free periods lasting 1 month.
2. Chronic: Attacks occur for more than 1 year without remission or with remission lasting less than 1 month.

Diagnostic Criteria for Paroxysmal Hemicrania
A. At least 20 attacks fulfilling criteria B–E.
B. Severe unilateral orbital, supraorbital, and/or temporal pain lasting 2–30 min.
C. At least one of the following symptoms or signs, ipsilateral to the headache:
   1. Conjunctival injection and/or lacrimation
   2. Nasal congestion and/or rhinorrhea
   3. Eyelid edema
   4. Forehead and facial sweating
   5. Forehead and facial flushing
   6. Sensation of fullness in the ear
   7. Miosis and/or ptosis

D. Attacks have a frequency above five per day for more than half of the time.
E. Attacks are absolutely prevented by therapeutic doses of indomethacin.
F. Not better accounted for by another ICHD-3 diagnosis.

Pivotal questions to ask patients are whether they feel restlessness or agitation during attacks and what is the duration of their headaches. Duration may last up to 5 hours in CPH and 3 hours or less in cluster. Thus, it may be difficult to distinguish between the two based solely on duration. The other tool that can help to distinguish CPH from chronic cluster is an adequate trial of indomethacin. However, there are a few case reports of cluster patients responding to indomethacin, particularly in women. There are also reports of CPH patients being only partially responsive to indomethacin. In cases where indomethacin is contraindicated, e.g., gastrointestinal issues, this is less helpful.

Hemicrania continua is a continuous side-locked unilateral headache that is indomethacin-responsive. However, chronic cluster patients may have allodynia around the eye involved with attacks and may have some unilateral, continuous, baseline pain symptoms, which could confuse the diagnosis. As a general rule, for any case of unilateral side-locked headache, an adequate trial of indomethacin should be considered.

Diagnostic Criteria for Hemicrania Continua
A. Unilateral headache fulfilling criteria B–D
B. Present for >3 months, with exacerbations of moderate or greater intensity
C. Either or both of the following:
  1. At least one of the following symptoms or signs, ipsilateral to the headache:
    a. Conjunctival injection and/or lacrimation
    b. Nasal congestion and/or rhinorrhea
    c. Eyelid edema

    d. Forehead and facial sweating
    e. Forehead and facial flushing
    f. Sensation of fullness in the ear
    g. Miosis and/or ptosis
  2. A sense of restlessness or agitation or aggravation of pain by movement
D. Responds absolutely to therapeutic doses of indomethacin
E. Not better accounted for by another ICHD-3 diagnosis

Short-lasting unilateral neuralgiform headaches include attacks of moderate to severe strictly unilateral head pain at least once a day and can mimic chronic cluster headaches due to prominent lacrimation and redness of eye unilaterally with attacks.

Short-Lasting Unilateral Neuralgiform Headache Attacks Have Two Subforms
1. Chronic SUNCT: Occurs in periods lasting 7 days to 1 year separated by pain-free periods lasting 1 month.
2. Chronic SUNA: attacks occur for more than 1 year without remission or with remission lasting Less than 1 month.

Diagnostic Criteria
A. At least 20 attacks fulfilling criteria B–D.
B. Moderate or severe unilateral head pain, with orbital, supraorbital, temporal, and/or other trigeminal distribution lasting 1–600 s and occurring as single stabs, series of stabs, or in a sawtooth pattern.
C. At least one of the following symptoms or signs, ipsilateral to the headache:
  1. Conjunctival injection and/or lacrimation
  2. Nasal congestion and/or rhinorrhea
  3. Eyelid edema
  4. Forehead and facial sweating
  5. Forehead and facial flushing

6. Sensation of fullness in the ear
7. Miosis and/or ptosis
D. Attacks have a frequency of at least one a day per day for more than half of the time when the disorder is active.
E. Not better accounted for by another ICHD-3 diagnosis.

The two subtypes are chronic SUNCT (short-lasting unilateral neuralgiform headache with conjunctival injection and tearing) and chronic SUNA (short-lasting unilateral neuralgiform headache with cranial autonomic symptoms). Both these subtypes have short forms and present with dramatically painful sharp stabs that last seconds, along with autonomic features, but no sense of agitation or restlessness. SUNCT has both conjunctival injection and tearing, along with other autonomic symptoms criteria, whereas SUNA has other autonomic symptoms but not the conjunctival injection and tearing. The key to this condition is the recognition that there are hundreds of attacks in a day that may last no more than seconds.

These types of headaches can be triggered without a refractory period. The main difference from cluster headaches is the duration of pain which lasts seconds (1–600) in SUNCT/SUNA. This can be difficult clinically to distinguish if patients are having attacks lasting 10 minutes or longer. Among the TACs, the seven cranial autonomic symptoms are common to all, but the "sense of restlessness and agitation" is specific to cluster headaches and hemicrania continua and is absent in CPH, SUNCT, and SUNA.

Persistent idiopathic facial pain (PIFP), previously termed "atypical facial pain", is a disorder of the face that is often in the differential diagnosis of trigeminal neuralgia [33, 34]. In some cases of chronic cluster headaches, where patients report residual and persistent mild periorbital pain between cluster attacks in the setting of secondary problems like temporomandibular joint dysfunction, there may be a concern for PIFP. PIFP symptoms are persistent rather than intermittent, and the pain is usually unilateral without autonomic signs or symptoms.

Chronic cluster patients may overuse symptomatic medications to treat their attacks and may develop medication-overuse headache (MOH). MOH further complicates chronic cluster headaches and may present with the development of a background headache. This may be either featureless or have some migrainous quality. MOH, in these cases, is described as a bilateral, dull, and featureless daily headache resulting from a wide range of monotherapies or varying combinations of simple analgesics, caffeine, opioids, ergotamine, or triptans [35]. A personal or familial history of migraine appears to be strongly associated with the development of MOH in cluster headache, and patients with a this history of migraine must be carefully monitored for MOH. Medication withdrawal should be considered in every chronic cluster headache patient [36]. Because MOH can add a bilateral, featureless, or migrainous element when superimposed on cluster, it is important to ask every patient to describe the headache as it was before the offending analgesic was started.

Secondary Cluster Headaches

Cluster headaches may be triggered by eye trauma, orbital pathology, cataract surgery, or even injections in the trigeminal sensory distribution, e.g., by palatal injections for dental procedures [37]. Several cases of cluster headaches have been reported in men and, in one case, a woman with multiple sclerosis. MR imaging for one of these cases showed a pontine demyelinating lesion involving the trigeminal nerve root inlet area on the same side as the pain [38–40]. Vascular pathology, e.g., aneurysms of the anterior [41] or posterior circulation or arteriovenous malformations [42–44], can cause cluster-like attacks that may be indistinguishable from primary cluster headaches [45].

Structural pathology in the cervical spinal cord in the lower brain stem, e.g., meningioma [46] or infarction [47, 48], can mimic cluster headache attacks. Sellar or parasellar pathology, e.g., pituitary adenoma or parasellar meningioma, can also mimic clusters [49, 50]. It may be clinically impossible to distinguish between primary and secondary cluster headaches. Every chronic cluster patient should have at least one brain imaging in his or her lifetime, preferably an MRI of the brain with orbital views, and also an MR angiogram to exclude secondary causes, e.g., lesions of the cerebral blood vessels or posterior fossa lesions.

Pathophysiology and Imaging Studies

Previously, the pathophysiological basis for cluster headaches was considered to be vascular: Inflammation of the walls of the cavernous sinus was thought to explain all the autonomic symptoms associated with cluster. The cavernous sinus has a convergence of both C-fibers transmitting pain and the sympathetic nerve fibers. Angiograms done on patients while having cluster headaches showed vasodilation of the ophthalmic artery or engorgement of the venous plexuses in this area. Other findings include superior ophthalmic vein narrowing and localized narrowing of the internal carotid artery during an acute attack followed by dilation. Increased corneal indentation and intraocular pressure and skin temperature around the eye during painful attacks have also been reported.

The advent of functional neuroimaging has debunked the vascular theory, in favor of the neurovascular theory, which is driven by a central hypothalamic generator, causing a release of proinflammatory vasodilators, e.g., calcitonin gene-related peptide (CGRP), vasoactive intestinal peptide (VIP), neurokinins, and histamine, with resultant neurogenic inflammation of the vasculature. The activation of the trigeminal system during cluster attacks is indicated by the elevation of CGRP plasma levels in the external jugular vein [51]. CGRP is a potent vasodilator and neurotransmitter, and plasma levels are elevated during and between cycles of episodic cluster headache [52]. The vascular events are, therefore, a marker of brain activation and not the driver. May et al. first demonstrated activation in acute attacks of cluster headache and

mapped them in color on T1-weighted MR scans of the brain in the areas of ipsilateral hypothalamus, anterior cingulate cortex, and other areas involved in the common pain matrix. Activation was observed in three broad categories: (1) areas known to be involved in pain processing, such as cingulate, insula, prefrontal cortex, and contralateral thalamus, (2) areas activated specifically in cluster headache but not in other head pain, and (3) extra-cerebral areas consistent with large intracranial blood vessels. Basal ganglia and cerebellum activation may be accounted for by preparation for movement, since patients typically like to pace during a cluster. Hypothalamic hyperactivity ipsilateral to the headache side in CH was observed during the attacks in all the PET and fMRI studies [53]. Furthermore, voxel-based morphometry (VBM) structural imaging shows structural changes in cluster patients [54, 55]. NAA/Cr ratio is reduced, and this is a permanent feature of cluster which is an expression of neuronal dysfunction, the mechanism of which is yet unknown. Episodic clusters seem to originate in the hypothalamus, and many studies have shown hypothalamic hypometabolism [56]. Persistent hypothalamic activation may be the factor that contributes to generate a central permissive state, which predisposes to activation of the trigeminal system, mediating pain, and of the parasympathetic reflex, producing the autonomic symptoms [57].

Chronic cluster functional neuroimaging seems to suggest that the thalamus may be central to the refractory nature of these headaches. A PET-CT study with six chronic cluster patients showed hypometabolism at the level of the thalamus ipsilateral to the cluster pain, suggesting that a thalamic genesis is a possible origin of refractory cluster headache [58]. May and colleagues scanned nine chronic cluster patients with H215O PET during nitroglycerine-induced attacks and were the first to clearly demonstrate inferior hypothalamic gray matter activation ipsilateral to the headache side. Moreover, they observed an increased regional cerebral blood flow in the contralateral ventroposterior thalamus, the anterior cingulate cortex, and in the insulae bilaterally as well [59]. Following this observation, others confirmed these data in a spontaneous headache attack of a chronic CH patient during an ongoing H2150 PET study [60]. In refractory chronic cluster patients treated with invasive occipital nerve stimulation, the hypothalamic hyperactivation still persists during the stimulator-on condition and despite its clinical efficacy [61].

Another important neuroimaging finding is the presence of hypometabolism in the perigenual anterior cingulate cortex (ACC) of episodic cluster patients scanned interictally. Perigenual ACC plays a major role in the central descending opiatergic pain control system, and its deficiency may be a mechanism that predisposes to the disorder and to its recurrence [52]. The involvement of the opiatergic system in cluster headache pathophysiology and opioid receptor availability in the rostral ACC and hypothalamus decreases with the duration of CH [62], and low-dosage opioid (levomethadone) induces complete and long-lasting CH remission [63]. Moreover, in refractory chronic cluster patients who responded to occipital nerve stimulation, an increased metabolism was observed in perigenual ACC in comparison to nonresponders [61], further underscoring the fact that one of the pathophysiological mechanisms of treatment efficacy in CH is the restoration of normal opioid analgesia. Initial cerebral blood flow studies done with SPECT imaging showed variable results, perhaps due to differences in methodology [64, 65].

In conclusion, the most striking neuroimaging findings in cluster headache are the posterior hypothalamic activation during the attacks, with concomitant pain neuromatrix activation and opioid system involvement as underlined by changes in perigenual ACC.

Treatment

Management of chronic cluster headache is broadly divided into treating acute attacks, adding long-term preventative treatment to decrease the frequency and intensity of daily attacks, and treatment of comorbidities, e.g., insomnia and sleep apnea. It is fortunate that in other than oxygen therapy that sets cluster headache apart from

migraine, many of the acute and preventative treatments for migraine are potentially effective for cluster treatment.

Management of Acute Attacks

The American Academy of Neurology has published evidence-based guidelines for the treatment of chronic cluster [66]. Acute abortive treatment should be prescribed to chronic cluster patients to treat individual attacks, which often occur many times daily. All the abortive treatments for episodic type may remain effective for chronic cluster headaches. Since cluster headaches are rapid onset and short-lasting, the ideal abortive agent is parenteral, intranasal, or inhaled.

Oxygen

Oxygen responsiveness is the "sine qua non" of clusters, and barring rare cases can be used to some degree as a clinical diagnostic test to separate cluster from other unilateral short-duration headaches. Oxygen responsiveness is, however, not a diagnostic criterion for clusters, according to the ICHD-3, even though no other headache disorder responds to oxygen administration. The pitfall in assessing oxygen responsiveness is not administering it at a sufficient flow rate, sufficient duration, and with an appropriate mask. Inhalation of 100% oxygen, at 7–15 L/min, for 15 minutes by a non-rebreather mask is an effective method to abort cluster attacks [67, 68]. If the cluster is oxygen-responsive, then it is an effective means to reduce the need for multiple daily doses of other acute abortive medications, e.g., triptans, therefore avoiding the issue of rebound analgesic headache. It is this author's opinion that every strictly unilateral headache patient should be given at least one oxygen trial during an acute attack of pain. Sometimes when patients report being unresponsive to oxygen, it is because they have not received an adequate flow rate or high oxygen percentage or a nasal cannula was used instead of a non-rebreather mask. Oxygen is effective in 70% or more of patients and may start working within 5 minutes [69]. However, in others, it may take up to 15 minutes to work and may decrease the impending attack or decrease the intensity of pain. The author considers a 50% reduction in pain level, a good indicator that oxygen therapy can be used for acute attacks in those patients. A chronic cluster patient may report an improvement in the continuous "shadow or aura" discomfort, which may then indicate oxygen responsiveness during an acute cluster attack. Hyperbaric oxygen has also been shown to interrupt a cluster cycle, but in clinical practice, the cost may be a limiting factor [70]. While there have been no placebo-controlled, double-blinded studies of oxygen in the cluster population, it is universally recognized by headache specialists as first-line treatment, based on nearly 75 years of clinical experience.

Triptans

Sumatriptan: Subcutaneous sumatriptan 3–6 mg is a first-line treatment for acute cluster attacks. It has a rapid effect, within 5–7 minutes and high response rate of about 75% of all cluster headache patients (i.e., pain-free within 20 minutes) [71]. In cluster headache, subcutaneous sumatriptan can be prescribed at a frequency of twice daily, on a long-term basis if necessary without risk of tachyphylaxis or rebound [72, 73]. Clinical trials are underway to assess the efficacy of sumatriptan 4 mg subcutaneously, which may allow for three times daily dosing [74]. There are auto-injectors and a needle-free device that are simple to use, especially for patients who find it difficult to prepare the injection in the midst of severe eye pain [75]. Chronic cluster patients generally need to take abortive treatment several times daily. Fortunately, sumatriptan continues to be effective for years and generally is well tolerated. Sumatriptan 20 mg nasal spray is another option for patients who may prefer a non-injectable and less painful treatment option [76]. Sumatriptan 100 mg oral tablets three times daily taken prior to an anticipated onset of an attack or at regular times does not prevent the attack, and regular oral triptans may induce medication-overuse headache in susceptible patients, so this approach is generally not recommended [77].

Zolmitriptan is an additional medication with a fairly rapid onset of action that is very well tolerated by patients. Oral zolmitriptan (2.5 or 5 mg) and the 5 mg nasal spray are both more effective than placebo [78–80].

Ergotamine Derivatives

Dihydroergotamine (DHE) nasal spray can also be effective in the treatment of acute attacks of cluster headache [81]. The intranasal option of both triptans and ergotamine derivatives may be useful for chronic cluster patients who are treating multiple attacks daily for many years. However, with frequent use of DHE, drug holidays are recommended, as there is a risk of fibrotic complications affecting the heart, lungs, and retroperitoneum. Parenteral DHE given either intramuscularly (0.5–1 mg dose) or by intravenous route can be effective, which may provide rapid relief within a few minutes; however there have not been clinical trials on this compound for cluster headaches [82, 83]. Oral ergotamine is generally too slow in onset to provide meaningful relief in a timely manner. Some patients may benefit from rectal ergotamine, but this method is cumbersome and unpopular.

Lidocaine

Intranasal application of 1 ml of 4–6% lidocaine solution ipsilateral to the pain or a spray deep in the nostril on the painful side results in mild to moderate relief in most patients, though only a few patients obtain complete pain relief [84]. Intranasal lidocaine serves as a useful adjunct to other abortive treatments but is rarely adequate on its own. Intranasal cocaine was historically used several decades ago, when there were few other choices for treatment, and is not used by clinicians anymore [85]. The aim of intranasal applications is to block the sphenopalatine ganglion, which controls the activation of the cranial parasympathetic outflow from the superior salivary nucleus of the facial nerve and is responsible for the autonomic features of cluster headache [86].

Octreotide

Matharu et al. showed that octreotide 100 µg when administered subcutaneously is effective in aborting an acute attack with the headache response rate of 52%, whereas that with placebo was 36% [87].

Indomethacin

Cluster headache is one of the TACs that does not respond to indomethacin; however, there have been some case reports of chronic cluster headaches responding to either 50 mg intravenous indomethacin [88] or oral indomethacin [89]. It is unclear whether these patients had undiagnosed CPH which can mimic cluster and response to indomethacin is typical.

Other Drugs

Opiates, nonsteroidal anti-inflammatory drugs (NSAIDs), and combination analgesics have no role in the acute management of cluster headache.

Greater Occipital Nerve (GON) Injection

There are consistent data that support the use of GON injections of steroids to abort an acute cluster attack; however, they generally provide only temporary relief in chronic cluster [90]. Anthony reported that cluster attacks could be arrested by GON injections in 1985, using a mixture of short- and long-acting corticosteroids [91]. Subsequently this has been confirmed by many studies on episodic cluster and a double-blind, placebo-controlled trial with a mixture of short- and long-acting steroids on cluster patients [92, 93]. Lambru et al. performed GON unilaterally in an open-label prospective study on 83 chronic cluster patients at 3-monthly intervals and showed an overall positive response in 57% patients after the first injection of a combination of steroids and lidocaine [94]. There has been debate however as to why these blocks work and whether their effect is due to steroids, anesthetic, or both. Busch et al. performed suboccipital injections of 1% lidocaine on cluster patients and found that local anesthetic alone was not effective in terminating cluster headache attacks [95]. Clinical studies have had mixed results perhaps due to the variations in types of steroids and anesthetics used and also differing injection techniques. With regard to the possible mechanism of action of GON in cluster, it is still unclear whether it is a systemic steroid effect or due to inhibition of central pain-processing mechanisms at the brainstem level. Using occipital nerve blockade and nociceptive blink reflexes,

Busch has demonstrated functional connectivity between the ophthalmic branch of the trigeminal and sensory occipital nerves in humans, but it is still unclear as to which level in this pathway the GON produces its inhibitory effect. Our recommendation for clinicians is similar to that of the expert consensus, to use corticosteroids in combination with a local anesthetic [96].

Long-Term Prophylactic Treatments

The aim of long-term preventive therapy in chronic cluster patients is to decrease the frequency and intensity of daily attacks, to shorten a cluster cycle and to maintain remission with minimal side effects for a longer period. There is very little data on the use of preventative agents in chronic cluster patients, and most of the information below pertains to the episodic patient. The lack of data for chronic cluster should not prevent the clinician from trying preventative agents that have shown effectiveness in episodic cluster headaches.

Verapamil

Currently, verapamil is the preventative drug of choice in both episodic and chronic cluster headache [28–30]. Clinical experience has demonstrated that higher doses are needed than those typically used in cardiologic indications. The most common side effects include constipation, dizziness, nausea, hypotension, pedal edema, and fatigue. Verapamil can cause heart block by slowing conduction in the atrioventricular node. About 20% of cluster headache patients on verapamil have cardiac conduction problems, and these can develop after months of stable dosing and are not dose-dependent [31]. Observing for PR interval prolongation on ECG can monitor for the potential development of heart block. After performing a baseline ECG, patients are usually started on 80 mg three times daily, and thereafter the total daily dose is increased in increments of 80 mg every 10–14 days. Dosages commonly employed range from 240 to 960 mg daily in divided doses. The author usually switches to the long-acting version of verapamil, after the effective daily dose of the shorter-acting version is reached. An ECG is performed prior to each dose increment. The dose is increased until the cluster attacks are suppressed, significant side effects intervene, or the maximum dose of 960 mg daily is achieved. ECGs should be performed periodically with long-term therapy.

Lithium

Lithium is an effective agent for cluster headache prophylaxis, with 78% of chronic cluster patients achieving remission of attacks, and some consider a first-line treatment for chronic cluster headache [97, 98]. Since it is effective at lower doses than typically needed for bipolar disorder, it can be used very successfully to treat chronic clusters. Typical starting dose is 150 mg twice daily, and the dose can be titrated up to 1200 mg daily. Lithium has a long half-life and may take up to 1 week to become effective, at which time serum level should be checked. The therapeutic range for chronic cluster is likely lower (0.4–0.8 mol/L) than for mania (0.8–1.1 mol/L) [99], but the therapeutic level in cluster headache has not been established. Side effects of lithium are dose-dependent and include nausea, tremor, lethargy, blurred vision, and diarrhea at lower doses and confusion, ataxia, extrapyramidal signs, and seizures at higher doses. Side effects from long-term use include hypothyroidism and nephrogenic diabetes insipidus. Therefore renal and thyroid function tests should be performed prior to initiation of therapy and at least on a 3-monthly basis. The concomitant use of NSAIDs, diuretics, verapamil, and carbamazepine requires careful monitoring, as they can increase the serum levels of lithium.

Melatonin

In cluster patients, there is disruption of the biological clock in the suprachiasmatic nucleus (SCN) of the hypothalamus, which regulates the circadian secretion of melatonin from the pineal gland, mostly at night. Hypothalamic dysfunction in cluster is reflected by altered melatonin production in patients during an attack cycle, as well as between cycles [100, 101]. Melatonin supplementation can be effective in reducing the number of nighttime attacks and can be used at doses between 1 and 10 mg depending on the patient preference. Several double-blind clinical trials have shown melatonin to be effective [102, 103].

Corticosteroids

Corticosteroids are highly effective and the most rapid-acting agent for achieving remission during an acute episodic cluster period but not useful, for safety reasons, in chronic cluster headaches. They are widely used for episodic cluster to terminate a cycle and achieve remission; however there are no clinical trials. Treatment should be limited to a short intensive course of a tapering dose because of the potential for side effects. The starting dose of oral prednisolone 1 mg/kg to a maximum of 60 mg once daily for 5 days is an acceptable dose widely used by neurologists. Treatment should be limited to 2–4 weeks and tapered down by 5–10 mg every 3–5 days. In this way, the risk of side effects due to long-term steroid use (diabetes, hypertension, avascular necrosis of femoral heads) is minimized. Unfortunately, recurrence often occurs as the dose is tapered. For this reason, corticosteroids are used as an initial therapy in conjunction with preventives, until the latter are effective. Oral and intravenous formulations have also been successfully used in combination [104].

A recently study showed that in parallel with the decrease in cluster frequency after corticosteroid administration, there was decrease in plasma CGRP levels and an increase in the urinary excretion of melatonin metabolites [105], which is indirect evidence that steroids decrease the activation of the trigeminal system and modulate the hypothalamic pathways.

Triptans

Whereas the short-acting triptans are used for acute abortive treatment of cluster attacks, several long-lasting triptans may produce a longer duration of therapeutic action, with the potential for use as prophylactic agents [106]. *Frovatriptan*, the triptan with the longest half-life (about 26 h) [107], has been used to prevent nighttime cluster attacks [108]. Another relatively longer-acting triptan, *naratriptan*, has also been used for preventative treatment, though mostly in the setting of acute clusters [109–111]. Short-term prophylaxis can be provided with other longer-acting triptans like *eletriptan*, but its long-term use in chronic cluster headache remains to be seen [112]. These triptans may be useful as add-on to other preventative treatment, reducing the number of daily attacks in the chronic cluster patients, assuming that the acute medications being used can be used concomitantly.

Antiepileptics

In the last decade, tremendous experience has been gained in treating migraine headaches with antiepileptics. They have been utilized to treat clusters, and this class of agents has emerged as an option for chronic cluster patients. The dosing of antiepileptics is the same as typically used for migraine headaches.

Topiramate is an FDA-approved migraine preventative agent and is generally well tolerated. Topiramate was effective in achieving remission of two chronic cluster patients [113]. There are several studies that show its effectiveness as a preventative agent in episodic cluster [114–117]. Starting dose of 25 mg at bedtime and titrating up gradually to a dose of 100–200 mg is recommended. There is a long-acting version of topiramate now available, which may be better tolerated. Well-known side effects include a small risk of kidney stones, paresthesias, weight loss, and cognitive side effects. Topiramate can also sometimes heighten anxiety, which is already heightened in many cluster patients.

Gabapentin has also been shown to be effective in treating chronic cluster patients in several small series [118–120]. There is a long-acting version of gabapentin, which has not been tested for cluster headaches but might provide some benefit, especially with nighttime dosing.

Divalproex sodium has the advantage of an intravenous formulation and therefore can be used in an acute setting, for example, in a headache infusion center, to provide a rapid loading dose, which can be maintained orally on a long-term basis for prevention, but there is very little evidence to support its intravenous use at this time. Intravenous valproate is very well tolerated, and the author has used it to achieve remission of cluster attacks in two episodic cluster patients. Oral sodium valproate can be an effective preventative treatment to achieve pain remission in episodic cluster patients [121, 122]. There are several boxed warnings for this drug, including hepatotoxicity, pancytopenia, and pancreatitis, and there is a risk of fetal malformations. Baseline liver function testing should be obtained, and a thorough discussion regarding effects on fetus and potential for polycystic ovary disease is mandated in females of child-bearing age. The extended release version is very useful, with starting dose of 250 mg, titrating weekly to 1000–1500 mg.

Zonisamide has been used in both episodic and chronic cluster patients with good response. It is generally very well tolerated with minimal side effects. Recommended doses are similar to those for epilepsy, and once nightly dose of 100 mg can be titrated up every 2 weeks to 600 mg daily. Due to very long half-life, effective levels may take several weeks to be achieved.

S-lysergic acid diethylamide (LSD) and *psilocybin*, which are controlled hallucinogen drugs, may abort an acute cluster attack, terminate the cluster cycle, and delay the next expected cluster period [123]. Interestingly, these drugs were effective at subhallucinogenic doses, and effective treatment required only 1–3 doses [124]. A 2006 survey of 53 cluster headache reported that psilocybin extended remission periods in 10% cases [125]. However, controlled trials of these agents are lacking.

Calcitonin gene-related peptide (CGRP) is a marker of trigeminal system activation and plays an important role in the pathogenesis of migraine and likely of cluster. Therapeutic blockade of this peptide has emerged as an important target in the treatment of migraine [126–128]. There are now results from randomized controlled phase III trials using monoclonal antibodies specifically for chronic cluster headache which are strongly positive [129], but these agents are not yet commercially available.

Methysergide was one of the few drugs available in the 1960s and the 1970s for migraine prevention and has shown to be effective in preventing cluster attacks [130]. It is a consideration in patients with short cluster periods that last less than 4–5 months. Because methysergide is an ergot, if used for prevention, triptans and similar agents cannot be used for rescue. It is rarely used by clinicians because of potentially serious side effects; prolonged treatment has been associated with rare fibrotic reactions (retroperitoneal, pulmonary, pleural, and cardiac). Methysergide is administered at a daily dose of 4–8 mg and can be increased up to 12 mg (starting with 1 mg/day). A drug holiday of 1 month, after every 6 months of methysergide treatment, is required, along with imaging for evidence of pulmonary, cardiac, renal, or abdominal pathology yearly in patients on prolonged methysergide therapy. Methysergide is now no longer available in the United States.

Clomiphene citrate is another agent which in three case reports has been shown to achieve complete remission of headache attacks, at 100 mg/day dose in chronic cluster headaches [131, 132]. The mechanism of action of clomiphene in cluster headache may be due to its ability to enhance testosterone production and to bind to hypothalamic estrogen receptors. In chronic cluster patients, it may be useful to check serum testosterone levels, since testosterone replacement therapy given to supplement low serum levels can result in remission of refractory cluster headaches [133].

Pizotifen is widely used in Europe but is not available for use in the United States. The typical dose is 3 mg/day. Side effects commonly seen are fatigue and weight gain.

Antihistaminics

Histamine has been implicated in the pathogenesis of cluster. Spontaneous cluster attacks in some patients are associated with increased urinary excretion of histamine [134], and whole blood histamine levels show a statistically significant rise during attack [135]. However double-blind controlled trials of histamine antagonists were ineffective in treating cluster headaches [136, 137].

Intranasal Agents

Intranasal application of capsaicin cream has been shown in three studies to be effective in preventing episodic cluster attacks [138–140]. A single study has also shown that intranasal application of civamide is effective in preventing episodic cluster attacks [141].

Interventional and Surgical Treatment

Refractory cluster patients who have failed medical treatment may be candidates for neurosurgical procedures or, more recently, for neurostimulation. The main targets of destructive procedures or neurostimulation include the sphenopalatine ganglion, trigeminal ganglion, occipital nerve, vagus nerve, and hypothalamus.

Sphenopalatine Ganglion (SPG)-Targeted Procedures

The SPG can be blocked only temporarily by intranasal topical application of local anesthetic, and the aim of invasive procedures is to permanently destroy the SPG by surgery or radiofrequency ablation. The most invasive procedure on the SPG, *ganglionectomy*, was reported in 1970 on a series of 13 refractory cluster patients, of which only 2 patients achieved pain remission [142]. In 2009, a study reported *percutaneous radiofrequency ablation* of the SPG via the infrazygomatic approach under fluoroscopic guidance on 15 refractory chronic cluster headache patients. There was a significant improvement in mean attack intensity, mean attack frequency, and pain disability index up to 18 months after procedure. The authors noted that precise needle placement with the use of real-time fluoroscopy and electrical stimulation prior to attempting radiofrequency ablation may reduce the incidence of adverse events [143]. The side effects from these destructive procedures of the SPG include permanent hypesthesia or dysesthesia in the palate, maxilla, or posterior pharynx, and therefore these are not commonly recommended.

Recently, however, there is emerging evidence that stimulation, rather than ablative procedures on the SPG, may be more effective in long-term therapy. Initial studies used temporary electrical stimulation. Electrical stimulation using a temporary stimulating electrode and a standard percutaneous infrazygomatic approach with a needle placed in the ipsilateral SPG in the pterygopalatine fossa under fluoroscopic guidance was used to abort an acute cluster attack in five refractory chronic cluster patients [144]. Shytz reported for the first time that low-frequency SPG stimulation might induce cluster-like attacks with autonomic features, which can subsequently be treated by high-frequency SPG stimulation. Efferent parasympathetic outflow from the SPG may initiate autonomic symptoms and activate trigeminovascular sensory afferents, which may initiate the onset of pain associated with cluster headache [145].

The authors suggested that high-frequency SPG stimulation might exert its effect by physiologically blocking parasympathetic outflow. This led to the Pathway CH-1 study, which is a randomized, sham-controlled study of implantable on-demand SPG neurostimulator in patients with refractory chronic cluster headaches. Twenty-eight patients completed the randomized experimental period, and pain relief was achieved in 67% of stimulation-treated attacks compared to 7.4% of sham-treated ($p < 0.0001$). Nineteen of 28 (68%) patients experienced a clinically significant improvement. Five adverse events were reported that included transient, mild/moderate loss of sensation within distinct maxillary nerve regions. This implantable on-demand SPG stimulation using the ATI Neurostimulation System is now approved in Europe and has dual beneficial effects, acute pain relief and attack prevention, with an acceptable safety profile compared to similar surgical procedures [146].

Trigeminal Ganglion-Targeted Therapy
In one clinical series reported in 1987, seven therapy-resistant patients with cluster headache (six of whom were chronic) were treated by percutaneous retro-gasserian *glycerol injections* under general anesthesia. Cluster attacks did cease but only temporarily [147]. Injection of glycerol in the trigeminal ganglion has been

abandoned due to risk of corneal injury and the dreaded pain of anesthesia dolorosa.

Taha et al. reviewed a series of seven patients with chronic cluster headache refractory to medical treatment who received percutaneous *stereotactic radiofrequency rhizotomy* and reported variable effects ranging from no relief to pain-free at 20 years follow-up [148]. Destructive surgery block trigeminal sensory or autonomic pathways should only be considered in patients with strictly unilateral attacks, as those whose attacks alternate sides may find an upsurge of attacks on the side contralateral to surgery. Sometimes, cluster attacks persist even after complete destruction of the trigeminal sensory pathway [149]. Ford et al. reported on a series of six who were treated for refractory cluster headache by *Gamma Knife radiosurgery* of the trigeminal nerve root entry zone. The maximum dose of radiation was 70 Gy to the isocenter. Pain-free state was obtained in four of the patients with minimal side effects, and the onset of action was a few days to a week. The main drawback of Gamma Knife radiosurgery is the unpredictability of the degree, the duration, and even the likelihood of a positive response.

Occipital Nerve-Targeted Therapy
Since 2007, occipital nerve stimulation has been used in treating refractory chronic migraines [150, 151] and used to successfully treat refractory chronic cluster headaches as well [152]. Burns et al. reported a retrospective assessment of 14 patients with medically intractable CCH, implanted with bilateral electrodes in the suboccipital region for occipital nerve stimulation, and at a median follow-up of 17.5 months, 10 of 14 patients reported improvement in the number of daily cluster attacks [153]. Fontaine et al. reported a series of 13 patients with medically refractory chronic cluster, of whom 10/13 showed improvement in their daily attack rate by >50% that was sustained beyond 12 months [154]. More recently, Miller et al. reported a cohort of 51 chronic cluster headaches, which decreased daily attacks by 46% and reduced triptan use by 65% [155]. There is one case of successful treatment of chronic refractory drug-resistant cluster headaches with a combined supraorbital and occipital

nerve stimulator [156]. Stimulator placement is an invasive procedure that requires general anesthesia, and long-term adverse events of concern include lead migration and battery depletion.

Vagus Nerve-Targeted Therapy

Noninvasive VNS (nVNS), which stimulates the carotid vagus nerve with the use of a personal handheld device, has been tested for chronic migraine and showed promising results [157]. Recently, the US Food and Drug Administration (FDA) has approved a handheld, neck-applied noninvasive vagus nerve stimulation device (gamma*Core*) for the treatment of pain from episodic cluster headache in adults. The FDA release was based on the prospective, placebo-controlled ACT1 and ACT2 trials. In ACT1, Silberstein et al. enrolled 85 participants with episodic cluster headache; 34% of those in the vagus nerve stimulation group reported pain reduction after treatment vs. 11% of the placebo group [158]. ACT2 assessed 27 patients, with 182 total attacks. Results showed 47.5% of those treated with the active device were pain-free 15 min later vs. 6.2% of those receiving placebo [159]. Gaul et al. showed that prophylactic treatment with VNS can lead to rapid, significant, and sustained reductions in chronic cluster headache attack frequency within 2 weeks after its addition to usual standard of care [160]. Since the nVNS device is safe with no major side effects, once available in the market, it may be considered for treatment of acute attacks in chronic cluster patients.

Hypothalamic-Targeted Therapy

Stereotactic stimulation of posterior hypothalamic gray matter in a patient with intractable cluster headache was first performed in Italy [161]. Subsequently *hypothalamic neurostimulators* implanted by Franzini's group were successful in treating refractory chronic clusters; however, this treatment was stopped when one patient died of hemorrhagic complications of implantation [162, 163]. This is the most invasive of neurostimulator devices, and given the expanded experience with occipital neurostimulation in migraines patients, it is reasonable to consider the occipital neurostimulators first as an invasive option.

The Cluster Patient Perspective

The European Headache Alliance collected a list of recommendations from cluster patient associations with the purpose of improving overall cluster headache management. The seven recommendations that have emerged for physicians taking care of clusters include the following:

1. Cluster headache diagnosis is easy if you consider few clinical clues.
2. Prescribe sumatriptan and oxygen.
3. Suggest patient avoid hiding and be active in a patients' support group.
4. Take patient seriously and listen to him/her.
5. Provide quality information and address myths about cluster treatment.
6. Be sensitive to cluster impact on the patient's significant other.
7. Acknowledge that cluster is a serious medical disorder that can have a significant impact on the person and support him/her [164].

In summary, chronic cluster headaches are debilitating and challenging for the clinician and patient. However, there is more awareness now within the medical community and among the general public, and the chances of early recognition are higher. Functional imaging modalities have made it possible to better understand the neuroanatomy and pathophysiology of chronic cluster headaches. A larger repertoire of medications and surgical options are available for the clinician. There is a need for randomized clinical trials to test many of the treatments that have anecdotally been effective in treating these patients.

References

1. Horton BT. Histaminic cephalgia (Horton's headache or syndrome). Md State Med J. 1961;10:178–203.
2. Kunkle EC, Pfeiffer JB, Hamrick LW. Brief headaches in a "cluster" pattern. Trans Am Neuro Assoc. 1952;77:240–3.
3. Isler H. Episodic cluster headache from a textbook of 1745: van Swieten's classic description. Cephalalgia. 1993;13:172–4.

4. Koehler PJ. Prevalence of headache in Tulp's "Observationes medicae" 1641 with a description of cluster headache. Cephalalgia. 1993;13:318–20.

5. Lambru G, Andreou AP, de la Torre ER, Martelletti P. Tackling the perils of unawareness: the cluster headache case. J Headache Pain. 2017;18(1):49.

6. Fischera M, Marziniak M, Gralow I, Evers S. The incidence and prevalence of cluster headache: a meta-analysis of population-based studies. Cephalalgia. 2008;28:614–8.

7. Sjaastad O. Cluster headache syndrome. London: WB Saunders; 1992.

8. Katsavara Z, et al. Prevalence of cluster headache in a population based sample in Germany. Cephalalgia. 2007;27:1014–9.

9. Jaastad O, Bakketeig LP. CH prevalence. Vaga study of headache epidemiology. Cephalalgia. 2003;23:528–33.

10. D'Alessandro R, Gamberini G, Bessani G. Cluster headache in the Republic of San Marino. Cephalalgia. 1986;6:189–92.

11. Voiticovschi-Iosob C, Allena M, De Cillis I, Nappi G, Sjaastad O, Antonaci F. Diagnostic and therapeutic errors in cluster headache: a hospital-based study. J Headache Pain. 2014;15:56.

12. Rozen TD, Fishman RS. Female cluster headache in the United States of America: what are the gender differences? Results from the United States Cluster Headache Survey. J Neurol Sci. 2012;317(1–2):17–28.

13. Headache Classification Committee of the International Headache Society (HIS). The international classification of headache disorders, (beta version). Cephalalgia. 2013;33(9):629–808.

14. Mitsikostas DD, Edvinsson L, Jensen RH, Katsarava Z, Lampl C, Negro A, Martelletti P. Refractory chronic cluster headache: a consensus statement on clinical definition from the European Headache Federation. J Headache Pain. 2014;15(1):79. https://doi.org/10.1186/1129-2377-15-79.

15. Lund N, Barloese M, Petersen A, Haddock B, Jensen R. Chronobiology differs between men and women with cluster headache, clinical phenotype does not. Neurology. 2017;88(11):1069–76.

16. Taga A, Russo M, Manzoni GC, Torelli P. Cluster headache with accompanying migraine-like features: a possible clinical phenotype. Headache. 2017;57:290–7.

17. Zidverc-Trajkovic J, Podgorac A, Radojicic A, Sternic N. Migraine-like accompanying features in patients with cluster headache. How important are they? Headache. 2013;53:1464–9.

18. Silberstein SD, Niknam R, Rozen TD, Young WB. Cluster headache with aura. Neurology. 2000;54(1):219.

19. Siow HC, Young WB, Peres MF, Rozen TD, Silberstein SD. Hemiplegic cluster. Headache. 2002;42(2):136–9.

20. Wilbrink LA, Louter MA, Teernstra OP, van Zwet EW, et al. Allodynia in cluster headache. Pain. 2017;158(6):1113–7.

21. Dousset V, Laporte A, Legoff M, Traineau MH, Dartigues JF, Brochet B. Validation of a brief self-administered questionnaire for cluster headache screening in a tertiary center. Headache. 2009;49:64–70.

22. Manzoni GC, Terzano MG, Bono G, Micieli G, Martucci N, Nappi G. Cluster headache – clinical findings in 180 patients. Cephalalgia. 1983;3:21–30.

23. Russell D. Cluster headache: severity and temporal profiles of attacks and patient activity prior to and during attacks. Cephalalgia. 1981;1:209–16.

24. Bahra A, May A, Goadsby PJ. Cluster headache: a prospective clinical study with diagnostic implications. Neurology. 2002;58:354–61.

25. Ekbom K. Patterns of cluster headache with a note on the relations to angina pectoris and peptic ulcer. Acta Neurol Scand. 1970;46:225–37.

26. Jürgens TP, Koch HJ, May A. Ten years of chronic cluster–attacks still cluster. Cephalalgia. 2010;30(9):1123–6.

27. Lee MJ, Choi HA, Shin JH, Park HR, Chung CS. Natural course of untreated cluster headache: a retrospective cohort study. Cephalalgia. 2017 1:333102417706350.

28. Torkamani M, Ernst L, Cheung LS, Lambru G, Matharu M, Jahanshahi M. The neuropsychology of cluster headache: cognition, mood, disability, and quality of life of patients with chronic and episodic cluster headache. Headache. 2015;55(2):287–300. https://doi.org/10.1111/head.12486.

29. Jensen RM, Lyngberg A, Jensen RH. Burden of cluster headache. Cephalalgia. 2007;27:535–41.

30. Obermann M, Yoon MS, Dommes P, et al. Prevalence of trigeminal autonomic symptoms in migraine. Cephalalgia. 2007;27:504–9.

31. Nappi G, Micieli G, Cavallini A, Zanferrari C, Sandrini G, Manzoni GC. Accompanying symptoms of cluster attacks: their relevance to the diagnostic criteria. Cephalalgia. 1992;12:165–8.

32. Van Vliet JA, Eekers PJ, Haan J, Ferrari M. Features involved in the diagnostic delay of cluster headache. J Neurol Neurosurg Psychiatry. 2003;74:1123–5.

33. Obermann M, Holle D, Katsarava Z. Trigeminal neuralgia and persistent idiopathic facial pain. Expert Rev Neurother. 2011;11(11):1619–29.

34. Mueller D, Obermann M, Yoon MS, et al. Prevalence of trigeminal neuralgia and persistent idiopathic facial pain: a population-based study. Cephalalgia. 2011;31(15):1542–8.

35. Paemeleire K, Bahra A, Evers S, Matharu MS, Goadsby PJ. Medication-overuse headache in patients with cluster headache. Neurology. 2006;67(1):109–13.

36. Paemeleire K, Evers S, Goadsby PJ. Medication-overuse headache in patients with cluster headache. Curr Pain Headache Rep. 2008;12(2):122–7.

37. Sahai-Srivastava S, Hartunian G. Onset of cluster headache after cataract surgery. Cephalalgia. 2011;31(1 Suppl):1–216.

38. Sahai-Srivastava S, Khan KJ. Rare presentation of cluster headaches in multiple sclerosis patient. Headache. 2014;54(S1):38.

39. Gentile S, Ferrero M, Vaula G, Rainero I, Pinessi L. Cluster headache attacks and multiple sclerosis. J Headache Pain. 2007;8(4):245–7. PubMed PMID: 17901919; PubMed Central PMCID: PMC3451675

40. Leandri M, Cruccu G, Gottlieb A. Cluster headache-like pain in multiple sclerosis. Cephalalgia. 1999;19(8):732–4. PubMed PMID: 10570729

41. Greve E, Mai J. Cluster headache like headaches: a symptomatic feature? Cephalalgia. 1988;8:79–82.

42. West P, Todman D. Chronic cluster headache associated with vertebral artery aneurysm. Headache. 1991;31:210–2.

43. Mani S, Deeter J. Arteriovenous malformation of the brain presenting as cluster headache – a case report. Headache. 1982;22:184–5.

44. Muoz C, Tejedor ED, Frank A, Barreiro P. Cluster headache syndrome associated with middle cerebral artery arteriovenous malformation. Cephalalgia. 1996;16:202–5.

45. Cremer P, Halmagyi GM, Goadsby PJ. Secondary cluster headache responsive to Sumatriptan. J Neurol Neurosurg Psychiatry. 1995;59:633–4.

46. Kuritzky A. Cluster headache-like pain caused by an upper cervical meningioma. Cephalalgia. 1984;4:185–6.

47. Cid C, Berciano J, Pascual J. Retroocular headache with autonomic features resembling 'continuous' cluster headache in a lateral medullary infarction. J Neurol Neurosurg Psychiatry. 2000;69:134–41.

48. de la Sayette V, Schaeffer S, Coskun O, et al. Cluster headache-like attack as an opening symptom of a unilateral infarction of the cervical cord: persistent anaesthesia and dysaesthesia to cold stimuli. J Neurol Neurosurg Psychiatry. 1999;66:397–400.

49. Tfelt-Hansen P, Paulson OB, Krabbe AE. Invasive adenoma of the pituitary gland and chronic migrainous neuralgia. A rare coincidence or a causal relationship? Cephalalgia. 1982;2:25–8.

50. Hannerz J. A case of parasellar meningioma mimicking cluster headache. Cephalalgia. 1989;9: 265–9.

51. Goadsby PJ, Edvinsson L. Human in vivo evidence for trigeminovascular activation in cluster headache. Neuropeptide changes and effects of acute attacks therapies. Brain. 1994;117(Pt 3):427–34.

52. Fanciullacci M, Alessandri M, Sicuteri R, et al. Responsiveness of the trigeminovascular system to nitroglycerine in cluster headache patients. Brain. 1997;120(Pt 2):283–8.

53. Sprenger T, Ruether KV, Boecker H, Valet M, Berthele A, Pfaffenrath V, Wöller A, Tölle TR. Altered metabolism in frontal brain circuits in cluster headache. Cephalalgia. 2007;27:1033–42. https://doi.org/10.1111/j.1468-2982.2007.

54. Goadsby PJ. Pathophysiology of cluster headache: a trigeminal autonomic cephalalgia. Lancet Neurol. 2002 Aug;1(4):251–7.

55. DaSilva AF, Goadsby PJ, Borsook D. Cluster headache: a review of neuroimaging findings. Curr Pain Headache Rep (Review). 2007;11(2):131–6.

https://doi.org/10.1007/s11916-007-0010-1. PMID 17367592

56. May A, Goasdby PJ. Hypothalamic involvement and activation in cluster headache. Curr Pain Headache Rep. 2001;5(1):60–6. https://doi.org/10.1007/s11916-001-0011-4.

57. Leone M, Bussone G. Pathophysiology of trigeminal autonomic cephalalgias. Lancet Neurol. 2009;8:755–64. https://doi.org/10.1016/S1474-4422(09)70133-4.

58. Nicolodi M, Torrini A, Sandoval V, Fanfani M, Taddei I. O013. Neuro-imaging and history of cases of refractory chronic cluster headache in young patients: a hint for reflections. J Headache Pain. 2015; 16(Suppl 1):A95. https://doi.org/10.1186/1129-2377-16-S1-A95.

59. May A, Bahra A, Büchel C, Frackowiak RSJ, Goadsby PJ. Hypothalamic activation in cluster headache attacks. Lancet. 1998;352:275–8. https://doi.org/10.1016/S0140-6736(98)02470-2.

60. Sprenger T, Boecker H, Tolle TR, Bussone G, May A, Leone M. Specific hypothalamic activation during a spontaneous cluster headache attack. Neurology. 2004;62:516–7.

61. Magis D, Bruno MA, Fumal A, Gérardy PY, Hustinx R, Laureys S, Schoenen J. Central modulation in cluster headache patients treated with occipital nerve stimulation: an FDG-PET study. BMC Neurol. 2011;24:11–25.

62. Sprenger T, Willoch F, Miederer M, Schindler F, Valet M, Berthele A, Spilker ME, Förderreuther S, Straube A, Stangier I, Wester HJ, Tölle TR. Opioidergic changes in the pineal gland and hypothalamus in cluster headache: a ligand PET study. Neurology. 2006;66:1108–10. https://doi.org/10.1212/01.wnl.0000204225.15947.f8.

63. Sprenger T, Seifert CL, Miederer M, Valet M, Tolle TR. Successful prophylactic treatment of chronic cluster headache with low-dose levomethadone. J Neurol. 2008;255:1832–3. https://doi.org/10.1007/s00415-008-0992-6.

64. Norris JW, Hachinski VC, Cooper PW. Cerebral blood flow changes in cluster headache. Acta Neurol Scand. 1976;54:371–4. https://doi.org/10.1111/j.1600-0404.1976.tb04367.x.

65. Krabbe AA, Henriksen L, Olesen J. Tomographic determination of cerebral blood flow during attacks of cluster headache. Cephalalgia. 1984;4:17–23. https://doi.org/10.1046/j.1468-2982.1984.0401017.x.

66. Robbins MS, Starling AJ, Pringsheim TM, Becker WJ, Schwedt TJ. Treatment of cluster headache: the American Headache Society Evidence-Based guidelines. Headache. 2016;56:1093–106. https://doi.org/10.1111/head.12866.

67. Cohen AS, Burns B, Goadsby PJ. High flow oxygen for treatment of cluster headache. A randomized trial. JAMA. 2009;302:2451–7.

68. Fogan L. Treatment of cluster headache. A double-blind comparison of oxygen v air inhalation. Arch Neurol. 1985;42(4):362–3. https://doi.org/10.1001/archneur.1985.04060040072015.

69. Kudrow L. Response of cluster headache attacks to oxygen inhalation. Headache. 1981;21:1–4.
70. DiSAbato F, Fusco BM, Pelaia P, Giacovazzo M. Hyperbaric therapy in cluster headache. Pain. 1993;52:243–5.
71. Cohen AS, Matharu MS, Goadsby PJ. Trigeminal autonomic cephalalgias: current and future treatments. Headache. 2007;47:969–80. https://doi.org/10.1111/j.1526-4610.2007.00839.x.
72. Leone M, Cecchini AP. Long-term use of daily sumatriptan injections in severe drug-resistant chronic cluster headache. Neurology. 2016;86(2):194–5.
73. Verslegers WR, Leone M, Cecchini AP. Long-term use of daily sumatriptan injections in severe drug-resistant chronic cluster headache. Neurology. 2016;87(14):1522–3.
74. Diamond Headache Clinic. Sumatriptan 4 mg stat-dose in the acute treatment of cluster headache. http://www.clinicaltrials.gov/show/NCT00399243
75. Diamond S, Robbins L, Freitag FG. 52nd Annual Scientific Meeting of the American Headache Society, Los Angeles, California, June 24–27, 2010.
76. van Vliet JA, Bahra A, Martin V, Aurora SK, Mathew NT, Ferrari MD, et al. Intranasal sumatriptan in cluster headache- randomized placebo-controlled double-blind study. Neurology. 2003;60:630–3.
77. Monstad I, Krabbe A, Micieli G. Preemptive oral treatment of Sumatriptan during a cluster period. Headache. 1995;35:607–13.
78. Bahra A, Gawel MJ, Hardebo J-E, Millson D, Brean SA, Goadsby PJ. Oral zolmitriptan is effective in the acute treatment of cluster headache. Neurology. 2000;54:1832–9.
79. Cittadini E, May A, Straube A, Evers S, Bussone G, Goadsby PJ. Effectiveness of intranasal zolmitriptan in acute cluster headache. A randomized, placebo-controlled, double-blind crossover study. Arch Neurol. 2006;63:1537–42.
80. Rapoport AM, Mathew NT, Silberstein SD, Dodick D, Tepper SJ, Sheftell FD, et al. Zolmitriptan nasal spray in the acute treatment of cluster headache: a double-blind study. Neurology. 2007;69:821–6.
81. Andersson PG, Jespersen LT. Dihydroergotamine nasal spray in the treatment of attacks of cluster headache. Cephalalgia. 1986;6:51–4.
82. Horton BT. Histaminergic cephalalgia. Lancet. 1952;2:92–8.
83. Magnoux E, Zlotnik G. Outpatient intravenous dihydroergotamine for refractory cluster headache. Headache. 2004;44:249–55.
84. Costa A, Pucci E, Antonaci F, Sances G, Granella F, Broich G, Nappi G. The effect of intranasal cocaine and lidocaine on nitroglycerin-induced attacks in cluster headache. Cephalalgia. 2000;20(2):85–91.
85. Barre F. Cocaine and an abortive agent in cluster headache. Headache. 1982;22:69–73.
86. Narouze SN. Role of sphenopalatine ganglion neuroablation in the management of cluster headache. Curr Pain Headache Rep. 2010;14(2):160–3.
87. Matharu MS, Levy MJ, Meeran K, Goadsby PJ. Subcutaneous octreotide in cluster headache: randomized placebo-controlled double-blind crossover study. Ann Neurol. 2004;56:488–94. https://doi.org/10.1002/ana.20210.
88. Lisotto C, Mainardi F, Maggioni F, Zanchin G. O004. Refractory chronic cluster headache responding absolutely to indomethacin. J Headache Pain. 2015;16(Suppl 1):A96. https://doi.org/10.1186/1129-2377-16-S1-A96.
89. Buzzi MG, Formisano R. A patient with cluster headache responsive to indomethacin: any relationship with chronic paroxysmal hemicrania? Cephalalgia. 2003;23:401–4. https://doi.org/10.1046/j.1468-2982.2003.00558.x.
90. Leroux E, Valade D, Taifas I, et al. Suboccipital steroid injections for transitional treatment of patients with more than two cluster headache attacks per day: a randomised, double-blind, placebo controlled trial. Lancet Neurol. 2011;10:891–7.
91. Anthony M. Arrest of attacks of cluster headache by local steroid injection of the occipital nerve. In: Rose C, editor. Migraine. Karger: Basel; 1985. p. 169–73.
92. Peres MF, Stiles MA, Siow HC, Rozen TD, Young WB, Silberstein SD. Greater occipital nerve blockade for cluster headache. Cephalalgia. 2002;22:520–2.
93. Ambrosini A, Vandenheede M, Rossi P, et al. Suboccipital injection with a mixture of rapid- and long-acting steroids in cluster headache: a double-blind placebo-controlled study. Pain. 2005;118:92–6.
94. Lambru G, Abu Bakar N, Stahlhut L, McCulloch S, Miller S, Shanahan P, Matharu MS. Greater occipital nerve blocks in chronic cluster headache: a prospective open-label study. Eur J Neurol. 2014;21(2):338–43.
95. Busch V, Jakob W, Juergens T, Schulte-Mattler W, Kaube H, May A. Occipital nerve blockade in chronic cluster headache patients and functional connectivity between trigeminal and occipital nerves. Cephalalgia. 2007;27(11):1206–14.
96. Blumenfeld A, Ashkenazi A, Napchan U, Bender SD, et al. Expert consensus recommendations for the performance of peripheral nerve blocks for headaches–a narrative review. Headache. 2013;53(3):437–46.
97. Matthew NT. Clinical subtypes of cluster headaches and response to Lithium therapy. Headache. 1978;18:26–30.
98. Ekbom K. Lithium for cluster headache: review of literature and preliminary results of long term treatment. Headache. 1981;21:132–9.
99. Silberstein SD, Lipton RB, Goadsby PJ. Headache in clinical practice. 2nd ed. London: Martin Dunitz; 2002.
100. Waldenlind E, Ekbom K, Wetterberg L, et al. Lowered circannual urinary melatonin concentrations in episodic cluster headache. Cephalalgia. 1994;14:199–204.
101. Chazot G, Claustrat B, Brun J, et al. A chronobiological study of melatonin, cortisol growth hormone

and prolactin secretion in cluster headache. Cephalalgia. 1984;4:213–20.

102. Leone M, D'Amico D, Moschiano F, Fraschini F, Bussone G. Melatonin vs. placebo in the prophylaxis of cluster headache: a double-blind pilot study with parallel groups. Cephalalgia. 1996;16:494–6.

103. Pringsheim T, Magnoux E, Dobson CF, Hamel E, Aube M. Melatonin as adjunctive therapy in the prophylaxis of cluster headache: a pilot study. Headache. 2002;42:787–92.

104. Mir P, Alberca R, Navarro A, et al. Prophylactic treatment of episodic cluster headache with intravenous bolus of methylprednisolone. Neurol Sci. 2003;24:318–21.

105. Neeb L, Anders L, Euskirchen P, Hoffmann J, Israel H, Reuter U. Corticosteroids alter CGRP and melatonin release in cluster headache episodes. Cephalalgia. 2015;35(4):317–26.

106. Rapoport AM, Tepper SJ. Triptans are all different. Arch Neurol. 2001;58(9):1479–80.

107. Buchan P, Keywood C, Wade A, Ward C. Clinical pharmacokinetics of frovatriptan. Headache. 2002;42(s2):54–62.

108. Siow HC, Pozo-Rosich P, Silberstein SD. Frovatriptan for the treatment of cluster headaches. Cephalalgia. 2004;24(12):1045–8.

109. Eekers PJE, Koehler PJ. Naratriptan prophylactic treatment in cluster headache. Cephalalgia. 2001;21:75–6.

110. Mulder LJMM, Spierings ELH. Naratriptan in the preventive treatment of cluster headache. Cephalalgia. 2002;22(10):815–7.

111. Loder E. Naratriptan in the prophylaxis of cluster headache. Headache. 2002;42(1):56–7.

112. Zebenholzer K, Wober C, Vigl M, Wessely P. Eletriptan for the short-term prophylaxis of cluster headache. Headache. 2004;44:361–4.

113. Wheeler SD, Carrazana EJ. Topiramate-treated cluster headache. Neurology. 1999;53(1):234.

114. Lainez MJ, Pascual J, Santonta JM, et al. Topiramate in the prophylactic treatment of cluster headache. Cephalalgia. 2001;21:500(abstract).

115. McGeeney BE. Topiramate in the treatment of cluster headache. Curr Pain Headache Rep. 2003;7:135–8.

116. Forderreuther S, Mayer M, Straube A. Treatment of cluster headache with topiramate: effects and side-effects in five patients. Cephalalgia. 2002;22:186–9.

117. Leone M, Dodick D, Rigamonti A, et al. Topiramate in cluster headache prophylaxis: an open trial. Cephalalgia. 2003;23:1001–2.

118. Ahmed F. Chronic cluster headache responding to gabapentin: a case report. Cephalalgia. 2000;20(4):252–3.

119. Schuh-Hofer S, Israel H, Neeb L, Reuter U, Arnold G. The use of gabapentin in chronic cluster headache patients refractory to first-line therapy. Eur J Neurol. 2007;14(6):694–6.

120. Leandri M, Luzzani M, Cruccu G, Gottlieb A. Drug-resistant cluster headache responding to gabapentin: a pilot study. Cephalalgia. 2001;21(7):744–6.

121. Hering R, Kuritzky A. Sodium valproate in the treatment of cluster headache: an open clinical trial. Cephalalgia. 1989;9:195–8.

122. Gallagher RM, Mueller LL, Freitag FG. Divalproex sodium in the treatment of migraine and cluster headaches. J Am Osteopath Assoc. 2002;102(2):92–4.

123. Sewell RA, Halpern JH, Pope HG. Response of cluster headache to psilocybin and LSD. Neurology. 2006;66:1920–2.

124. Sun-Edelstein C, Mauskop A. Alternative headache treatments: nutraceuticals, behavioral and physical treatments. Headache. 2011;51(3):469–83. https://doi.org/10.1111/j.1526-4610.2011.01846.x.

125. Vollenweider FX, Kometer M. The neurobiology of psychedelic drugs: implications for the treatment of mood disorders. Nat Rev Neurosci. 2010;11(9):642–51. https://doi.org/10.1038/nrn2884.

126. Jensen RH. The most important advances in headache research in 2016. Lancet Neurol. 2017;16(1):5.

127. Benemei S, Nicoletti P, Capone JG, Geppetti P. CGRP receptors in the control of pain and inflammation. Curr Opin Pharmacol. 2009;9(1):9–14.

128. Doods H, Arndt K, Rudolf K, Just S. CGRP antagonists: unravelling the role of CGRP in migraine. Trends Pharmacol Sci. 2007;28(11):580–7.

129. US National Library of Medicine (2016) ClinicalTrials.gov https://clinicaltrials.gov/ct2/show/NCT02438826. Accessed 21 Mar 2017.

130. Graham JR. Methysergide for prevention of headache: experience in five hundred patients over three years. N Engl J Med. 1964;270(2):67–72.

131. Rozen T. Clomiphene citrate for treatment refractory chronic cluster headache. Headache. 2008;48:286–90. https://doi.org/10.1111/j.1526-4610.2007.00995.

132. Rozen TD. Clomiphene citrate as a preventive treatment for intractable chronic cluster headache: a second reported case with long-term follow-up. Headache. 2015;55(4):571–4. https://doi.org/10.1111/head.12491.

133. Stillman MJ. Testosterone replacement therapy for treatment refractory cluster headache. Headache. 2006;46:925–33. https://doi.org/10.1111/j.1526-4610.2006.00436.x.

134. Sjaastad O, Sjaastad OV. The histaminuria in vascular headache. Acta Neurol Scand. 1970;46A:331–42.

135. Anthony M, Lance JW. Histamine and serotonin in cluster headache. Arch Neurol (Chicago). 1971;25:225–31.

136. Anthony M, Lord GDA, Lance JW. Controlled trials of cimetidine in migraine and cluster headache. Headache. 1978;18(5):261–4.

137. Russell DA. Cluster headache: trial of a combined histamine H1 and H2 antagonist treatment. J Neurol Neurosurg Psychiatry. 1979;42(7):668–9.

138. Sicuteri F, Fusco BM, Marabini S, et al. Beneficial effect of capsaicin application to the nasal mucosa in cluster headache. Clin J Pain. 1989;5:49–53.

139. Fusco BM, Marabini S, Maggi CA, Fiore G, Geppetti P. Preventative effect of repeated nasal applications of capsaicin in cluster headache. Pain. 1994;59:321–5.

140. Marks DR, Rapoport A, Padla D, et al. A double-blind placebo-controlled trial of intranasal capsaicin for cluster headache. Cephalalgia. 1993;13:114–6.

141. Saper JR, Klapper J, Mathew NT, Rapoport A, Phillips SB, Bernstein JE. Intranasal civamide for the treatment of episodic cluster headaches. Arch Neurol. 2002;59:990–4.

142. Mayer JS, Binns PM, Ericsson AD. Sphenopalatine ganglionectomy for cluster headache. Arch Otolaryngol. 1970;92:475–84.

143. Narouze S, Kapural L, Casanova J. Sphenopalatine ganglion radiofrequency ablation for the management of chronic cluster headache. Headache. 2009;49:571–7.

144. Ansarinia M, Rezai A, Tepper SJ. Electrical stimulation of sphenopalatine ganglion for acute treatment of cluster headaches. Headache. 2010;50:1164–74.

145. Schytz HW, Barløse M, Guo S, Selb J, Caparso A, Jensen R, Ashina M. Experimental activation of the sphenopalatine ganglion provokes cluster-like attacks in humans. Cephalalgia. 2013;33(10): 831–41.

146. Jurgens TP, Schoenen J, Rostgaard J, Hillerup S, Láinez MJ, Assaf AT, May A, Jensen RH. Stimulation of the sphenopalatine ganglion in intractable cluster headache: expert consensus on patient selection and standards of care. Cephalalgia. 2014;34:1100–10.

147. Ekbom K, Lindgren L, Nilsson BY, Hardebo JE, Waldenlind E. Retro-Gasserian glycerol injection in the treatment of chronic cluster headache. Cephalalgia. 1987;7:21–7.

148. Taha JM, Tew JM Jr. Long-term results of radiofrequency rhizotomy in the treatment of cluster headache. Headache. 1995;35:193–6.

149. Matharu MS, Goadsby PJ. Persistence of attacks of cluster headache after trigeminal nerve root section. Brain. 2002;125:976–84.

150. Saper JR, Dodick DW, Silberstein SD. Occipital nerve stimulation for the treatment of intractable chronic migraine headache: ONSTIM feasibility study. Cephalalgia. 2011;31:271–85.

151. Schwedt TJ, Green AL, Dodick DW. Occipital nerve stimulation for migraine: update from recent multicenter trials. Prog Neurol Surg. 2015;29:117–26. https://doi.org/10.1159/000434662.

152. Ambrosini A. Occipital nerve stimulation for intractable cluster headache. Lancet. 2007;369:1063–5.

153. Burns B, Watkins L, Goadsby PJ. Treatment of intractable chronic cluster headache by occipital nerve stimulation in 14 patients. Neurology. 2009;72:341–5.

154. Fontaine D, Christophe Sol J, Raoul S. Treatment of refractory chronic cluster headache by chronic occipital nerve stimulation. Cephalalgia. 2011;31:1101–5.

155. Miller S, Watkins L, Matharu M. Treatment of intractable chronic cluster headache by occipital nerve stimulation: a cohort of 51 patients. Eur J Neurol. 2017;24(2):381–90. https://doi.org/10.1111/ene.13215.

156. Mercieri M, Negro A, Silvestri B, D'Alonzo L, Tigano S, Arcioni R, Martelletti P. Drug-resistant chronic cluster headache successfully treated with supraorbital plus occipital nerve stimulation. A rare case report. J Headache Pain. 2015;16(Suppl 1):A97. https://doi.org/10.1186/1129-2377-16-S1-A97.

157. Silberstein SD, Calhoun AH, Lipton RB, Grosberg BM, et al., On behalf of the EVENT Study Group. Chronic migraine headache prevention with noninvasive vagus nerve stimulation: the EVENT study. Neurology. 2016;87(5):529–538. https://doi.org/10.1212/WNL.0000000000002918.

158. Silberstein SD, Mechtler LL, Kudrow DB, Calhoun AH, McClure C, Saper JR, Liebler EJ, Rubenstein Engel E, Tepper SJ, ACT1 Study Group. Non-invasive vagus nerve stimulation for the acute treatment of cluster headache: findings from the randomized, double-blind, sham-controlled ACT1 study. Headache. 2016;56(8):1317–32.

159. Goadsby P. Non-invasive vagus nerve stimulation for the acute treatment of episodic and chronic cluster headache: findings from the randomized, double-blind, sham-controlled ACT2 study. AAN annual meeting; 2017.

160. Gaul C, Magis D, Liebler E, Straube A. Effects of non-invasive vagus nerve stimulation on attack frequency over time and, expanded response rates in patients with chronic cluster headache: a post hoc analysis of the randomized, controlled PREVA study. J Headache Pain. 2017;18(1):22. https://doi.org/10.1186/s10194-017-0731-4.

161. Leone M, Franzini A, Bussone G. Stereotactic stimulation of posterior hypothalamic gray matter in a patient with intractable cluster headache. N Engl J Med. 2001;345:1428–9.

162. Leone M, Franzini A, Broggi G, Bussone G. Hypothalamic deep brain stimulation for intractable chronic cluster headache: a 3-year follow-up. Neurol Sci. 2003;24(Suppl 2):s143–5.

163. Leone M, Franzini A, Cecchini AP, Bussone G. Success, failure, and putative mechanisms in hypothalamic stimulation for drug-resistant chronic cluster headache. Pain. 2013;154:89–94.

164. Rossi P, Ruiz De La Torre E, Tassorelli C, the European Headache Alliance. O029. Lessons from the expert patients. Advice for the physician to improve the care of cluster headache patients. J Headache Pain. 2015;16(Suppl 1):A94. https://doi.org/10.1186/1129-2377-16-S1-A94.

New Daily Persistent Headache

7

LaurenLauren R. Natbony, Huma U. Sheikh,
and Mark W. Green

Introduction

New daily persistent headache (NDPH) was first described by Vanast in 1986 as a "benign syndrome, combining features of common migraine and tension headache and occurs (sic) daily from the first day the headache begins" [1]. It is currently classified as a type of primary long-duration chronic daily headache (CDH), of which there are three additional types: chronic migraine (CM), chronic tension-type headache (CTTH), and hemicrania continua (HC). What makes NDPH unique is that it starts abruptly and is daily from onset. Many patients will remember the exact day of onset, and some will be able to describe exactly what they were doing at the time the headache started. The pain of NDPH lacks characteristic features and may have elements of

migrainemigraine and/or tension-type headache [2]. Most patients have mild to moderate pain intensity which is bilateral, although there can be variations. It typically presents in individuals with no prior headache history.

Epidemiology

There have been only a handful of studies to help determine epidemiology, although most of them have similar results. Castillo et al. in 1999 looked at 2252 subjects in Spain and found that the prevalence of NDPH was around 0.1% [3]. In 2002, Bigal reported NDPH to be about 10% of patients who presented to a headache specialty clinic, as a subset of patients with chronic daily headache [4]. Most recently in 2009, Grande et al. determined a 1-year prevalence of 0.03% [5]. NDPH also appears to be slightly more prevalent in the pediatric population, with 13% of pediatric patients with CDH having a diagnosis of NDPH [6]. Other reports have confirmed this slightly higher prevalence among the adolescent population [7].

The most common age of onset of NDPH appears to be in the third and fourth decades. In Vanast's 1986 study, the age of onset was reported to be between 16 and 35, with earlier onset in women [1]. In 2002, Li and Rozen conducted a retrospective review over a 3-year period with a total of 56 patients diagnosed with primary NPDH. They found the peak age of onset in the teens and 20s for women and in the 40s for

L. R. Natbony (✉)
Neurology, Center for Headache and Facial Pain,
Icahn School of Medicine at Mount Sinai,
New York, NY, USA
e-mail: lauren.natbony@mountsinai.org

H. U. Sheikh
Neurology, Mount Sinai, New York, NY, USA

M. W. Green
Neurology, Icahn School of Medicine at Mt. Sinai,
New York, NY, USA

Anesthesiology, Icahn School of Medicine at Mt.
Sinai, New York, NY, USA

Rehabilitation Medicine, Icahn School of Medicine at
Mt. Sinai, New York, NY, USA

© Springer International Publishing AG, part of Springer Nature 2019
M. W. Green et al. (eds.), *Chronic Headache*, https://doi.org/10.1007/978-3-319-91491-6_7

97

men [8]. Other studies have shown that the age range for onset can be from 6 to 70, with a mean of 35 years of age [9]. In the cohort by Robbins et al. of 71 patients, the median age of onset was 26 in women and 28 in men. They also noted that most patients were female (71.8%) and Caucasian (80.3%) [10]. In the latest study published by Rozen in 2016, the average age of onset was reported to be in the mid-30s [11].

Diagnostic Criteria

The diagnostic criteria have evolved over time. While the first diagnostic criteria for NDPH were proposed in 1994 in the Silberstein-Lipton classification of CDH, the condition was not included in the International Classification of Headache Disorders (ICHD) until 2004 with the publication of ICHD, 2nd edition (ICHD-2). In the Silberstein-Lipton criteria, the components needed to diagnose NDPH included (1) headache for 15 or more days per month, (2) for more than 3 months, (3) lasting more than 4 h/day, and (4) beginning abruptly over fewer than 3 days without being preceded by increasing frequency of migraine or tension-type headache. A subdivision of NDPH was also proposed based on the presence of medication overuse [12]. In the ICHD-2, the diagnostic criterion was phenotypically a tension-type headache that started abruptly and was continuous from onset [13]. It excluded patients with prominent migraine features. In 2008, Kung et al. proposed a more simplified criteria that did not include the presence or absence of migrainous features [14].

In the newest edition of ICHD, ICHD-3 beta, NDPH is an abrupt onset of primary chronic daily headache at a specific time remembered by the patient. The onset of CDH occurs within 24 hours and remains continuous from onset with no remissions and no pain-free periods. Headache must be continuous for more than 3 months. Secondary causes first need to be ruled out. The key to diagnosis lies in the patient's recollection of abrupt onset of headache. The latest version now has two subtypes, one that is self-limited and usually resolves without treatment and one that

is more persistent and refractory [2]. There is the possibility to diagnose someone with "probable NDPH," if the 3-month timeline has not been met; however, this is put in place to prevent misdiagnosis [15].

The latest diagnostic criteria do not mention any particular phenotype of the headache. This was updated after much controversy regarding the diagnostic criteria, which previously did not allow for the presence of migrainous features [16]. The ICHD-3 does not preclude a diagnosis of NDPH in those with history of headache, even those with CM or CTTH. It specifies that, if a prior headache history does exist, the patient must not report an increasing frequency of that headache prior to onset of NDPH. Moreover, patients should not describe an exacerbation followed by a period of medication overuse [2].

ICHD-3 Diagnostic Criteria for NDPH

A. Persistent headache fulfilling criteria B and C

B. Distinct and clearly remembered onset, with pain becoming continuous and unremitting within 24 h

C. Present for >3 months

D. Not better accounted for by another ICHD-3 diagnosis

Clinical Features

The most prominent clinical feature is continuous pain from onset [10]. Most patients identify the day or month when the headache first began. Some are even able to remember the exact time the headache started and exactly what they were doing. Grande and Aseth conducted a cross-sectional study of the Norwegian population using a headache questionnaire and follow-up interview. Headaches were classified according to ICHD-2 criteria. In the total of four patients who were classified as having NDPH, all of them were able to recall the exact day of onset of their headache, and all previously recalled infrequent tension-type headaches [5]. In the retrospective review by Li and Rozen, 82% of the 56 patients could point to the exact day when headache symptoms began [8]. This percentage was lower in another study, showing about 42.3% of 71 patients with NDPH recalled the day of onset of headache, with almost double remembering the month of onset [10]. Grengs and Mack described NDPH in a population of children. They reviewed 104 patients with NDPH, and 92 of them were able to remember the month of onset [17].

Multiple studies consistently show that patients with a diagnosis of NDPH commonly have associated features that are typical of migraine, including nausea, photophobia, and phonophobia [8]. These symptoms are typically intermittent and may occur with exacerbations of baseline pain. There are also rare case reports that describe a visual aura or bilateral facial flushing [10]. Even in the first case series described by Vanast, some of the patients had migrainous features though many of the patients also reported other neurological symptoms, including dizziness, diplopia, or tinnitus [1]. The prognosis in this first case series was different from subsequent studies, and, therefore, it was unclear if these were all truly primary NDPH. In an epidemiological study by Grande and Aaseth, they detected a total of four patients from the general population with NDPH, two of whom had migrainous features including photophobia and nausea [5].

Robbins et al. studied a group of 71 patients with daily headaches using ICHD-2 criteria for NDPH. They compared this group to another group labeled NDPH-R, in whom migrainous features were not excluded. NDPH diagnosis was made using revised ICHD-2 criteria, according to Kung et al., and designated as NDPH-R. They found that there were 40 extra patients that would be classified with NDPH if migrainous features were included in the diagnostic criteria [14]. The majority of patients described bilateral pain, and the baseline pain was in the range of 4–6/10. Including all patients, according to both criteria, 45.1% of patients described throbbing pain, and almost 90% described bilateral pain. Nausea, photophobia, and phonophobia were present in about half of patients. Medication overuse was present in about 45% of patients [10]. Grande and Aaseth also found that three of the four patients in their study with NDPH were believed to have an element of medication-overuse headaches [5].

A large percentage of patients with NDPH have a prior history of headache. In the case series from Robbins et al., about 25% had another primary headache disorder prior to the onset of NDPH, most commonly either tension-type or migraine [10]. In Li and Rozen's 2002 study, about 38% of patients noted that they had a previous history of episodic headaches, either migraine or tension-type headaches. None reported chronic daily headaches in the past or escalation of headache frequency prior to the onset of NDPH [8]. Thus, abrupt onset of continuous daily headache in a patient with a history of episodic headache is suspicious for NDPH.

Comorbidities are common in NDPH patients. A recent article by Uniyal et al. assessed 55 patients with NDPH compared to age- and sex-matched healthy individuals with chronic low back pain. They found significantly higher rates of psychiatric comorbidities, including anxiety, depression, somatoform disorders, and pain catastrophization in patients with NDPH [18]. In a cohort of 71 NDPH patients, about a third of patients also reported a history of either anxiety or depression [19]. Other frequent comorbidities were hypertension and hyperlipidemia [10].

Etiology and Pathophysiology

Currently, the exact pathogenic mechanism that underlies NDPH is unknown though there are several proposed etiologies. Some of the confusion arises because it is not clear whether this is a single type of headache disorder or there are multiple pathologies with a similar presenting phenotype [11]. Some have argued that NDPH is a syndrome and not a discrete disorder [20]. Rozen did a retrospective analysis of medical records of patients who were diagnosed with NDPH. A headache specialist saw all the patients at a headache clinic from 2009 to 2013, and secondary

NDPH was ruled out by imaging and history. These patients were asked about a triggering event prior to the onset of their NDPH. Ninety-seven patients were identified in this study with NDPH. Of those, 65 were women and most were Caucasian. A little more than half could not recognize a triggering event. For those who could, 22% remembered a flu-like illness prior to NDPH, 9% remembered a stressful event, 9% recalled surgical procedure prior to onset of their NDPH, and the rest (about 7%) recognized some other event, including medication exposure or a syncopal event [21]. Further studies have verified these results along with pointing out a few other triggers including tapering of SSRIs, exposure to the HPV vaccine, and menarche [10]. There was not much difference in the triggering events across genders [8].

Triggering Events

Flu-Like Illness or Infection

A flu-like illness or infection has been postulated in many case series as a triggering event. This finding has led to the theory of increased inflammation of the central nervous system as a possible causative factor. In the series by Li and Rozen in 2002, about a third of patients noted that their headaches started in relation to a flu-like or other infection [8]. A study by Rozen and Swidan found that a significant percentage of patients (19/20) with primary NDPH had elevated tumor necrosis factor alpha (TNFα) (a cytokine believed to be involved in inflammation) in the cerebrospinal fluid (CSF) [22]. Since a viral illness is frequently thought to be a triggering event, some surmise that the initial inflammation becomes ongoing in these patients, leading to the chronic headache of NDPH [23]. TNFα has been known to induce calcitonin gene-related peptide production, a factor in the development of pain syndromes based in the trigeminal pathway [24]. In the initial case series by Vanast, 84% had elevated EBV titers out of 32 patients described to have NDPH [1]. This finding has added to the theory that a viral infection may bring on this headache disorder.

Stressful Event

In the Li and Rozen series, 12% of patients attributed onset of headache to a stressful life event [8]. Stress is thought to be a causative factor for the development of chronic headaches in general.

Surgical Procedure

In the 2002 review by Li and Rozen, about 12% attributed the onset of their headaches to a surgical procedure [8]. In Rozen's 2016 retrospective analysis, about 9% of patients with NDPH had onset of their headache after a surgical procedure. Most of the patients who had onset of NDPH after a surgical procedure were intubated, and all of them also had associated greater occipital nerve and upper cervical facet irritation during their exam on initial visit [21]. This finding has led to a hypothesis that cervical arthritis and upper cervical facet irritation may be a risk factor for the development of NDPH [8].

While not a triggering event, per se, cervical joint hypermobility has been postulated to be a potential cause of NDPH. Rozen and colleagues noticed similar physical characteristics of tall stature with thin body habitus and long necks in 12 patients with NDPH. Hypermobility of the cervical region was noticed to be a pervasive sign on exam in 11 of the 12 NDPH patients. Widespread systemic joint hypermobility was seen in 10 of the 12 patients [25]. As joint hypermobility is a risk factor for the development of chronic pain in the rheumatology literature, the authors concluded that cervical spine hypermobility might be a predisposing factor for the development of NDPH. It is thought that cervical hypermobility can bring on headaches since there is a convergence of trigeminal and cervical afferents in the trigeminal nucleus caudalis [26]. Of course, spontaneous CSF leak can result in a phenotypically similar headache and is more common in this same population.

Differential Diagnosis

The differential diagnosis for new daily headaches is broad and includes both primary and secondary headache types (Table 7.1).

Table 7.1 Differential diagnosis of new daily headaches present for >3 months

Primary headaches	Secondary headaches
New daily persistent headache	Intracranial hypotension
Chronic migraine	Intracranial hypertension
Chronic tension-type headache	Cerebral venous sinus thrombosis
Hemicrania continua	Postmeningitis/chronic meningitis
	Medication overuse
	Sphenoid sinusitis
	Posttraumatic headache
	Chronic subdural hematoma
	Neoplasm/mass lesion
	Giant cell arteritis
	Carotid/vertebral artery dissection
	Cervical facet syndrome (cervicogenic)
	Intranasal contact point headache
	Arteriovenous malformation
	Dural arteriovenous fistula
	Chiari malformation
	Temporomandibular joint dysfunction

Adapted from Evans [9]

Primary Headache Disorders

NDPH is one of four headache types in the CDH category that also includes CM, CTTH, and HC. It is possible that many NDPH patients have one of these disorders and are misclassified.

CM is fairly prevalent in the population and develops in persons who have a history of episodic migraine (EM) in the setting of increasing attack frequency [2]. The process of transformation from EM to CM is typically gradual over several weeks to months or even years [27]. This gradual transformation distinguishes CM from NDPH. It is possible that patients with NDPH simply have CM with an abrupt onset in the setting of an environmental trigger. In a study by Mack of a group of pediatric patients with CDH, he found that 30% of patients with CM reported an abrupt transition from EM. He concluded that pediatric patients with or without a headache history could develop an acute CDH [28].

CTTH, like CM, develops in a minority of episodic tension-type headache (ETTH) patients in the setting of escalating attack frequency. Just like in CM, the diagnosis of CTTH may be missed in patients diagnosed with NDPH due to underestimation or under-recognition of preexisting ETTH attacks.

HC is a strictly unilateral, continuous head pain accompanied by ipsilateral cranial autonomic signs during periods of headache exacerbation. It responds absolutely to therapeutic doses of indomethacin [2]. Like NDPH, HC typically starts as daily and continuous from onset. While HC was previously diagnosed only with ipsilateral head pain, many cases of HC featuring bilateral head pain responding definitively to indomethacin have now been reported [29]. Additionally, 11% of cases of NDPH may be unilateral, and cranial autonomic symptoms may be present with exacerbations in 26% of patients [9]. Thus, symptom overlap between these two syndromes can occur, and a trial of indomethacin may be needed to rule out HC. In NDPH, pain may improve temporarily with indomethacin; however it will not be abolished.

Secondary Headaches (NDPH Mimics)

A diagnosis of NDPH can be made only after secondary causes are excluded. The more recent the onset of NDPH, the more concern there should be for secondary causes. Secondary pathology should be especially considered when NDPH occurs over the age of 50. New-onset daily headaches with a normal neurologic examination can be due to various other causes especially when seen within the first 2 months after onset. When headaches have been present for more than 3 months with a normal neurologic examination, the yield of testing is low. Two disorders in particular that can mimic the presentation of NDPH are spontaneous CSF leak and cerebral venous sinus thrombosis. Additional secondary causes are discussed below.

Spontaneous Intracranial Hypotension
Spontaneous intracranial hypotension (SIH) from a spinal CSF leak typically presents as daily headache with a positional component. The

pain is generally not present on waking, worsens during the day, and is relieved by lying down. However, the longer a patient has a CSF leak-induced headache, the less pronounced the positional component becomes. Thus, since patients who are ultimately diagnosed with NDPH present to headache centers months to years after headache onset, care should be taken to explicitly delineate the initial headache characteristics or else the diagnosis of spontaneous intracranial hypotension can easily be missed. Magnetic resonance imaging (MRI) abnormalities of the brain and spine are present in about 90% of cases and may reveal diffuse pachymeningeal enhancement with gadolinium and in some cases subdural fluid collections [30]. Tonsillar descent and posterior fossa crowding may also be seen. It is important to note however that a slow-flow CSF leak may have less prominent MRI abnormalities. Low pressures, such as 0–5 cm H_2O, are usually identified with lumbar puncture; however higher pressures have been recorded with a documented leak. While opening pressures are increasingly recognized as unreliable markers, elevated protein and prolactin are suspicious for SIH in selected patients. In cases where SIH is suspected, spinal myelography with MRI or CT should be considered.

Cerebral Venous Thrombosis

Cerebral venous thrombosis (CVT) can present with headache in up to 90% of cases and is often the initial symptom. Headache can be the only symptom with a normal neurological examination in 32% of cases [31]. The headache can be hemicranial, bilateral, or poorly localized, constant or intermittent with exacerbations. The onset is typically gradual over several days but also can be thunderclap and then become chronic. Focal neurologic signs such as papilledema, cranial nerve palsies, decreased level of consciousness, and seizure can accompany headache.

Idiopathic Intracranial Hypertension

Idiopathic intracranial hypertension (IIH) can present with a daily headache. While this syndrome is often accompanied by neuro-ophthalmological symptoms including transient visual obscurations, pulsatile tinnitus, abducens nerve palsies, and varying visual field defects, it can also present with severe daily headache without evolution. Neurologic examination typically shows papilledema in IIH; however, IIH without papilledema is an increasingly recognized entity [15]. The headache of both IIH and NDPH is often bilateral, daily, continuous, throbbing, and accompanied by nausea. Both may respond to migraine prophylactic medications, especially topiramate [32]. Patients with IIH may have normal brain imaging or nonspecific abnormalities such as an empty sella and partial or complete obstruction of one or both transverse sinuses; thus lumbar puncture and measurement of opening pressure are needed for diagnosis. An opening pressure of greater than 25 cm H_2O in adults and 28 cm H_2O in children is diagnostic [2].

Viral Meningitis

Viral meningitis and a chronic post-viral headache may be misclassified as NDPH. Almazov and Brand evaluated children and adolescents at a pediatric neurology clinic in Israel and found that patients suffering from headache that mostly fit a chronic tension-type headache pattern had an extremely high prevalence of meningismus. Additionally, most experienced the onset of headache in the setting of an upper respiratory infection [33]. It is therefore important to look for signs and symptoms of underlying infection before diagnosing NDPH. For diagnosis of viral meningitis, CSF analysis must be performed during the acute period.

Reversible Cerebral Vasoconstriction Syndrome

Reversible cerebral vasoconstriction syndrome (RCVS) is an acute disorder characterized by severe headache and other neurological symptoms in the setting of multifocal, segmental vasospasm that is reversible [34]. There can be multiple thunderclap headaches at the onset of or during the acute period of this disorder. MRI scans are typically normal, and a vascular study done during the first few weeks after headache onset should show vasoconstriction. However, since vasospasm typically resolves after a few weeks, vascular imaging may be normal if obtained well after the onset [35]. Thus, it is important to get a thorough history of the headache pattern at onset, or the initial thunderclap headache pattern may be missed.

The long-term headache prognosis of RCVS is variable, and the phenotypic headache may mimic NDPH. One large prospective study of 67 patients in France with RCVS demonstrated a 35.8% presence of mild persistent headache at follow-up visits 3–6 weeks after hospital discharge [36]. More recently, 16 patients with RCVS were followed over 99 weeks. 42.9% of patients not lost to follow-up developed a persistent headache after RCVS despite no further thunderclap attacks and radiologic resolution of vasospasm [37].

Sphenoid Sinusitis

Sphenoid sinusitis may cause a severe intractable, new onset daily headache that interferes with sleep and is not relieved by simple analgesics. The headache is not specific in location; it often occurs in the vertex. There may be pain or paresthesia in the distribution of the fifth cranial nerve, photophobia, lacrimation, fever, and nasal drainage [38].

Cervical and Vertebral Artery Dissections

Dissections can present with headache or neck pain alone [39]. Occasionally, the headache can last for months or years and lead to a pattern of chronic daily headache. Conventional angiogram is the gold standard for diagnosis; however magnetic resonance imaging (MRI) with dissection protocol or computerized tomography angiogram (CTA) can visualize a dissection in most cases.

Giant Cell Arteritis

Approximately half of giant cell arteritis (GCA) patients can present with an unremitting, persistent headache reminiscent of NDPH. However, the pattern of GCA is typically unilateral, unlike that of NDPH and can be associated with other neurological or ophthalmological signs and symptoms. Features that further suggest this diagnosis include jaw pain/fatigue with chewing and ipsilateral visual deficits. GCA rarely occurs under the age of 50 with most biopsy proven large series having no patients under the age of 50 [40]. An elevated erythrocyte sedimentation rate (ESR) helps to diagnose GCA; however a normal ESR does not rule it out. A case series of 167 patients with GCA was undertaken at the Mayo Clinic, 90.4% of whom had positive temporal artery biopsies. Nine (5.4%) of the patients had a normal ESR, all of whom had a positive temporal artery biopsy. Of those nine patients, eight had either a new headache or prominent scalp tenderness, and in two patients, headache was the only presenting symptom [41].

Contact Point Headache

Contact point headache is thought to be due to contact between the lateral nasal wall and the nasal septum. It typically presents with periorbital pain and has been noted to respond to a septoplasty [42]. The diagnosis is frequently established by the application of local anesthetic agent and a vasoconstrictor to the identified potential contact point, which temporarily alleviates the headache.

Systemic Illness

A daily continuous headache can be the presenting feature of a systemic illness thereby mimicking NDPH. Bechet's disease (BD), for example, can present with a chronic headache even without signs of central nervous system involvement such as meningitis and venous sinus thrombosis [43]. Human immunodeficiency virus (HIV) infection is a rare cause of chronic daily headache, and HIV risk factors should routinely be queried. Hypothyroidism can produce headache in about 14% of patients [44].

Other

Other mimics include dural arteriovenous fistula, unruptured intracranial saccular aneurysms, Chiari malformation, posttraumatic headache, temporomandibular joint dysfunction, cervical facet syndrome, intracranial neoplasm or mass lesion, primary or secondary CNS angiitis [45].

Evaluation

NDPH is a diagnosis of exclusion. Initial investigations should include MRI of the brain with and without contrast, magnetic resonance venogram (MRV), and magnetic resonance angiography (MRA) of the head and neck (if headache presents with a thunderclap onset). Gadolinium contrast must be given to look for the pachymeningeal enhancement associated with CSF hypotension. While diagnosis of cerebral venous thrombosis (CVT) is best made with an MRV, the highest sensitivity is within the first 5 days of onset or after 6 weeks. If suspicion remains high for CVT and the MRV normal, digital subtraction venography can be performed. Further imaging can be considered based on the presenting symptoms.

Laboratory screening should include ESR, antinuclear antibody (ANA), Lyme antibody, viral titers including Epstein-Barr virus (EBV), human herpes virus 6 (HHV6), parvovirus and cytomegalovirus (CMV), thyroid function, complete blood count (CBC), and serum chemistries (Table 7.2). HIV and syphilis testing can be considered based on patient risk factors. A lumbar puncture should be considered if the above studies are negative and for patients refractory to

Table 7.2 Laboratory studies

CBC	Headache may be a symptom of decreased hemoglobin concentration (seen in thrombotic thrombocytopenic purpura)
TSH	Headache may be a symptom in 14% of cases of hypothyroidism
Chemistry profile	Renal failure and hypercalcemia can cause headaches
ESR	Elevated in (giant cell) arteritis
ANA	Headache with clinical signs of lupus or autoimmune disease
Lyme antibody	Lyme disease frequently presents with headache
HIV antibody and polymerase chain reaction	Upper respiratory symptoms at onset and daily generalized headache; test all patients with risk factors
Viral titers (IgM, IgG) for EBV, CMV, HHV6, parvovirus	Possible precipitants of NDPH

treatment. The lumbar puncture can rule out indolent infection and also determine CSF pressures. Given that patients may have a CSF leak without typical MRI changes or positional headache, an opening pressure, while helpful if low, does not rule the entity out, and further spine imaging may be necessary. Additionally, while TNFα levels may be elevated in the CSF, in NDPH, this level is not routinely checked as it does not change treatment or outcome and the original report has not been successfully replicated by other studies.

In most instances, laboratory and neuroimaging studies are normal. Elevated EBV titers have been identified, but the significance of this is unknown [46]. Li and Rozen investigated 49 patients who received either brain MRI or CT. Sixty-six percent had normal studies, while the remainder had nonspecific imaging findings felt not to be related to headache [8]. Data of CSF analysis in NDPH is sparse. Rozen et al. reported on CSF from adolescents with NDPH. A low and almost nonexistent CSF protein level was documented in four out of four of the adolescent patients with NDPH. Serum protein was normal in all patients. The cause of the low CSF protein level was unknown [8]. Additionally, clinical series of NDPH do not typically report the timing of CSF analysis with regard to headache onset or opening pressure measurements. In the Li and Rozen series, 41% of patients had CSF analysis at some point after headache onset. While no patients had elevated opening pressures, there was no mention of low opening pressures [8].

Treatment

Primary NDPH is felt to be the most treatment refractory of all headache disorders by many headache specialists. Treatment is rarely fully effective, and the goal, as in many primary headache disorders, is at least 50% reduction in headache days. Even with aggressive treatment, many patients do not improve. Patients may start to overuse medications (in up to 45% of NDPH patients) though correction of overuse does not seem to alter the course of NDPH as it can in chronic migraine [10].

Pharmacologic Treatment

Takase et al. published the largest uncontrolled series of 30 patients in Japan who met ICHD-2 criteria for NDPH. Patients were first administered a muscle relaxant (tizanidine or baclofen). If no effect was observed, tricyclic antidepressants (amitriptyline), selective serotonin reuptake inhibitors (SSRIs) (fluvoxamine or paroxetine), valproic acid, and beta-blockers were then administered. Twenty-seven percent of patients rated drug treatment as very effective, 3% rated as moderately effective, 20% rated as mildly effective, and 50% rated as ineffective [47]. The authors concluded that NDPH has a poor prognosis and is resistant to currently available treatment. In a retrospective study by Meineri et al., 18 NDPH patients were tried on amitriptyline, fluoxetine, and valproic acid. No drug was reported as effective [48].

At present, there is very limited peer-reviewed evidence for pharmacologic treatment of NDPH and no formal evidence-based guidelines. Most therapies that are reported to show benefit are presented in either abstracts or case reports. Thus, most headache specialists select therapy based on NDPH phenotype (migrainous or tension type). Muscle relaxants such as tizanidine and baclofen may be helpful [47]. Some patients may respond to triptans for headache escalations [8]. In children and adolescents, the most commonly used medications include the tricyclic antidepressants (amitriptyline) and antiepileptics (topiramate, gabapentin, valproic acid) [49]. A review of therapies that has been presented in the literature can be found below as well as in Table 7.2.

Antiepileptics

Rozen presented five patients in whom successful treatment was obtained with topiramate or gabapentin. In two cases, a topiramate dose of 75 mg twice a day was used. For gabapentin, there is no consistent dose recommended. One patient received 2700 mg/day and a second 1800 mg/day [50].

Antidepressants

There are case reports and small series of efficacy of venlafaxine (75 mg/day) and nortriptyline (100 mg/day) [51].

Tetracycline Derivatives

Rozen reported on the use of doxycycline (a TNFα inhibitor) 100 mg twice a day for 3 months in four patients with treatment-resistant NDPH and elevated CSF TNFα levels (>8.2 pg/ml). All patients had failed at least five preventative agents, three of four patients failed inpatient headache treatment, and another failed outpatient infusion therapy. Duration of NDPH ranged from 8 months to 3 years. An infection preceded the onset of daily headache in three of four patients. All patients had a positive response to doxycycline, and two patients became pain-free (those with the highest CSF TNFα levels). Average time to improvement on doxycycline was after 2 months of therapy; however, one patient responded within 2 weeks [52]. Given that time of onset to action is about 2 months, Rozen recommended a 3-month treatment trial for all patients.

Leukotriene Antagonists

The use of montelukast in NDPH is not actually documented in the literature. Rozen anecdotally found symptom improvement when montelukast 10 mg twice a day was used along with doxycycline [53].

Sodium Channel Blockers

Mexiletine (1050–1200 mg/day) showed some benefit in a report of three patients refractory to multiple preventative treatments. There was improvement in pain severity but limited reduction in headache frequency. All patients had side effects such as nausea, fatigue, tremor, and dizziness, which were dose dependent [54].

Corticosteroids

Prakash and Shah reported on nine patients with "postinfectious" NDPH. All patients were given high-dose intravenous methylprednisolone for

5 days, while six patients were given oral steroids for 2–3 weeks. All patients improved with seven patients getting almost complete pain relief within 2 weeks and two patients needing 6–8 weeks of treatment [55]. Of note, five out of the nine patients in this study did not technically meet the ICHD-3 criteria for NDPH at time of treatment as steroids were initiated several weeks after the headaches began (ICHD criteria necessitates 3 months of headache [2]). Thus, while high-dose steroids might be effective early in the course of presumed NDPH, those with established diagnoses of NDPH and more prolonged cases may not respond.

Prakash et al. subsequently studied 37 patients in India with a diagnosis of NDPH treated with a combination of intravenous methylprednisolone for 3–5 days (followed by oral therapy for 7–10 days), intravenous sodium valproate for 3–5 days (followed by oral valproate for 3–12 months), and an antidepressant for 2–12 months (amitriptyline or doxepin) with or without naprosyn for 1–3 weeks. Forty-six percent of patients showed an excellent response (no or less than one headache per month), 30% had a good response (>50% reduction in headache frequency or days per month), and 14% had a poor response. Those with shorter duration of headache had a better outcome [56]. It is unclear whether the positive response was due to the initial course of steroids or the medications that followed.

Dihydroergotamine
There has been limited data to support the use of intravenous dihydroergotamine (DHE). A retrospective review of CDH patients showed at least temporary improvement in some cases of NDPH [57]. A second retrospective review of IV DHE use in 31 NDPH patients with migrainous phenotype demonstrated medium-term headache benefit in two-thirds of patients [58]. Nagy et al. found that in 11 patients with NDPH, only those with migrainous symptoms responded to IV DHE and that response was less robust when compared to those patients with chronic migraine [59].

Interventional Procedures

Nerve Blocks
Given that some NDPH patients appear to have cervicogenic signs on examination, nerve blocks and/or facet blocks should be considered in selected patients. Robbins et al. reported on peripheral nerve block responses in patients with NDPH. 0.5% bupivacaine was used to block the greater and lesser occipital, auriculotemporal, supraorbital, and supratrochlear nerves. Fifty-four percent of patients had an acute response to nerve blockade; however this correlated to only 1 day of pain relief. No semipermanent procedures such as nerve ablation were tried [10]. Afridi et al. reported benefit of greater occipital nerve blocks in ten patients with NDPH. Of ten patients, four had complete but temporary response, and six had partial response. Sensitivity around the greater occipital nerve was associated with a response to injection [60].

Botulinum Toxin
There are three case reports of good to response to onabotulinumtoxinA (BTX). Spears documented a case of a 67-year-old man who had complete response to three rounds of 100 units of BTX [61]. Tsakadze and Wilson presented an abstract of three patients treated with 100 units of BTX every 3 months. All three patients had >75% relief and one patient had 100% relief [62]. Trucco and Ruiz reported on a 19-year-old patient treated with 195 units of BTX every 3 months for NDPH. The pain was partially relieved after the first cycle and subsided almost completely after the third cycle. While the pain became tolerable, the patient never became headache-free [63].

Other Agents
In a small series of four patients, clonazepam was found to be effective at dose of 0.5 mg nightly up to 1 mg twice a day with an extra 0.5–1 mg as needed for breakthrough pain [64]. A single case report suggests using nimodipine for NDPH with thunderclap onset [65]. There is a case report on the utility of mirtazapine for NDPH-associated chronic nausea at a dose of 15 mg nightly. Though there was complete remission in chronic nausea, no improvement in headache was seen (Table 7.3).

Table 7.3 Literature review of NDPH therapies

Medication	Dosage	Evidence
Oral therapy		
Topiramate	75 mg twice a day	Two case reports
Gabapentin	No consistent dose Consider 1800–1700 mg/day	Two case reports
Venlafaxine	75 mg/day	One case report
Nortriptyline	100 mg/day	One case report
Doxycycline	100 mg twice a day for 3 months	One abstract
Montelukast	10 mg twice a day, used concurrently with doxycycline	Anecdotal only, not actually documented in literature
Mexiletine	1050–1200 mg/day	One case report
Clonazepam	0.5 mg nightly up to 1 mg twice daily + 0.5–1 mg as needed for breakthrough pain	One case report
IV therapy		
Methylprednisolone	1 g IV for 5 days ± 60 mg prednisone daily for 2–3 weeks	One case report, not all patients met NDPH criteria
Dihydroergotamine	No standardized dose; authors suggest 5-day course	Three retrospective reviews
Interventional procedures		
0.5% bupivacaine block	No standard dose	Two case reports
onabotulinumtoxinA	100–195 units every 3 months	Three case reports

Emerging Therapies

Naltrexone

Joshi et al. proposed the potential of naltrexone as a therapeutic agent for NDPH. The use of naltrexone in fibromyalgia (FM) has been shown to be effective. Fibromyalgia is a chronic pain disorder due to chronic central sensitization of the nervous system. In a placebo crossover study, ten patients with FM were given low-dose naltrexone, 4.5 mg/day for 9 weeks. The patients showed a 30% reduction in pain scores compared with 23% reduction in the placebo group [60]. Another small trial of low-dose naltrexone in 27 FM patients showed an almost 50% reduction in pain scored compared to placebo [62].

Naratriptan

Naratriptan 2.5 mg twice daily has been proposed as treatment of refractory CDH. Rapoport et al. retrospectively reviewed 27 cases of patients with CDH (many of whom may have had NDPH [62]) who had received 2.5 mg naratriptan BID for more than 2 consecutive months. Sixty-five percent of 20 patients who took naratriptan for 6 months transformed to an episodic headache pattern. At 12-month follow-up, 55% continued

to have episodic headache [66]. These findings were further supported by a prospective pilot study with 30 intractable CDH patients treated with naratriptan 2.5 mg BID for 3 months. There was a reduction in mean headache frequency at 3 months from 27.1 to 19.0 days. Of the 22 patients who completed the protocol, 54% converted to an episodic headache pattern [67]. Gallagher and Mueller documented excellent response to daily naratriptan, especially a 1-year treatment, in intractable migraine patients [68]. These findings, though documented for the treatment of CDH (some cases might have been NDPH) may suggest naratriptan as a potentially useful agent for NDPH.

Prazosin

Prazosin is an alpha-adrenergic antagonist typically used to manage hypertension. It has been used by psychiatrists to treat anxiety, insomnia, and posttraumatic stress disorder. In a study by Ruff et al., treatment with prazosin resulted in long-term improvement of headache in 126 veterans with mild traumatic head injury caused by a blast injury [69]. Both peak headache pain and the number of headaches per month decreased. The authors speculated that prazosin, through alpha-adrenergic antagonism, may decrease sympathetically maintained pain, the postulated cause of chronification of posttraumatic headache. Thus, prazosin could also potentially be effective for the treatment of NDPH [62].

Diet and Lifestyle

Given similarities in phenotype with migraine, NDPH patients should be counseled about similar lifestyle adjustments that have been beneficial in decreasing migraine frequency including regular sleep, exercise, and meal schedules.

Treatment Approach

Rozen outlined a treatment approach based on symptom duration, triggering factors, and the available literature. He found that the success with intravenous therapy was highest in the 1 year following onset of NDPH and dropped off precipitously after that. Thus, he suggested treating early onset NDPH with intravenous therapy similar to that used in treating chronic migraine. Suggestions for treatment based on triggering factors can be seen in Table 7.4 [53]. In all subgroups, if outpatient therapy fails, it is recommended to consider use of daily mexiletine, according to that author.

Table 7.4 Treatment suggestions for NDPH based on triggering event

Postinfectious	If caught early: IV methylprednisolone up to 1 g/day for 2–3 days If believed to be post-viral with high serum viral titers: IV acyclovir for 3–5 days ± IV methylprednisolone ± IV doxycycline for several days then oral doxycycline If no elevated viral titers: tetracycline derivative (minocycline or doxycycline) 100 mg twice daily ± montelukast 10 mg for 3 months
Post-stressful life event	Tetracycline derivative ± montelukast for 3 months Evaluate for cervical hypermobility syndrome and cervical irritation on exam. If present, suggest physical therapy for neck-strengthening exercises and possibly anesthetic blockade
Postsurgical	Evaluate neck for upper cervical facet inflammation and greater occipital nerve irritation; consider nerve block Medications: Muscle relaxant + NSAID or tetracycline derivative ± montelukast or antiepileptic (topiramate or gabapentin)
Unknown trigger	Tetracycline derivative ± montelukast or antiepileptic (topiramate or gabapentin) If cervical issues consider nerve blockage and/or combination of muscle relaxant + NSAID

Prognosis

Vanast first described NDPH as a benign chronic daily headache that spontaneously regressed within 2 years without any treatment in 86% of 19 male patients and 73% of 26 female patients [1]. However, in headache specialty clinics, NDPH is not benign and is recognized as one of the most difficult headache syndromes to treat.

Robbins et al. proposed categorizing NDPH patients into three prognostic categories. Out of 71 patients, 76.1% had persisting form with continuous headache from onset, 15% had remitting form, and 8% had relapsing-remitting form. Over half of the patients with the persisting subform had daily headaches for longer than 2 years. Of those patients who remitted, 63.6% did so within 24 months. In the relapsing-remitting subgroup, all patients remitted for the first time within 24 months; however relapses inevitably occurred [10].

As previously stated, only two subforms of NDPH have been included in the ICHD-3: a self-limiting subform that typically resolves within several months without therapy and a refractory form that is resistant to aggressive treatment regimens [2]. The self-limiting form of NDPH has a good prognosis, as patients appear to improve without any intervention. In patients who have the refractory form of NDPH, their symptoms can go on for years to decades even with aggressive treatment. A 5-year study of 30 patients found a poor prognosis for recovery when patients had headache for a longer duration of time with a mean of 3.3 years and up to 27 years [47]. Children and adolescents seem to have more disability from NDPH. In a study of 28 children and adolescents, 20 out of 28 continued to have headache 6 months to 2 years later. Only 8 out of 28 were headache-free within 1–2 years [70].

Conclusion

New daily persistent headache is a unique form of primary chronic daily headache. NDPH is marked by headache that is continuous from onset with patients often being able to recall the exact date their headache started. The first step in managing a patient with suspected NDPH is to rule out secondary causes. Once a diagnosis of primary NDPH is made, we recommend initiating treatment based on (1) time course of symptom onset and (2) triggering event. Prognosis of NDPH is poor with most patients failing to improve despite aggressive medication therapy. Further research is needed given the increasing prevalence of NDPH and its refractory nature.

References

1. Vanast W. New daily-persistent headaches: definition of a benign syndrome. Headache. 1986;26:318.
2. Headache Classification Committee of the International Headache Society. The international classification of headache disorders, 3rd edition (beta version). Cephalalgia. 2013;33(9):629–808.
3. Castillo J, Munoz P, Guitera V, Pascual J. Kaplan Award 1998. Epidemiology of chronic daily headache in the general population. Headache. 1999;39(3):190–6.
4. Bigal ME, Sheftell FD, Rapoport AM, Lipton RB, Tepper SJ. Chronic daily headache in a tertiary care population: correlation between the International Headache Society diagnostic criteria and proposed revisions of criteria for chronic daily headache. Cephalalgia. 2002;22(6):432–8.
5. Grande RB, Aaseth K, Lundqvist C, Russell MB. Prevalence of new daily persistent headache in the general population. The Akershus study of chronic headache. Cephalalgia. 2009;29(11):1149–55.
6. Koenig MA, Gladstein J, McCarter RJ, Hershey AD, Wasiewski W. Pediatric Committee of the American Headache Society. Chronic daily headache in children and adolescents presenting to tertiary headache clinics. Headache. 2002;42(6):491–500.
7. Bigal ME, Lipton RB, Tepper SJ, Rapoport AM, Sheftell FD. Primary chronic daily headache and its subtypes in adolescents and adults. Neurology. 2004;63(5):843–7.
8. Li D, Rozen TD. The clinical characteristics of new daily persistent headache. Cephalalgia. 2002;22(1):66–9.
9. Evans RW. New daily persistent headache. Headache. 2012;52(Suppl 1):40–4.
10. Robbins MS, Grosberg BM, Napchan U, Crystal SC, Lipton RB. Clinical and prognostic subforms of new daily-persistent headache. Neurology. 2010;74(17):1358–64.
11. Rozen TD. New daily persistent headache: a lack of an association with white matter abnormalities on neuroimaging. Cephalalgia. 2016;36(10):987–92.
12. Siberstein SD, Lipton RB, Solomon S, Mathew NT. Classification of daily and near-daily headaches: proposed revisions to the IHS criteria. Headache. 1994;34(1):1–7.
13. Headache Classification Subcommittee of the International Headache Society. The international classification of headache disorders: 2nd edition. Cephalalgia. 2004;24(Suppl 1):9–160.
14. Kung E, Tepper SJ, Rapoport AM, Sheftell FD, Bigal ME. New daily persistent headache in the paediatric population. Cephalalgia. 2009;29(1):17–22.
15. Robbins MS, Evans RW. The heterogeneity of new daily persistent headache. Headache. 2012;52(10):1579–89.
16. Young WB. New daily persistent headache: controversy in the diagnostic criteria. Curr Pain Headache Rep. 2011;15(1):47–50.
17. Grengs LR, Mack KJ. New daily persistent headache is most likely to begin at the start of school. J Child Neurol. 2016;31(7):864–8.
18. Uniyal R, Paliwal VK, Tripathi A. Psychiatric comorbidity in new daily persistent headache: a cross-sectional study. Eur J Pain. 2017;21:1031.
19. Robbins MS. New daily-persistent headache and anxiety. Cephalalgia. 2011;31(7):875–6.
20. Goadsby PJ. New daily persistent headache: a syndrome, not a discrete disorder. Headache. 2011;51(4):650–3.
21. Rozen TD. Triggering events and new daily persistent headache: age and gender differences and insights on pathogenesis-a clinic-based study. Headache. 2016;56(1):164–73.
22. Rozen T, Swidan SZ. Elevation of CSF tumor necrosis factor alpha levels in new daily persistent headache and treatment refractory chronic migraine. Headache. 2007;47(7):1050–5.
23. Rozen TD. New daily persistent headache: an update. Curr Pain Headache Rep. 2014;18(7):431.

24. Durham PL. Calcitonin gene-related peptide (CGRP) and migraine. Headache. 2006;46(Suppl 1):S3–8.

25. Rozen T, Roth J, Denenberg N. Joint hypermobility as a predisposing factor for the development of new daily persistent headache. Headache. 2005;45:828–9.

26. Piovesan EJ, Kowacs PA, Oshinsky ML. Convergence of cervical and trigeminal sensory afferents. Curr Pain Headache Rep. 2003;7(5):377–83.

27. Bigal ME, Lipton RB. Clinical course in migraine: conceptualizing migraine transformation. Neurology. 2008;71(11):848–55.

28. Mack KJ. New daily persistent headache in children and adults. Curr Pain Headache Rep. 2009;13(1):47–51.

29. Southerland AM, Login IS. Rigorously defined hemicrania continua presenting bilaterally. Cephalalgia. 2011;31(14):1490–2.

30. Schievink WI. Spontaneous spinal cerebrospinal fluid leaks and intracranial hypotension. JAMA. 2006;295(19):2286–96.

31. Cumurciuc R, Crassard I, Sarov M, Valade D, Bousser MG. Headache as the only neurological sign of cerebral venous thrombosis: a series of 17 cases. J Neurol Neurosurg Psychiatry. 2005;76(8):1084–7.

32. Digre KB. Idiopathic intracranial hypertension headache. Curr Pain Headache Rep. 2002;6(3):217–25.

33. Almazov I, Brand N. Meningismus is a commonly overlooked finding in tension-type headache in children and adolescents. J Child Neurol. 2006;21(5):423–5.

34. Calabrese LH, Dodick DW, Schwedt TJ, Singhal AB. Narrative review: reversible cerebral vasoconstriction syndromes. Ann Intern Med. 2007;146(1):34–44.

35. Chen SP, Fuh JL, Wang SJ, Chang FC, Lirng JF, Fang YC, et al. Magnetic resonance angiography in reversible cerebral vasoconstriction syndromes. Ann Neurol. 2010;67(5):648–56.

36. Ducros A, Boukobza M, Porcher R, Sarov M, Valade D, Bousser MG. The clinical and radiological spectrum of reversible cerebral vasoconstriction syndrome. A prospective series of 67 patients. Brain. 2007;130(Pt 12):3091–101.

37. Hastriter E, Halker R, Vargas B, Dodick D. Headache prognosis in reversible cerebral vasoconstriction syndrome (RCVS) (abstract). Headache. 2011;51:49.

38. Silberstein SD. Headaches due to nasal and paranasal sinus disease. Neurol Clin. 2004;22(1):1–19, v.

39. Mokri B. Headaches in cervical artery dissections. Curr Pain Headache Rep. 2002;6(3):209–16.

40. Lee JL, Naguwa SM, Cheema GS, Gershwin ME. The geo-epidemiology of temporal (giant cell) arteritis. Clin Rev Allergy Immunol. 2008;35(1–2):88–95.

41. Salvarani C, Hunder GG. Giant cell arteritis with low erythrocyte sedimentation rate: frequency of occurrence in a population-based study. Arthritis Rheum. 2001;45(2):140–5.

42. Rozen TD. Intranasal contact point headache: missing the "point" on brain MRI. Neurology. 2009;72(12):1107.

43. Al-Araji A, Kidd DP. Neuro-Behcet's disease: epidemiology, clinical characteristics, and management. Lancet Neurol. 2009;8(2):192–204.

44. Evans RW, Seifert TD. The challenge of new daily persistent headache. Headache. 2011;51(1):145–54.

45. Nierenburg H, Newman LC. Update on new daily persistent headache. Curr Treat Options Neurol. 2016;18(6):25.

46. Hamada T, Ohshima K, Ide Y, Sakato S, Takamori M. A case of new daily persistent headache with elevated antibodies to Epstein-Barr virus. Jpn J Med. 1991;30(2):161–3.

47. Takase Y, Nakano M, Tatsumi C, Matsuyama T. Clinical features, effectiveness of drug-based treatment, and prognosis of new daily persistent headache (NDPH): 30 cases in Japan. Cephalalgia. 2004;24(11):955–9.

48. Meineri P, Torre E, Rota E, Grasso E. New daily persistent headache: clinical and serological characteristics in a retrospective study. Neurol Sci. 2004;25(Suppl 3):S281–2.

49. Baron EP, Rothner AD. New daily persistent headache in children and adolescents. Curr Neurol Neurosci Rep. 2010;10(2):127–32.

50. Rozen T. Successful treatment of new daily persistent headache with gabapentin and topiramate. Headache. 2002;42(4):389.

51. Evans RW, Rozen TD. Etiology and treatment of new daily persistent headache. Headache. 2001;41(8):830–2.

52. Rozen T. Doxycycline for treatment resistant new daily persistent headache. Neurology. 2008;70(Suppl 1):A348.

53. Rozen TD. New daily persistent headache: clinical perspective. Headache. 2011;51(4):641–9.

54. Marmura MJ, Passero FC Jr, Young WB. Mexiletine for refractory chronic daily headache: a report of nine cases. Headache. 2008;48(10):1506–10.

55. Prakash S, Shah ND. Post-infectious new daily persistent headache may respond to intravenous methylprednisolone. J Headache Pain. 2010;11(1):59–66.

56. Prakash S, Saini S, Rana KR, Mahato P. Refining clinical features and therapeutic options of new daily persistent headache: a retrospective study of 63 patients in India. J Headache Pain. 2012;13(6):477–85.

57. Silberstein SD, Silberstein JR. Chronic daily headache: long-term prognosis following inpatient treatment with repetitive IV DHE. Headache. 1992;32(9):439–45.

58. Eller M, Gelfand A, Riggins N, Goadsby P. An inpatient course of intravenous dihydroergotamine use for new daily persistent headache. Neurology. 2014;82(10 Suppl):P7.180.

59. Nagy AJ, Gandhi S, Bhola R, Goadsby PJ. Intravenous dihydroergotamine for inpatient management of refractory primary headaches. Neurology. 2011;77(20):1827–32.

60. Afridi SK, Shields KG, Bhola R, Goadsby PJ. Greater occipital nerve injection in primary headache syndromes--prolonged effects from a single injection. Pain. 2006;122(1–2):126–9.

61. Spears RC. Efficacy of botulinum toxin type A in new daily persistent headache. J Headache Pain. 2008;9(6):405–6.

62. Joshi SG, Mathew PG, Markley HG. New daily persistent headache and potential new therapeutic agents. Curr Neurol Neurosci Rep. 2014;14(2):425.

63. Trucco M, Ruiz L. P009. A case of new daily persistent headache treated with botulinum toxin type A. J Headache Pain. 2015;16(Suppl 1):A119.

64. Tarshish S, Robbins M, Napchan U, Buse D, Grosberg B. Prophylaxis of new daily persistent headache (NDPH): response to clonazepam in four patients [abstract]. Cephalalgia. 2009;29(Suppl. 1):49.

65. Rozen TD, Beams JL. New daily persistent headache with a thunderclap headache onset and complete response to nimodipine (a new distinct subtype of NDPH). J Headache Pain. 2013;14:100.

66. Rapoport AM, Bigal ME, Volcy M, Sheftell FD, Feleppa M, Tepper SJ. Naratriptan in the preventive treatment of refractory chronic migraine: a review of 27 cases. Headache. 2003;43(5):482–9.

67. Sheftell FD, Rapoport AM, Tepper SJ, Bigal ME. Naratriptan in the preventive treatment of refractory transformed migraine: a prospective pilot study. Headache. 2005;45(10):1400–6.

68. Gallagher RM, Mueller L. Managing intractable migraine with naratriptan. Headache. 2003;43(9):991–3.

69. Ruff RL, Ruff SS, Wang XF. Improving sleep: initial headache treatment in OIF/OEF veterans with blast-induced mild traumatic brain injury. J Rehabil Res Dev. 2009;46(9):1071–84.

70. Wintrich S, Rothner D. New daily persistent headaches-follow up and outcome in children and adolescents. Headache. 2010;50(Suppl. 1):s23.

Chronic Secondary Headaches

8

Robert Kaniecki

Overview and Clinical Assessment

Headache may result from intrinsic biological dysfunction of the nervous system or from activation of nociceptors from an identifiable organic process. These nociceptors may be found in intracranial structures or extracranial tissues of the head and neck. Intracranial pain may result from irritation of nociceptive neurons arising largely from the ophthalmic branch of the trigeminal nerve and terminating in the dura, meningeal or proximal cerebral arteries, dural sinuses, or periosteum. Additional innervation is seen from cranial nerves IX and X and the second cervical root. Extracranial tissues are innervated by all three branches of the trigeminal nerve; cranial nerves VII, IX, and X (largely the auricle); and the second and third cervical roots. The *International Classification of Headache Disorders* 3rd edition beta version (ICHD-3 beta) recognizes three headache subtypes: primary headaches, secondary headaches, and painful cranial neuralgias [1]. Primary headaches are organized by clinical criteria, while secondary headaches are categorized on the basis of contributory pathology. Suspicion for secondary headache should be heightened in the setting of clinical "red flags."

Secondary Headache Disorders
Post-traumatic headache
  Head injury
  Whiplash injury
  Headache attributed to cranial or cervical vascular disorder
  Ischemic stroke or transient ischemic attack
  Parenchymal or subarachnoid hemorrhage
  Unruptured vascular malformation or aneurysm
  Intracranial or extracranial arteritis
  Arterial dissection
  Venous or sinus thrombosis
  Headache attributed to nonvascular intracranial disorders
  Intracranial hypertension or hypotension
  Brain neoplasia
  Noninfectious inflammatory disorders (sarcoidosis)
  Chiari malformation
  Headache attributed to substance use or withdrawal
  Medication adverse event (nitrates)
  Alcohol
  Caffeine withdrawal
  Medication overuse headache
  Headache attributed to infection
  Intracranial infection (meningitis, encephalitis, brain abscess)

R. Kaniecki
Headache Division, Department of Neurology,
UPMC Headache Center, University of Pittsburgh
School of Medicine, Pittsburgh, PA, USA
e-mail: kanieckirg@upmc.edu

© Springer International Publishing AG, part of Springer Nature 2019
M. W. Green et al. (eds.), *Chronic Headache*, https://doi.org/10.1007/978-3-319-91491-6_8

Extracranial infection (systemic bacterial infection, viral syndrome)

Headache attributed to disorder of homeostasis

Hypertensive crisis, dialysis, hypoxia, hypercapnia, hypothyroidism

Headache attributed to disorder of the neck, eyes, ears, nose, sinuses, teeth, or mouth

Headache attributed to psychiatric disorder

Data from: Headache Classification Committee of the International Headache Society (IHS). The International Classification of Headache Disorders, 3rd edition (beta version). Cephalalgia. 2013;33:683.

Red Flags for Secondary Headache Disorders

First or worst severe headache

Abrupt or thunderclap-onset headache

Progressive or fundamental change in headache pattern

Abnormal physical examination findings

Neurologic symptoms lasting greater than 1 h

New headache in persons younger than 5 years or older than 50 years

New headache in patients with cancer, immunosuppression, or pregnancy

Headache associated with alteration in or loss of consciousness

Headache triggered by exertion, sexual activity, or Valsalva maneuvers

---

A detailed headache history outlining the temporal pattern of past and present headache occurrences is essential. Age of onset, attack frequency and duration, and associated features should be documented. Identification of the timing and circumstances of transition into a daily or near-daily headache pattern in those with chronic headache

is imperative. Recent changes in headache quantity or quality must always be explored. General physical and complete neurological examinations with detailed cranial nerve and fundoscopic evaluation are essential.

Diagnostic studies are typically necessary in the evaluation of patients with chronic headache. Brain imaging is the most valuable diagnostic study despite yielding abnormalities in only 1–3% of those with chronic headaches [2, 3]. Guidelines recommend head CT scan when headache is acute and severe and brain MRI when headaches are subacute or chronic [4]. Noninvasive and occasionally invasive vascular imaging modalities are required in the setting of potential vascular etiologies. Lumbar puncture with opening pressure assessment may be helpful in the workup of intracranial pressure disorders and suspected meningitis. Serum chemistries, erythrocyte sedimentation rate and C-reactive protein, and thyroid function studies are sometimes helpful. Tissue biopsy (brain mass lesion, temporal artery) may be required in select circumstances. Electroencephalography has no role in the assessment of headache disorders unless suspicion for seizure activity is also present.

Secondary Chronic Headache Disorders

Headache Attributed to Trauma or Injury to the Head and/or Neck

Trauma to the head and neck frequently results in acute headache and sometimes chronic headache. ICHD classification applies the term "acute" to those subjects reporting headache within the first 3 months following the injury and "persistent" to those extending beyond that time point. Criteria require development of headache within 7 days of one of the following: trauma, regaining consciousness following the injury, or discontinuation of medications that might impair headache recognition. Diagnostic subcategories include headaches from head trauma, whiplash injuries, and craniotomy procedures [1].

Headaches Following Head Injury

Traumatic brain injury (TBI) may result from nervous system exposure to either blunt or penetrating trauma. Fractures of the skull or facial bones and intracranial hemorrhages are potential complications. Most patients with serious intracranial structural lesions, such as epidural or parenchymal hemorrhages, will present acutely. Subdural hematomas (SDH) may present either acutely or with more chronic complaints [5]. The elderly, those with a history of alcohol abuse, and those receiving anticoagulation may be at particular risk. SDH may occur in the setting of relatively insignificant trauma and are occasionally spontaneous. The interval between trauma and symptom development may extend from hours to weeks. Headaches are typically global, progressive, and with variable intensity. Other common symptoms include somnolence, confusion, dizziness, hemiparesis, and seizure. Diagnosis is typically made following brain MRI. Blood under venous pressure accumulates between the dura and meninges, resulting in a crescent-shaped extracerebral imaging abnormality. Small subdural hematomas are often followed conservatively. Indications for surgical drainage include hematoma thickness greater than 10 mm, a midline shift greater than 5 mm, and significant neurological compromise [6].

The terms concussion and mild TBI are often used interchangeably. Approximately 75% of TBI is classified as mild. The most common causes of mild TBI in the civilian population are motor vehicle or recreational accidents, falls, competitive athletics, occupational hazards, and assaults [7]. The incidence in the US military population has increased dramatically in the past two decades, primarily through blast exposure during conflicts in the Middle East [8].

Post-traumatic headache (PTH) is the most common symptom after mild TBI, and it is often the most lasting and most disabling complaint. There is no direct correlation between the degree of trauma and either the duration or severity of the subsequent headache condition [9]. The pathophysiology of PTH likely involves multiple mechanisms including neuroinflammation, disruption of blood-brain barrier, and release of migraine-associated neuropeptides such as calcitonin gene-related peptide (CGRP) and pituitary adenylate cyclase-activating polypeptide (PACAP) [10]. Headache is reported by over 90% of athletes after sports-related concussion, with the majority improving within several days to several weeks [11]. From 8 to 35% may experience persistent headaches at 1 year and perhaps 25% at 4 years [12]. Nearly 80% of those with combat-related TBI will report episodic headache and 20% chronic daily headache following return from military theater [13]. Risk factors for the development of PTH include preexisting headaches, family history of headache disorder, female sex, and, in the military population, the presence of post-traumatic stress disorder [14]. Age under 60 was recently shown to be an additional risk factor [15]. The presence of a continuous headache appears to be associated with negative occupational outcomes in the military population [16].

Additional complaints of those with post-concussion syndrome include cognitive impairment, fatigue, dizziness, blurred vision, and disturbances of sleep or mood. Management of the assorted symptoms of the post-concussion syndrome is largely rehabilitative and symptomatic and extends beyond PTH. Visual therapy may help address convergence insufficiency, which commonly provokes or aggravates headaches. Vestibular-balance therapy is also a valuable ally in the management of dizziness following TBI. Specific therapies for insomnia or depression may be necessary. Cognitive impairment may require specific attention, and it often affects therapeutic choices aimed at other post-concussion complaints. Nonpharmacological steps such as regulation of sleep, nutrition, and hydration, combined with a graduated exercise program, are essential in recovery [17]. There are no large-scale studies on the management of headaches following TBI [18]. The majority of patients rely on nonprescription analgesics, but many presenting to clinical attention will require prescription medication [19]. Pharmacologic management is typically tailored to the phenotype of the headache disorder. The most common headache subtype appears to possess migraine characteristics, but many possess traits similar to tension-type headaches and trigeminal autonomic cephalalgias (TACs) or are unclassifiable [20]. Acetaminophen, aspirin, NSAIDs, and triptans are effective acute therapies for severe breakthrough headaches, while opioids and butalbital products should be avoided. Certain β-blockers, antidepressants (tricyclic antidepressants and venlafaxine), and antiepileptic drugs (sodium valproate and topiramate) may be useful for headache prevention in those with persistent post-traumatic migraines. Only topiramate and onabotulinumtoxin A have substantial data in the setting of chronic migraine. Those with chronic tension-type or TAC phenotypes should be managed like their primary headache counterparts.

Headaches Following Neck Injury

Whiplash is defined as a sudden acceleration/deceleration movement of the head, typically with extension and then flexion of the cervical spine. This may involve either high- or low-impact forces. Similar to TBI, whiplash injuries are most commonly classified as mild to moderate, and no correlation is apparent between the degree of injury and the extent of post-traumatic symptomatology. Persistent headache attributed to whiplash is defined by ICHD-3 beta criteria requiring development of headache within 7 days of the injury and persistence of discomfort for >3 months [1]. Neck and shoulder pain are common. Many report features of the post-concussion syndrome such as dizziness, fatigue, and disturbances of sleep or mood. Exam may be normal or reveal tightness or spasm of the paraspinal cervical muscles [21]. Imaging is typically only indicated in the presence of signs of cervical radiculopathy or myelopathy. Cervical MRI may be normal or reveal loss of cervical lordosis or occasionally a disc bulge or herniation. Management is typically symptomatic and usually involves a combination of NSAID analgesics, muscle relaxants, and physiotherapy.

Occipital nerve blocks or cervical trigger point injections may be helpful and are usually well-tolerated. No specific guidelines for management are available, with controlled clinical trials failing to show benefit of any active treatment over conservative care [22]. Recovery is seen in the majority of patients over several weeks to months, with only 12% reporting persistent symptoms at 6 months. Risk factors for a more prolonged course include advanced age, female sex, pain or numbness in the upper extremities, severe headaches, or prior history of concussion or mental health disorder [23]. Ongoing legal issues may contribute to delayed recovery in some cases.

Headaches Following Craniotomy

Persistent headache attributed to craniotomy is defined as >3 months of headache discomfort following a craniotomy performed for non-traumatic reasons. Like other forms of post-traumatic headache, ICHD-3 beta criteria require the headache develop within 7 days of the procedure or either the restoration of consciousness or elimination of pain-modifying medication [1]. At least 50% of patients experience acute headache, while 25–30% appear to develop the persistent form [24]. Larger craniotomies and those performed in the posterior fossa appear more likely to result in persistent headaches [25]. Pathophysiology of persistent post-craniotomy headache may involve a number of mechanisms including pericranial nerve injury or neuroma development, scar tissue adhering muscular tissue to dura mater, or central sensitization [26]. Although postoperative headaches often exhibit features of migraine, the most frequent phenotypical description of persistent post-craniotomy headache is a tension-type pattern [27]. Local tenderness or allodynia at the scar site tends to persist for up to 1 year [28]. In the absence of empiric data, most use the headache characteristics as a guide to preventive and symptomatic medications. Pericranial nerve blocks may also be of some utility.

Headache Attributed to Cranial or Cervical Vascular Disorder

Ischemic or Hemorrhagic Stroke

Headaches of cerebrovascular origin will most often present acutely. Headache may be a transient symptom of ischemic or hemorrhagic stroke, while some may continue to experience chronic headaches [29]. Studies indicate 10–23% will continue report headaches at 2 years [30]. One report at 3 years of follow-up documented new headaches following prior stroke persisting in over 7%, with the majority displaying tension-type features. Approximately 20% described chronic headaches occurring 15 or more days per month [31]. A minority present with a constant, unrelenting headache that is refractory to treatment and may continue for months or years. Management of poststroke headache is symptomatic and based on phenotype. Triptans are contraindicated in the presence of known ischemic cerebrovascular disease.

Cerebral Venous Thrombosis

Thrombosis of the cerebral veins or sinuses may present acutely or with a pattern of chronic head discomfort. Headache is the most common symptom, seen in 80–90%, and is the most common presenting symptom. The pain is frequently unrelenting from onset and exhibits mixed tension-type and migraine features. The majority of cases are associated with papilledema or focal neurological findings. The triad of findings of increased intracranial pressure, focal neurological deficits, and encephalopathy is characteristic, at least early in the course [32]. Focal symptoms and signs are highly variable and dependent on the location of thrombosis. Seizures occur in up to 40% [33]. Those with isolated headache often go undetected. Suspicion should be raised in the presence of certain prothrombotic conditions such as the use of oral contraceptives, pregnancy, or malignancy. Imaging with brain MRI and MRV is more sensitive than head CT [34]. Catheter-based angiography is the gold standard, but due to the risks of this invasive procedure, it is reserved for cases where MRI and MRV are inconclusive [35]. Management steps include symptomatic care and heparin in the acute setting, followed by oral anticoagulation for 3–6 months. Those with identified hereditary hypercoagulable states receive long-term anticoagulation [36]. Management of headache is generally symptomatic.

Cerebral Aneurysm

The most well-known headache associated with cerebral aneurysm is the severe thunderclap attack associated with leak or rupture. Chronic headaches may persist following subarachnoid hemorrhage, may follow interventional procedures for aneurysm, or may be associated with unruptured cerebral aneurysms [37]. Cerebral aneurysms are present in 0.4–3.6% of the population. Headache has been reported in up to 20% but is not well defined. In one trial 68% of patients experienced headache frequency reduction, while 9% of patients had new or worsened headaches following aneurysm treatment [38].

Vascular Malformation

Vascular malformations of the brain or dura may be linked with recurrent headaches. Developmental venous anomalies (DVAs), also known as venous angiomas, account for 60% of cerebral vascular malformations. DVAs are best visualized on contrast-enhanced T1-weighted brain MRI scans. Acute or chronic headache may result from a complication of DVA such as ischemic infarction or hemorrhage. Annual risk of hemorrhage is approximately 0.2% and most are followed conservatively. Any link between chronic headaches and uncomplicated DVA is uncertain [39]. Arteriovenous malformations (AVMs) may present with headaches in approximately 15% of cases. Headache may be persistent but is often episodic. Atypical presentations of migraine and cluster have been reported. Side-locked headache with contralateral neurological symptoms is common in symptomatic cases [40]. Diagnosis may be made by head CT angiography or brain MR angiography, but digital subtraction angiography remains the gold standard imaging technique. Risk of hemorrhage is 2–4% in those with unruptured and 4.5% ruptured AVMs. Older patients, those with asymptomatic or unruptured AVMs, and those with low risk of rupture (absence of deep location/drainage or associated aneurysm) are treated conservatively [41]. Observation is also recommended for very large lesions or those located in surgically challenging areas. Headache management typically follows migraine protocols. Cavernous malformations or angiomas are present in 0.5% of the population and may be associated with headache in up to 40% of cases. Most may mimic but will not meet diagnostic criteria for any specific primary headache disorder [42]. Many only become symptomatic at the time of hemorrhage. Conservative management may be superior to surgical excision or radiosurgical procedures in most settings [43]. Headache treatment is symptomatic. Dural or pial arteriovenous fistulas may also mimic any of the primary headache disorders. Risk of hemorrhage varies widely with the type of venous drainage pattern [44].

Cervicocephalic Artery Dissection

Dissections of the intracranial and extracranial cervicocephalic arteries commonly present with acute head or neck pain. Onset may be thunderclap. Focal neurological findings such as cranial nerve abnormalities or Horner syndrome are often noted. These are seen in younger individuals and sometimes are a consequence of trauma. A variety of headache phenotypes have been described, including migraine and trigeminal autonomic cephalalgia [45]. Diagnosis may be confirmed by MRA, CTA, or catheter-based angiography. Most are treated with aspirin. Evidence suggests some patients may develop long-term headaches, which are treated symptomatically [46].

Giant Cell Arteritis

Headache is the most common presenting symptom of giant cell arteritis (GCA). Incidence is nearly always after age 50 and peaks between 70 and 80 years of age. American College of Rheumatology criteria require fulfillment of three of the following five clinical attributes for diagnosis: a new headache, onset age 50 or older, elevated erythrocyte sedimentation rate (ESR) of >50 mm per hour, a clinical temporal artery abnormality,

and an abnormal temporal artery biopsy [47]. Headache is classically subacute in onset, temporal in location, with focal scalp tenderness, but is highly variable [48]. Persistent pain is more common than episodic, and pain may extend from mild to severe. Jaw claudication, pain in the muscles of mastication after a period of chewing, is nearly pathognomonic but present in only 25% of cases. Polymyalgia rheumatica is seen in nearly 50%, and other symptoms such as fatigue, malaise, fevers, anorexia, and weight loss are not uncommon. Cranial nerve palsies and stroke are additional potential complications. Visual loss from anterior ischemic optic neuropathy is the most common serious outcome and is typically permanent. It may occur in up to 20% of patients [49]. ESR is elevated in 95% of biopsy-proven GCA cases, with a mean value of 85 millimeters per hour. Diagnosis may require bilateral temporal artery biopsies of at least 2 cm in length. Prednisone at a daily dose of 1 mg/kg is the initial treatment of choice, and corticosteroids may be necessary for a period of 6–24 months. Headaches typically respond rapidly and completely. Guidelines also recommend addition of low-dose aspirin in the absence of contraindications. Those presenting with visual compromise or neurologic findings are best managed initially with intravenous methylprednisolone [50]. Introduction of alternate immunosuppressive agents such as methotrexate should be considered in patients with resistant disease or steroid-related complications. Both clinical and laboratory values are helpful in assessing improvement or relapse [51].

Nonvascular Intracranial Disorders

Intracranial Hypertension

Idiopathic intracranial hypertension (IIH), previously pseudotumor cerebri, involves CSF pressure elevation in the absence of an identifiable structural cause such as an intracranial mass lesion or hydrocephalus. Potential pathophysiologic mechanisms include excess CSF production, reduced CSF absorption, increased brain water content, and increased back pressure in the cerebral venous sinus drainage system [52]. Approximately 90%

of subjects are female, 90% of childbearing age, and 90% with elevations in body mass index. The main risk factor appears to be obesity [53]. Headache is present in the vast majority at time of diagnosis. It presents heterogeneously but tends to be daily and constant with fluctuations in pain intensity. Headache may be aggravated by Valsalva maneuvers. Migrainous features are not uncommon, while autonomic symptoms are rare. Blurring or episodic darkening of vision (visual obscurations), diplopia, pulsatile tinnitus, and neck pain are other frequent complaints. The hallmark finding of increased intracranial pressure, papilledema, is nearly universal [54]. Other potential causes of increased ICP must be considered in the history and examination.

> **Possible Causes of Increased Intracranial Pressure**
> **Intracranial mass lesion**
>   Neoplasm, abscess, hemorrhage
>   **Intracranial venous or sinus pressure elevation**
>   Venous or sinus thrombosis
>   Sinus stenosis
>   Dural fistula
>   Extracranial   obstruction—jugular vein occlusion, pulmonary hypertension, right heart failure
>   **Cerebrospinal fluid pressure elevation**
>   Hydrocephalus
>   CSF shunt obstruction
>   Meningeal   inflammation—malignant, infectious, autoimmune, granulomatous
>   Colloid cyst of 3rd ventricle
>   **Other causes**
>   Idiopathic intracranial hypertension
>   Hypervitaminosis A
>   Drug effect—tetracycline or similar antibiotics, isotretinoin
>   Uremia
>   Other—obstructive sleep apnea, carbon monoxide poisoning, hypoparathyroidism, Addison disease

Diagnostic evaluation should include brain MRI with magnetic resonance venography and lumbar puncture. Imaging may be normal or reveal distention of optic nerve sheaths, flattening of the posterior globe, empty sella, or transverse sinus stenosis [55]. Elevated CSF opening pressure (>250 mm H_2O in adults) in the absence of intracranial lesions confirms the diagnosis [1]. Visual perimetry is essential initially and is the most valuable test in the course of disease management. Enlargement of the blind spot and loss of peripheral fields are noted in 75–80% at diagnosis [56]. The focus of treatment is preservation of vision, with headache reduction a secondary goal. Lumbar puncture acutely reduces intracranial pressure. It is immediately and usually transiently helpful and at times may need to be repeated. Acetazolamide has been shown to improve visual field function and is the drug of choice [57]. Many now prescribe topiramate for the added benefit of weight loss. Weight reduction is an essential management step in those with elevated BMI. A program involving diet and exercise should be instituted and bariatric surgery considered when those steps have failed. Optic nerve fenestration or shunt procedures (ventriculoperitoneal or lumboperitoneal) may be required in refractory cases [58]. Any role of cerebral venous sinus stenting remains controversial.

Intracranial Hypotension

Headache from intracranial hypotension is most commonly seen in the setting of recent lumbar puncture. Risk factors for post-dural puncture headache include age under 60 years, female sex, low BMI, history of prior low-pressure headache, and use of a large-diameter traumatic needle [59]. Although 90% of patients develop headache within 72 h of the procedure, some may develop low-pressure headaches several weeks later. The headache may be generalized or focal and develops within 15 min upon assuming an upright posture. It may be worsened by physical activity or Valsalva maneuvers. Resolution of discomfort is typically within minutes of returning to the supine position. Neck pain or stiffness, nausea, vertigo, muffled hearing, and tinnitus are other common complaints. Neurological examination may show a 6th nerve palsy but is typically normal. Contrast-enhanced brain MRI may show diffuse non-nodular pachymeningeal enhancement and occasionally cerebellar tonsillar descent or subdural fluid collections. Spontaneous recovery is common, but 15% will still be symptomatic at 6 weeks. Bedrest and hydration are the first steps in management. Both caffeine and theophylline have data in headache reduction [60]. The use of an epidural blood patch is often curative in patients with symptoms persisting beyond the first several days [61]. Surgical intervention is rarely necessary.

Intracranial hypotension may also occur in the settings of mild or no trauma. Spontaneous intracranial hypotension (SIH) may present with the same clinical features and brain imaging findings seen with post-dural puncture headache [62]. Some with a prolonged course may develop non-orthostatic or reverse-orthostatic headache. Predisposing conditions for SIH include Marfan or Ehlers-Danlos syndromes, joint hypermobility, and neurofibromatosis. Microtrauma from osteophytes or disc herniations may be responsible in some cases of ventral dural leaks [63]. Identification of the presence and site of CSF leak in cases of SIH can be challenging. Normal CSF pressure may actually be noted on rare occasions [64]. CT myelography of the entire spine has been considered the gold standard technique, but spinal MRI is less invasive and may identify many patients with CSF leaks [65]. Radioisotope cisternography may be useful in patients with suspected CSF leaks without MRI or CT abnormalities [66]. Conservative and medical management is similar to that with post-dural puncture headache. Single or serial epidural blood patch procedures are associated with resolution of symptoms in 90% of cases. Blood patch "targeting" the defined site of CSF leak is more effective than empiric "blind" lumbar procedures [67]. Efficacy is approximately 90%, while rate of recurrence is approximately 10%. Additional invasive procedures such as direct surgical repair may be required in refractory cases.

Brain Tumor

Headache from intracranial neoplasm is highly variable. It may arise from mass effect or parenchymal hemorrhage in those with solid tumors or from disruption of cerebrospinal fluid flow in those with malignant meningitis. Brain tumors may aggravate an underlying primary headache condition or provoke a new headache profile. Only 2% will experience isolated headache on presentation. Approximately 20% of patients will present and 60% eventually develop headache linked to the malignancy [68]. Those with prior headache history and those with evidence of increased intracranial pressure, supratentorial mass location, and large tumor size are all associated with greater likelihood of headache development [69]. Patients at extremes of age appear to be less likely to develop headache. Symptoms typically arise from increased intracranial pressure from the mass lesion, associated edema, or obstructive hydrocephalus. The textbook presentation of headache worse in the morning with associated vomiting is present in approximately 10% of cases [70]. Instead the majority will describe headaches phenotypically similar to tension-type headache, while others may report migraine-like events [71]. Treatment strategies are aimed at tumor management and symptom control.

Chiari Malformation

Chiari I malformations involve downward displacement of the cerebellar tonsils through the foramen magnum. The majority are diagnosed following brain or cervical spine MRI. Present criteria require cerebellar tonsillar descent of >5 mm (below the line connecting the internal occipital protuberance to the basion) or descent of >3 mm with crowding of the subarachnoid space at the craniocervical junction [72]. Syringomyelia of the cervical cord may be seen in up to 40% of cases. Population prevalence of Chiari I malformation is nearly 1%, the majority apparently asymptomatic. It is congenital but may be acquired, with cerebellar tonsillar descent also seen in the setting of intracranial hypotension. Women are more often affected than men, and time of presentation seemingly extends from early childhood to mid-adulthood. Headache may be the sole symptom, part of a complicated symptom complex, or absent. In children it is the most common symptom [73]. An occipital or suboccipital location is most common [74]. By definition headache has at least one of the following three characteristics: triggered by cough or other Valsalva-like maneuver, occipital or suboccipital location, and duration <5 min [1]. Dizziness, ataxia, changes in hearing, and diplopia or transient visual phenomena are not unusual. Conversion from an asymptomatic to a symptomatic state has been reported to occur following minor head or neck trauma [75]. Neurological examinations are typically normal but may show brainstem or cerebellar findings. Cervical spine abnormalities may be seen when the Chiari is complicated by a syrinx or when there is cord compression from the tonsillar ectopia. There appears to be some correlation between obstructed CSF and occipital headaches, but the precise role of cine MRI CSF flow study is unclear [76]. Surgery should be reserved for those patients exhibiting abnormalities on physical exam or for those with refractory headaches meeting the previously outlined diagnostic criteria.

Substances

Headache may be associated with the use of multiple substances or their withdrawal. In most cases the headaches are acute and transient. Chronic headaches are less common but may arise with continued exposure to certain medications or substances administered on a regular basis. Food additives or preservatives, nitrates, phosphodiesterase inhibitors, alcohol, antidepressants, neurostimulants, endogenous hormones, and excessive caffeine are the agents most commonly indicted. A high index of suspicion is required. Treatment involves discontinuation of the offending agent when possible. Headaches linked to overtreatment with acute medication, now termed "medication overuse" headache (previously "rebound" headache), are covered separately.

Intracranial Infection

Headache may be a symptom of intracranial or systemic infection. Meningitis, encephalitis, and focal abscess or empyema are potential intracranial causes. In most settings these headaches are acute or subacute in onset and the history brief. Intracranial infection is a rare cause of chronic headache. Chronic meningitis is arbitrarily defined as meningitis lasting more than 4 weeks. It may have infectious and noninfectious causes, and the treatment depends upon the etiology. Headache management is otherwise symptomatic.

Possible Causes of Chronic Infectious Meningitis
Mycobacterium
Mycobacterium tuberculosis
Spirochete
Borrelia burgdorferi
Treponema pallidum
Leptospira
Bacteria
Listeria
Brucella
Actinomyces
Francisella tularensis
Other: *Erlichia*, *Nocardia*, Whipple disease
Virus
Human immunodeficiency virus
Cytomegalovirus
Epstein-Barr virus
Other: *Enterovirus*, Herpes simplex, Varicella zoster, HTLV I and II
Fungus
Cryptococcus
Histoplasma
Blastomyces
Other: *Sporothrix*, *Coccidioides*
Parasite
Toxoplasma
Schistosoma
Other: *Taenia solium* (cysticercosis), *Acanthamoeba*, *Angiostrongylus*

Miscellaneous

Disorders of homeostasis may occasionally provoke chronic headaches. Hypothyroidism and sleep apnea are two of the more common etiologies to consider [77]. Headaches respond to treatment of the underlying disorder. Structural disease of specific extracerebral structures may result in chronic head, neck, or face pain. Headache may be a symptom of conditions primarily affecting the eye, ear, or paranasal sinuses, bit it rarely is seen in isolation. In such settings referral to an ophthalmologist or otolaryngologist is indicated [78]. Cervicogenic headache arises from irritation of upper cervical nerve roots caused by bone, disc, or soft tissue pathology. Pain is frequently side-locked, worsened by neck motion, and associated with cervical abnormalities on examination or imaging. NSAIDs and muscle relaxants are often helpful acutely. Physical therapy or manipulation, preventive medications such as amitriptyline or gabapentin, and procedures such as occipital nerve or cervical facet blocks may be helpful in chronic cases [79]. Dysfunction of the temporomandibular joint may cause unilateral or bilateral pain that is typically temporal and aggravated by chewing. The appearance is similar to tension-type headache, and the pain often responds to local ice, NSAIDs, and a soft diet [80]. Referral to a dentist or maxillofacial specialist may be required in refractory cases. Chronic headache may also be reported by patients with mood, anxiety, or personality disorders. Given comorbidity associations with migraine and tension-type headache, these patients should receive management for the primary headache phenotype as well as psychiatric assessment and treatment [81].

References

1. Headache Classification Subcommittee of the International Headache Society. The international classification of headache disorders: 2nd edition. Cephalalgia. 2013;33:629–808.
2. Clarke CE, Edwards J, Nicholl DJ, Sivaguru A. Imaging results in a consecutive series of 530 new patients in the Birmingham headache service. J Neurol. 2010;257:1274–8.
3. Sempere AP, Porta-Etessam J, Medrano V, et al. Neuroimaging in the evaluation of patients with non-acute headache. Cephalalgia. 2005;25:30–5.
4. Loder E, Weizenbaum E, Frishberg B, Silberstein S, American Headache Society Choosing Wisely Task Force. Choosing wisely in headache medicine: the American headache Society's list of five things physicians and patients should question. Headache. 2013;53:1651–9.
5. Almenawer S, Farrokhyar F, Hong C, et al. Chronic subdural hematoma management: a systematic review and meta-analysis of 34,829 patients. Ann Surg. 2014;259:449–57.
6. Ducruet AF, Grobelny BT, Zacharia BE, et al. The surgical management of chronic subdural hematoma. Neurosurg Rev. 2012;35:155–69.
7. D'Onofrio F, Russo A, Conte F, et al. Post-traumatic headaches: an epidemiological overview. Neurol Sci. 2014;35(Suppl 1):203–6.
8. Theeler BJ, Flynn FG, Erickson JC. Headaches after concussion in US soldiers returning from Iraq or Afghanistan. Headache. 2010;50:1262–72.
9. Lucas S, Hoffman JM, Bell KR, et al. Characterization of headache after traumatic brain injury. Cephalalgia. 2012;32:600–6.
10. Moye LS, Pradhan AA. From blast to bench: a translational mini-review of post-traumatic headache. J Neurosci Res. 2017;95:1347–54.
11. Meehan WP, d'Hemecourt P, Comstock RD. High school concussion in the 2008–2009 academic year: mechanism, symptoms, and management. Am J Sports Med. 2010;38:2405–9.
12. Seifert TD, Evans RW. Posttraumatic headache: a review. Curr Pain Headache Rep. 2010;14:292–8.
13. Theeler B, Lucas S, Riechers R, Ruff R. Post-traumatic headaches in civilians and military personnel: a comparative, clinical review. Headache. 2013;53:881–900.
14. Walker WC, Marwitz JH, Wilk AR, et al. Prediction of headache severity (density and functional impact) after traumatic brain injury: a longitudinal multicenter study. Cephalalgia. 2013;33:998–1008.
15. Lucas S, Hoffman JM, Bell KR, Dikmen S. A prospective study of prevalence and characterization of headache following mild traumatic brain injury. Cephalalgia. 2014;34:93–102.
16. Finkel AG, Ivins BJ, Yerry JA, et al. What matters more? A retrospective cohort of headache characteristics and diagnosis type in soldiers with mTBI/concussion. Headache. 2017;57:719–28.
17. Seifert T. Post-traumatic headache therapy in the athlete. Curr Pain Headache Rep. 2016;20:41.
18. Monteith TS, Borsook D. Insights and advances in post-traumatic headache: research considerations. Curr Neurol Neurosci Rep. 2014;14:428.
19. Meehan WP. Medical therapies for concussion. Clin Sports Med. 2011;30:115–24.
20. Finkel AG, Yerry JA, Klaric JS, et al. Headache in military service members with a history of mild traumatic brain injury: a cohort study of diagnosis and classification. Cephalalgia. 2017;37:548–59.
21. Ferrari R. Whiplash–a review of a commonly misunderstood injury. Am J Med. 2002;112:162–3.
22. Michaleff Z, Maher C, Lin C, et al. Comprehensive physiotherapy exercise programme or advice for chronic whiplash (PROMISE): a pragmatic randomised controlled clinical trial. Lancet. 2014;384:133–41.
23. Suissa S. Risk factors of poor prognosis after whiplash injury. Pain Res Manag. 2003;8:69–75.
24. Magelhaes JE, Azevedo-Filho HR, Rocha-Filho PAS. The risk of headache attributed to surgical treatment of intracranial aneurysms: a cohort study. Headache. 2013;53:1613–23.
25. Thibault M, Girard F, Moumdjian R, et al. Craniotomy site influences postoperative pain following sur-

gical procedures: a retrospective study. Can J Anaesth. 2007;54:544–8.

26. Rocha-Filho PA. Post-craniotomy headache: a clinical view with a focus on the persistent form. Headache. 2015;55:733–8.

27. Schankin CJ, Gall C, Straube A. Headache syndromes after acoustic neuroma surgery and their implications for quality of life. Cephalalgia. 2009;29:760–71.

28. Mosek AC, Dodick DW, Ebersold MJ, Swanson JW. Headache after resection of acoustic neuroma. Headache. 1999;39:89–94.

29. Tentschert S, Wimmer R, Greisenegger S. Headache at stroke onset in 2196 patients with ischemic stroke or transient ischemic attack. Stroke. 2005;36:e1–3.

30. Naess H, Lunde L, Brogger J. Post-stroke pain on long-term follow-up: the Bergen stroke study. J Neurol. 2010;257:1446–52.

31. Hansen A, Marcusen N, Klit H, et al. Development of persistent headache following stroke: a 3-year follow-up. Cephalalgia. 2015;35:399–409.

32. Agrawal K, Burger K, Rothrock J. Cerebral sinus thrombosis. Headache. 2016;56:1380–9.

33. Ameri A, Bousser MG. Cerebral venous thrombosis. Neurol Clin. 1992;10:87–111.

34. Saposnik G, Barinagarrementeria F, Brown RD, et al. Diagnosis and management of cerebral venous thrombosis: a statement for healthcare professionals from the American Heart Association/American Stroke Association. Stroke. 2011;42:1158–92.

35. Leach J, Fortuna R, Jones B, et al. Imaging of cerebral venous thrombosis: current techniques, spectrum of findings, and diagnostic pitfalls. Radiographics. 2006;26:519–41.

36. Martinelli I, Bucciarelli P, Passamonti SM, et al. Long-term evaluation of the risk of recurrence after cerebral sinus-venous thrombosis. Circulation. 2010;121:2740–6.

37. Wardlaw JM, White PM. The detection and management of unruptured intracranial aneurysms. Brain. 2000;123:205–21.

38. Schwedt T, Gereau R, Frey K, Kharash E. Headache outcomes following treatment of unruptured intracranial aneurysms: a prospective analysis. Cephalalgia. 2011;31:1082–9.

39. Naff NJ, Wemmer J, Hoenig-Rigamonti K, Rigamonti DR. A longitudinal study of patients with venous malformations: documentation of a negligible hemorrhage risk and benign natural history. Neurology. 1998;50:1709–14.

40. Asif K, Leschke J, Lazzaro MA. Cerebral arteriovenous malformation diagnosis and management. Semin Neurol. 2013;3(3):468–75.

41. Mohr JP, Parides MK, Stapf C, et al. Medical management with or without interventional therapy for unruptured brain arteriovenous malformations (ARUBA): a multicentre, non-blinded, randomised trial. Lancet. 2014;383:614–21.

42. Epstein MA, Berman PH, Schut L. Cavernous angioma presenting as atypical facial and head pain. J Child Neurol. 1990;5:27–30.

43. Moultrie F, Horne MA, Josephson CB, et al. Outcome after surgical or conservative management of cerebral cavernous malformations. Neurology. 2014;83:582–9.

44. Kwon PM, Evans RW, Grosberg BM. Cerebral vascular malformations and headache. Headache. 2015;55:1133–42.

45. Silbert PL, Mokri B, Schievink WI. Headache and neck pain in spontaneous internal carotid and vertebral artery dissections. Neurology. 1995;45:1517–22.

46. Sheikh HU. Headache in intracranial and cervical artery dissections. Curr Pain Headache Rep. 2016;20(2):8.

47. Ninan J, Lester S, Hill C. Giant cell arteritis. Best Pract Res Clin Rheumatol. 2016;30:169–88.

48. Solomon S, Cappa KG. The headache of temporal arteritis. J Am Geriatr Soc. 1987;35:163–5.

49. Aiello PD, Trautmann JC, McPhee TJ, et al. Visual prognosis in giant cell arteritis. Ophthalmology. 1993;100:550–5.

50. Dasgupta B, Borg FA, Hassan N, et al. BSR and BHPR guidelines for the management of giant cell arteritis. Rheumatology. 2010;49:1594–7.

51. Smith J, Swanson J. Giant cell arteritis. Headache. 2014;54:1217–89.

52. McGeeney BE, Friedman DI. Pseudotumor cerebri pathophysiology. Headache. 2014;54:445–58.

53. Wall M, Kupersmith MJ, Kieburtz KD, the NORDIC Idiopathic Intracranial Hypertension Study Group. The idiopathic intracranial hypertension treatment trial: clinical profile at baseline. JAMA Neurol. 2014;71:693–701.

54. Friedman DL. Papilledema and idiopathic intracranial hypertension. Continuum. 2014;20:857–76.

55. Wakerly B, Tan M, Ting E. Idiopathic intracranial hypertension. Cephalalgia. 2015;35:248–61.

56. Markey KA, Mollan SP, Jensen RH, Sinclair AJ. Understanding idiopathic intracranial hypertension: mechanisms, management, and future directions. Lancet Neurol. 2016;15:78–91.

57. Wall M, McDermott MP, Kieburtz KD, NORDIC Idiopathic Intracranial Hypertension Study Group Writing Committee, et al. Effect of acetazolamide on visual function in patients with idiopathic intracranial hypertension and mild visual loss: the idiopathic intracranial hypertension treatment trial. JAMA. 2014;311:1641–51.

58. Graff-Radford SB, Schievink WI. High-pressure headaches, low-pressure syndromes, and CSF leaks: diagnosis and management. Headache. 2014;54:394–401.

59. Bezov D, Lipton RB, Ashina S. Post-dural puncture headache: part I diagnosis, epidemiology, etiology, and pathophysiology. Headache. 2010;50:1144–52.

60. Basurto Ona X, Osorio D, Bonfill CX. Drug therapy for treating post-dural puncture headache. Cochrane Database Syst Rev. 2015;7:CD007887.

61. Bezov D, AShina S, Lipton RB. Post-dural puncture headache: part II prevention, management, and prognosis. Headache. 2010;50:1482–98.

62. Mokri B. Spontaneous intracranial hypotension. Continuum. 2015;21:1086–108.
63. Beck J, Ulrich CT, Fung C, et al. Diskogenic microspurs as a major cause of intractable spontaneous intracranial hypotension. Neurology. 2016;87:1220–6.
64. Kranz PG, Tanpitukpongse TP, Choudhury KR, et al. How common is normal cerebrospinal fluid pressure in spontaneous intracranial hypotension. Cephalalgia. 2016;36:1209–17.
65. Starling A, Hernandez F, Hoxworth J, et al. Sensitivity of MRI of the spine compared with CT myelography in orthostatic headache with CSF leak. Neurology. 2013;81:1789–92.
66. Mokri B. Radioisotope cisternography in spontaneous CSF leaks: interpretations and misinterpretations. Headache. 2014;54:1358–68.
67. Cho K, Moon H, Jeon H, et al. Spontaneous intracranial hypotension. Efficacy of radiologic targeting vs blind blood patch. Neurology. 2011;76:1139–44.
68. Goffaux P, Fortin D. Brain tumor headaches: from bedside to bench. Neurosurgery. 2010;67:459–66.
69. Schankin CJ, Ferrari U, Reinisch VM, et al. Characteristics of brain tumour-associated headache. Cephalalgia. 2007;27:904–11.
70. Forsyth PA, Posner JB. Headaches in patients with brain tumors: a study of 111 patients. Neurology. 1993;43:1678–83.
71. Nelson S, Taylor L. Headaches in brain tumor patients: primary or secondary? Headache. 2014;54:776–85.
72. Taylor FR, Larkins MV. Headache and chiari I malformation: clinical presentation, diagnosis, and controversies in management. Curr Pain and Headache Rep. 2002;6:331–7.
73. Toldo I, Tangari M, Mardari R, et al. Headache in children with Chiari I malformation. Headache. 2014;54:899–908.
74. Pascual J, Oterino A, Berciano J. Headache in type I Chiari malformation. Neurology. 1992;42:1519–21.
75. Wan MJ, Nomura H, Tator CH. Conversion to symptomatic Chiari I malformation after minor head or neck trauma. Neurosurgery. 2008;63:748–53.
76. McGirt MJ, Nimjee SM, Floyd J, et al. Correlation of cerebrospinal fluid flow dynamics and headache in Chiari I malformation. Neurosurgery. 2005;56:716–21.
77. Tepper DE, Tepper SJ, Sheftell FD, Bigal ME. Headache attributed to hypothyroidism. Curr Pain Headache Rep. 2007;11:304–9.
78. Friedman D. The eye and headache. Continuum. 2015;21:1109–17.
79. Ng A, Wang D. Cervical facet injections in the management of cervicogenic headaches. Curr Pain Headache Rep. 2015;19(5):484. https://doi.org/10.1007/s11916-015-0484-1.
80. Bellegaard V, Thede-Schmidt-Hansen P, Svensson P, Jensen R. Are headache and temporomandibular disorders related? A blinded study. Cephalalgia. 2008;28:832–41.
81. da Silva A Jr, Costa EC, Gomes JB, et al. Chronic headache and comorbidities: a two-phase, population-based, cross-sectional study. Headache. 2010;50:1306–12.

Chronic Facial Pain and Other Chronic Neuralgias

Salman Farooq and Fallon C. Schloemer

The International Association for Study of Pain defines neuralgia as pain in the distribution of a nerve or nerves which are otherwise normal in function. Neuropathy is defined as a disturbance of function or pathologic change in a nerve or nerves. Neuropathic pain can be caused by a lesion or disease of the central or peripheral somatosensory system.

Facial pain is usually caused by a stimulation of afferent fibers in the trigeminal nerve (cranial nerve V), nervus intermedius (cranial nerve VII), glossopharyngeal nerve (cranial nerve IX), vagus nerve (cranial nerve X), and upper cervical spinal cord roots [1].

Trigeminal Neuralgia

Introduction

The International Classification of Headache Disorders (ICHD), 3rd edition defines trigeminal neuralgia *(also known as tic douloureux)* as a facial pain disorder characterized by paroxysms of recurrent, brief electric shock-like or stabbing

pain which are abrupt in onset and termination (lasting seconds to minutes). The painful paroxysms are limited to the distribution of one or more divisions of the trigeminal nerve which can arise spontaneously or triggered by trivial stimuli, including light touching, cold air, eating, drinking, washing, shaving, brushing the hair or teeth, and applying make-up [1–4].

Epidemiology

Trigeminal neuralgia is a rare condition but is also the most common and the most severe of all cranial neuralgias. The annual incidence of trigeminal neuralgia is 5–30 per 100,000 people [3, 5–7]. Peak age of onset is after 50 and the incidence increases with age. Women are 1.7 times more likely to be affected compared to men [3, 4, 6, 8–10].

Etiology

Most cases of trigeminal neuralgia are caused by compression of the trigeminal nerve root [3]. The compression is usually located within a few millimeters of entry into the pons and can extend several millimeters along the root without involving the peripheral trigeminal nerve [3, 8].

The compression is most commonly caused by an aberrant loop of an artery or vein (80–90% of cases) [3, 8, 11] but can also result from a

S. Farooq (✉)
Neurology, Medical College of Wisconsin,
Wauwatosa, WI, USA
e-mail: sfarooq@mcw.edu

F. C. Schloemer
Neurology, Froedtert and the Medical College
of Wisconsin, Milwaukee, WI, USA

vestibular schwannoma, meningioma, epidermoid cyst, saccular aneurysm, arteriovenous malformation, or rarely an osteoma [7, 12–18].

Trigeminal neuralgia can also be seen as a complication of multiple sclerosis where demyelination involves the root entry zone of the trigeminal nerve in the pons [3, 19]. This rarely (in 1% of cases) can be the initial manifestation of multiple sclerosis [20, 21]. Trigeminal neuralgia can also be seen in patients with peripheral demyelinating neuropathies such as Charcot-Marie-Tooth disease [22].

Other uncommonly reported causes of trigeminal neuralgia include infiltrative carcinomatous or amyloid deposits within the nerve root, Gasserian ganglion and/or the nerve itself [23, 24], as well as infarcts or angiomas involving the brainstem [25–27]. Some cases may even be idiopathic for which no identifiable cause is found.

Pathogenesis

Compression of trigeminal nerve from above-mentioned etiologies results in focal demyelination around the site of compression [28]. This focal demyelination then creates abnormal circuits between the exposed axons, resulting in generation of abnormal sensory impulses (termed "ephaptic transmission") which are carried along the pathways involved in the perception of pain and light touch from specific areas of face. This is the proposed mechanism resulting in generation of the painful paroxysms by touching the trigger areas on the face [3, 29]. The same mechanism of ephaptic transmission also applies to trigeminal neuralgia resulting from demyelinating disorders described above.

Classification and Clinical Presentation:

The ICHD-3 has broadly divided trigeminal neuralgia into *classical trigeminal neuralgia* and *painful trigeminal neuropathy* [1].

Classical trigeminal neuralgia is caused by neurovascular compression until proven other-

wise, and the superior cerebellar artery is most frequently the cause of compression. The pain most commonly involves the second or third divisions of the trigeminal nerve and is typically unilateral, and the right side of the face is affected more commonly than the left side [4, 8, 10, 30]. Following a painful paroxysm, there is usually a refractory period during which pain cannot be triggered and patients are mostly asymptomatic in between the paroxysms. Severe attacks may cause ipsilateral contraction of facial muscles (*hence the term tic douloureux*) and also can be associated with mild autonomic symptoms such as lacrimation and/or conjunctival injection [4, 9]. The duration and intensity of these painful attacks can increase over time, significantly affecting patients' quality of life.

The ICHD-3 has defined the following criteria for the clinical diagnosis of classical trigeminal neuralgia [1]:

ICHD Criteria for Classical Trigeminal Neuralgia

Classical Trigeminal Neuralgia

A. At least three attacks of unilateral facial pain fulfilling criteria B and C.

B. Occurring in one or more divisions of the trigeminal nerve, with no radiation beyond the trigeminal distribution.

C. Pain has at least three of the following four characteristics:
1. Recurring in paroxysmal attacks lasting from a fraction of a second to 2 min.
2. Severe intensity.
3. Electric shock-like, shooting, stabbing, or sharp in quality.
4. Precipitated by innocuous stimuli to the affected side of the face.

D. No clinically evident neurological deficit.

E. Not better accounted for by another ICHD-3 diagnosis.

Classical trigeminal neuralgia is further subdivided into:

a) *Purely paroxysmal classical trigeminal neuralgia* which is defined as recurrent paroxysms of unilateral facial pain fulfilling criteria for classical trigeminal neuralgia but without persistent facial pain between attacks. This subtype is usually responsive to pharmacotherapy.

b) *Classical trigeminal neuralgia with concomitant persistent facial pain (aka atypical trigeminal neuralgia or trigeminal neuralgia type 2)* which is defined as recurrent paroxysms of unilateral facial pain fulfilling criteria for classical trigeminal neuralgia with persistent facial pain of moderate intensity in the affected area. Unlike the former subtype, this subtype is less likely to respond to medical or surgical therapy and is usually not triggered by innocuous stimuli.

Painful trigeminal neuropathy (previously known as secondary trigeminal neuralgia) is head, facial, and/or oral pain in the distribution of one or more branches of the trigeminal nerve that fulfills criterion C of classical trigeminal neuralgia but is caused by lesions other than vascular compression [1].

a) *Painful trigeminal neuropathy attributed to acute herpes zoster* usually precedes the herpetic eruptions by <7 days, lasts for less than 3 months, and is localized to the territory of the same trigeminal nerve branch or branches affected by such eruptions/rash [31]. Ophthalmic division is the most commonly involved (80% of cases). Rarely, however, the pain is not followed by the eruption or rash and diagnosis in such cases is confirmed by polymerase chain reaction (PCR) detection of varicella zoster virus DNA in the cerebrospinal fluid (CSF).

b) *Postherpetic trigeminal neuralgia* is defined as unilateral head and/or facial pain following acute herpes zoster that persists or recurs for at least 3 months in the distribution of the same trigeminal nerve branch or branches affected by herpes zoster eruptions [31]. It is more prevalent in the elderly and ophthalmic division of trigeminal nerve is the most commonly involved.

c) *Painful post-traumatic trigeminal neuropathy* is defined as constant unilateral facial or oral severe burning/aching pain that develops within 3–6 months following trauma to the trigeminal nerve. The pain is located in the distribution of the same trigeminal nerve branch or branches affected by trauma. The trauma can be mechanical, chemical, and thermal or caused by radiation [32].

d) *Painful trigeminal neuropathy attributed to multiple sclerosis (MS) plaque* is defined as unilateral or bilateral head and/or facial pain in the distribution of trigeminal nerve in a patient who has been diagnosed with MS and with MRI evidence of an MS plaque affecting the trigeminal nerve root [18, 19]. This subtype of trigeminal neuralgia is less likely to respond to pharmacotherapy.

e) *Painful trigeminal neuropathy attributed to space-occupying lesion* is defined as unilateral head and/or facial pain in the distribution of a trigeminal nerve in a patient with radiologic evidence of a space-occupying lesion affecting the trigeminal nerve [15, 17].

f) *Painful trigeminal neuropathy attributed to other disorders* is defined as unilateral or bilateral head, facial, and/or oral pain with the characteristics of trigeminal neuralgia caused by disorders other than those described above.

An important differential diagnosis: *Short-lasting unilateral neuralgiform headache attacks*, because of their overlapping clinical presentation, can often be misdiagnosed as trigeminal neuralgia or vice versa [33]. ICHD-3 have classified them separately under the category of trigeminal autonomic cephalalgias and established the following criteria for their diagnosis and differentiation from trigeminal neuralgia and other headache disorders [1]:

them apart. It is important to note that these too can become chronic defined by occurring without a remission period or with remissions lasting <1 month for at least 1 year [Table 9.1] [1].

Medical Management

The best and initial approach for the management of trigeminal neuralgia is pharmacotherapy. Various classes of medication have been used, most commonly the antiepileptics, for the treatment of trigeminal neuralgia. We will individually discuss the commonly used drugs and their efficacy for the treatment of this disorder.

Carbamazepine is the most studied drug for the management of trigeminal neuralgia (Class I and II evidence from four randomized, controlled trials including a total of 147 patients), making it the drug of choice for the management of this condition [34–42]. The commonly reported side effects include drowsiness, dizziness, and nausea which can be controlled by slow titration of the drug. Leukopenia and in rare cases aplastic anemia can be seen as a complication of trigeminal neuralgia. Another serious side effect, however, is the development Stevens-Johnson syndrome (SJS) which should be an indication for stopping the drug. Asian patients who are positive for HLA-B 15:02 allele are more prone to the development of SJS secondary to carbamazepine [43].

Dosing (orally):

Initial: 200 mg daily in two divided doses, gradually increasing by 200 mg/day as needed.

Maintenance: 400–800 mg daily in two divided doses.

Maximum dose: 1200 mg daily in two divided doses.

Oxcarbazepine has shown to be equally effective to carbamazepine for the management trigeminal neuralgia (Class II evidence from two randomized, controlled trials including a total of 130 patients) [37, 40, 42]. Unfortunately, it carries the same risk as carbamazepine for the development of rash in Asian patients who are positive for HLA-B 15:02 allele [43].

Dosing (orally):

Initial: 600 mg daily in two divided doses; gradually increasing by 300 mg every 5 days as needed.

ICHD Criteria for Short-Lasting Unilateral Neuralgiform Headache

Short-Lasting Unilateral Neuralgiform Headache

A. At least 20 attacks fulfilling criteria B–D.
B. Moderate or severe unilateral head pain, with orbital, supraorbital, temporal, and/or other trigeminal distribution, lasting for 1–600 s and occurring as single stabs, series of stabs, or in a sawtooth pattern.
C. At least one of the following cranial autonomic symptoms or signs, ipsilateral to the pain:
   1. Conjunctival injection and/or lacrimation.
   2. Nasal congestion and/or rhinorrhea.
   3. Eyelid edema.
   4. Forehead and facial sweating.
   5. Forehead and facial flushing.
   6. Sensation of fullness in the ear.
   7. Miosis and/or ptosis.
D. Attacks have a frequency of at least 1 day for more than half of the time when the disorder is active.
E. Not better accounted for by another ICHD-3 diagnosis.

Short-lasting unilateral neuralgiform headache attacks are further subclassified by ICHD-3 as short-lasting unilateral neuralgiform headache attacks with conjunctival injection and tearing (SUNCT) and short-lasting unilateral neuralgiform headache attacks with cranial autonomic symptoms (SUNA). The two subtypes are clinically differentiated by the presence (SUNCT) or absence (SUNA) of conjunctival injection and/or lacrimation [1, 33].

Chronic cluster headache, which was covered in chapter 6 also falls under the umbrella of the trigeminal autonomic cephalalgias. Others in this category that are often confused with cluster headache include paroxysmal hemicrania and hemicrania continua. While each is very similar, frequency and duration of attacks, circadian periodicity, and responsiveness to indomethacin are what separates

Table 9.1 Characteristics of the trigeminal autonomic cephalalgias

	Characteristic	Cluster	Paroxysmal hemicrania	SUNCT/ SUNA	Hemicrania continua
Similarities	Pain quality	Stabbing	Throbbing, stabbing	Burning, stabbing	Baseline steady ache with stabbing attacks
	Pain severity	Severe	Severe	Severe	Baseline mild-to-moderate pain with moderate-to-severe attacks
	Typical site of pain	Orbit, temple	Orbit, temple	Orbit, temple	Orbit, temple
	Autonomic features	Yes	Yes	Yes	Present with attacks
	Response to indomethacin	Occasionally	Yes	No	Yes
Distinguishing features	Duration of attacks	15–180 min	2–30 min	1–600 s	Constant pain with variable attack duration
	Correlation with circadian rhythm	Yes	No	No	No
	Nocturnal attacks	Yes	No	No	No
	Triggers	Alcohol	Alcohol, cervical nerve root pressure/ neck movement	Cutaneous pressure	No specific triggers

Maximum dose: 1200–1800 mg daily in two divided doses.

Baclofen has limited evidence in the management of trigeminal neuralgia (Class II evidence from a single double-blind crossover study including a total of ten patients) [37, 44]. Drowsiness, dizziness, and dyspepsia are the commonly reported side effects.

Dosing (orally):

Initial: 15–30 mg daily in three divided doses, gradually increasing by 10 mg every other day over 1–2 weeks.

Maximum dose: 50–60 mg daily in three divided doses.

Lamotrigine has been studied as an adjuvant therapy to carbamazepine for trigeminal neuralgia (Class II evidence from a double-blind crossover study including a total of 14 patients) [7, 37, 45, 46].

Dosing (orally):

For patients not taking other anticonvulsants: initial dose of 25 mg daily for the first 2 weeks, gradually increasing as needed to 50 mg daily for weeks 3 and 4 and then by 50 mg daily every 2 weeks to a maximum dose of 400 mg daily.

For patients taking carbamazepine, phenytoin, or primidone (CYP450 enzymes, enzyme inducers): initial dose of 50 mg once daily, gradually increasing as needed to 100 mg once daily

at week 3, 200 mg once daily at week 5, 300 mg once daily at week 6, and 400 mg once daily at week 7.

For patients taking valproate (Depakote): initial dose of 12.5–25 mg every other day, gradually increasing by 25 mg every 2 weeks as needed to a maximum of 400 mg daily.

Pimozide has been shown to be more effective than carbamazepine (Class II evidence from a double-blind crossover trial including a total of 48 patients). However, because of limited evidence of its efficacy and safety compared to carbamazepine, pimozide is rarely used for trigeminal neuralgia [7, 37, 47].

Tizanidine was found to be more effective than placebo in a small 3-week double-blind crossover trial including 12 patients (Class III evidence), but because of limited evidence and short-term benefits, it is not commonly used for the treatment of trigeminal neuralgia [7, 37, 48].

Tocainide was found to be as effective as carbamazepine in a small 2-week double-blind crossover study including 12 patients (Class III evidence), but because of limited evidence and side effect profile (nausea, distal paresthesias and skin rash), it is rarely used [7, 37, 49].

Topical   ophthalmic   anesthesia (Proparacaine hydrochloride 0.5%) was found to ineffective in a randomized double-blind placebo-controlled trial including 47 patients (Class I evidence) [7, 37, 50].

Phenytoin, clonazepam, gabapentin, and valproate have shown therapeutic benefits in small open-label studies (Class IV evidence), but because of lack of controlled trials, their role is limited in the management of trigeminal neuralgia [37, 51].

Botulinum toxin injections which are commonly used for chronic migraine prevention have shown limited evidence (two double-blind, placebo-controlled trials and five prospective case series) for the treatment of trigeminal neuralgia in patients who have either failed or are intolerant of oral medications [52, 53]. Techniques and dose of the neurotoxins varied in these studies. Some authors mapped out a grid of the painful area and injected at various cross points, while others injected trigger points. Often the same technique was done bilaterally to achieve facial asymmetry. While the exact mechanism of how botulinum toxin injections work for trigeminal neuralgia is unknown, it is thought to be due to inhibition of the release of pain-related mediators [42].

Surgical Management

Surgical management is usually reserved for patients who are refractory to medical management. The commonly used surgical techniques for the management of trigeminal neuralgia include microvascular decompression and ablative therapy.

Microvascular decompression is an invasive neurosurgical procedure that involves separation of compressing vascular structures away from the trigeminal nerve through craniotomy to reach the posterior fossa [8]. The efficacy of this procedure has been demonstrated by five major prospective studies (Class III evidence) which showed an initial relief following the procedure in 90% of patient which then decreased to 80% at 1 year, 75% at 3 years, and 73% at 5 years [36, 37, 40]. The most commonly reported complication was aseptic meningitis, followed by severe hearing loss, CSF leak, and trigeminal distribution sensory loss. Only two procedure-related deaths were reported in these studies [54].

Rhizotomy is also an invasive procedure that involves penetration of the foramen ovale with a cannula, followed by controlled lesion of the trigeminal ganglion or root by following means:

(a) Radiofrequency thermocoagulation: uses heat to lesion trigeminal root.
(b) Mechanical balloon compression: uses balloon inflated into Meckel's cave to compress the trigeminal nerve root.
(c) Chemical rhizolysis: produces chemical lesion of trigeminal nerve root by injection of 0.1–0.4 mL of glycerol.

The efficacy of these rhizotomy procedure is demonstrated by only four uncontrolled case series (Class III evidence) which showed an initial relief following the procedure in 90% of patients which then decreased to 68–85% at 1 year, 54–64% at 3 years, and 50% at 5 years [37, 40]. Aseptic meningitis was reported in 0.2% of patients, trigeminal-distribution sensory loss was reported in almost half of patients, 12% developed dysesthesias, 4% developed anesthesia dolorosa, and 4% developed corneal numbness. Transient jaw weakness was reported in 50% of patients undergoing balloon compression. No procedure-related deaths were reported [36, 37].

Gamma knife surgery is a noninvasive procedure which uses a stereotactic frame and MRI to target a focused beam of radiation at the trigeminal root in the posterior fossa [36, 55]. The efficacy of this procedure is demonstrated by three case series (Class III evidence) which showed a complete relief at 1 year following the procedure in 90% of patient which then dropped to 52% at 3 years. Pain relief following this procedure can be delayed by 1 month at an average. The most commonly reported complication was facial numbness (9–37% of patients) [37, 40].

Peripheral denervation techniques involve focal destruction of trigeminal nerve distal to the Gasserian ganglia and include cryotherapy, neurectomies, alcohol injection, phenol injection, peripheral acupuncture, radiofrequency, and thermocoagulation, but the evidence supporting these techniques is very weak (Class IV) [37, 40].

Glossopharyngeal Neuralgia

Introduction

The ICHD-3 defines glossopharyngeal neuralgia (previously known as vagoglossopharyngeal neuralgia) as a facial pain disorder characterized by paroxysms of severe, stabbing pain in the ear, base of the tongue, tonsillar fossa, and/or underneath the angle of the jaw. It is commonly triggered by innocuous stimuli, including swallowing, talking, yawning, coughing, or manipulation of external auditory canal and usually lasts seconds or minutes [1]. The pain is unilateral in most of the cases, but bilateral involvement has been reported more often than in trigeminal neuralgia [56, 57].

Epidemiology

Glossopharyngeal neuralgia is a rare disease; annual incidence is 0.4–0.8 per 100,000 populations. It affects both sexes almost equally and the risk increase with age [5, 6, 56, 57].

Etiology

Most of the cases of glossopharyngeal neuralgia are idiopathic, but it can be caused by compression of cranial nerves IX and X at the nerve root entry zone, commonly by the vertebral artery or posterior inferior cerebellar artery [58]. Other secondary causes of glossopharyngeal neuralgia include neck trauma, demyelinating diseases, tonsillar or regional abscesses/tumors, cerebellopontine angle tumors, Arnold-Chiari malformation, and Eagle syndrome (an elongated or calcified stylohyoid ligament compressing the cranial nerve IX) [1, 5, 59].

Clinical Presentation and Diagnostic Criteria

Glossopharyngeal neuralgia is less severe than the classical trigeminal neuralgia, but the two disorders can often coexist. Pain from glossopharyngeal neuralgia occurs in the distribution of the auricular and pharyngeal branches of the vagus nerve (X) as well as branches of the glossopharyngeal nerve (IX). The development of overt glossopharyngeal neuralgic pain attacks can often be preceded by an aura consisting of an uncomfortable sensation in the affected area, lasting for weeks to months [1].

Paroxysms of pain can rarely be associated with vagal symptoms such as cough, hoarseness, syncope, and/or bradycardia (*hence the old term vagoglossopharyngeal neuralgia*), likely because of close connections between the vagus nerve and glossopharyngeal nerve. The afferent impulses from glossopharyngeal nerve may reach the dorsal nucleus of the vagus nerve (via collaterals from the tractus solitarius nucleus of the midbrain) which supplies parasympathetic fibers to the heart, bronchi, and abdominal nerve [59].

The ICHD-3 has defined the following criteria for the clinical diagnosis of glossopharyngeal neuralgia [1]:

> **ICHD Criteria for Glossopharyngeal Neuralgia**
> **Glossopharyngeal Neuralgia**
>
> A. At least three attacks of unilateral pain fulfilling criteria B and C.
> B. Pain is located in the posterior part of the tongue, tonsillar fossa, pharynx, beneath the angle of the lower jaw, and/or in the ear.
> C. Pain has at least three of the following four characteristics:
>   1. Recurring in paroxysmal attacks lasting from a few seconds to 2 min.
>   2. Severe intensity.
>   3. Shooting, stabbing, or sharp in quality.
>   4. Precipitated by swallowing, coughing, talking, or yawning.
> D. No clinically evident neurological deficit.
> E. Not better accounted for by another ICHD-3 diagnosis.

Pain attacks from glossopharyngeal neuralgia can occur in clusters lasting weeks to months, alternating with longer periods of remission, ranging from months to years [59].

Medical Management

Like trigeminal neuralgia, the best and initial approach for the management of glossopharyngeal neuralgia is medical management with drugs. The medical management is essentially the same as for trigeminal neuralgia and has been discussed in detail in the section of trigeminal neuralgia.

Surgical Management

Surgical management is usually reserved for patients who are refractory to medical management. The commonly used surgical techniques for the management of glossopharyngeal neuralgia include microvascular decompression and intracranial suctioning.

Microvascular decompression of the cranial nerve IX and cranial nerve X is an effective treatment strategy for patients refractory to maximal medical therapy and had shown to provide complete and long-lasting relief ~80% of patients treated [58]. Although this is an invasive procedure, only a small percentage of complications have been reported from the procedure, including cerebrospinal fluid leaks (<2% of patients) and postoperative cranial nerve palsies (<3% of patients) [58, 60].

Intracranial sectioning of cranial nerve IX and the upper three to four rootlets of cranial nerve X at the jugular foramen has also been used for the management of glossopharyngeal neuralgia. Because of comparatively more risk of complications and less long-term benefits, microvascular decompression is the procedure of choice for the management of refractory glossopharyngeal neuralgia [57, 58].

Nervus Intermedius Neuralgia

Introduction

The ICHD-3 defines nervus intermedius neuralgia (also known as facial nerve or geniculate neuralgia) as a rare facial pain disorder characterized by brief paroxysms of unilateral pain felt deeply in the auditory canal which can sometimes radiate to the parieto-occipital region [1]. It is occasionally associated with a trigger zone in the posterior wall of auditory canal; however, presence of trigger is not a characteristic feature of nervus intermedius neuralgia [61].

Classification

The ICHD-3 classifies trigeminal neuralgia into *classical nervus intermedius neuralgia* and *secondary nervus intermedius neuropathy*.

Epidemiology, Etiology, and Clinical Diagnostic Criteria

Classical nervus intermedius neuralgia is nervus intermedius neuralgia developing without an apparent cause. Most of the cases are idiopathic, but like other cranial neuralgias, possible vascular compression has been proposed as a possible etiology, although evidence is limited and controversial. Classical nervus intermedius neuralgia is an extremely rare condition. It affects women more commonly than men and the average age of onset is ~40 years [61].

The ICHD-3 has defined the following criteria for the clinical diagnosis of classical nervus intermedius neuralgia [1]:

ICHD Criteria for Nervus Intermedius Neuralgia

Nervus Intermedius Neuralgia

A. At least three attacks of unilateral pain fulfilling criteria B and C.
B. Pain is located in the auditory canal, sometimes radiating to the parieto-occipital region.
C. Pain has at least three of the following four characteristics:
　　1. Recurring in paroxysmal attacks lasting from a few seconds to minutes.

2. Severe intensity.
3. Shooting, stabbing, or sharp in quality.
4. Precipitated by stimulation of a trigger area in the posterior wall of the auditory canal and/or periauricular region.
D. No clinically evident neurological deficit.
E. Not better accounted for by another ICHD-3 diagnosis.

Secondary nervus intermedius neuropathy (*also known as Ramsay Hunt syndrome*) is nervus intermedius neuralgia attributed to acute herpes zoster of the nervus intermedius. It is associated with facial paresis and zoster lesions in the ear or oral mucosa. Additionally reported associated symptoms in this disorder include taste, lacrimation/salivation, and acoustic disturbances [61]. Secondary nervus intermedius neuralgia is also a rare disease but more common compared to classic nerve intermedius neuralgia and also affects women more commonly than men, and the average age of onset is ~50 years [5, 62].

The ICHD-3 has defined the following criteria for the clinical diagnosis of nervus intermedius neuralgia attributed to herpes zoster neuralgia [1]:

ICHD Criteria for Nervus Intermedius Neuropathy Attributed to Herpes Zoster Nervus Intermedius Neuropathy Attributed to Herpes Zoster

A. Unilateral facial pain fulfilling criterion C.
B. Herpetic eruption has occurred in the ear and/or oral mucosa, in the territory of the nervus intermedius.
C. Evidence of causation demonstrated by both of the following:
   1. Pain has preceded the herpetic eruption by <7 days.
   2. Pain is localized to the distribution of the nervus intermedius.
D. Clinical features of peripheral facial paresis.
E. Not better accounted for by another ICHD-3 diagnosis.

Medical Management

The best and initial approach for the management of nervus intermedius neuralgia is pharmacotherapy. The medical management is essentially the same as for trigeminal neuralgia with carbamazepine being the initial drug of choice and has been discussed in detail in the section of trigeminal neuralgia. However, in secondary nervus intermedius neuropathy attributed to Herpes zoster, treatment should be initiated with steroids and acyclovir as early as possible.

Surgical Management

Surgical management is reserved as the last resort when medical management fails. The commonly used surgical techniques for the management of nervus intermedius neuralgia include microvascular decompression and excision of involved nerve and its ganglion.

Excision of the nervus intermedius and geniculate ganglion is an invasive neurosurgical procedure that involves exposing the motor component of the facial nerve, geniculate ganglion, greater superficial petrosal nerve, and nervus intermedius from the cochleariformis process to the cerebellopontine angle and then excising the segment of nervus intermedius at the internal auditory canal before it joins the facial nerve. The geniculate ganglion is also excised from the internal genu of the facial nerve along with a segment of the greater superficial petrosal nerve. The efficacy of this procedure has been demonstrated by a case series of 64 patients which showed an excellent relief following the procedure in 98% of patients. The most commonly reported complication was permanent ipsilateral xerophthalmia in all the patients (100%), followed by temporary partial facial paralysis in 11 patients (17%) [63].

The procedure can also involve exploration and/or transection of multiple cranial nerves as well as microvascular vascular decompression (if a potential offending vessel is seen during exploration) as demonstrated by Rupa et al. in a series of 18 patients which showed pain relief following the procedure in 72% of the patient. Post-op complications included sensorineural hearing loss (two patients), CSF leak (one patient), aseptic meningitis (one patient), and transient facial paresis (one patient) [64].

Microvascular decompression of cranial nerves V, IX, and X with or without section of the nervus intermedius is also an invasive procedure used in patients with medically refractory nervus intermedius neuralgia. Its efficacy was demonstrated in a series of 14 patients (and a few other case reports) with long-term relief in 90% of the patients. Post-op complications were similar to those reported by Rupa et al. [64–66].

Extracranial intratemporal division of the cutaneous branches of the facial nerve has shown to offer a safer treatment (no complication reported over 1 year) with similar effectiveness in a series of three cases. Because of small sample sizes, relatively short follow-up, and poor study design, further research is needed to confirm the effectiveness and safety of this procedure [66].

Occipital Neuralgia

Introduction

The ICHD-3 defines occipital neuralgia as a headache disorder characterized by unilateral or bilateral paroxysmal, shooting or stabbing pain in the posterior part of the scalp. It is sometimes accompanied by diminished sensation or dysesthesia in the affected area and is commonly associated with tenderness over the involved nerve(s) [1].

Epidemiology

The actual incidence and prevalence of occipital neuralgia are unknown.

Etiology

Most of the cases are idiopathic. Uncommonly reported etiologies include posterior head trauma and whiplash injuries, chronic entrapment of the occipital nerves by the posterior neck and scalp muscles, and vascular compression of the nerve by the occipital artery, posterior inferior cerebellar artery, and arteriovenous fistulas [67].

Clinical Presentation and Diagnostic Criteria

Pain from occipital neuralgia occurs in the distribution of the greater, lesser, or third occipital nerves which are branches off of the upper cervical nerve roots. Each episode is sudden in onset, originates in the nuchal region, and immediately spreads toward the vertex, lasting for seconds to minutes. Pain from the lesser occipital nerve is felt laterally, while pain from the greater and third occipital nerves is felt medially. In some cases the pain may radiate to the ipsilateral fronto-orbital region. The paroxysms can start spontaneously or be provoked by specific maneuvers such as brushing the hair or moving the neck. The pain is unilateral in 85% of the cases, but bilateral involvement had also been reported. Physical examination of affected area reveals tenderness and might trigger a painful paroxysm [67].

The ICHD-3 has defined the following criteria for the diagnosis of occipital neuralgia [1]:

ICHD Criteria for Occipital Neuralgia
Occipital Neuralgia

A. Unilateral or bilateral pain fulfilling criteria B-E.
B. Pain is located in the distribution of the greater, lesser, and/or third occipital nerves.
C. Pain has two of the following three characteristics:
  1. Recurring in paroxysmal attacks lasting from a few seconds to minutes.

2. Severe intensity.
3. Shooting, stabbing, or sharp in quality.
D. Pain is associated with both of the following:
   1. Dysesthesia and/or allodynia apparent during innocuous stimulation of the scalp and/or hair.
   2. Either or both of the following:
      (a) Tenderness over the affected nerve branches.
      (b) Trigger points at the emergence of the greater occipital nerve or in the area of distribution of C2.
E. Pain is eased temporarily by local anesthetic block of the affected nerve.
F. Not better accounted for by another ICHD-3 diagnosis.

Management

Conservative management, including rest, periodic application of warm or cold compresses, massage, and physical therapy directed at improving posture, may improve symptoms in some patients and should be tried initially [67].

Block of the greater or lesser occipital nerves is often the treatment of choice for occipital neuralgia as it also has diagnostic potential (Fig. 9.1).

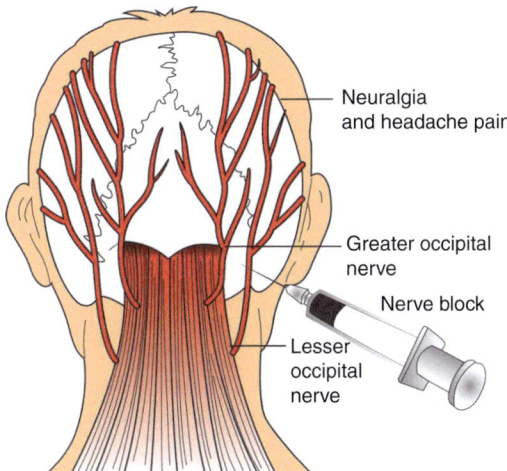

Fig. 9.1 Block of the greater occipital nerve. From Anesthesia Key with permission from Lucas Clelemo. [Accessed at: https://aneskey.com/occipital-nerve-block/]

It provides immediate relief which may last for several weeks to a couple of months and can be repeated as it is a relatively safe procedure with fewer, if any, complications. Knowing the anatomical landmarks and course of the nerves helps guide where to perform the injections. Various local anesthetics such as lidocaine, and bupivacaine have been used alone and in combination with each other (often in a 1:1 ratio) or with a corticosteroid such as methylprednisolone or triamcinolone to achieve the blockade [67, 68].

Alternate strategies: Carbamazepine, gabapentin, nonsteroidal anti-inflammatory medications, or tricyclic antidepressants may be used if the pain is paroxysmal in nature or the patient is not tolerant/hesitant of repeated nerve blocks.

Limited evidence suggests that neuromodulation with pulsed radiofrequency and implanted occipital nerve stimulators may be effective in refractory cases [67, 69]. This will be discussed in detail in Chapter 25.

Optic Neuritis

Introduction

Optic neuritis is an acute inflammatory, demyelinating condition that is characterized by pain behind one or both eyes and is accompanied by impairment of central vision.

Epidemiology

The annual incidence of acute demyelinating optic neuritis is ~6 per 100,000 people and is more common in the northern United States and Western Europe. The age of onset is between the 20 and 40 and two-thirds of the cases occur in women compared to men [70, 71].

Etiology

The most etiology for optic neuritis is immune-mediated inflammatory demyelination of the optic nerve, but the specific mechanism and target antigens are unknown [72].

Clinical Presentation and Diagnostic Criteria

Optic neuritis usually presents with retro-orbital pain which worsens with movement and is associated with progressively worsening visual loss over a period of hours to days and peaking within 1 to 2 weeks. Visual loss is usually monocular and bilateral involvement is more common in children. The clinical features of optic neuritis have been systematically characterized in the Optic Neuritis Treatment Trial (ONTT), and the most commonly reported symptoms are visual loss and eye pain [73, 74]. One-third of patients have visible optic nerve inflammation on funduscopic examination, while in the remainder, the inflammation is retrobulbar. Optic neuritis can present as an isolated syndrome or as a manifestation of multiple sclerosis or neuromyelitis optica. Diagnosis of optic neuritis is based on history and clinical features, but an MRI of the brain and orbit and CSF evaluation are commonly used to aide in diagnosis when in doubt [72, 74, 75].

The ICHD-3 has defined the following criteria for the diagnosis of optic neuritis [1]:

ICHD Criteria for Optic Neuritis
Optic Neuritis

A. Unilateral or bilateral headache fulfilling criterion C.
B. Clinical, electrophysiological, imaging, and/or laboratory evidence confirming the presence of optic neuritis.
C. Evidence of causation demonstrated by both of the following:
   1. Headache has developed in temporal relationship to optic neuritis.
   2. Headache has either or both of the following features:
      (a) Localized in retro-orbital, orbital, frontal, and/or temporal regions.
      (b) Aggravated by eye movement.
D. Not better accounted for by another ICHD-3 diagnosis.

Management

Visual recovery from optic neuritis usually begins within the first 2–4 weeks of symptom onset and usually reaches 20/20 or better in 75% of patients who have normal vision at baseline. Thirty percent of adults will eventually develop multiple sclerosis (MS) at 5 years; however, children are less likely than adults to develop MS. Treatment with intravenous methylprednisolone hastens recovery of vision and delays onset of MS but does not impact long-term visual function (Class I evidence from several studies including ONTT) [73–75].

Headache Attributed to Ischemic Ocular Motor Nerve Palsy

Introduction

The ICHD-3 defines this disorder as unilateral frontal and/or periorbital pain caused by ischemic paresis of the ipsilateral third, fourth or sixth cranial nerve and associated with other symptoms and/or clinical signs of cranial nerve paresis [1, 76].

Etiology

The most common risk factor for ischemic ocular motor nerve palsy is diabetes mellitus. Other risk factors include left ventricular hypertrophy, elevated hematocrit, hypercholesterolemia, coronary artery disease, and smoking. Cranial nerve III is affected more commonly followed in order by cranial nerves IV and VI [77, 78].

Clinical Presentation and Diagnostic Criteria

Most cases of ischemic ocular motor nerve palsy are associated with pain, regardless of the etiology, but pain is more frequently seen with CN III palsies followed by cranial nerves VI and IV palsies. The pain is mostly unilateral and is mainly localized to ipsilateral brow and eye (presenting as unilateral frontal headache). The pain usually precedes the onset of visual symptoms by a few weeks but can occur concurrently with diplopia [76].

The ICHD-3 has defined the following criteria for the diagnosis of headache attributed to ischemic ocular motor nerve palsy [1]:

ICHD Criteria for Headache Attributed to Ischemic Ocular Motor Nerve Palsy
Headache Attributed to Ischemic Ocular Motor Nerve Palsy

A. Unilateral headache fulfilling criterion C.
B. Clinical and imaging findings confirming an ischemic ocular motor nerve palsy.
C. Evidence of causation demonstrated by both of the following:
1. Headache has developed in temporal relation to the motor nerve palsy.
2. Headache is localized around the ipsilateral brow and eye.
D. Not better accounted for by another ICHD-3 diagnosis.

Management

Treatment is aimed at modifying the risk factors and treating the underlying etiologies (antiplatelet therapy is usually recommended). Patients with ischemic ocular motor nerve palsies frequently recover, regardless of nerve affected. The pain usually resolves within a few days to a few months depending on the intensity of pain. The visual symptoms also recover over several weeks to months; however, if they persist beyond 6 months, prism therapy or surgical interventions are indicated to alleviate disabling diplopia and/or ptosis [76, 78, 79].

Recurrent Painful Ophthalmoplegic Neuropathy

Introduction

Recurrent painful ophthalmoplegic neuropathy (previously known as ophthalmoplegic migraine) is a rare condition, characterized by recurrent attacks of paresis of one or more ocular cranial nerves (commonly the cranial nerve III), with associated ipsilateral headache [1, 80].

Epidemiology

Recurrent painful ophthalmoplegic neuropathy is a rarely encountered headache syndrome; annual incidence is estimated at 0.7 per million populations. It most commonly affects the children and young adults with a mean age of onset at ~4–5. Females are affected more commonly [81, 82].

Etiology

Although the exact etiology of this disorder is controversial, MRI of the brain demonstrates gadolinium enhancement or thickening of the cisternal segment of the affected cranial nerve (in a ~75% of cases) suggesting a demyelinating or inflammatory etiology [81, 82].

Clinical Presentation and Diagnostic Criteria

It was previously known as ophthalmoplegic migraine, but ICHD reclassified the syndrome as a cranial neuralgia by ICHD because of its non-migrainous character and associated MRI findings. The onset of headache can precede ophthalmoplegia by up to 2 weeks [80, 81]. The third cranial nerve is most commonly affected, in which case mydriasis and ptosis can also be observed [80].

The ICHD-3 has defined the following criteria for the diagnosis of recurrent painful ophthalmoplegic neuropathy [1]:

ICHD Criteria for Other Causes of Painful Ophthalmoplegia
Recurrent Painful Ophthalmoplegic Neuropathy

A. At least two attacks fulfilling criterion B.
B. Unilateral headache accompanied by ipsilateral paresis of one, two, or all three ocular motor nerves.
C. Orbital, parasellar, or posterior fossa lesion has been excluded by appropriate investigation.

D. Not better accounted for by another ICHD-3 diagnosis.
   Tolosa-Hunt Syndrome

A. Unilateral headache fulfilling criterion C.
B. Both of the following:
   1. Granulomatous inflammation of the cavernous sinus, superior orbital fissure, or orbit, demonstrated by MRI or biopsy.
   2. Paresis of one or more of the ipsilateral third, fourth and/or sixth cranial nerves.
C. Evidence of causation demonstrated by both of the following:

1. Headache has preceded paresis of the third, fourth and/or sixth nerves by less than or equal to 2 weeks or developed with it.
2. Headache is localized around the ipsilateral brow and eye.

D. Not better accounted for by another ICHD-3 diagnosis.
   Paratrigeminal   Oculosympathetic (Raeder's) Syndrome

A. Constant, unilateral headache fulfilling criterion C.
B. Imaging evidence of underlying disease of either the middle cranial fossa or of the ipsilateral carotid artery.
C. Evidence of causation demonstrated by both of the following:

1. Headache has developed in temporal relation to the onset of the underlying disorder.
2. Headache has either or both of the following features:
   (a) Localized to the distribution of the ophthalmic division of the trigeminal nerve, with or without spread to the maxillary division.
   (b) Aggravated by eye movement.

D. Ipsilateral Horner's syndrome.
E. Not better accounted for by another ICHD-3 diagnosis.

Similar causes of painful ophthalmoplegias are included for comparison and should be considered on the differential diagnosis. Tolosa-Hunt and Raeder's syndrome are further discussed in detail below.

Management

Treatment with corticosteroids has shown to be beneficial in some patients; however, the evidence is limited, and further trials are indicated to confirm the efficacy of steroids in this syndrome [1, 80].

Tolosa-Hunt Syndrome

Introduction

Tolosa-Hunt syndrome is an extremely rare facial pain syndrome which consists of unilateral orbital pain associated with ophthalmoplegia caused by a granulomatous inflammation in the cavernous sinus, superior orbital fissure, or orbit [1, 83, 84].

Epidemiology

Annual incidence is estimated at one to two per million populations. Any age group can be affected from the first to eighth decade of life, and men and women are equally affected [85].

Etiology

The Tolosa-Hunt syndrome is caused by granulomatous inflammatory process of unknown etiology in the region of the cavernous sinus, superior orbital fissure, or orbit which may spread intra-cranially in rare cases [83, 85].

Clinical Presentation and Diagnostic Criteria

It is characterized by episodic, unilateral orbital pain associated with paresis of one or more of the third (most common), fourth, and/or sixth cranial nerves (see ICHD Criteria above). Additional involvement of the cranial nerves II, V1, V2, VII, or VIII has also been uncommonly reported, suggesting that inflammation can extend beyond the cavernous sinus in some cases [83, 85]. The pain is usually constant and retro-orbital with frequent extension to frontal and temporal regions. The onset of pain usually precedes the ophthalmoplegia by several days, but their onset can also coincide. Bilateral involvement has also been reported although it is less common. There can also be associated sympathetic/parasympathetic involvement of pupil and sensory loss in the division of cranial nerve V1 [85]. Tolosa-Hunt syndrome is diagnosed on the basis of clinical presentation in conjunction with neuroimaging findings (enlarged cavernous sinus, isointense on T1-weighted images with marked enhancement with gadolinium) and also a clinical response to corticosteroids [84].

Management

Tolosa-Hunt syndrome is a benign syndrome. Pain and paresis usually resolve within 72 h of adequate treatment with systemic corticosteroids [85] but may take up to 8 weeks in some cases [83]. The steroid regimens for treatment of Tolosa-Hunt syndrome vary with institutions and providers, but we recommend an additional dose of prednisone 80 mg for 3 days and if the symptoms have resolved, then a slow taper over 8 weeks.

Even if untreated, the episode usually resolves spontaneously after a couple of months, but recurrences are common at an interval of months or years. However, follow-up is indicated to exclude other causes of persistent painful ophthalmoplegia such as tumors, vasculitis, basal meningitis, sarcoidosis, or diabetes mellitus [1, 84, 85].

Paratrigeminal Oculosympathetic (Raeder's) Syndrome

Introduction

Paratrigeminal oculosympathetic syndrome (also known as Raeder's syndrome) is characterized by constant, unilateral pain in the distribution of the ophthalmic division of the trigeminal nerve, along with ipsilateral Horner's syndrome [1].

Epidemiology

Paratrigeminal oculosympathetic syndrome is a rare facial pain syndrome. Males are affected more commonly then females, and onset is usually between the fourth and fifth decade of life [86].

Etiology

It is commonly caused by lesions involving the middle cranial fossa (particularly neoplasm) or the carotid artery (particularly dissection) [86].

Clinical Presentation and Diagnostic Criteria

Patients mostly complain of constant, unilateral, burning pain (often with hypesthesia and/or dysesthesia) in the distribution of the ophthalmic division of the trigeminal nerve which may sometimes extend to the maxillary division of the trigeminal nerve (see ICHD Criteria above). Associated ptosis and miosis are seen in almost all the cases; however, anhidrosis is not a common association (seen in lesions involving common carotid artery). Some authors also use the term "painful Horner's syndrome" as a diagnostically useful indication of a middle cranial fossa lesion or of carotid artery dissection. An MRI of the brain and angiogram of carotid vessels are indicated to rule out/confirm carotid or middle cranial fossa lesions and also to confirm the clinical diagnosis [1, 86].

Management

Treatment is aimed at treating the underlying etiology. Systemic steroids have been occasionally used to hasten the recovery [87]. The headache usually resolves spontaneously in 1–3 months, but the residual features of Horner's syndrome may persist. Recurrences are uncommon [86].

Burning Mouth Syndrome

Introduction

Burning mouth syndrome *(previously known as stomatodynia, or glossodynia when confined to the tongue)* is characterized by recurrent intraoral burning or dysesthetic sensation without clinically evident causative lesions [1].

Epidemiology

The prevalence of burning mouth syndrome in US population is estimated at 0.7% of all adults (0.8% of women and 0.6% of men). It most commonly affects middle-aged women, and the incidence increases with age in both sexes [88, 89].

Etiology

Although the exact etiology of burning mouth syndrome is unclear, trigeminal small-fiber sensory neuropathy, presynaptic dysfunction of the nigrostriatal dopaminergic pathway of central pain modulation, salivary gland dysfunction, and alteration of oral mucosal blood flow have been proposed as possible etiologies [89, 90].

Clinical Presentation and Diagnostic Criteria

The pain of burning mouth syndrome is usually bilateral, recurring daily for more than 2 h per day over more than 3 months. The most common site for pain is the tip of the tongue, and it may be associated with dysesthesia, altered taste sensation, and/or subjective dryness of the mouth. Comorbid psychosocial and psychiatric disorders have been commonly reported in these patients [88, 89].

Oral mucosal diseases, such as herpes simplex and aphthous stomatitis, can often be associated with burning mouth pain. Other commonly associated conditions include psychiatric disorders, xerostomia (drug, connective tissue disease, or age related), nutritional deficiencies (vitamin B12, iron, folate, zinc, vitamin B6), allergic contact stomatitis, candidiasis, diabetes, denture-related pain, thyroid abnormalities, and menopause. These secondarily associated conditions should be ruled out before making the diagnosis of idiopathic burning mouth syndrome [90, 91].

The ICHD-3 has defined the following criteria for the clinical diagnosis of burning mouth syndrome [1]:

ICHD Criteria for Burning Mouth Syndrome
Burning Mouth Syndrome

A. Oral pain fulfilling criteria B and C.
B. Recurring daily for >2 h per day for >3 months.
C. Pain has both of the following characteristics:

1. Burning quality.
2. Felt superficially in the oral mucosa.

D. Oral mucosa is of normal appearance and clinical examination including sensory testing is normal.
E. Not better accounted for by another ICHD-3 diagnosis.

Management

In cases of burning mouth pain secondary to above-mentioned etiologies, treating the underlying cause usually results in the remission of the symptoms [91]. However, when no secondary cause of symptoms is found, the condition is considered idiopathic burning mouth syndrome. Research evidence providing guidance for the treatment of idiopathic burning mouth syndrome is limited. Based on the systematic review of several clinical trials, three interventions have shown a reduction in symptoms compared with placebo, including alpha-lipoic acid, clonazepam, and cognitive behavioral therapy. However, credibility of most these trials is limited by methodological errors, low quality, and greater bias risk; hence, caution and clinical judgment are warranted while interpreting results of these treatment trials [90]. On the basis of available date and our clinical practice, we recommend tricyclic antidepressants as first-line agents for the treatment of idiopathic burning mouth syndrome. Gabapentin, pregabalin, clonazepam, and alpha-lipoic acid are suitable alternatives for those intolerant/unresponsive to tricyclic antidepressants [89].

Pain

Introduction

Persistent idiopathic facial pain (previously known as atypical facial pain) is defined as persistent and recurrent facial and/or oral pain in the absence of clinical neurological deficit [1].

Epidemiology

The actual incidence and prevalence of persistent idiopathic facial pain are unknown, but the prevalence of orofacial pain has been estimated at 25% of the general population. Women are affected more commonly then men [92, 93].

Etiology

The exact etiology of persistent idiopathic facial pain is unknown. Although injury to the face, maxillae, teeth, or gums from minor procedures or trauma may trigger the pain; the symptoms usually persist even after healing of the presumed initial noxious trigger and without any demonstrable local cause. Psychogenic factors and peripheral nerve dysfunction have been proposed as possible etiologies, but such hypothesis lacks sufficient evidence at this time [92].

Clinical Presentation and Diagnostic Criteria

The pain is commonly described as dull, nagging, or aching and is usually located in the nasolabial fold or upper jaw and may spread to region of the eyes, nose, cheek, and temple. Patients experience daily recurrences, lasting more than 2 hours, over more than 3 months. It is often associated with comorbid chronic pain syndromes, irritable bowel syndrome, and various psychiatric and psychosocial disorders. Persistent idiopathic facial pain is mainly a diagnosis of exclusion [1, 92].

The ICHD-3 has defined the following criteria for the diagnosis of persistent idiopathic facial pain [1]:

ICHD Criteria for Persistent Idiopathic Facial Pain

Persistent Idiopathic Facial Pain

A. Facial and/or oral pain fulfilling criteria B and C.
B. Recurring daily for >2 h per day for >3 months.
C. Pain has both of the following characteristics:

1. Poorly localized and not following the distribution of a peripheral nerve.
2. Dull, aching, or nagging quality.

D. Clinical neurological examination is normal.
E. A dental cause has been excluded by appropriate investigations.
F. Not better accounted for by another ICHD-3 diagnosis.

Management

On the basis of available date and our clinical practice, we recommend tricyclic antidepressants as first-line agents for the treatment of persistent idiopathic facial pain. Gabapentin, pregabalin, and topiramate, with or without behavioral therapy, are suitable alternatives; however, clinicians should be aware of the fact that no Class I or Class II evidence is available for any of these treatments and further randomized controlled trials are needed [92].

Central Neuropathic Pain

Introduction

Central neuropathic pain is defined as unilateral or bilateral craniocervical pain, caused by lesions involving the central nervous system. The pain can have a variable presentation, depending on the cause; it may be constant or remitting and relapsing [1, 94].

Pathogenesis

The exact pathophysiology of central neuropathic pain is not entirely understood but may multiple mechanisms including central neuronal hyperexcitability, loss of inhibition, and alterations in the processing of incoming noxious and non-noxious stimuli [94–96].

Classification

The ICHD-3 classifies central neuropathic pain, on the basis of etiology, as central neuropathic pain attributed to multiple sclerosis or central poststroke pain [1].

Epidemiology, Etiology, and Clinical Presentation and Diagnostic Criteria

Central neuropathic pain attributed to multiple sclerosis is defined as a unilateral or bilateral craniocervical pain with variable presentation, attributed to a demyelinating lesion in the brain stem or ascending projections of the trigeminal nuclei in a person with multiple sclerosis. Its prevalence is estimated between 12% and 28% in multiple sclerosis patients; however, it rarely is the presenting symptoms of multiple sclerosis. The pain commonly remits and relapses, with or without sensory changes (usually dysesthesia but also hypoesthesia, anesthesia, hypoalgesia, paresthesia) but may be continuous in some cases [1, 97].

The ICHD-3 has defined the following criteria for the diagnosis of central neuropathic pain attributed to multiple sclerosis [1]:

ICHD Criteria for Central Neuropathic Pain Attributed to Multiple Sclerosis
Central Neuropathic Pain Attributed to Multiple Sclerosis

A. Facial and/or head pain fulfilling criterion C.
B. Multiple sclerosis (MS) has been diagnosed, with MRI demonstration of a demyelinating lesion in the brain stem or ascending projections of the trigeminal nuclei.
C. Pain has developed in temporal relation to the demyelinating lesion or led to its discovery.
D. Not better accounted for by another ICHD-3 diagnosis.

Central poststroke pain is defined as facial and/or head pain with varying presentations involving parts or the entire craniocervical region and associated with impaired sensation which occurs within 6 months of an ischemic or hemorrhagic stroke and is not explicable by a lesion involving peripheral trigeminal or other cranial or cervical nerves. The pain is unilateral and persistent in most of the cases and is seen in approximately 8% of poststroke patients. Central poststroke pain has varying characteristics, and the most commonly reported characters of pain include cramping, dysesthetic, hyperpathic (heightened response to noxious stimuli), allodynic, shooting/lancinating, and jabbing (pin/needles sensation) [94, 95].

Central poststroke pain is attributed to a lesion of the ascending projections of the trigeminal nuclei. Symptoms may also involve the trunk and limbs of the affected side, indicating possible involvement of cervical spinothalamic pathways and their cortical processing. The pain develops in about 8% of poststroke patients [1, 94].

The ICHD-3 has defined the following criteria for the diagnosis of central poststroke pain [1]:

ICHD Criteria for Central Poststroke Pain
Central Poststroke Pain

A. Facial and/or head pain fulfilling criterion C.
B. Ischemic or hemorrhagic stroke has occurred.
C. Evidence of causation demonstrated by both of the following:

1. Pain has developed within 6 months after the stroke.
2. Imaging (usually MRI) has demonstrated a vascular lesion in an appropriate site.

D. Not better accounted for by another ICHD-3 diagnosis.

Management

Amitriptyline (Class II, level B evidence from a double-blind, placebo-controlled crossover study) and **lamotrigine** (Class I, level B evidence from a double-blind, randomized, placebo-controlled crossover study and two case series) are first-line drugs for the treatment of central neuropathic pain. However, the prophylactic role of amitriptyline has been evaluated to be ineffective in preventing central poststroke pain in a double-blind, placebo-controlled study [94–96].

Dosing (orally):
Amitriptyline: Initial 25 mg daily may increase as tolerated to 75 mg daily.
Lamotrigine: Initial 25 mg daily may increase as tolerated to 200 mg daily.

Carbamazepine has been evaluated to be ineffective as monotherapy (Class II, level B evidence from a placebo-controlled crossover study); however, it may be used as adjuvant therapy if desired response is not achieved from recommended agents. Other alternative/adjuvant agents for the treatment of central neuropathic pain include gabapentin, pregabalin, and fluvoxamine; however, their efficacy has not been proven in clinical trials [95–97].

Conclusion

Cranial neuralgias are characterized by craniofacial pain of varying character and distribution and are usually associated with, at least, some neurologic symptoms/deficits.

Trigeminal neuralgia is the most common of all cranial neuralgias, and most cases are caused by compression of the trigeminal nerve root. The best initial approach for the management of trigeminal neuralgia is pharmacotherapy with carbamazepine being the most effective initial therapy. Most cases of glossopharyngeal neuralgia are idiopathic, but it can be caused by vascular compression of cranial nerves IX and X at the nerve root entry zone. Nervus intermedius neuralgia is classified into classic (mostly idiopathic) and secondary (caused by acute herpes zoster) types.

The medical management of glossopharyngeal and nervus intermedius neuralgias is essentially the same as for trigeminal neuralgia with carbamazepine being the initial drug of choice.

Greater or lesser occipital nerve block is the treatment (and also diagnostic test) of choice for occipital neuralgias. In patients with optic neuritis, treatment with intravenous steroids hastens recovery of vision and delays onset of MS but does not impact long-term visual function. For ischemic ocular motor nerve palsy, risk factor modification and treating the underlying etiologies is recommended.

Tricyclic antidepressants are the recommended first-line agents for treatment of idiopathic burning mouth syndrome.

Other rare chronic facial pain disorders and their initial treatments include recurrent painful ophthalmoplegic neuropathy (corticosteroids may be beneficial), Tolosa-Hunt syndrome (systemic corticosteroids), Raeder's syndrome (treating the underlying etiology), persistent idiopathic facial pain (tricyclic antidepressants), and central neuropathic pain (amitriptyline or lamotrigine). For all of these headache disorders, the history is key to determine the diagnosis and imaging, or other diagnostic tests may be indicated to rule out secondary causes.

References

1. Headache Classification Committee of the International Headache Society (IHS). The international classification of headache disorders, 3rd edition (beta version). Cephalalgia. 2013;33(9):629–808.
2. Cruccu G, et al. Trigeminal neuralgia: new classification and diagnostic grading for practice and research. Neurology. 2016;87(2):220–8.
3. Love S, Coakham HB. Trigeminal neuralgia: pathology and pathogenesis. Brain. 2001;124(Pt 12):2347–60.
4. Maarbjerg S, et al. Trigeminal neuralgia–a prospective systematic study of clinical characteristics in 158 patients. Headache. 2014;54(10):1574–82.
5. van Hecke O, et al. Neuropathic pain in the general population: a systematic review of epidemiological studies. Pain. 2014;155(4):654–62.
6. Katusic S, et al. Incidence and clinical features of trigeminal neuralgia, Rochester, Minnesota, 1945–1984. Ann Neurol. 1990;27(1):89–95.
7. Zhang J, et al. Non-antiepileptic drugs for trigeminal neuralgia. Cochrane Database Syst Rev. 2013;12:Cd004029.
8. Bowsher D. Trigeminal neuralgia: an anatomically oriented review. Clin Anat. 1997;10(6):409–15.
9. Sjaastad O, et al. Trigeminal neuralgia. Clinical manifestations of first division involvement. Headache. 1997;37(6):346–57.
10. Rasmussen P. Facial pain. III. A prospective study of the localization of facial pain in 1052 patients. Acta Neurochir. 1991;108(1–2):53–63.
11. Linskey ME, Jho HD, Jannetta PJ. Microvascular decompression for trigeminal neuralgia caused by vertebrobasilar compression. J Neurosurg. 1994;81(1):1–9.
12. Cheng TM, Cascino TL, Onofrio BM. Comprehensive study of diagnosis and treatment of trigemi-

nal neuralgia secondary to tumors. Neurology. 1993;43(11):2298–302.
13. Ildan F, et al. Isolated trigeminal neuralgia secondary to distal anterior inferior cerebellar artery aneurysm. Neurosurg Rev. 1996;19(1):43–6.
14. Figueiredo PC, et al. Arteriovenous malformation in the cerebellopontine angle presenting as trigeminal neuralgia. Arq Neuropsiquiatr. 1989;47(1):61–71.
15. Matthies C, Samii M. Management of 1000 vestibular schwannomas (acoustic neuromas): clinical presentation. Neurosurgery. 1997;40(1):1–9. discussion 9-10
16. Haddad FS, Taha JM. An unusual cause for trigeminal neuralgia: contralateral meningioma of the posterior fossa. Neurosurgery. 1990;26(6):1033–8.
17. Mohanty A, et al. Experience with cerebellopontine angle epidermoids. Neurosurgery. 1997;40(1):24–9. discussion 29-30
18. Leclercq D, Thiebaut JB, Heran F. Trigeminal neuralgia. Diagn Interv Imaging. 2013;94(10):993–1001.
19. Lazar ML, Kirkpatrick JB. Trigeminal neuralgia and multiple sclerosis: demonstration of the plaque in an operative case. Neurosurgery. 1979;5(6):711–7.
20. Jensen TS, Rasmussen P, Reske-Nielsen E. Association of trigeminal neuralgia with multiple sclerosis: clinical and pathological features. Acta Neurol Scand. 1982;65(3):182–9.
21. Moulin DE, Foley KM, Ebers GC. Pain syndromes in multiple sclerosis. Neurology. 1988;38(12):1830–4.
22. Coffey RJ, Fromm GH. Familial trigeminal neuralgia and Charcot-Marie-tooth neuropathy. Report of two families and review. Surg Neurol. 1991;35(1):49–53.
23. Chong VF. Trigeminal neuralgia in nasopharyngeal carcinoma. J Laryngol Otol. 1996;110(4):394–6.
24. Bornemann A, et al. Amyloidoma of the gasserian ganglion as a cause of symptomatic neuralgia of the trigeminal nerve: report of three cases. J Neurol. 1993;241(1):10–4.
25. Katsuno M, Teramoto A. Secondary trigeminal neuropathy and neuralgia resulting from pontine infarction. J Stroke Cerebrovasc Dis. 2010;19(3):251–2.
26. Saito N, et al. Intramedullary cavernous angioma with trigeminal neuralgia: a case report and review of the literature. Neurosurgery. 1989;25(1):97–101.
27. Nakamura K, Yamamoto T, Yamashita M. Small medullary infarction presenting as painful trigeminal sensory neuropathy. J Neurol Neurosurg Psychiatry. 1996;61(2):138.
28. Love S, Hilton DA, Coakham HB. Central demyelination of the Vth nerve root in trigeminal neuralgia associated with vascular compression. Brain Pathol. 1998;8(1):1–11. discussion 11-2
29. Hilton DA, et al. Pathological findings associated with trigeminal neuralgia caused by vascular compression. Neurosurgery. 1994;35(2):299–303. discussion 303
30. Braga FM, et al. Familial trigeminal neuralgia. Surg Neurol. 1986;26(4):405–8.
31. Dworkin RH, et al. Diagnosis and assessment of pain associated with herpes zoster and postherpetic neuralgia. J Pain. 2008;9(1 Suppl 1):S37–44.
32. Benoliel R, et al. Peripheral painful traumatic trigeminal neuropathy: clinical features in 91 cases and

proposal of novel diagnostic criteria. J Orofac Pain. 2012;26(1):49–58.

33. Lambru G, Matharu MS. SUNCT, SUNA and trigeminal neuralgia: different disorders or variants of the same disorder? Curr Opin Neurol. 2014;27(3):325–31.

34. Campbell FG, Graham JG, Zilkha KJ. Clinical trial of carbazepine (tegretol) in trigeminal neuralgia. J Neurol Neurosurg Psychiatry. 1966;29(3):265–7.

35. Rockliff BW, Davis EH. Controlled sequential trials of carbamazepine in trigeminal neuralgia. Arch Neurol. 1966;15(2):129–36.

36. Bennetto L, Patel NK, Fuller G. Trigeminal neuralgia and its management. BMJ. 2007;334(7586):201–5.

37. Gronseth G, et al. Practice parameter: the diagnostic evaluation and treatment of trigeminal neuralgia (an evidence-based review): report of the quality standards Subcommittee of the American Academy of neurology and the European Federation of Neurological Societies. Neurology. 2008;71(15):1183–90.

38. Nicol CF. A four year double-blind study of tegretol in facial pain. Headache. 1969;9(1):54–7.

39. Killian JM, Fromm GH. Carbamazepine in the treatment of neuralgia. Use of side effects. Arch Neurol. 1968;19(2):129–36.

40. Cruccu G, et al. AAN-EFNS guidelines on trigeminal neuralgia management. Eur J Neurol. 2008;15(10):1013–28.

41. Wiffen PJ, McQuay HJ, Moore RA. Carbamazepine for acute and chronic pain. Cochrane Database Syst Rev. 2005;3:Cd005451.

42. Beydoun A. Clinical use of tricyclic anticonvulsants in painful neuropathies and bipolar disorders. Epilepsy Behav. 2002;3s(3):S18–s22.

43. Sun D, et al. Association of HLA-B*1502 and *1511 allele with antiepileptic drug-induced Stevens-Johnson syndrome in Central China. J Huazhong Univ Sci Technolog Med Sci. 2014;34(1):146–50.

44. Fromm GH, Terrence CF, Chattha AS. Baclofen in the treatment of trigeminal neuralgia: double-blind study and long-term follow-up. Ann Neurol. 1984;15(3):240–4.

45. Zakrzewska JM, et al. Lamotrigine (lamictal) in refractory trigeminal neuralgia: results from a double-blind placebo controlled crossover trial. Pain. 1997;73(2):223–30.

46. Lunardi G, et al. Clinical effectiveness of lamotrigine and plasma levels in essential and symptomatic trigeminal neuralgia. Neurology. 1997;48(6):1714–7.

47. Lechin F, et al. Pimozide therapy for trigeminal neuralgia. Arch Neurol. 1989;46(9):960–3.

48. Fromm GH, Aumentado D, Terrence CF. A clinical and experimental investigation of the effects of tizanidine in trigeminal neuralgia. Pain. 1993;53(3):265–71.

49. Lindstrom P, Lindblom U. The analgesic effect of tocainide in trigeminal neuralgia. Pain. 1987;28(1):45–50.

50. Kondziolka D, et al. The effect of single-application topical ophthalmic anesthesia in patients with trigeminal neuralgia. A randomized double-blind placebo-controlled trial. J Neurosurg. 1994;80(6):993–7.

51. Sindrup SH, Jensen TS. Pharmacotherapy of trigeminal neuralgia. Clin J Pain. 2002;18(1):22–7.

52. Guardiani E, et al. A new treatment paradigm for trigeminal neuralgia using Botulinum toxin type a. Laryngoscope. 2014;124(2):413–7.

53. Wu CJ, et al. Botulinum toxin type a for the treatment of trigeminal neuralgia: results from a randomized, double-blind, placebo-controlled trial. Cephalalgia. 2012;32(6):443–50.

54. Barker FG 2nd, et al. The long-term outcome of microvascular decompression for trigeminal neuralgia. N Engl J Med. 1996;334(17):1077–83.

55. Flickinger JC, et al. Does increased nerve length within the treatment volume improve trigeminal neuralgia radiosurgery? A prospective double-blind, randomized study. Int J Radiat Oncol Biol Phys. 2001;51(2):449–54.

56. Katusic S, et al. Incidence and clinical features of glossopharyngeal neuralgia, Rochester, Minnesota, 1945–1984. Neuroepidemiology. 1991;10(5–6):266–75.

57. Rushton JG, Stevens JC, Miller RH. Glossopharyngeal (vagoglossopharyngeal) neuralgia: a study of 217 cases. Arch Neurol. 1981;38(4):201–5.

58. Resnick DK, et al. Microvascular decompression for glossopharyngeal neuralgia. Neurosurgery. 1995;36(1):64–8. discussion 68-9

59. Elias J, et al. Glossopharyngeal neuralgia associated with cardiac syncope. Arq Bras Cardiol. 2002;78(5):510–9.

60. Patel A, et al. Microvascular decompression in the management of glossopharyngeal neuralgia: analysis of 217 cases. Neurosurgery. 2002;50(4):705–10. discussion 710-1

61. Smith JH, et al. Triggerless neuralgic otalgia: a case series and systematic literature review. Cephalalgia. 2013;33(11):914–23.

62. Lee HL, et al. Clinical characteristics of headache or facial pain prior to the development of acute herpes zoster of the head. Clin Neurol Neurosurg. 2017;152:90–4.

63. Pulec JL. Geniculate neuralgia: long-term results of surgical treatment. Ear Nose Throat J. 2002;81(1):30–3.

64. Rupa V, Saunders RL, Weider DJ. Geniculate neuralgia: the surgical management of primary otalgia. J Neurosurg. 1991;75(4):505–11.

65. Lovely TJ, Jannetta PJ. Surgical management of geniculate neuralgia. Am J Otol. 1997;18(4):512–7.

66. Tang IP, et al. Geniculate neuralgia: a systematic review. J Laryngol Otol. 2014;128(5):394–9.

67. Dougherty C. Occipital neuralgia. Curr Pain Headache Rep. 2014;18(5):411.

68. Anthony M. Headache and the greater occipital nerve. Clin Neurol Neurosurg. 1992;94(4):297–301.

69. Jasper JF, Hayek SM. Implanted occipital nerve stimulators. Pain Physician. 2008;11(2):187–200.

70. Rodriguez M, et al. Optic neuritis: a population-based study in Olmsted County, Minnesota. Neurology. 1995;45(2):244–50.

71. Percy AK, Nobrega FT, Kurland LT. Optic neuritis and multiple sclerosis. An epidemiologic study. Arch Ophthalmol. 1972;87(2):135–9.

72. Roed H, et al. Systemic T-cell activation in acute clinically isolated optic neuritis. J Neuroimmunol. 2005;162(1–2):165–72.
73. The clinical profile of optic neuritis. Experience of the optic neuritis treatment trial. Optic neuritis study group. Arch Ophthalmol. 1991;109(12):1673–8.
74. Balcer LJ. Clinical practice. Optic neuritis. N Engl J Med. 2006;354(12):1273–80.
75. Toosy AT, Mason DF, Miller DH. Optic neuritis. Lancet Neurol. 2014;13(1):83–99.
76. Wilker SC, et al. Pain in ischemic ocular motor cranial nerve palsies. Br J Ophthalmol. 2009;93(12):1657–9.
77. Jacobson DM, McCanna TD, Layde PM. Risk factors for ischemic ocular motor nerve palsies. Arch Ophthalmol. 1994;112(7):961–6.
78. Berlit P. Isolated and combined pareses of cranial nerves III, IV and VI. A retrospective study of 412 patients. J Neurol Sci. 1991;103(1):10–5.
79. Rush JA, Younge BR. Paralysis of cranial nerves III, IV, and VI. Cause and prognosis in 1,000 cases. Arch Ophthalmol. 1981;99(1):76–9.
80. Gelfand AA, et al. Ophthalmoplegic "migraine" or recurrent ophthalmoplegic cranial neuropathy: new cases and a systematic review. J Child Neurol. 2012;27(6):759–66.
81. Lance JW, Zagami AS. Ophthalmoplegic migraine: a recurrent demyelinating neuropathy? Cephalalgia. 2001;21(2):84–9.
82. McMillan HJ, et al. Ophthalmoplegic migraine: inflammatory neuropathy with secondary migraine? Can J Neurol Sci. 2007;34(3):349–55.
83. Cakirer S. MRI findings in Tolosa-hunt syndrome before and after systemic corticosteroid therapy. Eur J Radiol. 2003;45(2):83–90.
84. La Mantia L, et al. Tolosa-hunt syndrome: critical literature review based on IHS 2004 criteria. Cephalalgia. 2006;26(7):772–81.
85. Iaconetta G, et al. Tolosa-hunt syndrome extending in the cerebello-pontine angle. Cephalalgia. 2005;25(9):746–50.
86. Solomon S, Lustig JP. Benign Raeder's syndrome is probably a manifestation of carotid artery disease. Cephalalgia. 2001;21(1):1–11.
87. Ikeuchi T, et al. Progression of cluster headache to Raeder's syndrome with marked response to corticosteroid therapy: a case report. Rinsho Shinkeigaku. 2005;45(4):321–3.
88. Bergdahl M, Bergdahl J. Burning mouth syndrome: prevalence and associated factors. J Oral Pathol Med. 1999;28(8):350–4.
89. Patton LL, et al. Management of burning mouth syndrome: systematic review and management recommendations. Oral Surg Oral Med Oral Pathol Oral Radiol Endod. 2007;103(Suppl):S39.e1–13.
90. Zakrzewska JM, Forssell H, Glenny AM. Interventions for the treatment of burning mouth syndrome. Cochrane Database Syst Rev. 2005;1:Cd002779.
91. Evans RW, Drage LA. Burning mouth syndrome. Headache. 2005;45(8):1079–81.
92. Sardella A, et al. An up-to-date view on persistent idiopathic facial pain. Minerva Stomatol. 2009;58(6):289–99.
93. Manzoni GC, Torelli P. Epidemiology of typical and atypical craniofacial neuralgias. Neurol Sci. 2005;26(Suppl 2):s65–7.
94. Nicholson BD. Evaluation and treatment of central pain syndromes. Neurology. 2004;62(5 Suppl 2):S30–6.
95. Kim JS. Pharmacological management of central post-stroke pain: a practical guide. CNS Drugs. 2014;28(9):787–97.
96. Kumar B, et al. Central poststroke pain: a review of pathophysiology and treatment. Anesth Analg. 2009;108(5):1645–57.
97. Nurmikko TJ, Gupta S, Maclver K. Multiple sclerosis-related central pain disorders. Curr Pain Headache Rep. 2010;14(3):189–95.

CDH in Pediatric and Adolescent Patients

10

Andrew D. Hershey and Shannon Babineau

Introduction

Headache is a common complaint in children. It is one of the primary reasons for visits to the pediatrician and emergency room as either a problem by itself or as a symptomatic feature of another disease process. Headache is often a symptom of infection and usually resolves with effective treatment [1, 2]. However, a significant portion of the pediatric population suffers with recurrent headache. These episodic, recurrent headaches and its associated features should then be considered a primary headache disorder. Primary headache disorders, like migraine and tension-type headache, occur in all ages but increase in frequency as children age. Epidemiologic data shows that migraine occurs in 1.2–3.2% of 3–7-year-olds, 4–11% of 7–11-year-olds, and in 8–23% of those aged 15 [3]. The epidemiology of tension-type headache is more variable, secondary to differences in populations, study design methods, and inclusion of migraine, but studies show it to be present in 10–72% of the pediatric population [4]. To address some of these variations, the latest version of the International Classification of Headache Disorders (ICHD) [8] specifies that all headache types should be classified but that if a diagnosis of migraine is suspected for any of the headaches, the migraine diagnosis should trump classification as tension-type headache. Historically, this variation in nomenclature has made comparisons and conclusions difficult, and this chapter will include the original authors' nomenclature but in general chronic headaches and chronic daily headaches (CDH) can be equated to chronic migraine (CM), although it can sometimes include chronic tension-type headaches (CTTH).

When headaches become frequent, they have been generically called "chronic daily headaches" (CDH). CDH are broadly defined as 15 headache days per month for at least 3 months. It should be defined by the predominant primary headache semiology. Although CDH may only occur in 1% of children and adolescents, they make up a large portion of patients seen in specialty clinics [5]. Chronic pain in children causes significant disability and not only impacts their lives but the lives of their caregivers [6, 7]. In addition, it is very challenging to treat chronic pain, and while there have been some recent high-quality studies on treatment methods, evidence-based data and guidance are lacking for these patients.

CDH in children and adolescents is divided into the same categories as adults with the primary headache driving the nosology (i.e., when the headaches have a migraine phenotype at least some of the time, they should be called chronic

A. D. Hershey (✉)
Department of Pediatrics, Division of Neurology, Cincinnati Children's Hospital Medical Center, University of Cincinnati College of Medicine, Cincinnati, OH, USA
e-mail: andrew.hershey@cchmc.org

S. Babineau
Pediatrics, Goryeb Children's Hospital, Morristown, NJ, USA

migraine (CM), while if they lack this phenotype completely and meet the features of tension-type headache, they should be called chronic tension-type headache (CTTH)). In addition to CM and CTTH, children may have new daily persistent headache (NDPH) and hemicrania continua. Hemicrania continua is rare in children and will not be reviewed in this chapter. The ICHD-3 suggests that migraine in children and adolescents may differ slightly from adults, headaches may be of shorter duration, and location may be more likely frontotemporal. The onset of an attack is often more rapid. In addition, parental observation may play a role in identifying associated features [8]. At this time there is insufficient data to support that there is need for a different classification syndrome. Although knowing that there are some differences in presentation in children, it would be interesting to continue to pursue the possible need for modifications to the criteria for CM, CTTH, and NDPH for children.

Epidemiology

The prevalence of CDH in two population-based studies of adolescents was shown to be 1.5–1.7% [9, 10]. There is less known about CDH in those younger than 12 years. One large headache center reported that over a 6-year period, 4.8% of their patients were children under 6 years with daily headache [11]. Arruda et al. also looked specifically at a population-based sample of children between 5 and 12 years and identified that 1.68% had CDH [12].

The adult prevalence of CM is about 2–3% of the population. In a large population survey of adolescents, CM was identified in 0.79% not including those with medication-overuse headaches (MOH) and 1.75% if MOH was included [13]. This data has been supported by other population-based studies showing rates of 1.5% [14] in Turkish adolescents and a slightly lower rate in a Norwegian population of 0.8% [15]. CM, like in adults, is more likely to be an issue for girls than boys than the other subtypes of CDH [16]. CM also carries the highest disability of all the subtypes of CDH [15] and is more

likely to be associated with medication overuse than other types [16], although MOH is less likely to be an issue in adolescents than in the adult population.

Rates of CTTH have been identified as around 0.1–5.9% [4]. There are no large population studies for NDPH. In studies that look at the percent of each subtype in children/adolescents with CDH, CM is shown to be the most common. However, a relatively higher percent of the adolescent population versus the adult population has CTTH or NDPH. NDPH is the second most common CDH type in adolescents [17–19]. NDPH occurs in 1.7–10.8% of adults with daily headaches, and in those under 18 years, it occurs in 13–35% of those with daily headaches [19].

Risk Factors for Chronification/ Progression

Most children with CDH (80%) have transformed from episodic headache [20]. This happens, on average, over about 2 years from onset of headaches [21]. With any progression of headache frequency, secondary causes certainly need to be ruled out. There are also some conditions that increase the risk of the transformation from episodic to chronic. Lu showed in 63 kids with CDH independent risk factors for CDH including female gender, family financial distress, obesity, higher-frequency headache at baseline, and baseline diagnosis of migraine [22].

Medication overuse is one reason adults with episodic headaches, particularly migraine, progress to CM. MOH is less common in children and adolescents than adults, but it still represents an issue and a risk factor for progression to CM [9]. In a patient with CDH, particularly relatively new onset, it is important to ask about frequency of use of pain relieving medication including over-the-counter agents and dietary caffeine. Identifying overuse of medication and counseling about MOH can result in a significant decrease in headache frequency. Hering-Hanit et al. showed that cessation of overused medications completely stopped headaches in 20 out of

26 pediatric patients with CDH and MOH and reduced the frequency significantly in another 5 children [23].

Family history of headaches seems to be associated with CM and less likely to be a factor in those with NDPH [16]. Frequency of headaches in the mother can predict the frequency of headaches in her children; when a mother has CDH, the risk of CDH in her children increases by almost 13-fold [24]. It is unknown if this is a genetic contribution of frequency, shared environment, or co-dependence.

The relationship between psychiatric comorbidities and CDH in children is less clear, with some studies showing rates that are equal to the general population and other showing rates that are much higher. In a study of children under 6 years of age with CDH, authors identified psychiatric comorbidity in 80% of the kids including anxiety, adjustment disorder, sleep disorders, and hyperactivity [11]. In Taiwanese adolescents with CDH, not followed at a headache clinic, 47% were identified as having at least one psychiatric comorbidity. The two most common comorbidities were depression (21%) and panic disorder (19%). Interestingly, there was a stronger association with depression and suicidal risk in those with migraine with aura [25]. In a separate study in a pediatric headache clinic population, of those with daily headache, about 30% met criteria for a psychiatric disorder. This number was similar to general population rate of 36% in children and adolescents [26], although those with psychiatric comorbidity did have increased disability from migraine. A different study also looking at pediatric patients from a headache center showed that there was a higher percentage of CDH sufferers with clinically significant anxiety than population norms (11% vs. 5%), but this did not occur with depression. Most children/adolescents with CDH did not have clinically significant depression (93%) or anxiety (88.7%) [27]. In a study of children with migraine, CM, and controls, the children with CM had significantly higher scores on social anxiety inventories [28].

Adult data shows that childhood abuse and PTSD are risk factors for CM; however it is unclear if this is a later effect or if the onset of daily headache occurs while the child is still under 18 years. A limited set of a long-term longitudinal study on children of abuse did not see an increased risk of CM. Conversely, in one study of children and adolescents, the rate of child abuse was 6.5% which is significantly higher than the rate in the general population (0.012%) [29, 30].

Mild traumatic brain injury and its short- and long-term effects on brain health are increasingly being recognized in the lay and medical population. The majority of children who suffer a concussion will recover in a few weeks, but a significant minority will have symptoms persisting beyond 3 months. Headache is the most common symptom of concussion, and in one longitudinal study of children presenting with concussion, 7.8% had persisting headaches after 3 months with about 50% of those patients having daily headache [31].

Impact

Daily headache impacts not only the child but also the family. The Pediatric Migraine Disability Assessment (PedMIDAS) is a validated questionnaire for children and adolescents to help assess disability from migraine. PedMIDAS has three significant domains—impact on school, home, and social functioning – and is helpful for tracking success/worsening over time in a clinic population [5]. It is important to focus beyond just school days missed because of headache but also on days present at school with pain where the child cannot function optimally. Children that attend school with pain often struggle with focus and attention. In a study of functional ability at school, children with CM were shown to have significantly increased struggles compared to healthy children [7], and in a study of children with CDH, half reported that school performance was influenced moderately (48%) or severely (21%) by their headaches [9].

Often during periods of more intense pain, the child or adolescent will miss school, which leads to a disruption in their education. The missed school can also cause a vicious cycle of falling behind and increased stress about catching up, all leading to amplification of symptoms and worsened disability from the headaches. There are some children whose headaches, and the subsequent disruption they cause, make them stop attending school altogether. This withdrawal from the regular schedule of the day as well as socialization with peers leads to further disability, depression, and worsening of lifestyle habits. The impact in these circumstances extends beyond the child to impact caregivers as well, who not only have to watch the child suffer with pain but have to cope with disruption in their own lives as they have to stay home from work to attend to the child and accompany him/her to doctor's visits.

Treatment

The majority of patients suffering with CDH do not seek treatment right away, and when they do seek treatment, they often do not see a neurologist [32], meaning that this population of patients is tremendously underserved.

Treatment of chronic pain has to have a different focus than treatment of episodic pain. When headache is only a few days a month, it is helpful to keep track of the circumstances under which the headache occurs. While triggers are notoriously inaccurate and inconsistent, awareness of possible triggers can help modify certain daily activities and focus on adoption of healthy lifestyle habits including adequate hydration, exercise, healthy eating, and regular, adequate sleep. Patients with migraine are encouraged to be treated early in the attack. However, when pain is daily, it may be difficult to identify a beginning, especially when continuous. In these instances, advice to treat at the beginning of an attack or at the onset of worsening on three specific school days (Monday, Wednesday, and Friday) can simplify the treatment regimen and improve compliance while avoiding medication-overuse headache.

It is important that the child and caregivers are ready to treat the child for the pain, rather than continue to spend efforts finding a "cause" or overly worry about specific triggers. Patients

and caregivers should be confident of the diagnosis through appropriate history and any testing to ensure there isn't a secondary cause of the headaches. This may be accomplished through a detailed explanation of the differences among common etiologies of chronic and acute pain. They should be educated that pain is a signal that usually identifies when something is wrong with the body, but in chronic pain the body has started to misinterpret those pain signals making it think there is something causing pain even when there is not. Caregivers and patients should be prepared that many of the treatment methods are going to ask them to work with some degree of discomfort. It's also important to ensure them that they will not have to go through this process alone and that the goal is to manage and function with the pain, rather than eliminate it. They need to feel that they can control how they perceive the pain and how they let the pain affect their lives. And, rather than feeling that there is nothing that can be done to cure the pain, they should learn to focus on the power of positive, active, and internally motivated solutions to live, despite the pain.

The beginning goal of CDH management is to help a child or adolescent assume some semblance of normalcy in their daily life. Chronic pain is exhausting, and while it is best for a child to maintain a normal schedule attending school and participating in activities after school, they are unlikely to be able to maintain the breakneck pace that many children keep up. They may be able to participate in one after school activity, but not multiple ones. This is further complicated by the observation that many of these children and adolescents are overachievers with a degree of anxiety about their immediate and long-term success. Taking care of one's body and mental health become priorities. Sleep needs to be emphasized as does making time to relax/destress, including unstructured time as well as fitting in some physical exercise. It is also helpful to establish a relationship with the school, making sure they understand the child's needs. It is helpful to work with the school and caregivers to create reasonable accommodations, particularly in those children with high-frequency absences, to help the child be successful academically.

As with most conditions in pediatrics, there is insufficient research done on interventional treatments for migraine, let alone CM and other subtypes of CDH. There have been a few papers in the past 10 years that have started to work on identifying approaches, but there is still a lack of guidance, although the inclusion of cognitive behavioral therapy (CBT) should be considered an essential component of treatment. In general, it is best to break treatment modalities into lifestyle modifications, non-medication-based therapies, and medications. The children that do the best employ treatments from all categories. It is helpful to think of all components of treatment to be part of a multidisciplinary, multimodality treatment plan with no one treatment or therapy that is going to be 100% effective. Also, it is important to emphasize that therapies will need to be tried for an adequate time period. Often it has taken at least a year to reach a point of daily pain and longer still to seek the advice of a physician, so the pain is not going to resolve overnight. Setting expectations with the family and patient of a slow steady improvement will help avoid giving up on effective therapies too soon. It is also helpful not to be prescriptive, because there is not overwhelming evidence that any one method of treatment is the best and having the family and older children/adolescents help guide which therapies they want to start with will improve compliance.

Lifestyle Modifications

There is only a modest amount of data about use of lifestyle measures in treatment of CDH, but the general consensus in reports on CDH in children and adolescents is that there are certain behaviors that are better for chronic pain than others. One of the biggest areas of focus is on sleep and sleep hygiene. There is often a significant issue with sleep deprivation in children and adolescents. About 70% of adolescents do not get the recommended 8–10 h of sleep that is needed [33]. This is because of the teenager's natural tendency to phase shift to later bedtimes/later wake times compounded by early school start times. This has been recognized by the Center for Disease Control (CDC) but remains inadequately addressed by states and school systems. Also, there is frequent practice of sacrificing sleep to allow more time to do homework or extracurricular activities. It is often unfathomable to teenagers, and their caregivers, that sleep may need to take priority over after school activities including homework. It may be helpful to review that studies show those with more sleep do better in athletic competitions and academically than those with less sleep [34, 35]. In addition, it is helpful to emphasize that those with chronic pain often need more sleep to feel rested and the quality of sleep with chronic pain can be lower, meaning longer nighttime stretches and dedicated sleep are important [36]. It is helpful to review the sleep requirements based on age with the family, as there are many young children who are getting insufficient sleep (National Sleep Foundation Sleep Poll 2014 [37]). Then, some time spent on sleep hygiene with take home resources can help start the family in the right direction. Also, if sleep is a big struggle for the patient, you may need to look into sleep disorders, like sleep apnea, which occur more commonly in migraine sufferers [38–40].

It is important for chronic pain sufferers to ensure that they are eating regularly, as skipping meals is one of the more reproducible triggers for migraine. Patients with CDH should not be skipping meals and should try to eat regular protein with each meal. Caregivers should ensure that the child/adolescent is actually eating the lunch provided to them and that they have access to a snack if needed. Also, children should have adequate hydration, particularly in children that are also suffering with dizziness. Intake should approximate one cup of liquid for each year of age with additional cups when the child participates in physical activity. It is important to review caffeine use in all children. Often people do not realize that the iced tea or the soda they are drinking contains caffeine, and subsequently there are some children who intake a fair amount of daily caffeine. This high rate of caffeine intake can lead to medication-overuse headache [41] and worsen dehydration, as caffeine is a natural diuretic.

In addition to these lifestyle measures, high-frequency exercise is also helpful. Exercise is excellent as a stress reliever and can help with mood and sleep difficulties. The tendency in children with chronic pain is to stop moving because it can make pain worse; however this will only lead to deconditioning and worsening of the pain as well as amplify mood symptoms and worsen symptoms of fatigue and dizziness. CDH is a pain amplification syndrome, and other pain amplification syndromes like fibromyalgia and amplified musculoskeletal pain respond very well to physical activity. In the beginning, patients may not be able to work to a full aerobic level and may need to use lower impact activities to avoid aggravating head pain with bouncing. Activities that combine some posture and core strengthening as well as low impact aerobics can be very helpful. Physical therapy may be beneficial to get people started, particularly those who are very disabled or who have not done a lot of sports/activities in the past. Physical therapy can help them feel safe in an observed environment, but the goal should be to help set up a home regimen that can be continued long term [36].

Non-medication Therapies

Addressing stress as well as identifying and managing the mood comorbidities in CDH is very important. It is helpful to have a mental health professional assess the patient with CDH at least once to help identify comorbid psychiatric issues and screen for PTSD and trauma. Although this rarely reaches the level of a disease state, it may be a contributing comorbidity. Many of the non-medication-based therapies do focus on both pain and stress reduction. These methods are some of the best studied, with the best evidence. However, they are significantly underused.

One of the most effective treatments for CDH in children is cognitive behavioral therapy (CBT). CBT is helpful in teaching the patient to take control over and stop catastrophizing the pain. It can also be effective in helping with anxi-ety issues that amplify or trigger headaches [42]. Powers et al. randomized children between 10 and 17 years old with CM to amitriptyline plus CBT or amitriptyline with regular headache education. There was a significant reduction in headache days (average decrease of 11 days in CBT group vs. 6 days in medication alone group) and disability in the children provided with CBT and amitriptyline [43].

There are many barriers to the use of CBT. There is often a negative perception associated with going to see a therapist. Emphasizing that this is behavioral medicine and not a mental health issue in which the child or adolescent is using their own brain power to control their behavioral response to pain can be quite successful in persuading the family of its usefulness. CBT can be thought of as a method of coping with pain and the impact of chronic pain on one's life regardless of whether it has affected mental health or not [44]. Many patients struggle to find a practitioner that is familiar with CBT that accepts insurance or who can see new patients in a timely fashion. In addition, there are even fewer available CBT practitioners that are familiar with the use of CBT for pain management. However, many CBT practitioners are open to the use of CBT for pain after a conversation with the treating practitioner who can familiarize them with the concept of using it for pain. Some programs have designed online–/computer-based CBT, and while this certainly needs further study and standardization, this option would likely greatly improve compliance and provide a more readily accessible service.

Other less rigorously studied non-medication options that can also be helpful in the management of CDH include biofeedback, mindfulness meditation, and acupuncture [45–49].

Medication

The use of medication can be effective in the management of CM, although the effect may be largely driven by the placebo response and the expectation of benefit. The management of

CTTH and NDPH has a true dearth of information in the pediatric literature. Many of the same medications used for migraine are used in these conditions, but there are not specific recommendations in management, so the below discussion will focus on CM. In addition, a recent seminal paper of randomized 361 children and adolescents with migraine (a portion of which had CM, but not continuous headache) to treatment with either amitriptyline, topiramate, or placebo showed no difference in outcomes between the three groups, and those treated with medication had more adverse events, leading to early termination of the study [50]. It is important to note that this was not due to a lack of efficacy; it was due to the fact that all arms, including the placebo arm, were very effective. This called into question whether there is a role for medication at all in treatment of CM. Most practitioners would agree this study highlighted that medication should not be the sole or go-to treatment, but likely there is still benefit in some patients. It is also very likely that the method of presentation and allowing the child or adolescent to choose can enhance the expectation of response and ultimately a superior outcome. Trying to understand what type of patient, and at what point in the course of treatment medication should be offered, is certainly a large question that needs to be answered.

Medication can be broken down into rescue and preventive. Typically, most of the focus in CDH is placed on preventive therapy. The medications used for adults, topiramate, propranolol, valproate, and amitriptyline, are the medications also typically used in children. None of these medications have US FDA approval for use in pediatrics for CM; however topiramate does have FDA approval for use in episodic migraine in teenagers (age 12–17 years old). Propranolol and topiramate are used in very young children for other conditions, and there are studies in episodic migraine, so there are dosing guidelines for a variety of weights. Propranolol must be used with caution as it can exacerbate asthma and oftentimes can make children and adolescents feel depressed, worsening this anxiety and depression of CM. Valproate is also used in all ages of children for other indications, with caution in those under 2 years of age and with studies for episodic migraine to guide dosing. There is not high utility of the tricyclic antidepressants in those under the age of 5, so typically this is listed as a lower age cut point; however this has also been studied widely in migraine, so dosing is available for those over that age [5]. If preventive medicine is deemed appropriate, a review of the side effect profile, with attention to a child's comorbid conditions that may be made worse/better, should be taken into consideration. Also, in younger children, the method of administration should also be taken into account, as some medications come in a liquid or sprinkle, making it easier to take if pills cannot be swallowed. OnabotulinumtoxinA, in a single study for CM in 45 children, showed a change from severe to moderate disability, a statistical drop in headache frequency from 27 days to 21 days/month. It was well tolerated [51]. There was one other series of ten patients aged 11–17 years with medically refractory daily headache. Forty percent had subjective but meaningful relief (decreased intensity and some had decrease in frequency) and improved quality of life after repeated administration of onabotulinumtoxinA [52]. While there certainly needs to be more research in this population, if a patient can tolerate the injections, it is worth considering.

The supplements such as magnesium, butterbur, coenzyme q10, vitamin B2, and melatonin do not have any studies for use in CDHs in children. However, they are safe and are often well tolerated. It is reasonable to try them either as a first-line treatment while other lifestyle habits and/or biobehavioral methods are being established or as an add-on to the medication to help with overall percent reduction in pain and severity [53].

Rescue medicine can provide some benefit for breakthrough pain. NSAIDS and acetaminophen are used frequently in the pediatric population and can be used in this setting. Guidance on appropriate dosing should be reviewed, recognizing that over-the-counter directions often underdose children. Some of the triptans have US FDA approval for episodic migraine in the pediatric population including rizatriptan for those older than 6 years and zolmitriptan/almotriptan and combined sumatriptan/naproxen for those over 12 years. There are a few ways to use rescue medicine in those with daily headache. Many patients with CDH will have days where the pain is more intense. In this instance, they can be instructed to use the rescue medication as soon as the escalation of pain can be recognized. Or, if it is related to a certain environmental factor that can be predicted (a menstrual period or change in the weather) as associated with more intense headache, when that trigger has occurred, the patient is instructed to use the rescue medicine as soon as pain begins. The patient can use the medication on days where the pain is likely to be disruptive, like a day when there is a test at school or an anticipated social event. Continued counseling on avoiding MOH should be provided at every visit.

Additional Interventions

Nerve blocks have been used in children with CDH and can be used in different ways. They can help as a bridge therapy to mitigate pain as a person is trying to discontinue an overused medication. In addition, during periods of worsening, they can help more immediately than preventive therapies to mitigate an attack. Gelfand et al. found that on a retrospective chart review of 46 patients under 18 with a CDH syndrome and tenderness over the greater occipital nerve (CM, NDPH) who received a onetime treatment of greater occipital nerve blockade, 53% benefitted from it, of which those 52% benefitted significantly. The treatment typically helped for about 5.4 weeks and seemed to be more effective in CM [54]. Some people do use repetitive nerve blocks over time as management for CDH [55].

Hospitalizations for repetitive dihydroergotamine have been used for migraine in children, typically to help periods of status migrainosus or also to help in bridging off overused medications [56]. It can be considered as an option, particularly for children that are severely disabled and missing school secondary to CM.

Prognosis

There are some long-term follow-up studies of children with CDH that in general are positive. In most studies over time, the headaches become less frequent, and the percentage of children/adolescents/young adults still suffering with high-frequency or chronic pain dramatically improves over a 5–10-year period.

In a study of 103 children/adolescents with daily headaches followed over 8 years, 12% still met criteria for CDH, with CM as the most common subtype. The presence of migraine at baseline predicted poorer outcome as well as CDH onset at <13 years, duration of more than 2 years, and presence of medication overuse. While only 11% had no headaches at the long-term follow-up point, the majority only had episodic headaches [32].

Another study with a 4-year follow-up of children with CDH showed that 29% were headache-free. The others still had headaches, but 60% had improvement in frequency of attacks. The presence of a psychiatric disorder at the first-time point was related to persistence of headaches as was the total number of psychiatric disorders per patient [57].

Conclusion

CDH affects those of all ages, including those in their preschool years. CDH causes disability and impacts families in the same way it does for the adult population. There is significant overlap in the treatments used for this population and the adult CDH population partly because the lack of specific studies in children has led to extrapolation from adult data and also because many of the adult measures seem to work in pediatrics. Of note, the data that is specific to childhood CDH points away from use of medication and encourages practitioners to emphasize non-medication approaches. With the advent of newer, migraine-specific drugs, this will need to be reevaluated.

These youngest patients may represent those with the highest penetrance of a genetic predisposition to headache, and it is helpful to identify them and involve them in research about the underlying pathophysiology of headache as well as mechanisms for high frequency/CDH. It is also important to involve children in therapeutic trials, to help identify mechanisms that can help with treatment and possibly reverse the course of what can be a very disabling condition.

While most children with CDH will "outgrow" the high-frequency nature, the majority will still have episodic headaches. The hope is that by identifying and educating these children early, one can help modify the course of the disease. Hopefully the burden of the disease can be lessened, impacting not only the individual's life but lessening the lifelong impact migraine and other CDHs have on the economic and health-care system.

References

1. Conicella E, et al. The child with headache in a pediatric emergency department. Headache. 2008;48(7):1005–11.
2. Gelfand AA, Goadsby PJ. Treatment of pediatric migraine in the emergency room. Pediatr Neurol. 2012;47(4):233–41.
3. Lewis DW. Pediatric migraine. Pediatr Rev. 2007;28:43–53.
4. Seshia SS, Abu-Arafeh I, Hershey AD. Tension-type headache in children: the Cinderella of headache disorders! Can J Neurol Sci. 2009;36(6):687–95.
5. Özge A, Yalın OÖ. Chronic migraine in children and adolescents. Curr Pain Headache Rep. 2016;20:14.
6. Perquin CW, et al. Pain in children and adolescents: a common experience. Pain. 2000;87(1):51–8.
7. Kashikar-Zuck S, et al. Quality of life and emotional functioning in youth with chronic migraine and juvenile fibromyalgia. Clin J Pain. 2013;29(12):1066–72.
8. Headache Classification Committee of the International Headache Society (IHS). The international classification of headache disorders. 3rd ed (beta version). Cephalalgia. 2013;33(9):629–808.
9. Wang S-J, et al. Chronic daily headache in adolescents prevalence, impact, and medication overuse. Neurology. 2006;66(2):193–7.
10. Arruda MA, et al. Primary headaches in childhood–a population-based study. Cephalalgia. 2010;30(9):1056–64.
11. Raieli V, et al. Recurrent and chronic headaches in children below 6 years of age. J Headache Pain. 2005;6(3):135–42.
12. Arruda MA, et al. Frequent headaches in the preadolescent pediatric population a population-based study. Neurology. 2010;74(11):903–8.
13. Lipton RB, et al. Prevalence and burden of chronic migraine in adolescents: results of the chronic daily headache in adolescents study (C-dAS). Headache. 2011;51(5):693–706.
14. Özge A, et al. The prevalence of chronic and episodic migraine in children and adolescents. Eur J Neurol. 2013;20(1):95–101.
15. Krogh A-B, Larsson B, Linde M. Prevalence and disability of headache among Norwegian adolescents: a cross-sectional school-based study. Cephalalgia. 2015;35(13):1181–91.
16. Cuvellier J-C, et al. Chronic daily headache in French children and adolescents. Pediatr Neurol. 2008;38(2):93–8.
17. Kung E, et al. New daily persistent headache in the paediatric population. Cephalalgia. 2009;29(1):17–22.
18. Bigal ME, et al. Primary chronic daily headache and its subtypes in adolescents and adults. Neurology. 2004;63(5):843–7.
19. Baron EP, David Rothner A. New daily persistent headache in children and adolescents. Curr Neurol Neurosci Rep. 2010;10(2):127–32.
20. Seshia SS, et al. Chronic daily headache in children and adolescents: a multi-faceted syndrome. Can J Neurol Sci. 2010;37(6):769–78.
21. Koenig MA, et al. Chronic daily headache in children and adolescents presenting to tertiary headache clinics. Headache. 2002;42(6):491–500.
22. Lu S-R, et al. Incidence and risk factors of chronic daily headache in young adolescents: a school cohort study. Pediatrics. 2013;132(1):e9–e16.
23. Hering-Hanit R, Cohen A, Horev Z. Successful withdrawal from analgesic abuse in a group of youngsters with chronic daily headache. J Child Neurol. 2001;16(6):448–9.
24. Arruda MA, et al. Frequency of headaches in children is influenced by headache status in the mother. Headache. 2010;50(6):973–80.
25. Wang S-J, et al. Psychiatric comorbidity and suicide risk in adolescents with chronic daily headache. Neurology. 2007;68(18):1468–73.
26. Slater SK, et al. Psychiatric comorbidity in pediatric chronic daily headache. Cephalalgia. 2012;32(15):1116–22.
27. Rousseau-Salvador C, et al. Anxiety, depression and school absenteeism in youth with chronic or episodic headache. Pain Res Manag. 2014;19(5):235–40.
28. Masruha MR, et al. Social anxiety score is high in adolescents with chronic migraine. Pediatr Int. 2012;54(3):393–6.
29. Zafar M, et al. Childhood abuse in pediatric patients with chronic daily headache. Clin Pediatr. 2012;51(6):590–3.
30. Juang KD, et al. Association between adolescent chronic daily headache and childhood adversity: a community-based study. Cephalalgia. 2004;24(1):54–9.

31. Kuczynski A, et al. Characteristics of post-traumatic headaches in children following mild traumatic brain injury and their response to treatment: a prospective cohort. Dev Med Child Neurol. 2013;55(7):636–41.

32. Wang S-J, Fuh J-L, Shiang-Ru L. Chronic daily headache in adolescents an 8-year follow-up study. Neurology. 2009;73(6):416–22.

33. CDC website: "Teen Sleep Habits" Found February 2018 https://www.cdc.gov/media/subtopic/matte/pdf/2011/teen_sleep.pdf.

34. Copenhaver EA, Diamond AB. The value of sleep on athletic performance, injury, and recovery in the young athlete. Pediatr Ann. 2017;46(3):e106–11.

35. Shochat T, Cohen-Zion M, Tzischinsky O. Functional consequences of inadequate sleep in adolescents: a systematic review. Sleep Med Rev. 2014;18(1):75–87.

36. Friedrichsdorf SJ, et al. Chronic pain in children and adolescents: diagnosis and treatment of primary pain disorders in head, abdomen, muscles and joints. Children. 2016;3(4):42.

37. National Sleep Foundation. 2014 Sleep in America® Poll–sleep in the modern family. [Online at: https://sleepfoundation.org/sites/default/files/2014-NSF-Sleep-in-America-poll-summary-of-findings---FINAL-Updated-3-26-14-.pdf] Accessed 5 Mar 2018.

38. Freedom T. Headaches and sleep disorders. Dis Mon. 2015;61(6):240–8.

39. Dosi C, et al. Sleep and headache. In: Seminars in pediatric neurology. Vol. 22, No. 2. New York: Elsevier; 2015.

40. Bruni O, Galli F, Guidetti V. Sleep hygiene and migraine in children and adolescents. Cephalalgia. 1999;19(25_suppl):57–9.

41. Hering-Hanit R, Gadoth N. Caffeine-induced headache in children and adolescents. Cephalalgia. 2003;23(5):332–5.

42. Ernst MM, O'brien HL, Powers SW. Cognitive-behavioral therapy: how medical providers can increase patient and family openness and access to evidence-based multimodal therapy for pediatric migraine. Headache. 2015;55(10):1382–96.

43. Powers SW, et al. Cognitive behavioral therapy plus amitriptyline for chronic migraine in children and adolescents: a randomized clinical trial. JAMA. 2013;310(24):2622–30.

44. Hickman C, Jacobson D, Melnyk BM. Randomized controlled trial of the acceptability, feasibility, and preliminary effects of a cognitive behavioral skills building intervention in adolescents with chronic daily headaches: a pilot study. J Pediatr Health Care. 2015;29(1):5–16.

45. Powers SCOTTW, Hershey AD. Biofeedback for childhood migraine. In: Current management in child neurology. 2nd ed. Hamilton, Ontario: BC Decker, Inc; 2002. p. 83–5.

46. Mullally WJ, Hall K, Goldstein R. Efficacy of biofeedback in the treatment of migraine and tension type headaches. Pain Physician. 2009;12(6):1005–11.

47. Blume HK, Brockman LN, Breuner CC. Biofeedback therapy for pediatric headache: factors associated with response. Headache. 2012;52(9):1377–86.

48. Palermo TM, et al. Randomized controlled trials of psychological therapies for management of chronic pain in children and adolescents: an updated meta-analytic review. Pain. 2010;148(3):387–97.

49. Gottschling S, et al. Laser acupuncture in children with headache: a double-blind, randomized, bicenter, placebo-controlled trial. Pain. 2008;137(2):405–12.

50. Powers SW, et al. Trial of amitriptyline, topiramate, and placebo for pediatric migraine. N Engl J Med. 2017;376(2):115–24.

51. Kabbouche M, O'Brien H, Hershey AD. OnabotulinumtoxinA in pediatric chronic daily headache. Curr Neurol Neurosci Rep. 2012;12(2):114–7.

52. Ahmed K, et al. Experience with botulinum toxin type a in medically intractable pediatric chronic daily headache. Pediatr Neurol. 2010;43(5):316–9.

53. Gelfand AA, Qubty W, Goadsby PJ. Pediatric migraine prevention—first, do no harm. JAMA Neurol. 2017;74(8):893–4.

54. Gelfand AA, Reider AC, Goadsby PJ. Outcomes of greater occipital nerve injections in pediatric patients with chronic primary headache disorders. Pediatr Neurol. 2014;50(2):135–9.

55. Dubrovsky AS. Nerve blocks in pediatric and adolescent headache disorders. Curr Pain Headache Rep. 2017;21(12):50.

56. Gelfand AA, Goadsby PJ. Medication overuse in children and adolescents. Curr Pain Headache Rep. 2014;18(7):428.

57. Galli F, et al. Chronic daily headache in childhood and adolescence: clinical aspects and a 4-year follow-up. Cephalalgia. 2004;24(10):850–8.

Imaging in CDH

11

Danielle D. DeSouza and Anton Rogachov

Introduction

Over the past few decades, our understanding of brain abnormalities in headache syndromes has greatly improved with the use of advanced neuroimaging methods. Neuroimaging allows for the noninvasive examination of brain structure and function using modalities such as magnetic resonance imaging (MRI), positron emission tomography (PET), magnetoencephalography (MEG), and magnetic resonance spectroscopy (MRS), among others. While the majority of studies in the headache literature have examined episodic headache disorders, the most common being migraine (for reviews on this topic, see [1–4]), there has been a recent push toward understanding neuroimaging-based brain abnormalities associated with chronic headache, with the goals of gaining insight into its pathophysiological underpinnings and improving treatment strategies.

In this chapter, we will discuss studies focused on MRI methods to assess structural and functional brain abnormalities in chronic daily headache (CDH). We will end with a discussion on future directions for neuroimaging research in CDH.

D. D. DeSouza (✉)
Neurology and Neurological Sciences, Stanford University, Palo Alto, CA, USA
e-mail: desouzad@stanford.edu

A. Rogachov
Institute of Medical Science, Krembil Research Institute, Toronto Western Hospital, Toronto, ON, Canada

MRI Approaches to Study CDH

MRI uses strong magnets and radiofrequency pulses to collect information about atomic nuclei within tissues of the body [5]. Unlike other forms of imaging, it does not require the use of ionizing radiation to obtain images. MRI approaches can largely be divided into two broad categories: (1) structural (to assess brain gray matter (GM) and white matter (WM)) and (2) functional (to assess activity in the brain associated with hemodynamic and metabolic changes).

Multiple structural approaches are available to assess brain GM and WM structure in CDH patients using T1-weighted MRI and diffusion tensor imaging (DTI), respectively. For these approaches, data are first preprocessed to distinguish and classify brain tissues into GM, WM, and cerebrospinal fluid (CSF) components. To measure GM, a number of automated and semi-automated techniques are available, with the two most common methods being voxel-based morphometry (VBM) [6] and cortical thickness analysis (CTA) [7]. VBM can assess both subcortical and cortical GM density and volume; however, CTA was developed to measure the thickness of cortical GM on a submillimeter scale [7]. This precision is important since the cortex is highly convoluted and measuring thickness based on volume measurements can result in overestimations of GM [7]. Since many disease processes involve subtle cortical changes, the submillimeter accuracy of CTA is advantageous.

© Springer International Publishing AG, part of Springer Nature 2019
M. W. Green et al. (eds.), *Chronic Headache*, https://doi.org/10.1007/978-3-319-91491-6_11

For WM methods, analyses are typically based on MR-diffusion-weighted imaging (DWI), which is sensitized to the random Brownian motion of hydrogen protons, mainly in water molecules [8, 9]. DWI requires the acquisition of multiple images so that the signal can be sensitized to diffusion in many directions, allowing multiple measurements for each voxel comprising the brain images [8]. The diffusion of water in body tissues occurs inside, outside, around, and through cellular structures [10]. Some structural barriers can hinder diffusion. For example, diffusion in WM is more restricted across an axon than along it due to structural barriers such as myelin, axonal membranes, microtubules, and neurofilaments [11]. Importantly, regional diffusion may be lessened or exacerbated by certain pathological conditions [10, 12]. To obtain meaningful measures from diffusion scans, mathematical models can be fit to each voxel to derive information about the directionality of the diffusion and presumably underlying tissue microstructure within that voxel. The most common model is the diffusion tensor model. DTI involves fitting a tensor, which is an ellipsoid-shaped mathematical model, at each brain voxel of a DWI scan. In general, the shape of the tensor carries information about the three-dimensional character of the water molecules' diffusion [8]. For example, diffusion is isotropic, with the tensor model being roughly spherical in shape, when it is not hindered and molecules can flow equally in all directions (e.g., within CSF). In contrast, diffusion is anisotropic when there are barriers to diffusion (e.g., within WM), making diffusion along the length of the axis greater than across it. Using the tensor model, the degree of anisotropy can be captured by the parameter fractional anisotropy (FA), which ranges from zero (completely isotropic) to one (completely anisotropic). However, FA alone does not fully capture the tensor shape. Measuring FA in combination with other DTI metrics such as mean, axial, and radial diffusivity can provide more information about the tensor shape and potentially reflect certain pathophysiological processes [10–12].

Functional MRI methods rely on blood oxygen level-dependent (BOLD) signals that are related to the proportion of oxy- to deoxy-hemoglobin in the blood [13]. Physiological events (e.g., changes in neural activity) that change the oxy- to deoxy-hemoglobin ratio can be detected noninvasively as a change in BOLD response [13]. Recently, fMRI studies of functional connectivity, which refers to the examination of temporally correlated activity of remote brain regions, have become increasingly popular to study headache disorders [14]. Connectivity can be assessed in both task-based and resting-state fMRI experimental conditions.

In the following sections, recent literature using these described MRI methods to examine brain structure and function in patients with CDH will be reviewed.

Structural MRI Reveals Abnormalities in the Brain Structure of CDH Patients

CDH is a descriptive term whereby headaches occur on 15 days or more per month for at least 3 months [15]. Given the incessant and disabling nature of CDH, there has been a recent push toward understanding structural brain abnormalities that may be associated with these conditions to both understand CDH pathophysiology and develop and improve treatment strategies. CDH encompasses several types of headache including chronic migraine (CM), chronic tension-type headache (CTTH), new daily persistent headache (NDPH), and hemicrania continua. Medication overuse can often be a key contributing factor to the transformation of EM into chronic daily headache, a phenomenon known as "medication overuse headache" (MOH) [16]. Most studies in the CDH literature have focused on patients with CM (with or without MOH); however, in some cases, mixed groups were included. In this section, the main findings from these studies will be reviewed in the context of other pain and neuroimaging studies.

In general, pain is a multidimensional experience involving many brain structures as revealed by MRI among other methods. Neuroimaging has revealed that many of the brain regions are involved in acute pain function abnormally and/or have abnormal structure in patients with chronic pain disorders. Nociceptive stimuli can evoke changes in brain activity associated with the sensory-discriminative, affective, motor, and/or pain modulatory dimensions of pain. These brain regions include the primary and secondary somatosensory cortices (S1, S2), the anterior and midcingulate cortices (ACC, MCC), insula, amygdala, prefrontal cortex (PFC), primary and supplementary motor areas (M1, SMA), thalamus, basal ganglia, cerebellum, and brainstem structures such as the periaqueductal gray (PAG) [17–21] (Fig. 11.1). In studies of episodic migraine (EM), structural abnormalities have

Fig. 11.1 Schematic representation of gray matter regions contributing to the multidimensional experience of pain. Several cortical and subcortical brain areas contribute to the multidimensional experience of pain. These regions include the dorsolateral prefrontal cortex (DLPFC), primary motor and somatosensory cortices (M1, S1), brainstem periaqueductal gray (PAG), anterior and midcingulate cortices (ACC, MCC), supplementary motor area (SMA), insula, basal ganglia, and thalamus. Other gray matter regions frequently implicated in pain perception but not pictured here include the amygdala and cerebellum

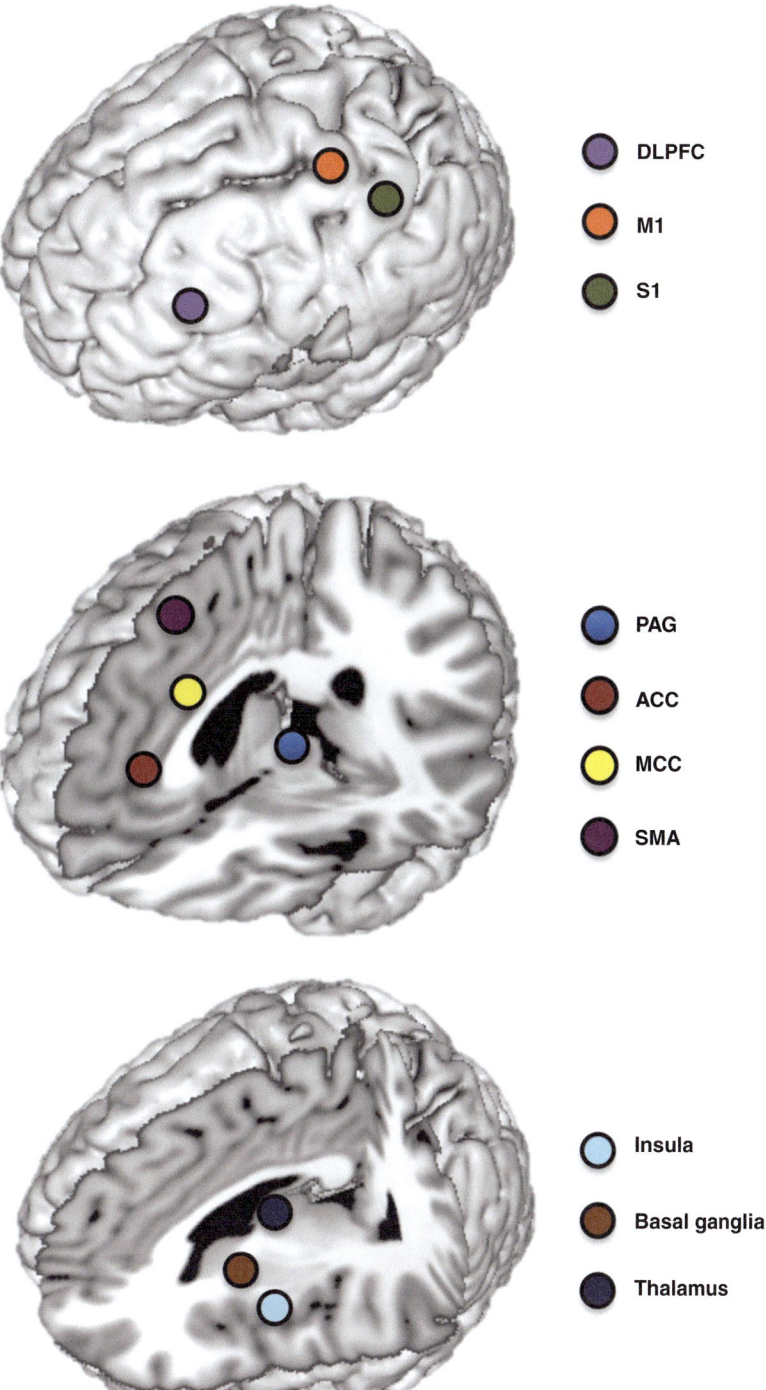

been reported in many of these regions [1, 4]. Likewise, the WM connecting these brain regions may also present with gross or microstructural abnormalities [4]. In CDH, structural abnormalities are also evident in these areas; however, there is some evidence to support a greater severity of abnormality compared to their episodic counterparts. This may be indicative of disease progression, as epidemiological studies report that approximately 14% of individuals with migraine may progress to CDH [22] and/or differentiate CDH pathophysiological mechanisms. The shift from episodic to chronic headache has been proposed to involve progressive changes in the central nociceptive system; however for some types of CDH, additional mechanisms are likely [23].

One of the major brain regions implicated in pain disorders, including headache, is the PAG, a brainstem structure known for its role in pain modulation, among other functions. Some evidence suggests that repeated migraine attacks result in free radical formation in the PAG, resulting in a lowered threshold for additional migraine attacks [24]. In one study, Welch and colleagues compared mean values of specific MRI relaxation time ratios, indicative of iron levels, in the PAG, red nucleus, and substantia nigra of patients with EM, CDH (patients with near daily headaches due to medication overuse), and healthy controls [24]. Each group consisted of 17 participants. The results indicated that both the EM and CDH groups had higher levels of iron in the PAG compared to controls, and for both groups, these levels increased with illness duration. It has been previously described that elevations in tissue iron are markers of disturbed neuronal function [25]. Since this finding was ubiquitous across headache groups, the authors suggested a role for the PAG as a potential "generator" of migraine. Interestingly, when comparing the intercept values of the correlations with disease duration, tissue iron values were higher than normal at the outset in migraine-susceptible individuals. This suggests that in addition to iron levels rising as a consequence of migraine, it may also contribute to its etiology.

Tepper and colleagues conducted another study aimed at evaluating structural differences in patients with CDH [26]. In this study, a mixed group of patients with CDH, including two with CM, one with CTTH, and eight with medication overuse headache (MOH), was compared to patients with EM ($n = 10$) with or without aura and to controls with or without infrequent episodic tension-type headaches ($n = 12$). They used T2-weighted MRI to assess local iron concentrations, as done previously in patients with episodic migraine [24, 27]. Tissue iron levels have been shown to be associated with cellular function, and as such, measures of tissue iron may provide insight into disease pathophysiology [23]. They restricted their analyses to the basal ganglia and red nucleus, structures previously shown to have decreased T2 signal intensity, consistent with increased iron, in patients with migraine with longer migraine histories [27]. The results of the study by Tepper and group showed that when all migraine patients were compared to controls, patients had significantly lower T2 values in the globus pallidus of the basal ganglia and in the red nucleus, in line with the results of Kruit and colleagues. However, when episodic migraine patients were compared to CDH patients, only T2 values in the globus pallidus were significantly different. Therefore, this study provides evidence that T2-weighted MRI can differentiate structural differences in the globus pallidus between patients who have episodic migraine and those who have CDH [26]. The authors suggest this finding may reflect differences in headache frequency and/or pathophysiology between episodic and chronic headache groups.

In a recent paper with a larger sample size ($n = 63$), a VBM approach was used to compare GM in groups of patients with EM, CM (including MOH), and healthy controls without any history of primary or secondary headache [28]. Patients who had migraine diagnoses were excluded if they had aura. Participants were age- and sex-matched between groups. The results of the whole-brain analyses revealed that compared to controls, patients with CM had significantly larger right amygdala and right putamen volumes. In contrast, patients with EM did not demonstrate any significant volume differences compared to controls. Additionally, regression analyses of GM volume and headache frequency (headache days/month) showed significant positive correlations in the temporal gyrus bilaterally, right putamen, and inferior frontal gyrus and a significant negative correlation with the left cuneus and headache frequency. These progressive changes suggest that at least some observed structural GM abnormalities may be the consequence of repetitive attacks over time. Interestingly, all associations with headache frequency did not overlap with the areas of significant differences compared to controls. This corroborates another recent VBM study demonstrating significant interactions between affective measures and amygdala volume in CM in the absence of group volumetric differences [29] and highlights the importance of examining abnormal associations in CDH in addition to group differences.

Since many of the previous neuroimaging studies described included patients with MOH in their CDH cohorts, Lai and colleagues [30] sought to specifically compare GM volumes in CM patients with medication overuse (MO) and those without. The results of their whole-brain VBM analysis revealed that CM patients with MO had decreased GM volumes in the orbitofrontal cortex and left middle occipital gyrus and increased GM volumes in the left temporal pole and parahippocampal gyrus. These GM volume differences explained approximately 31% of variance in analgesics use frequency and orbitofrontal GM volume was predictive of MO treatment response. These results suggest that CM with MO and CM without MO are reflected differently in brain GM and provide insight into a potential source of variation between brain imaging studies that have mixed CM cohorts.

Cortical thickness has also been assessed in patients with MOH. In a study by Riederer et al. [31], 29 patients with MOH who had on average approximately 25 headache days per month were compared to 29 sex-matched healthy control participants. Compared to controls, MOH patients had thinner cortex in the left PFC and higher local gyrification in a region encompassing the fusiform cortex and in the right occipital pole. Since cortical thickness better estimates cortical GM compared to VBM, these findings

provide additional insight into the putative neurobiological underpinnings involved in MOH, specifically.

In a study combining cortical thickness and volume measures of GM, Schwedt et al. used machine learning to classify CM patients compared to controls, with approximately 86% accuracy [32]. The GM regions that contributed to this classification included most of the cingulate gyrus, the lateral and medial prefrontal regions, the superior temporal lobe, the parahippocampal cortex, the entorhinal cortex, and the insula. Average classifier accuracies were only 67% for EM patients versus controls. When classifying EM versus CM patients directly, GM regions that contributed to the classification accuracy of 84% included the S1, cingulate gyrus, lateral and medial PFC, insula, and temporal pole, among other regions. These results provide further support that subtle differences in MRI-derived structural GM measures can reflect headache chronicity and potentially CDH pathophysiology.

Others have shown that abnormalities in WM microstructure may be predominant in individuals with long-term CM. In a recent study, Gomez-Beldarrain and colleagues [33] examined structural abnormalities in WM using tract-based spatial statistics (TBSS), an automated method that allows for the comparison of WM tracts between groups [34]. They used a region of interest (ROI) approach to specifically examine FA in WM underlying the cingulate and insular gyri, in addition to the uncinate fasciculus. Patients with CM ($n = 18$) and EM ($n = -19$) were assessed at baseline compared to controls ($n = 15$), and patients were again assessed at a 3-month and 6-month post-baseline. At the 3-month time point, patients maintained the same diagnoses, and no differences in FA were evident. However, at the 6-month time point, only nine patients still met diagnostic criteria for CM (i.e., more than 15 days of migraine pain per month) and were labeled the long-term CM group. Only this group demonstrated significantly lower FA values in the regions examined, which were also more pronounced on the right side and associated with headache frequency. The authors discussed that these structural WM abnormalities may reflect migraine pain chronification and as they were only evident in patients that maintained a CM diagnosis over time. These results contrast earlier work by Neeb and colleagues [35] that found no WM microstructural abnormalities in patients with EM and CM using a whole-brain TBSS approach. The differences between study results may reflect methodological considerations such as using an ROI versus a whole-brain approach to examine WM microstructure, differences in patient sampling, medication use, and/or other factors.

Taken together, these findings support a role for structural abnormalities in the progression of CDH and, in some cases, may even predispose individuals to developing CDH.

Functional Brain Abnormalities in CDH as Assessed by fMRI

Functional activity in the brain can be associated with electromagnetic, hemodynamic, and metabolic changes [14]. fMRI methods are most commonly used capture brain hemodynamics, which serves as a proxy for functional activity and connectivity measures in the brain. There are numerous ways to assess brain function using fMRI. One option is to use a hypothesis-driven approach (e.g., general linear model regression), whereby signal time courses are extracted from specific seeds or ROIs based on a priori hypotheses. Alternately, a whole-brain approach may be used when hypotheses about specific brain area involvement are lacking. Data-driven approaches (e.g., independent component analysis) can additionally identify networks of activity (e.g., default mode network, salience network, central executive network, sensorimotor network) (Fig. 11.2) that may not have been predicted [14, 36]. While these options allow for flexibility when designing a study, they can also be the source of heterogeneity between study results. In recent years, there have been important advances in our understanding of brain activity in CDH. Some of these prominent findings will be discussed.

In a study by Chen and colleagues [37], resting-state fMRI scans were acquired for 18 patients with EM, 16 patients with CM, 44 patients with CM and MOH, and 32 normal control participants. The authors were specifically interested in examining functional connectivity of the marginal division of neostriatum, a flat, pan-shaped zone between the neostriatum and the globus pallidus, which has been implicated in learning, memory, and pain modulation. They employed an ROI approach to examine marginal division connectivity with the rest of the brain. The results of their study indicated that functional connectivity of the marginal division of neostriatum could not only differentiate patients from controls but also patient subtypes. Specifically, when compared to controls, EM patients showed altered connectivity between the marginal division and the right insula, right precentral gyrus, and ACC. For the CM group, altered connectivity occurred between the marginal division and brain regions including the right cuneus, left MCC, bilateral middle frontal gyri, and left hippocampus. The patients that had CM and MOH demonstrated altered connectivity only between the marginal division and the left parahippocampus, right middle frontal gyrus, and inferior temporal gyrus. The authors concluded that the marginal division of neostriatum is an important structure to understand pain modulation and migraine chronification, as connectivity of this structure could differentiate headache subtypes [37].

Chen and colleagues again used an ROI resting-state fMRI approach to study amygdala connectivity in patients with EM, CM, and controls [38]. Patients with EM had increased functional connectivity between the left amygdala and the left MCC and left precuneus, compared to controls. No functional connectivity differences were observed for the right amygdala in EM patients. In contrast, patients with CM had significantly lower functional connectivity between the right amygdala and regions of the occipital lobe, compared to controls, but no connectivity differences of the left amygdala. This right lateralized amygdala finding in CDH

Fig. 11.2 Brain networks implicated in chronic pain. (**a**) DMN: medial prefrontal cortex (mPFC), left and right lateral parietal cortex, left and right lateral temporal cortex, and posterior cingulate cortex. (**b**) SN: right and left temporoparietal junction, midcingulate cortex, left and right anterior insula, and left and right dorsolateral prefrontal cortex (dlPFC). (**c**) Central executive network: mPFC, dlPFC, and posterior parietal cortex. (**d**) Sensorimotor cortex: left and right primary motor cortex and left and right primary somatosensory cortex

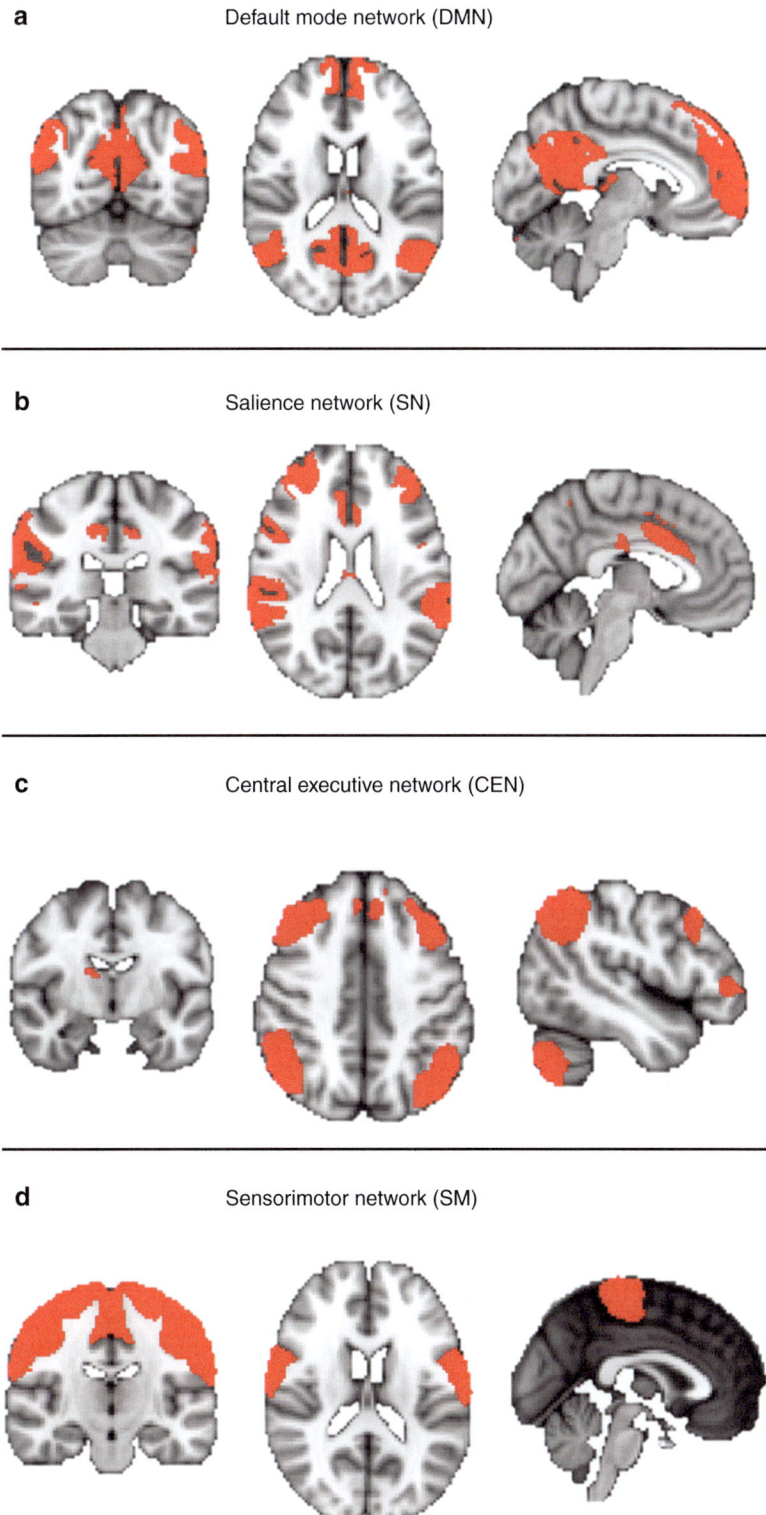

a   Default mode network (DMN)

b   Salience network (SN)

c   Central executive network (CEN)

d   Sensorimotor network (SM)

patients has also been demonstrated using structural MRI [29, 39]. The animal literature has shown right lateralized pain-related activity in animal models of inflammatory pain [40, 41]. Moreover, transient increases in amygdala activity were observed only acutely in the left amygdala in a neuropathic pain model, whereas activity in the right amygdala became predominant at 2 weeks post-surgery and persisted [42]. While these amygdala findings may not be specific to CDH, they may serve as a useful biomarker of pain chronicity and the heavy affective burden it imparts, in general.

In another study, Schulte and colleagues [43] used a standardized trigeminal nociceptive stimulation task to examine brainstem activity of patients with EM ($n = 20$), CM ($n = 22$), and healthy controls ($n = 21$). Typically, the spatial resolution of conventional whole-brain fMRI protocols does not allow for the detailed differentiation of brainstem structures. As such, the authors used a specialized fMRI sequence to specifically examine the brainstem, as they have done previously [44]. The fMRI task involved the application of either gaseous ammonia, an activator of nociceptive fibers, or air to the left nostril of participants using an olfactometer with a Teflon tube. The results showed that in patients with CM, activity within the right anterior hypothalamus was higher compared to controls when the ammonia and air conditions were compared. Additionally, it was demonstrated that this anterior hypothalamus region showed greater activity in patients with CM who had a headache at the time of scanning compared to EMs with headaches at the time of scanning. Because a larger subgroup of CM patients had headache at the time of scanning, a secondary analysis was conducted to exclude headache chronicity as a variable. This time, significant activity in the posterior hypothalamus in migraineurs with headache at the time of the scan was observed, compared to migraineurs without headache and controls. These findings suggest an important role for the hypothalamus in the pathophysiology of migraine chronification and provide evidence for differential roles of the anterior and posterior hypothalamus in migraine. The authors concluded that the posterior hypothalamus appears to play a role in the acute stage pain, while the anterior hypothalamus seems to be more involved in attack generation and migraine chronification.

A recent study carried out by Androulakis et al. [45] sought to evaluate resting-state functional connectivity of women with CM (including those with MOH) in three major intrinsic brain networks: the default mode network (DMN), salience network (SN), and the central executive network (CEN) (Fig. 11.2a–c). Previous work on patients with EM demonstrated abnormal connectivity within these networks [46–48]; however, their connectivity patterns in CM had not previously been characterized. Compared to controls, all three networks were less coherent in CM patients compared to age- and sex-matched controls. When CM patients were stratified based on MOH status, each group remained less coherent in the resting-state networks examined compared to controls. No significant differences in network connectivity were found between the patient subtypes. Importantly, significant associations were also found for the SN and clinical variables such that decreased SN activity was associated with the frequency of moderate and severe headache days and increased SN activity was associated with cutaneous allodynia, providing potential pathophysiologic underpinnings for these findings.

As discussed in the structural imaging section, machine learning has been used to classify CM from EM patients and controls using GM thickness and volume measures with high accuracy. In their recent paper, Chong et al. demonstrated that resting-state functional connectivity could also discriminate patients with migraine from healthy controls [32]. Connectivity of the right middle temporal, posterior insula, MCC, left ventromedial PFC, and amygdala bilaterally contributed to this discrimination. While this analysis combined patients with EM and CM, it was demonstrated that classification accuracy was higher (~97% accuracy) for migraineurs with longer disease duration (>14 years) compared to migraineurs with shorter disease duration (~82% accuracy), suggesting that greater functional reorganization occurs over time in patients with migraine.

Several recent studies have started to employ fMRI methods to elucidate CDH pathophysiology; however, differences between imaging methods and participant samples make it difficult to generalize findings. These studies nonetheless provide significant insight into how brain activity and connectivity differs in patients with CDH compared to episodic headache and controls and set the foundation for future studies to build upon.

What Other Neuroimaging Modalities Reveal About CDH

In addition to structural and functional MRI, other neuroimaging modalities, such as PET, have been used to investigate functional abnormalities in CDH patients. Unlike MRI, PET is an invasive procedure that involves the administration of a biologically active molecule tagged with a radioactive tracer into the bloodstream. Using advanced kinetic modeling, the decay of the radioactive tracer can be used to image synaptic activity or the tissue concentration of a molecule of interest (i.e., membrane-bound receptors). Given its invasive nature, PET represents a sensitive technique for assessing in vivo changes in cerebral blood flow (CBF) during pathological conditions in humans [49].

Many patients suffering from EM often resort to a multitude of analgesics to manage their symptoms, which can result in MOH. To investigate patients with MOH, Fumal and colleagues [50] used PET imaging to examine the functional properties of the brain in chronic migraineurs ($n = 16$) with analgesic overuse before and 3 weeks following medication withdrawal. Before withdrawal, chronic migraineurs exhibited aberrant activity across many pain processing structures, including the thalamus, ACC, insula, orbitofrontal cortex (OFC), and cerebellum. Interestingly, these aberrations were effectively reversed in all of these regions 3 weeks after medication discontinuation, with the exception of the OFC which continued to show abnormal activity. The inability to restore activity in the OFC, a region of the brain implicated in drug dependence, to normal levels of function could predispose these patients to recurring analgesic overuse. Nevertheless, because MOH appears to be largely reversible following medication withdrawal, a failure to halt medication overuse is believed to contribute to the chronification of headaches.

Another common modality used to study pathological brain function is MEG, a highly sensitive brain imaging tool capable of recording the magnetic fields produced by neural activity and has greater temporal resolution than fMRI methods. Its noninvasive nature permits its utility in many different patient populations, including pediatric populations. A study by Leiken and colleagues [51] used MEG to assess the spatial and temporal properties of brain activity during a finger tapping motor task in a pediatric cohort of patients suffering from acute ($n = 27$) and chronic ($n = 27$) migraine. While healthy subjects ($n = 27$) displayed the expected activation of primary motor region contralateral to the finger performing the tapping motion, this pattern of activity extended beyond the primary motor regions in acute migraine patients into sensorimotor regions, SMA, premotor regions, and occipital cortex. This effect was even more prominent in the CM group, suggesting that cortical excitability is elevated in migraine and the degree of excitability tracks the severity of the migraine (i.e., greater excitability in chronic migraine than in acute migraine). In addition to heightened cortical excitability, this study also demonstrated that CM patients were at significantly higher odds for engaging deep brain (subcortical) areas in comparison to acute migraine and controls. Together, these findings suggest that pediatric chronic migraine patients experience elevated activation of cortical-subcortical networks and recruit abnormally large neural network to perform a basic motor task.

Other neuroimaging modalities can serve as powerful tools to assess brain function in different ways than MRI approaches. The use of alternate imaging modalities in conjunction with MRI can provide valuable opportunities to fully characterize brain function associated with CDH.

Future Directions for Neuroimaging Research in CDH

There are several exciting opportunities for future neuroimaging research in CDH. As previously mentioned, CDH is a descriptive term encompassing several types of chronic headache. To date, the neuroimaging literature has primarily focused on CDH patients with CM or MOH, likely due to their higher prevalence in the population. A large literature now exists to suggest that structural and functional brain abnormalities may reflect specific clinical features of chronic pain disorders and/or their underlying pathophysiology [12, 52]. The ability to differentiate CDH subtypes based on neuroimaging-derived biomarkers would be highly beneficial toward understanding the neural underpinnings of chronic headache subtypes and provide insight into the mechanisms of action of effective treatments. Neuroimaging-based biomarkers have previously been used to differentiate subtypes of depression with varying clinical symptoms with high accuracy and even predict which patients would benefit from repetitive transcranial magnetic stimulation therapy [53]. Knowing in advance which CDH patients would be responsive to specific therapeutic strategies could greatly decrease both the patient and economic burden of these disorders.

While recent studies have begun to employ individual neuroimaging approaches to advance our understanding of brain abnormalities in CDH, multimodal neuroimaging approaches may offer new insights into how different structural of functional abnormalities relate to each other, allowing for a more comprehensive understanding of CDH pathophysiology. Multimodal neuroimaging can allow for the joint analysis of brain structure and function by combining PET and MRI, or MRI and MEG [54]. This would allow for the limitation of one imaging modality to be compensated by another. For example, MRI methods allow for high spatial resolution but are limited in temporal resolution. On the other hand, MEG acquires data with much higher temporal resolution compared to fMRI. By combining these methods, one could overcome each modality's specific limitation and cross-validate findings from different sources.

There remains an opportunity for future research to understand the cellular and molecular underpinnings of structural and functional brain abnormalities as detected by neuroimaging. Several candidate mechanisms exist to account for these findings including changes in axon sprouting, dendritic branching, neurogenesis, glial changes, angiogenesis, fiber organization, myelin remodeling, and astrocyte changes, among others [55]. However, their precise roles in CDH neuroimaging findings remain to be determined. Knowing which cellular and molecular processes contribute to alterations in GM thickness and volume, WM microstructure, and function could potentially allow for the development of new therapeutic strategies aimed at limiting or reversing these abnormalities.

Conclusion

In summary, neuroimaging provides a valuable tool to gain insight into CDH pathophysiology. There are several modalities available to assess both brain structure and function in CDH patients. While great leaps have been made in our understanding of CDH, there are several opportunities for the future studies to use neuroimaging to develop biomarkers of CDH subtypes, cross-validate imaging modalities, and determine the cellular and molecular underpinnings of these imaging findings.

References

1. Sprenger T, Borsook D. Migraine changes the brain: neuroimaging makes its mark. Curr Opin Neurol. 2012;25(3):252–62.
2. Burstein R, Noseda R, Borsook D. Migraine: multiple processes, complex pathophysiology. J Neurosci. 2015;35(17):6619–29.
3. Schulte LH, May A. Functional neuroimaging in migraine: chances and challenges. Headache. 2016;56(9):1474–81.
4. Chong CD, Schwedt TJ, Dodick DW. Migraine: what imaging reveals. Curr Neurol Neurosci Rep. 2016;16(7):64.
5. van Geuns RJ, Wielopolski PA, de Bruin HG, Rensing BJ, van Ooijen PM, Hulshoff M, et al. Basic principles of magnetic resonance imaging. Prog Cardiovasc Dis. 1999;42(2):149–56.

6. Ashburner J, Friston KJ. Voxel-based morphometry–the methods. NeuroImage. 2000;11(6 Pt 1):805–21.

7. Fischl B, Dale AM. Measuring the thickness of the human cerebral cortex from magnetic resonance images. Proc Natl Acad Sci U S A. 2000;97(20):11050–5.

8. Johansen-Berg H, Rushworth MF. Using diffusion imaging to study human connectional anatomy. Annu Rev Neurosci. 2009;32:75–94.

9. Mori S, Zhang J. Principles of diffusion tensor imaging and its applications to basic neuroscience research. Neuron. 2006;51(5):527–39.

10. Alexander AL, Lee JE, Lazar M, Field AS. Diffusion tensor imaging of the brain. Neurotherapeutics. 2007;4(3):316–29.

11. Beaulieu C. The basis of anisotropic water diffusion in the nervous system - a technical review. NMR Biomed. 2002;15(7–8):435–55.

12. DeSouza DD, Hodaie M, Davis KD. Abnormal trigeminal nerve microstructure and brain white matter in idiopathic trigeminal neuralgia. Pain. 2014;155(1):37–44.

13. Ogawa S, Lee TM, Kay AR, Tank DW. Brain magnetic resonance imaging with contrast dependent on blood oxygenation. Proc Natl Acad Sci U S A. 1990;87(24):9868–72.

14. Maleki N, Gollub RL. What have we learned from brain functional connectivity studies in migraine headache? Headache. 2016;56(3):453–61.

15. (IHS) HCCotIHS. The international classification of headache disorders, 3rd edition (beta version). Cephalalgia. 2013;33(9):629–808.

16. Mathew NT, Stubits E, Nigam MP. Transformation of episodic migraine into daily headache: analysis of factors. Headache. 1982;22(2):66–8.

17. Apkarian AV, Bushnell MC, Treede RD, Zubieta JK. Human brain mechanisms of pain perception and regulation in health and disease. Eur J Pain. 2005;9(4):463–84.

18. Davis KD, Moayedi M. Central mechanisms of pain revealed through functional and structural MRI. J Neuroimmune Pharmacol. 2013;8(3):518–34.

19. Duerden EG, Albanese MC. Localization of pain-related brain activation: a meta-analysis of neuroimaging data. Hum Brain Mapp. 2013;34(1):109–49.

20. Peyron R, Laurent B, García-Larrea L. Functional imaging of brain responses to pain. A review and meta-analysis (2000). Neurophysiol Clin. 2000;30(5):263–88.

21. Tracey I. Nociceptive processing in the human brain. Curr Opin Neurobiol. 2005;15(4):478–87.

22. Katsarava Z, Schneeweiss S, Kurth T, Kroener U, Fritsche G, Eikermann A, et al. Incidence and predictors for chronicity of headache in patients with episodic migraine. Neurology. 2004;62(5):788–90.

23. Aurora SK. Spectrum of illness: understanding biological patterns and relationships in chronic migraine. Neurology. 2009;72(5 Suppl):S8–13.

24. Welch KM, Nagesh V, Aurora SK, Gelman N. Periaqueductal gray matter dysfunction in migraine: cause or the burden of illness? Headache. 2001;41(7):629–37.

25. Morris CM, Candy JM, Omar S, Bloxham CA, Edwardson JA. Transferrin receptors in the parkinsonian midbrain. Neuropathol Appl Neurobiol. 1994;20(5):468–72.

26. Tepper SJ, Lowe MJ, Beall E, Phillips MD, Liu K, Stillman MJ, et al. Iron deposition in pain-regulatory nuclei in episodic migraine and chronic daily headache by MRI. Headache. 2012;52(2):236–43.

27. Kruit MC, Launer LJ, Overbosch J, van Buchem MA, Ferrari MD. Iron accumulation in deep brain nuclei in migraine: a population-based magnetic resonance imaging study. Cephalalgia. 2009;29(3):351–9.

28. Neeb L, Bastian K, Villringer K, Israel H, Reuter U, Fiebach JB. Structural gray matter alterations in chronic migraine: implications for a progressive disease? Headache. 2017;57(3):400–16.

29. DeSouza DD, Woldeamanuel YW, Peretz AM, Sanjanwala BM, Cowan RP. Interactions between affective measures and amygdala volume in chronic migraine: associations in the absence of group volumetric differences. Cephalalgia. 2017;37:47–8.

30. Lai TH, Chou KH, Fuh JL, Lee PL, Kung YC, Lin CP, et al. Gray matter changes related to medication overuse in patients with chronic migraine. Cephalalgia. 2016;36(14):1324–33.

31. Riederer F, Schaer M, Gantenbein AR, Luechinger R, Michels L, Kaya M, et al. Cortical alterations in medication-overuse headache. Headache. 2017;57(2):255–65.

32. Schwedt TJ, Chong CD, Wu T, Gaw N, Fu Y, Li J. Accurate classification of chronic migraine via brain magnetic resonance imaging. Headache. 2015;55(6):762–77.

33. Gomez-Beldarrain M, Oroz I, Zapirain BG, Ruanova BF, Fernandez YG, Cabrera A, et al. Right fronto-insular white matter tracts link cognitive reserve and pain in migraine patients. J Headache Pain. 2015;17:4.

34. Smith SM, Jenkinson M, Johansen-Berg H, Rueckert D, Nichols TE, Mackay CE, et al. Tract-based spatial statistics: voxelwise analysis of multi-subject diffusion data. NeuroImage. 2006;31(4):1487–505.

35. Neeb L, Bastian K, Villringer K, Gits HC, Israel H, Reuter U, et al. No microstructural white matter alterations in chronic and episodic migraineurs: a case-control diffusion tensor magnetic resonance imaging study. Headache. 2015;55(2):241–51.

36. Hubbard CS, Khan SA, Keaser ML, Mathur VA, Goyal M, Seminowicz DA. Altered brain structure and function correlate with disease severity and pain catastrophizing in migraine patients. eNeuro. 2014;1(1):e20.14.

37. Chen Z, Chen X, Liu M, Liu S, Shu S, Ma L, et al. Altered functional connectivity of the marginal division in migraine: a resting-state fMRI study. J Headache Pain. 2016;17(1):89.

38. Chen Z, Chen X, Liu M, Dong Z, Ma L, Yu S. Altered functional connectivity of amygdala underlying the neuromechanism of migraine pathogenesis. J Headache Pain. 2017;18(1):7.

39. DeSouza DD, Woldeamanuel YW, O'Hare M, Sanjanwala BM, Cowan RP. Abnormal amygdala volumes predicted by behavioral measures in patients with chronic daily headache. Ann Neurol. 2016;80:S240–S1.

40. Carrasquillo Y, Gereau RW. Activation of the extracellular signal-regulated kinase in the amygdala modulates pain perception. J Neurosci. 2007;27(7):1543–51.

41. Ji G, Neugebauer V. Hemispheric lateralization of pain processing by amygdala neurons. J Neurophysiol. 2009;102(4):2253–64.

42. Gonçalves L, Dickenson AH. Asymmetric time-dependent activation of right central amygdala neurones in rats with peripheral neuropathy and pregabalin modulation. Eur J Neurosci. 2012;36(9):3204–13.

43. Schulte LH, Allers A, May A. Hypothalamus as a mediator of chronic migraine: evidence from high-resolution fMRI. Neurology. 2017;88(21):2011–6.

44. Schulte LH, Sprenger C, May A. Physiological brainstem mechanisms of trigeminal nociception: an fMRI study at 3T. NeuroImage. 2016;124(Pt A):518–25.

45. Androulakis XM, Krebs K, Peterlin BL, Zhang T, Maleki N, Sen S, et al. Modulation of intrinsic resting-state fMRI networks in women with chronic migraine. Neurology. 2017;89(2):163–9.

46. Schwedt TJ, Schlaggar BL, Mar S, Nolan T, Coalson RS, Nardos B, et al. Atypical resting-state functional connectivity of affective pain regions in chronic migraine. Headache. 2013;53(5):737–51.

47. Tessitore A, Russo A, Conte F, Giordano A, De Stefano M, Lavorgna L, et al. Abnormal connectivity within executive resting-state network in migraine with aura. Headache. 2015;55(6):794–805.

48. Amin FM, Hougaard A, Magon S, Asghar MS, Ahmad NN, Rostrup E, et al. Change in brain network connectivity during PACAP38-induced migraine attacks: a resting-state functional MRI study. Neurology. 2016;86(2):180–7.

49. Weiller C, May A, Limmroth V, Jüptner M, Kaube H, Schayck RV, et al. Brain stem activation in spontaneous human migraine attacks. Nat Med. 1995;1(7):658–60.

50. Fumal A, Laureys S, Di Clemente L, Boly M, Bohotin V, Vandenheede M, et al. Orbitofrontal cortex involvement in chronic analgesic-overuse headache evolving from episodic migraine. Brain. 2006;129(Pt 2):543–50.

51. Leiken KA, Xiang J, Curry E, Fujiwara H, Rose DF, Allen JR, et al. Quantitative neuromagnetic signatures of aberrant cortical excitability in pediatric chronic migraine. J Headache Pain. 2016;17:46.

52. Gustin SM, Peck CC, Wilcox SL, Nash PG, Murray GM, Henderson LA. Different pain, different brain: thalamic anatomy in neuropathic and non-neuropathic chronic pain syndromes. J Neurosci. 2011;31(16):5956–64.

53. Drysdale AT, Grosenick L, Downar J, Dunlop K, Mansouri F, Meng Y, et al. Resting-state connectivity biomarkers define neurophysiological subtypes of depression. Nat Med. 2017;23(1):28–38.

54. Liu S, Cai W, Zhang F, Fulham M, Feng D, Pujol S, et al. Multimodal neuroimaging computing: a review of the applications in neuropsychiatric disorders. Brain Inform. 2015;2(3):167–80.

55. Zatorre RJ, Fields RD, Johansen-Berg H. Plasticity in gray and white: neuroimaging changes in brain structure during learning. Nat Neurosci. 2012;15(4):528–36.

Laboratory Investigation in CDH

12

Benjamin J. Saunders, Iryna S. Aberkorn, and Barbara L. Nye

Introduction

The chronic daily headache patient will present in two distinct clinical settings: to the outpatient practitioner and to the emergency department for evaluation. The role of the provider in these diverse clinical settings is very different. The role of the emergency practitioner is to stabilize and exclude conditions that will lead to immediate morbidity, where the outpatient provider is tasked with the role of establishing a clear diagnosis and treating the patient appropriately for the condition. Both providers have the important task of evaluating for red flag signs and symptoms that may lead to the diagnosis of a secondary condition causing the patient's headaches.

In the previous chapters, you have read about how to take a headache history and about specific headache disorders that should be considered. In this chapter we will walk you through available laboratory testing that should be considered in each of the clinical scenarios. Finally, we will go through some special cases and considerations that can present to either the inpatient or outpatient setting. The focus will be to eliminate the suspicion for a secondary headache disorder,

remembering that just because a patient has a history of a primary headache disorder, it does *not* mean that they cannot develop a *new* secondary headache disorder.

The laboratory and neuroimaging evaluation of the patient is often preformed concurrently, and one can inform the other.

Serological Testing

Complete Blood Profile

A complete blood count includes white blood cell count, red blood cell count, platelets, as well as a differential.

White blood cell count and differential: Neutrophil count elevation with a left shift would be indicative of an infectious process. In patients that are immunocompromised, leukopenia and thrombocytopenia may be present. Elevation in the neutrophils vs lymphocytes can help differentiate between bacterial and viral etiologies, respectively.

Red blood cell, hemoglobin, and hematocrit: Relationships between anemia, myeloproliferative diseases such as polycythemia vera, and sickle cell disease with the development of headaches have also been described.

B. J. Saunders
Commonwealth of Massachusetts, Boston, MA, USA

I. S. Aberkorn · B. L. Nye (✉)
Dartmouth-Hitchcock Medical Center,
Lebanon, NH, USA
e-mail: Barbara.L.Nye@hitchcock.org

© Springer International Publishing AG, part of Springer Nature 2019
M. W. Green et al. (eds.), *Chronic Headache*, https://doi.org/10.1007/978-3-319-91491-6_12

Platelets: Thrombocytopenia can be found as a result of a medication reaction in headache patients. Medications that can cause this include but are not limited to acetaminophen, ibuprofen, naproxen, carbamazepine, and valproic acid. Drug-induced thrombocytopenia typically occurs within the first 2 weeks of drug exposure. Recovery starts 1 to 2 days following the discontinuation of the medication. Recovery to the patient's normal range typically occurs within 1 week [1].

Complete Metabolic Profile (CMP)

This study includes evaluation of liver function, renal function, as well as electrolytes and glucose.

CMP can be useful in the evaluation of the chronic daily headache patient for both the initial assessment and continued medical management and monitoring. Renal failure has been found to be a cause of headache. Dehydration is common in headache patients who frequently have associated symptoms of nausea, vomiting, gastroparesis, and decreased oral intake. This can lead to prerenal failure especially with the concomitant use of nonsteroidal anti-inflammatory drugs (NSAIDs). These have been linked to an increased risk for renal injury, causing parenchymal kidney disease.

Hypoglycemia can cause brain dysfunction and may be associated with headache; however there is no conclusive evidence to support this association.

The combination of the lactic acidosis in patients with migraine attacks and seizures or stroke-like episodes could be suspicious for MELAS (mitochondrial encephalopathy, lactic acidosis, and stroke-like episodes). In addition to elevated lactate level, there might be an elevated level of pyruvate in the serum. However these abnormalities are not confirmatory for the diagnosis. MELAS is covered in more details later in this chapter.

Liver function studies are used more for the monitoring of medication complications (Table 12.1).

Table 12.1 List of medications used for the treatment of headache disorders that cause drug-induced liver injury [2]

Type of liver toxicity	Medications
Acute injury	Acetaminophen, aspirin, bupropion, diclofenac, fluoxetine, lisinopril, losartan, NSAID, paroxetine, sertraline, trazodone, valproate, varenicline
Cholestasis	Carbamazepine, chlorpromazine, diclofenac, phenothiazine
Mixed liver injury	Amitriptyline, carbamazepine, cyproheptadine, ibuprofen, phenothiazines, trazadone, verapamil
Steatohepatitis and microvesicular steatosis	Valproic acid
Granulomas	Carbamazepine, diclofenac, diltiazem
Autoimmune hepatitis	Diclofenac
Chronic hepatitis	Diclofenac, Lisinopril, trazodone
Neoplasm	Carbamazepine
Ischemic necrosis	Ergot

Coagulation Studies

Coagulation studies are useful in evaluation of refractory headache in patients with suspected hypercoagulable disorders such as SLE, an antiphospholipid syndrome.

Current literature points to a connection between migraine, especially with aura, and elevated level of procoagulation factors [4].

Current evidence suggests checking:

1. Full hypercoagulable profile in patients with migraine with (1) aura and a personal history or family history of thrombosis or (2) MRI evidence of microvascular ischemia or of stroke.
2. Screen patients with migraine with aura for markers of endothelial activation (vWF, high-sensitivity C-reactive protein and fibrinogen) [3].

Patients taking oral contraceptives are also at risk for secondary headaches due to hypercoagulable state as estrogen-containing oral contraceptives are associated with elevated plasma concentrations of clotting factors II, VII, VII, X, and prothrombin, fibrinogen, and thrombin-activatable fibrinolysis inhibitor (TAFI), a procarboxypeptidase B- like proenzyme which inhibits fibrinolysis [4, 5].

Lupus Anticoagulant, Anticardiolipin Antibodies, Protein S, Protein C, Factor VIII, Antithrombin III, and Factor V Leiden

Antiphospholipid protein syndrome (APS) can be primary or secondary. The primary syndrome is present in the absence of other autoimmune diseases. Secondary forms include systemic lupus erythematous (SLE). Chronic headache or episodes of migraines are the most common neurological manifestation of APS [5].

Patients that have a history of headache, miscarriages, and venous thrombosis should be screened for hypercoagulable states.

D-Dimer

Cerebral venous thrombosis (CVT) is uncommon but should be suspected in a patient presenting with acute worsening headache symptoms. This is more common in women (3:1, female/male ratio) with some gender-specific risk factors, including the use of oral contraceptives, pregnancy, puerperium, and hormone replacement therapy [6]. The D-dimer study has not been shown to be clinically helpful in the assessment of CVT in most cases. Up to 26% of 73 patients in one study with a negative D-dimer had radiography-confirmed CVT [7]. A meta-analysis demonstrated that in low-risk patients (headache patients with normal neurological examination, normal standard CT head, and absence of risk factors), d-dimer has a high negative predictive value for excluding CVT. Sensitivity was low but comparable to values accepted in pulmonary embolism and deep venous thrombosis assessments [8].

Plasma Metanephrines

Catecholamine-secreting tumors can be considered with refractory chronic headache and his-

tory of hypertension. The most common tests for detection of this condition are 24-h urine collection for creatinine, total catecholamines, vanillyl-mandelic acid, and metanephrines. The most sensitive test is plasma metanephrine. Be aware that false-negative results can occur, and it is best to collect specimens during symptomatic periods [9, 10].

Markers of Inflammation

Vasculitis and giant cell arteritis may be causes of chronic daily headache. Erythrocyte sediment rate (ESR) and C-reactive protein (CRP), as well as platelet counts and iron studies, can be beneficial in identifying systemic inflammation. It should be noted that steroids as well as NSAIDs may artificially suppress ESR and CRP.

ESR

Erythrocyte sediment rate (ESR) is the rate at which red blood cells sediment in a period of 1 h. This is a very nonspecific test that requires a level of clinical suspicion to help guide the provider. It can be elevated in a variety of conditions including inflammation, pregnancy, anemia, autoimmune disorders, infections, kidney diseases, and some cancers—like lymphoma and multiple myeloma.

For patients that are over 50 years old and have headache, this can be useful in the identification or ruling out giant cell arteritis (GCA). ICHD-3 beta criteria for headache attributed to giant cell arteritis (GCA) include the development of headache in temporal relationship with clinical or biological signs of onset of GCA; this would include ESR, CRP, and temporal artery biopsy [11]. The American College of Rheumatology GCA diagnostic criteria include the elevation of ESR above 50 mm/hour by the Westergren method. Sensitivity of ESR alone is 86.5% and a specificity of 47.7% [12].

Normal clinical ESR value is anything less than age divided by 2 in men and age plus 10 divided by 2 in women [13]. An alternative formula uses a more complex method to determine a normal ESR based on age: $17.3 + (0.18 \yen age)$ for men and $22.1 + (0.18 \yen age)$ for women [14].

ESR result depends on multiple factors including age and medication use. Steroids and NSAIDs use could suppress the ESR value in GCA. It also could be normal in cases of biopsy-proven GCA [15, 16].

CRP

C-reactive protein (CRP) is an acute-phase reactant; levels rise in response to inflammation. CRP level is stable and does not depend on age or sex. A CRP value of 5 is considered elevated. The sensitivity of CRP in biopsy-proven GCA is 98.6%, and specificity is 75.7% [10, 17].

The combination of both ESR and CRP provides high sensitivity and specificity for a diagnosis of GCA. Per 1 study of 199 patients, only 1 patient had both a normal ESR and normal CRP in the presence of biopsy-proven GCA [10, 18].

ANA

Antinuclear antibodies (ANA) are autoantibodies that bind to the contents of the cell nucleus. There are many subtypes that can be found in specific autoimmune disorders including systemic lupus erythematosus (SLE)—both primary and drug induced—antiphospholipid syndrome (APS), Sjögren's syndrome, mixed connective tissue disease, scleroderma, polymyositis, dermatomyositis, and autoimmune hepatitis. Headache is one of the most often described neurologic manifestation in patients with APS, being presented either as a chronic headache or episodes of migraine [19].

There some evidence that about 1% of patients with SLE develop headaches due to idiopathic intracranial hypertension (IIH). Also, patients with polycystic ovary syndrome (POS) have shown abnormalities in coagulation cascade associated with IIH. Based on these findings, an ANA test and a lumbar puncture to evaluate an opening pressure should be included in an evaluation of patients with chronic refractory headache [20–24].

A diagnosis of antiphospholipid antibody syndrome should be considered in female patients with recurrent pregnancy loss or patients with unexplained vascular thrombosis. It is an autoimmune syndrome, and diagnosis requires evidence of antiphospholipid antibodies. It is appropriate to test for anti-beta-2- glycoprotein I antibodies or clot-based tests for the presence of the lupus anticoagulant [10, 25].

Primary angiitis of the central nervous system (PACNS)—normal serological markers but abnormal CSF (nonspecific elevation in total protein or WBC count).

Endocrine Testing

Thyroid Function Studies

There are multiple studies investigating the relationship between headache disorders and thyroid function. The relationship between headache and hypothyroidism has not been well established. Several small studies have shown a weak relationship between hypothyroidism and migraines. A small case control study published in 2002 suggested an association [26], and a small uncontrolled case series in 1998 showed resolution of headache in 31 of 102 patients treated for hypothyroidism [27]. A more recent article by Carvalho et al. described a cross-sectional study of overt hypothyroidism and subclinical hypothyroidism both with and without headache attributed to hypothyroidism [28]. The study showed similar frequencies of headache attributed to hypothyroidism in both overt and subclinical hypothyroidism. The study did also show that a history of migraine was more common in patients presenting with headache attributed to hypothyroidism. After levothyroxine treatment the study showed an improvement in 78% of cases. This study did have some limitations as it was a relatively small, cross-sectional study.

There have been some conflicting studies, which have shown that hypothyroidism is not prevalent among patients with chronic headaches or that there is no association between hypothyroidism and headache [29–31]. However, these studies too have their limitations, as they tend to be older studies and were on a small scale.

Martin et al. [32] report that patients with preexisting headache disorders had a 21% increased risk of developing new-onset hypothyroidism, while those with possible migraine showed an increased risk of 41%. One of the population-based studies reported that headache was 50% less likely in women with no history of thyroid dysfunction [31].

Based on growing evidence of relationship between headache disorders and thyroid abnormalities, we recommend checking serum TSH and a free T4 in all patients with chronic migraine to evaluate for hypo- and hyperthyroidism. Diagnostic TSH value for hypothyroidism is 10 mU/L with total serum thyroxine (T4) levels of 4.8 lg/dL. If TSH levels are elevated, a free T4 level should be checked. Some experts suggest checking total T4 level and thyroid-binding globulin level. Elevation of TSH levels in the setting of a low T4 is specific for primary hypothyroidism diagnosis. Elevated TSH in the presence of normal T4 levels is defined as subclinical hypothyroidism [33].

Hypothalamic or pituitary tumors, lymphocytic hypophysitis, and traumatic brain injury could present clinically with headache, and central hypothyroidism should be suspected when TSH levels are inappropriately low in relation to T4 level.

Prolactin, GH, and ACTH

Evaluation of pituitary hormonal function for patients with chronic headache is not recommended routinely. Headaches secondary to pituitary adenoma are usually diagnosed by radiological methods. Pituitary apoplexy, which is a life-threatening condition, can be diagnosed in ER based on clinical symptoms. Pituitary function tests can be abnormal in cases of pituitary apoplexy, but they usually do not play a critical role in the diagnosis.

Although not the part of diagnostic criteria, in cases of lymphocytic hypophysitis, prolactin level could be elevated in 50% of cases, or autoantibodies against hypophyseal cytosol protein could be detected in 20% [1].

Infectious

Lyme

Testing for Lyme disease is not recommended in patients with vague complaints, which may include but are not limited to headache, myalgia, arthralgias, fever, and fatigue, and who have no other clinical signs or symptoms of Lyme disease, particularly erythema migrans, and do not have a history of exposure to an arthropod vector and do not live or have not recently traveled to an endemic area [34].

The current CDC recommendation is for a two-tiered test for Lyme disease. At the current time, serologic testing is the only Lyme disease test method approved by the US FDA. The first test is performed using either an enzyme immunoassay (EIA) or immunofluorescence assay (IFA) [1]. Most commonly enzyme immunoassays are used, and measured total immunoglobulin G (IgG), immunoglobulin M (IgM), and, less commonly, immunofluorescence assays are used [34]. Enzyme immunoassays are quantitative tests, and they are diagnostically sensitive but not specific; specificity rates range only about 85% [34]. False-positive enzyme immunoassays may occur in the presence of multiple cross-reactive antibodies, some of which include but are not limited to *Helicobacter pylori*, some autoimmune disorders, syphilis, anaplasmosis, and others [35]. In the presence of a positive first-tier test, a second-tier test should be able to differentiate Lyme disease from other conditions, since second-tier testing has a higher diagnostic specificity [36]. Further testing is not performed if the first-tier test is negative, because doing so would reduce the test diagnostic specificity and could potentially yield a false positive.

Second-tier testing uses immunoblot tests; this consists of a Western blot for IGF and IgG which has a very high diagnostic specificity [34, 37]. Failing to follow the sequence outlined in the CDC recommendation increases the probability of a false-positive result, because of decreasing test specificity. Negative EIA testing is not sent for further testing and is considered negative. A positive or equivocal EIA with a negative Western blot is reported as negative, while a positive or equivocal EIA with a positive Western blot is reported as positive [38].

Unfortunately, two-tiered testing is relatively insensitive (<40%) during early illness which is characterized by erythema migrans rash; however it is reasonably sensitive (>87%) and very specific (99%) when used for diagnostic testing of disseminated Lyme disease [39]. During the first 30 days of the disease, when erythema migrans are most notably present, an IgM response is present, and an IgG response does not typically develop until after 30 days. If the patient has had signs and symptoms for less than 30 days, IgM and IgG Western blots should be performed; if symptoms are present for more than 30 days, only IgG Western blot should be performed. Both IgM and IgG can remain elevated for years after successful treatment; therefore IgM is not a dependable indicator of reinfection [34]; instead the clinician should rely on clinical signs and symptoms.

Negative testing during the early stages of Lyme disease does not completely eliminate the possibility of Lyme disease. If there is a high clinical suspicion of Lyme disease, a second specimen may be tested; it is also important keep in mind that antimicrobial therapy may decrease the main response and lead to negative testing at later dates [40, 41].

Lyme neuroborreliosis occurs in proximally 5–20% of Lyme disease cases in North America. Manifestations can include aseptic meningitis, encephalopathy, cranial nerve palsies, and peripheral neuropathies [34]. Aseptic meningitis produced by Lyme disease can manifest as headaches and neck pain with possibility of low-grade fever. Cerebrospinal fluid profile is similar to that of viral meningitis, with a mild to moderate lymphocytic pleocytosis, normal to slightly decreased glucose level, and a mild increase in protein. Approximately 5% of untreated patients went on to develop chronic neuroborreliosis which can manifest as encephalomyelitis and chronic axonal polyneuropathy which can present as radicular pain or paresthesias. In cases of suspected neuroborreliosis, CSF should be evaluated for the presence of antibodies by EIA and should have a higher titer in the CSF than in the serum (this seems to have fallen out of favor). Headache, fatigue, paresthesias, and mild stiff neck alone are not criteria for neurological involvement [42].

HIV

In patients with acute symptomatic HIV infection, the usual time from exposure to development of symptoms is typically 2–4 weeks, although incubation periods of up to 10 months have been observed [43]. Initial HIV infections can present with a variety of symptoms and are known as acute retroviral syndrome. Typical signs and symptoms include, but are not limited to, fever, sore throat, rash, arthralgias, lymphadenopathy, weight loss, diarrhea, and headaches [44]. The headache is often described as retro-orbital exacerbated by eye movement. With the onset of headache, one must be concerned about aseptic meningitis which is typically accompanied by photophobia. In addition to HIV testing, a lumbar puncture with cerebrospinal fluid analysis should be obtained [45]. In a study of 41 patients presenting with acute symptomatic HIV infection, approximately 24% had signs and symptoms that would be suggestive of an aseptic meningitis [46].

Thus, in high-risk populations, we recommend a very low threshold for HIV testing with new-onset chronic headache. High-risk populations include homosexual and bisexual men who engage in unprotected sex [47]; in particular, minorities appear to be more affected in this demographic. In addition certain minorities appear to have higher infection rates and higher percentage of infected individuals in their communities. These include African Americans and those of Latino descent [47]. Incarcerated individuals have also been shown to have an infection rate up to five times the rate of non-incarcerated individuals [47]. High-risk behaviors include but are not limited to IV drug use and having unprotected sex with multiple partners.

In patients with newly diagnosed HIV with signs and symptoms of aseptic meningitis, a lumbar puncture with appropriate CSF fluid studies should certainly be pursued. CSF studies of patients with later-stage HIV disease and suspected opportunistic infections will be covered in the cerebral spinal fluid analysis section.

Lumbar Puncture

Patients with chronic refractory headaches may require lumbar puncture as part of the workup; this may be pursued after imaging has been performed. Lumbar puncture may be used to evaluate for both high and low pressure headaches, as well as basic labs which may assess for signs of inflammation and infection. Every lumbar puncture should have an opening pressure measured; this should be done in the lateral decubitus position with the patient's legs extended. Normal CSF pressure should be 7–18 cm H_2O in adults [48], although some sources do report this as 5–25 cm H_2O [49, 50]. Certainly an opening pressure of less than 5 cm H_2O or greater than or equal to 25 cm H_2O is cause for concern (Table 12.2). Basic CSF labs should be sent with each lumbar puncture; this should include a cell count and differential, protein, and glucose.

Cell Count and Differential, Protein, and Glucose

Typical protein levels in CSF may vary by laboratory, but a typical CSF protein level for an adult is <45 mg/dl. Elevated CSF protein can be a sign of meningitis or tuberculosis, and low levels can be a sign of autoimmune disease or multiple sclerosis. Elevated protein can also raise suspicion of subarachnoid hemorrhage. Normal CSF glucose is approximately 60% of serum values. CSF glucose can be low in fungal and bacterial meningitis or in

cases of tuberculosis. Elevated CSF glucose is more often seen in cases of aseptic meningitis but if not can be <40% in cases of HSV. Cases of subarachnoid hemorrhage often have normal glucose levels. Nucleated cell counts will vary with laboratory, but elevated cell counts are often indicative of meningitis or multiple sclerosis. Typically, multiple sclerosis will have a normal to slightly elevated cell count, typically on the order or 0–20 cells/microliter with a lymphocyte predominance. Bacterial meningitis will typically a have cell count of >100 cells/microliter with a polymorphonuclear predominance. Typically, aseptic meningitis will have a lymphocyte predominance, and cell counts may range between 10 and 1000 cells/microliter. CSF typically has a clear color, and cloudiness or opacity may clue the clinician into possible infections.

Opening Pressure

Obtaining a close opening pressure when preforming a lumbar puncture can help guide the management of a headache patient. An elevated opening pressure ≥ 25 cmH_2O in adults or ≥ 28 cmH_2O in children will meet diagnostic criteria for idiopathic intracranial hypertension in the setting of a normal cerebrospinal fluid profile [11, 51].

ACE

Neurologic complications can occur in about 5% of patients with sarcoidosis [52], and the presenting manifestation of sarcoid can be neurological in up to half of those patients with neurosarcoidosis. Headache is one of the most common presenting symptoms of neurosarcoidosis [53]. In patients with or without isolated neurosarcoidosis, serum angiotensin-converting enzyme (ACE) may not always be elevated; in addition CSF ACE may either not be consistently elevated or may be falsely elevated. Both infection and carcinomatosis meningitis can cause elevated ACE. The most common CSF abnormalities in

Table 12.2 Conditions associated with headache categorized by opening pressure measurements

Low-pressure headaches	CSF leak, CSF flow obstruction
Normal pressure headaches	Aseptic meningitis, intracranial masses, cerebral epidural abscess
High-pressure headaches	IIH, meningitis, SAH (acute), abscess, intracranial vasculitis, encephalitis, meningeal carcinomatosis, intracranial mass, venous sinus thrombosis, GBS, jugular venous compression, choroid plexus papilloma

patients with diagnosed neurosarcoidosis were elevated CSF protein and/or pleocytosis, and elevated CSF ACE is a less common finding [54]. CSF ACE concentrations could also potentially be elevated if serum ACE elevations exist in addition to conditions which may cause a leaky blood-brain barrier. For this reason, CSF ACE testing should be pursued if there is a clinical suspicion of sarcoidosis.

Cytology

Although carcinomatous meningitis is a rare complication of cancer, it is often devastating. Headache is often the most common initial symptom and can present in up to 32% of patients [55]. CSF findings are typically high protein, low glucose, and lymphocytic pleocytosis. Cytology is the definitive diagnostic finding with a very high specificity. However the sensitivity has been reported between 80 and 95 percent. To minimize false negatives, a minimum of 10 ml should be sent for cytological analysis, specimens should be promptly processed, and the lumbar puncture should be repeated if there is high clinical suspicion. The optimal number of samples is unclear, but the rates of positive cytology approach 98% for more than three samples per patient; however this did vary with the volume of CSF as well as specimen processing and intervening treatment [56].

Infectious Workup

The infectious workup with regard to headache can be broad. Typically, the CSF results may point the clinician in the proper direction. CSF results showing meningitis will necessitate Gram stains and cultures in the case of bacterial meningitis. CSF consistent with aseptic meningitis should be sent for cultures, Gram stain, and PCR particularly for herpes simplex virus and varicella zoster. Cases of fungal meningitis will necessitate India ink stains, CSF, and blood cultures.

However, the infectious work may vary by the time of year. During the spring and summer months, the clinician should have a higher suspicion of arthropod-associated diseases and test accordingly based upon location and risk factors.

TNF-Alpha

Levels of tumor necrosis factor alpha (TNF-α) have been shown to be elevated in patients with new daily persistent headache (NDPH) [57]. TNF-α is a pro-inflammatory cytokine that is involved in immune and inflammatory activities as well as pain initiation. A 2007 study by Rozen et al. compared CSF TNF-α levels of 36 healthy volunteers with 38 patients with chronic daily headache [57]. The study evaluated 20 patients with new daily persistent headache as well as 16 chronic migraine patients and 2 posttraumatic headache patients. The study did demonstrate elevations and tumor necrosis factor alpha in 19 of the 20 new daily persistent headache patients, with levels above the upper limit of normal. The study did also demonstrate that all 16 chronic migraine patients had elevated levels of CSF tumor necrosis factor alpha above the upper limit of normal as defined by the testing laboratory. Serum TNF-α levels had also been tested in 14 NDPH patients as well as 5 chronic migraine patients, and these levels were only elevated in 3 of the NDPH patients. None of these patients demonstrated abnormal CSF cell counts, total protein, or glucose. Cultures were also done and negative. Seven patient's did have elevated spinal opening pressures (>20 cm H_2O), but none of which were deemed to have intracranial hypertension and all had normal funduscopic examinations. It is thought that pro-inflammatory cytokines in the CSF produce and enhance pain in animal models [57]. TNF-α has also been thought to induce calcitonin gene-related peptide production, and elevated levels of TNF-α in the CSF may explain why a certain percentage of hospitalized patients do not improve with standard headache therapy.

The overall role of TNF-α is unclear at this point, and even the methods used in the initial paper describing elevated TNF-α remain controversial [58, 59]. In 2013, Rozen et al. did publish a case report of a patient with NDPH that did respond to nimodipine. The proposed action of nimodipine in this case was inhibition of TNF-α [60]. However, at this time there is very little evidence to support this. Routinely measuring CSF TNF-α is not recommended, as there is no significant evidence for its use in directing management of such patients.

IGG Index and Oligoclonal Bands

The majority of studies reviewing the potential association between multiple sclerosis (MS) and migraine have not supported a definite link [61]. The overall incidence of headache in MS does not appear to be significantly higher than that of the general population. There is an association between MS and trigeminal neuralgia; in addition there may be atypical facial pain syndromes and neuralgias, associated with multiple sclerosis which may be referred for evaluation by headache specialist. Typically head imaging will assist in this diagnosis, if there is a high suspicion for a diagnosis of MS, and lumbar puncture might also be useful, testing for oligoclonal bands [62] as well as IgG index. However, we do not recommend routine testing for IgG index and oligoclonal bands without a clinical suspicion of multiple sclerosis, whether by history or by imaging. Although often times done, checking for myelin basic protein is not shown to be beneficial for a diagnosis of multiple sclerosis [63].

Genetic Testing

CADASIL

The stroke syndrome CADASIL (cerebral autosomal dominant arteriopathy with subcortical infarcts and leukoencephalopathy) is thought to be caused by mutations of the NOTCH3 gene on chromosome 19 [64]. This disorder results in a variety of symptoms, which most commonly include vascular degeneration, progressive cognitive decline, dementia, and subcortical ischemic strokes, in addition to migraine with aura [64]. Migraine with aura can occur in nearly one half of CADASIL patients [65, 66] and is often the initial manifestation of the disease. The average age of onset is approximately 30 years, and aura symptoms tend to involve the visual and sensory symptoms [66]. Isolated migraine aura (without headache) may represent up to 20% of patients with CADASIL [66]. Patients with a family history or personal history of multi-infarct dementia, vascular encephalopathy, or early-onset dementia in addition to chronic migraine with aura should certainly be tested for CADASIL.

At the current time, there are at least 200 mutations in the NOTCH3 gene, resulting in an odd number of residues which are known to be associated with CADASIL [64]. There are several ways of diagnosing CADASIL; traditionally skin biopsy with histological examination has been used. This evaluates two features which are highly specific of the condition: granular osmophilic material and deposition of the NOTCH3 receptor in the vascular media. However despite the use of biopsy testing, low sensitivity levels have been reported [64]. Genetic sequencing using a traditional Sanger sequencing system has been shown to be expensive and time-consuming because of the large number of axons combined with high GC content in the NOTCH3 gene [64]. Current recommendations are for next-generation sequencing (NGS) technologies to be used for genetic testing for NOTCH3 mutations associated with CADASIL [64].

MTHFR and ACE Polymorphisms

The mechanism of migraine is believed to involve the trigeminal cervicogenic complex which receives nociceptive information via afferent projections from the dura matter in large intracranial vessels. This information is then in turn passed up to higher processing centers within the brain. It is believed that vasoactive neuropeptides are released leading to neurogenic inflammation [67]. Based on this information, it has been theorized that the biochemical molecules disrupt endothelial function and may influence susceptibility to migraines. Two genes that are of interest are angiotensin-converting enzyme (ACE) and the C677T polymorphism in the homocysteine metabolism gene methylenetetrahydrofolate reductase (MTHFR). Although the exact role of these genes still remains controversial in this process, testing for polymorphisms in these genes has been suggested as a possible pathway to treatment, particularly with regard to supplementation of the MTHFR genotype [68].

Both the MTHFR and the ACE gene have been known to affect the vasculature in change regulation of cerebral blood flow. MTHFR in particular regulates circulating homocysteine levels which interact with epithelial cells. Experiments in animal models have suggested that hyperhomocysteinemia may cause persons with this polymorphism to be more susceptible to migraine. It is also been hypothesized that homocysteine-related endothelial dysfunction may play a role in initiation and maintenance of migraine attacks. ACE has been shown to play a role in blood pressure regulation and electrolyte balance and has been expressed in vascular endothelial cells among other cell types. ACE has also been shown to inactivate bradykinin which is a potent vasodilator [67]. To this date investigational efforts have not been shown to be able to demonstrate a reproducible and significant influence of a single genetic variant of these two genotypes on migraine. However, it is important to recognize that the interplay of multiple genetic variants likely contributes to a much greater extent than single variations by themselves.

In 2016, Essmeister et al. reviewed 420 patients with migraine for genotype frequencies of both the MTHFR and ACE variants. They were unable to show that polymorphisms in either of these two genes increase susceptibility to migraine alone. They also did not show any association between polymorphisms in the ACE

and the MTHFR gene with migraine [67]. This reinforces the idea that migraine is likely the result multiple genetic variances. At this time, we do not recommend routine testing for ACE or MTHFR polymorphisms in chronic migraine patients.

MELAS

Mitochondrial encephalomyelitis with lactic acidosis and stroke-like episodes (MELAS) is a multi-system disorder and is caused by mutations in mitochondrial DNA. This is a maternally inherited disorder and is caused by mutations in mitochondrial DNA [69–71]. The disorder is characterized by recurrence of stroke-like episodes with resultant hemiparesis, cortical blindness, or hemianopia. Other common features include generalized seizures, recurrent migraine-like headaches, vomiting, short stature, hearing loss, and muscle weakness [72, 73]. Stroke-like symptoms in MELAS are described as acute-onset neurological symptoms, and MRI imaging does show high signal on diffusion-weighted imaging. The term "stroke-like symptoms" is used for several reasons; as unlike typical embolic or thrombotic ischemic strokes, the brain lesions of MELAS do not follow vascular territories. The acute MRI signal changes may not be static and may actually fluctuate, migrate, or resolve quickly when compared to a typical ischemic stroke. Apparent diffusion coefficient on MRI is not always decreased as it is classically with ischemic strokes; it may also be increased or demonstrate a mixed-type pattern [72]. Typically MELAS manifests in childhood with a relapsing remitting course and progressive neurologic dysfunction and dementia [69, 73]. Patients with stroke-like episodes before age 40 in addition to encephalopathy and seizures or dementia should be tested for MELAS.

Testing for MELAS should include appropriate mitochondrial studies; approximately 80% of cases are related to the m.3243A>G mutation and 10% to the m.3271T>C mutation; however there are over 30 genetic variants that are described as being associated with MELAS [74]. Blood work should check for lactic acidosis and skeletal muscle biopsy for the presence of ragged red fibers which may aid in the diagnosis of MELAS. Genetic testing is typically done via molecular genetic testing of mitochondrial DNA. Patients with atypical presentations or inconclusive testing may benefit from an evaluation by a genetics counselor.

Familial Hemiplegic Migraine

Hemiplegic migraine is characterized by unilateral weakness that accompanies a migraine headache attack, which differentiates it from other types of migraine. This weakness is a manifestation of motor aura and occurs with other forms of aura that can impair visual, sensation, and speech. Familial hemiplegic migraine comes in three varieties; in addition sporadic hemiplegic migraine cases have also been documented.

Familial hemiplegic migraine is transmitted in an autosomal dominant pattern; however penetrance can be variable between the different types of familial hemiplegic migraine. Familial hemiplegic migraine type I is associated with mutations in the CACNA1A gene on chromosome 19p13. This encodes an alpha subunit of the P−/Q-type calcium channel [75]. This mutation, like all familial hemiplegic syndromes, lowers the susceptibility to cortical spreading depression. The estimated penetrance for familial hemiplegic migraine type 1 is somewhere between 67% and 89% [76–78].

Familial hemiplegic migraine type II is associated with mutations in the ATP1A2 gene on chromosome 1q23. This encodes a subunit of the sodium potassium ATPase; this mutation has also been associated with migraine with brainstem aura as well as several types of epilepsy [79, 80]. Familial hemiplegic migraine type II has a penetrance of between 63% and 87% [76, 77, 81].

Familial hemiplegic migraine type III is caused by mutation in the SCN1A gene on chromosome 2q24, which encodes the transmembrane alpha subunit of the sodium channel [82]. The esti-

mated penetrance of this mutation is upward of 100% [76]. This mutation has also been linked to several types of epilepsy.

Patients with first member of their family to have hemiplegic migraine are categorized as having the sporadic hemiplegic migraine variant. Both de novo mutations and inheritance from an asymptomatic parent could be the cause in these cases. The CACNA1A and ATP1A2 mutations have been demonstrated in patients with sporadic hemiplegic migraine [76, 83].

Although diagnosis of hemiplegic migraine remains a clinical diagnosis, the clinician should rely on a thorough history as well as a thorough family history; genetic testing may be useful, particularly in cases of early-onset sporadic hemiplegic migraine or in cases of familial hemiplegic migraine when the phenotype diverges from those of the affected relatives. Genetic testing for mutations involves testing for CACNA1A, ATP1A2, and SCN1A mutations.

Special Cases

Pregnancy

A change in headache pattern or new headaches during pregnancy is not uncommon and may be due to migraine- or tension-type headaches, but a variety of secondary causes may occur. This includes preeclampsia, postdural puncture headache, and cerebral venous thrombosis. Preeclampsia must be excluded in every pregnant woman over 20 week's gestation. Common laboratory studies include a complete blood cell count, complete metabolic panel to include liver function tests, and urine studies for protein, and a referral to maternal fetal medicine should be considered.

Immunocompromise

Daily headaches in patients who are immunocompromised, either by HIV infection, immunosuppression, or primary immunodeficiency, warrant extensive workup, as there are many opportunistic infections as well as tumors which may cause headaches. Workup should be extensive and include a lumbar puncture, which should include basic cell counts as well as protein and glucose; an elevated opening pressure may also be a clue as to the presence of a CNS infection. Tuberculosis is a concern at all CD4 counts, but if CD4 counts less than 250, coccidioidomycosis and pneumocystosis are of concern. With the lower CD4 counts, histoplasmosis, toxoplasma, and cryptococcus are of more concern. CSF fluid should be evaluated for these infections.

Traumatic Brain Injury

Headache may occur in as many as 78% of persons following mild traumatic brain injury. Typically, headache prevalence, as well as duration severity, is often more of an issue in patients with milder head injuries than those with more severe head injuries.

Hypercoagulability States

Overall, the pathogenesis of migraine is complex and multifaceted; the relationship of migraine to thrombophilia states is not fully understood. Most consistently positive are studies investigating estrogen, platelets, red blood cells, and markers of endothelial activation and dysfunction [3]. There are several hypotheses which link hypercoagulability to migraine; the first theorized mechanism is via ischemia-induced cortical spreading depression without infarction. This was supported by a 2010 study in which cortical spreading depression was triggered in a rodent model by injections of microspheres, air, and cholesterol crystals which induced hypoperfusion without infarct [33]. A second possible mechanism linking migraine with aura and hypercoagulability is that cortical spreading depression leads to endothelial damage and elicits an inflammatory cascade with subsequent activation of peripheral and central trigeminal vascular neurons. Other potential mechanisms may link migraine to hypercoagulability through stress, which is a common trigger and consequence of migraine.

Stroke in the general population is typically atherosclerotic in nature. Migraine-related stroke tends to be most prevalent in young persons, particularly women, and is likely in persons with low vascular risk factor profiles. This supports the hypothesis that migraine-related strokes are non-atherosclerotic in nature. This is also supported by several comorbid conditions that are often found with migraine including Raynaud's disease, non-atherogenic endotheliopathies, livedo reticularis, preeclampsia, and vasospastic angina [3]. The relationship between patent foramen ovale, thrombophilia states, and migraine with aura-associated stroke has been shown in several studies, but the management of these in migraine remains controversial.

Screening for hypercoagulable states and patent foramen ovale becomes important if one accepts that there's a spectrum between CSD-related ischemia without infarction and migraine-related stroke. Table 12.3 summarizes our recommendations for screening in patients with migraine with aura in addition to history of endotheliopathies, family history of thrombosis, white matter abnormalities, and stroke-like lesions on brain MRI. Management of patients with stroke symptoms or history of thrombosis in addition migraine with order should not only revolve around management of migraine but should also involve minimizing stroke risk factors.

Table 12.3 Headache in hypercoagulable state

Clinical presentation	Hypercoagulable evaluation	Evaluation of stroke risk factors
Migraine with aura with history of endotheliopathies	CBC, CRP, von Willebrand factor, fibrillation, homocysteine	HgbA1C Fasting lipid profile
Migraine with aura with a personal or family history of thrombosis	CBC, CRP, von Willebrand factor, fibrillation, homocysteine, glycosylated hemoglobin, fasting lipid profile, protein C, protein S, antithrombin deficiencies, prothrombin, antiphospholipid antibodies	HgbA1C Fasting lipid profile
Migraine with aura with subcortical white matter abnormalities on MRI	CBC, CRP, von Willebrand factor, fibrillation, homocysteine, glycosylated hemoglobin, fasting lipid profile, antiphospholipid antibodies, CADASIL	HgbA1C Fasting lipid profile
Migraine with aura with stroke-like lesions on MRI	CBC, CRP, von Willebrand factor, fibrillation, homocysteine, glycosylated hemoglobin, fasting lipid profile, protein C, protein S, antithrombin deficiencies, activated protein C, prothrombin, antiphospholipid antibody, evaluation for PFO (agitated saline TTE or TEE)	HgbA1C Fasting lipid profile

References

1. George JN, et al. Drug-induced thrombocytopenia: a systematic review of published case reports. Ann Intern Med. 1998;129(11):886–90.
2. Chang CY, Schiano TD. Review article: drug hepatotoxicity. Aliment Pharmacol Ther. 2007;25(10):1135–51.
3. Tietjen GE, Collins SA. Hypercoagulability and migraine. Headache. 2017;58(1):173–83.
4. Zakharova MY, et al. Risk factors for heart attack, stroke, and venous thrombosis associated with hormonal contraceptive use. Clin Appl Thromb Hemost. 2011;17(4):323–31.
5. Miyakis S, et al. International consensus statement on an update of the classification criteria for definite antiphospholipid syndrome (APS). J Thromb Haemost. 2006;4(2):295–306.
6. Coutinho JM, et al. Cerebral venous and sinus thrombosis in women. Stroke. 2009;40(7):2356–61.
7. Crassard I, et al. A negative D-dimer assay does not rule out cerebral venous thrombosis: a series of seventy-three patients. Stroke. 2005;36(8):1716–9.
8. Alons IM, et al. D-dimer for the exclusion of cerebral venous thrombosis: a meta-analysis of low risk patients with isolated headache. BMC Neurol. 2015;15:118.
9. Kudva YC, Sawka AM, Young WF Jr. Clinical review 164: the laboratory diagnosis of adrenal pheochromocytoma: the Mayo Clinic experience. J Clin Endocrinol Metab. 2003;88(10):4533–9.
10. Loder E, Cardona L. Evaluation for secondary causes of headache: the role of blood and urine testing. Headache. 2011;51(2):338–45.
11. Headache Classification Committee of the International Headache Society (IHS). The international classification of headache disorders, 3rd edition (beta version). Cephalalgia. 2013;33(9):629–808.
12. Hunder GG, et al. The American college of rheumatology 1990 criteria for the classification of giant cell arteritis. Arthritis Rheum. 1990;33(8):1122–8.
13. Miller A, Green M, Robinson D. Simple rule for calculating normal erythrocyte sedimentation rate. Br Med J (Clin Res Ed). 1983;286(6361):266.
14. Hayreh SS, et al. Giant cell arteritis: validity and reliability of various diagnostic criteria. Am J Ophthalmol. 1997;123(3):285–96.
15. Levin M, Ward TN. Horton's disease: past and present. Curr Pain Headache Rep. 2005;9(4):259–63.
16. Nye BL, Ward TN. Clinic and emergency room evaluation and testing of headache. Headache. 2015;55(9):1301–8.
17. Costello F, et al. Role of thrombocytosis in diagnosis of giant cell arteritis and differentiation of arteritic from non-arteritic anterior ischemic optic neuropathy. Eur J Ophthalmol. 2004;14(3):245–57.
18. Parikh M, et al. Prevalence of a normal C-reactive protein with an elevated erythrocyte sedimentation rate in biopsy-proven giant cell arteritis. Ophthalmology. 2006;113(10):1842–5.
19. Mayer M, et al. Antiphospholipid syndrome and central nervous system. Clin Neurol Neurosurg. 2010;112(7):602–8.
20. Glueck CJ, et al. Idiopathic intracranial hypertension: associations with coagulation disorders and polycystic-ovary syndrome. J Lab Clin Med. 2003;142(1):35–45.
21. Kim JM, et al. Idiopathic intracranial hypertension as a significant cause of intractable headache in patients

with systemic lupus erythematosus: a 15-year experience. Lupus. 2012;21(5):542–7.

22. Tse C, Klein R. Intracranial hypertension associated with systemic lupus erythematosus in a young male patient. Lupus. 2013;22(2):205–12.

23. Dhungana S, Sharrack B, Woodroofe N. Idiopathic intracranial hypertension. Acta Neurol Scand. 2010;121(2):71–82.

24. Hanly JG, et al. Headache in systemic lupus erythematosus: results from a prospective, international inception cohort study. Arthritis Rheum. 2013;65(11):2887–97.

25. Galli M. Clinical utility of laboratory tests used to identify antiphospholipid antibodies and to diagnose the antiphospholipid syndrome. Semin Thromb Hemost. 2008;34(4):329–34.

26. Singh SK. Prevalence of migraine in hypothyroidism. J Assoc Physicians India. 2002;50:1455–6.

27. Moreau T, et al. Headache in hypothyroidism. Prevalence and outcome under thyroid hormone therapy. Cephalalgia. 1998;18(10):687–9.

28. Lima Carvalho MF, de Medeiros JS, Valenca MM. Headache in recent onset hypothyroidism: prevalence, characteristics and outcome after treatment with levothyroxine. Cephalalgia. 2016;37(10):938–46.

29. Iwasaki Y, et al. Thyroid function in patients with chronic headache. Int J Neurosci. 1991;57(3–4):263–7.

30. Amy JR. Tests of thyroid function in chronic headache patients. Headache. 1987;27(6):351–3.

31. Hagen K, et al. Low headache prevalence amongst women with high TSH values. Eur J Neurol. 2001;8(6):693–9.

32. Martin AT, et al. Headache disorders may be a risk factor for the development of new onset hypothyroidism. Headache. 2017;57(1):21–30.

33. Surks MI, et al. Subclinical thyroid disease: scientific review and guidelines for diagnosis and management. JAMA. 2004;291(2):228–38.

34. Miraglia CM. A review of the centers for disease control and prevention's guidelines for the clinical laboratory diagnosis of Lyme disease. J Chiropr Med. 2016;15(4):272–80.

35. Understanding the EIA Test| Lyme Disease | CDC. [cited 2017 May 16]; Available from: https://www. cdc.gov/lyme/diagnosistesting/labtest/twostep/eia/ index.htm.

36. Dressler F, et al. Western blotting in the serodiagnosis of Lyme disease. J Infect Dis. 1993;167(2):392–400.

37. Two-step laboratory testing process| lyme disease | CDC. [cited 2017 May 16]; Available from: https:// www.cdc.gov/lyme/diagnosistesting/labtest/twostep/.

38. Notice to Readers Recommendations for Test Performance and Interpretation from the Second National Conference on Serologic Diagnosis of Lyme Disease. [cited 2017 May 16]; Available from: https:// www.cdc.gov/mmwr/preview/mmwrhtml/00038469. htm.

39. Hinckley AF, et al. Lyme disease testing by large commercial laboratories in the United States. Clin Infect Dis. 2014;59(5):676–81.

40. Aucott J, et al. Diagnostic challenges of early Lyme disease: lessons from a community case series. BMC Infect Dis. 2009;9:79.

41. Aguero-Rosenfeld ME, et al. Evolution of the serologic response to Borrelia burgdorferi in treated patients with culture-confirmed erythema migrans. J Clin Microbiol. 1996;34(1):1–9.

42. Lyme Disease | 2017 Case Definition. [cited 2017 May 16]; Available from: /nndss/conditions/lyme-disease/ case-definition/2017/.

43. Ridzon R, et al. Simultaneous transmission of human immunodeficiency virus and hepatitis C virus from a needle-stick injury. N Engl J Med. 1997;336(13):919–22.

44. Robb ML, et al. Prospective study of acute HIV-1 infection in adults in East Africa and Thailand. N Engl J Med. 2016;374(22):2120–30.

45. Ho DD, et al. Isolation of HTLV-III from cerebrospinal fluid and neural tissues of patients with neurologic syndromes related to the acquired immunodeficiency syndrome. N Engl J Med. 1985;313(24):1493–7.

46. Schacker T, et al. CLinical and epidemiologic features of primary hiv infection. Ann Intern Med. 1996;125(4):257–64.

47. HIV Among Gay and Bisexual Men. 2017; Available from: https://www.cdc.gov/hiv/group/msm/index. html.

48. Reichman EF, Polglaze K, Euerle B. Neurological and neurosurgical procedures: lumbar puncture. In: Emergency medicine procedures. New York: McGraw Hill; 2013. p. 747–61.

49. Lee SC, Lueck CJ. Cerebrospinal fluid pressure in adults. J Neuroophthalmol. 2014;34(3):278–83.

50. Whiteley W, et al. CSF opening pressure: reference interval and the effect of body mass index. Neurology. 2006;67(9):1690–1.

51. Friedman DI, Liu GT, Digre KB. Revised diagnostic criteria for the pseudotumor cerebri syndrome in adults and children. Neurology. 2013;81(13):1159–65.

52. Stern BJ, et al. Sarcoidosis and its neurological manifestations. Arch Neurol. 1985;42(9):909–17.

53. O'Connell K, et al. Neurosarcoidosis: clinical presentations and changing treatment patterns in an Irish Caucasian population. Ir J Med Sci. 2017;186(3):759–66.

54. Joseph FG, Scolding NJ. Neurosarcoidosis: a study of 30 new cases. J Neurol Neurosurg Psychiatry. 2009;80(3):297–304.

55. Kaplan JG, et al. Leptomeningeal metastases: comparison of clinical features and laboratory data of solid tumors, lymphomas and leukemias. J Neuro-Oncol. 1990;9(3):225–9.

56. Glantz MJ, et al. Cerebrospinal fluid cytology in patients with cancer: minimizing false-negative results. Cancer. 1998;82(4):733–9.

57. Rozen T, Swidan SZ. Elevation of CSF tumor necrosis factor alpha levels in new daily persistent headache and treatment refractory chronic migraine. Headache. 2007;47(7):1050–5.

58. Saxon A. CSF TNFalpha has not been shown to be elevated in headache patients. Headache. 2015;55(9):1266.
59. Rozen TD. TNF-alpha has not been shown to be elevated in headache patients: a response. Headache. 2015;55(9):1267.
60. Rozen TD, Beams JL. New daily persistent headache with a thunderclap headache onset and complete response to nimodipine (a new distinct subtype of NDPH). J Headache Pain. 2013;14:100.
61. Terlizzi R, et al. P037. Headache in multiple sclerosis: prevalence and clinical features in a case control-study. J Headache Pain. 2015;16(Suppl 1):A83.
62. Huss AM, et al. Importance of cerebrospinal fluid analysis in the era of McDonald 2010 criteria: a German-Austrian retrospective multicenter study in patients with a clinically isolated syndrome. J Neurol. 2016;263(12):2499–504.
63. Lim ET, et al. Anti-myelin antibodies do not allow earlier diagnosis of multiple sclerosis. Mult Scler. 2005;11(4):492–4.
64. Maksemous N, et al. Targeted next generation sequencing identifies novel NOTCH3 gene mutations in CADASIL diagnostics patients. Hum Genomics. 2016;10(1):38.
65. Liem MK, et al. CADASIL and migraine: a narrative review. Cephalalgia. 2010;30(11):1284–9.
66. Guey S, et al. Prevalence and characteristics of migraine in CADASIL. Cephalalgia. 2015;36(11):1038–47.
67. Essmeister R, et al. MTHFR and ACE polymorphisms do not increase susceptibility to migraine neither alone nor in combination. Headache. 2016;56(8):1267–73.
68. Lea RA, et al. Genetic variants of angiotensin converting enzyme and methylenetetrahydrofolate reductase may act in combination to increase migraine susceptibility. Brain Res Mol Brain Res. 2005;136(1–2):112–7.
69. Pavlakis SG, et al. Mitochondrial myopathy, encephalopathy, lactic acidosis, and strokelike episodes: a distinctive clinical syndrome. Ann Neurol. 1984;16(4):481–8.
70. Montagna P, et al. MELAS syndrome: characteristic migrainous and epileptic features and maternal transmission. Neurology. 1988;38(5):751–4.
71. Ohno K, Isotani E, Hirakawa K. MELAS presenting as migraine complicated by stroke: case report. Neuroradiology. 1997;39(11):781–4.
72. Koenig MK, et al. Recommendations for the management of strokelike episodes in patients with mitochondrial encephalomyopathy, lactic acidosis, and strokelike episodes. JAMA Neurol. 2016;73(5):591–4.
73. Kaufmann P, et al. Natural history of MELAS associated with mitochondrial DNA m.3243A>G genotype. Neurology. 2011;77(22):1965–71.
74. Sunde K, et al. Case report: 5 year follow-up of adult late-onset mitochondrial encephalomyopathy with lactic acid and stroke-like episodes (MELAS). Mol Genet Metab Rep. 2016;9:94–7.
75. Ophoff RA, et al. Familial hemiplegic migraine and episodic ataxia type-2 are caused by mutations in the Ca2+ channel gene CACNL1A4. Cell. 1996;87(3):543–52.
76. Russell MB, Ducros A. Sporadic and familial hemiplegic migraine: pathophysiological mechanisms, clinical characteristics, diagnosis, and management. Lancet Neurol. 2011;10(5):457–70.
77. Thomsen LL, et al. The genetic spectrum of a population-based sample of familial hemiplegic migraine. Brain. 2007;130(Pt 2):346–56.
78. Ducros A, et al. The clinical spectrum of familial hemiplegic migraine associated with mutations in a neuronal calcium channel. N Engl J Med. 2001;345(1):17–24.
79. De Fusco M, et al. Haploinsufficiency of ATP1A2 encoding the Na+/K+ pump alpha2 subunit associated with familial hemiplegic migraine type 2. Nat Genet. 2003;33(2):192–6.
80. Ambrosini A, et al. Familial basilar migraine associated with a new mutation in the ATP1A2 gene. Neurology. 2005;65(11):1826–8.
81. Jurkat-Rott K, et al. Variability of familial hemiplegic migraine with novel A1A2 Na+/K+-ATPase variants. Neurology. 2004;62(10):1857–61.
82. Dichgans M, et al. Mutation in the neuronal voltage-gated sodium channel SCN1A in familial hemiplegic migraine. Lancet. 2005;366(9483):371–7.
83. Thomsen LL, et al. Screen for CACNA1A and ATP1A2 mutations in sporadic hemiplegic migraine patients. Cephalalgia. 2008;28(9):914–21.

Monitoring of Chronic Daily Headaches

13

Sam Hooshmand and Fallon C. Schloemer

Introduction

In 1996, Silberstein and Lipton proposed their criteria which classified chronic daily headache (CDH) as a stand-alone diagnosis [1]. Since then the significant debate has occurred regarding CDH classification. The consensus today per the International Classification of Headache Disorders 3rd edition (ICHD-3) is that CDH is not a specific headache type but rather an encompassing term for several different specific headache types. In general, CDH refers to headaches that occur on more days than not (at least 15 or more days a month for longer than 3 months) [2]. Predominantly, clinicians attempt to divide CDH into primary versus secondary entities. This initial approach allows implementation of appropriate intervention or therapies as well as referrals. In regard to primary entities, one can divide CDH into long-duration headaches (>4 h) and short-duration headaches (<4 h). The five major subtypes of long-duration CDHs include chronic migraine, chronic tension-type headache, medication overuse headache, hemicrania continua, and new daily persistent headache. Subtypes of chronic daily headache of shorter duration include chronic cluster headache, chronic paroxysmal hemicrania, hypnic headache, and primary stabbing headache as well as the unilateral neuralgiform headache [2, 3].

While epidemiological data on CDH is limited, evidence suggests that US and worldwide prevalence is roughly 3–4%, with Central/South American content having the highest prevalence (5%) and the African continent having the smallest prevalence (1.7%) [4–8]. This prevalence translates into the US population having an estimated 11 million individuals suffering from CDH. In the USA, the most prevalent subtype of CDH is tension-type headache (TTH). Chronic tension-type headache is followed by chronic migraine [6]. It is no surprise that the prevalence of CDH as well as its debilitating effects has a tremendous societal cost through healthcare expenditures and loss of economic productivity. Patients with chronic headache utilize more healthcare resources and have healthcare claims for medication twice as much compared to patients with other diseases [9]. To date, no study provides the financial impact of all CDH subtypes, but when examining the two most frequent subtypes, it is estimated to be between 20 and 26 billion dollars annually [10, 11].

Caring for patients suffering from CDH is no easy task. While the diagnosis can often be made during the initial visit using ICHD-3 guidelines, the subsequent identification of subtype, treatment strategy, and risk reduction is a large undertaking.

S. Hooshmand (✉) · F. C. Schloemer
Department of Neurology, Froedtert and the Medical College of Wisconsin, Milwaukee, WI, USA
e-mail: shooshmand@mcw.edu

© Springer International Publishing AG, part of Springer Nature 2019
M. W. Green et al. (eds.), *Chronic Headache*, https://doi.org/10.1007/978-3-319-91491-6_13

The first step in the effective management of CDH starts with the monitoring of CDH. The information gained from monitoring CDH allows clinicians to exclude secondary causes, identify risk factors, recognize the specific CDH subtype, and ultimately identify the most beneficial therapy.

Office Visit

The outpatient visit is the cornerstone to monitoring any chronic condition, and CDH is no different. With the variety of pathology CDH encompasses and the multitude of treatment modalities, a shift from individual provider to multidisciplinary therapy (MDT) has occurred over the past few decades. This multidisciplinary focus adds CDH to the growing list of other neurological conditions such as muscular dystrophy, amyotrophic lateral sclerosis, dementia, and traumatic brain injury which already utilize this approach. Consideration of MDT is not a necessary first step in the care of CDH unless the patient's headaches are refractory.

The establishment of multidisciplinary headache programs began in the late 1990s and early 2000s, for patients with frequent refractory headaches [12–15]. There is limited data on comparing MDT to individual providers. Most of it covers a limited time span of 3 to 12 months. It showed that MDT is advantageous concerning a reduction in headache frequency [16, 17], a decrease in anxiety and depression [16], and a reduction in emergency room and clinic visits [14]. While MDT is not a novelty, what constitutes the team is under debate with notable differences between European versus North American health systems [12, 13, 16, 18–20].

Regarding CDH, MDT consists of a neurologist or headache specialist, occupational therapists (OTs), physical therapists (PTs), and psychologists. While each member of the team provides an essential role, the physician has remained responsible for establishing the correct headache diagnoses and developing therapy plans in collaboration with the patients and others on the team. Often, the roles of other members are in tiers with the idea that almost all

patients see that the first-tier providers and referrals are to be made on a case-by-case basis to the second tier. The first tier encompasses OTs, PTs, and psychologists, while the second tier includes but is not limited to neurosurgeons, pain management, nurse educators, nutritionist, personal trainers, various alternative healthcare practitioners, etc.

Out of the first-tier team members, the role of OTs has been the least researched. Overall, OTs help patients engage in meaningful activities of daily living through education and problem-solving through barriers. The Canadian Occupational Performance Measure (COPM) is a valid and reliable client-centered occupational therapy tool that allows patients to identify areas of occupational difficulty or deficit [20]. With data obtained from COPM, the OT can then implement desired treatment techniques that would be of the greatest benefit to CDH patients. OT serves to educate the patient about headache self-management, help the patient change his or her behaviors and lifestyle factors that could be influencing the frequency and intensity of headaches, and improve the patient's ability to function and participate in everyday life.

PTs are experts in identifying musculoskeletal dysfunction through their analysis of movement. PTs have a long established role in the treatment of various headache conditions. A PT monitoring of CDH consists of both subjective and objective measures that help identify abnormalities that could be causing or exacerbating patients' headaches. The subjective information includes the history of symptoms, pain location/description, and aggravating factors/triggers that help to guide and individualize the objective examination as well as supplement the clinician's history. Objectively they examine common areas associated with headaches such as the jaw and cervical spine.

Psychologists make up the third component in the first tier of providers for CDH. While recognized as a vital member of the CDH treatment team, historically they have been underutilized due to availability, providers' concerns over appropriate referrals, and patient hesitation for fear of being labeled. Due to the nature of CDH, afflicted individuals are similar to other chronic pain patients and therefore should be evaluated by a psychologist at least once. Psychologists utilize many mental health monitoring scales, which we review in the next section of this chapter. Many of these scales are quick to perform and do not require formal training. Conversely, one commonly used monitoring tool, the Minnesota Multiphasic Personality Inventory-II (MMPI-II), can take up to 90 min to perform and is difficult to interpret without training. This monitoring measure is useful in identifying personality types that tend to exaggerate psychopathology or adopt a sick role, which can influence treatment [21].

Overall the roles of the first-tier providers have significant overlap, but all have a unique value that can benefit patients with CDH. Not only can monitoring of CDH patients by first-tier providers supplement data, but it can also identify overlooked etiologies or barriers that may have prevented effective treatment. Additionally, the efforts of multiple providers allow a role in dealing with medication adherence and trigger management, sleep disturbances, and overall coping with headaches.

In the MDT, the second tier of providers can encompass almost any healthcare provider. The breath of integrating the varied expertise of such providers depends on the clinical presentation of the patient. In general, the second-tier goal is to provide disease interventions rather than clinical data through monitoring. It is up to the leader of the MDT to determine the utility of such a referral or integration within the treatment team.

The most obvious limitation in the MDT is the lack of available providers. Coordinating the expertise of a variety of practitioners outside large healthcare organizations or academic centers is extremely challenging. Besides logistical limitations, analyses of the studies examining MDT have raised concerns. First, it is not possible to evaluate by a randomized trial with a placebo condition due to the nature of the comparison groups. Second, the measurement of overall outcome does not allow conclusions about the efficacy of the implementation of different parts of MDT. Nonetheless, MDT has become more and more prevalent in the treatment of CDH, and

there is a consensus among headache specialists that this approach is particularly best for refractory patients [20, 22].

Mental Health Monitoring

Psychiatric disorders such as depression, anxiety, bipolar disorder, and obsessive-compulsive disorder are exceedingly common in CDH [23, 24]. In fact, some studies indicate psychiatric comorbidity rates as high as 90% in patients with primary CDH [25]. While clinicians are well aware of the need to evaluate CDH patients for the existence of comorbid psychiatric disorders, the abundance of different scales and metrics can make this a daunting task.

Selecting an appropriate screening tool starts with knowing whether or not you want breadth or depth in your coverage. If a patient is already known to have a specific psychiatric comorbidity, then disorder-specific measures should be utilized, as more information about the nature and severity of psychiatric symptoms can be gained. On the other hand, for patients that do not carry a diagnosis or whose psychiatric presentation is complex, a multidimensional screening measure would likely provide more diagnostic clarity.

While utilization of disorder-specific multidimensional measures provides the first step in psychiatric monitoring, clinicians need to be aware of the role of transdiagnostic symptoms (TDS) [26]. TDS are a disease characteristic that overlaps two processes. TDS may result in a false-positive screen, further complicating diagnosis and treatment of CDH. For example, changes in sleep patterns, issues with concentration, and changes in appetite occur in both CDH and depression. The complexity of TDS and limited time physicians have to treat patients raise the consideration of having a mental health professional involved in a CDH patient such as in an MDT setting, which we described in the above section.

Several multidimensional measures are available to screen patients for psychiatry conditions, which include the Brief Symptom Inventory (BSI), the Psychiatric Diagnostic Screening

Questionnaire (PDSQ), and the Pain Patient Profile (P-3). Each of these screening tools can provide valuable information; however, due to the ease in use and interpretation, the Primary Care Evaluation of Mental Disorders (PRIME-MD) is recommended for multidimensional screening over the previously mentioned tools. PRIME-MD has two components: (1) a 1-page self-report called the patient questionnaire (PQ) and (2) a 12-page provider-guided questionnaire referred to as Clinical Evaluation Guide (CEG). Once the patient has completed the PQ, the clinicians then utilize CEG to evaluate the initial positive responsiveness. Overall, PRIME-MD assesses five psychiatric categories: somatoform, depression, anxiety, substance use, and eating. Although PRIME-MD is administered and interpreted with relative ease, it is time-consuming. To reduce time burden, a purely self-reported derivative of PRIME-MD known as a primary health questionnaire (PHQ) was developed. PHQ requires less than 3 minutes of the clinicians' time for 85% of patients and has a sensitivity (75%) and specificity (90%) similar to PRIME-MD [27]. Pfizer developed both of these monitoring tools, and they are both freely available.

Depression has the most extensive variety of available monitoring tools regarding disease-specific screening instruments. Out of the many verified and researched instruments, preference is for the Beck Depression Inventory-II (BDI-II) and the Patient Health Questionnaire depression module (PHQ-9) for their brevity and sensitivity. Out of the two, BDI-II provides the most depth regarding depression data. The BDI-II accomplishes this by having patients rate on a 0–3 scale, 21 groups of symptoms [28]. These groups cover a broad range of depression symptomatology including psychological, cognitive, and physical manifestations. A derivative of BDI-II, Beck Depression Inventory for Primary Care (BDI-PC), has been implemented by some clinicians as a time-saving measure due to it containing only seven items, but the BDI-PC is limited in that it only evaluates for the psychological symptoms of depression [29]. If brevity is of primary importance, the PHQ-9 would be preferred over BDI-II

as it does include nonpsychological symptoms of depression. The PHQ-9 is a subsection of the previously mentioned PHQ. The PHQ-9 starts by screening for two sentinel symptoms of depression, anhedonia and depressed mood, and then testing for psychological and somatic symptoms. The PHQ-9 sensitivity and specificity for depression are both 88% [30].

Considerably less research exists on assessment of anxiety compared to depression, but there are still many various scales to assess for anxiety. Like depression, to evaluate the various scales, factors such as ease of use, interpretation, and brevity were considered, and this led to the identification of the Beck Anxiety Inventory (BAI) and the Generalized Anxiety Disorder 7-item scale (GAD-7) as the best two tools. The BAI provides a broad evaluation of anxiety rather than identify specific anxiety subtypes. Patients rate 21 symptoms on a 0 to 4 scale. The creator's goal was to assess only for anxiety rather than for both depression and anxiety. The questions include somatic symptom items that emphasize panic [31]. Unlike BAI, the GAD-7 is a disorder-specific anxiety measure. GAD-7 evaluates for generalized anxiety disorder and utilizes a seven-item questionnaire, which patients rate on a 0 to 3 scale. Completion takes approximately 2 min [32].

Overall, no single monitoring tool is the most suitable for screening CDH patients in regard to mental health. A consensus exists that CDH patients should have formal screening for depression and anxiety at a minimum, while some pursue a more comprehensive multidimensional psychiatric screening. Any clinician can utilize the above monitoring measures mentioned in this chapter, but particular attention to the interpretation of scores should consider the somatic items as these may indicate TDS rather than a psychiatric disorder.

Vitals

The monitoring of vital signs serves two major purposes for CDH patients. Firstly, vital signs are a primary indicator of medication side effects, and secondly, vitals can reveal various pathologies that can cause and exacerbate CDH. Assessment of the essential information obtained from blood pressure, heart rate, respiratory rate, temperature, and weight measurements occurs each clinical visit. The variety of effects headache medications can have on the above-mentioned vital signs is beyond the scope of this section and will be discussed with specific drugs in other chapters.

The evidence is clear that headache patients, in general, have increased risk of stroke or cardiovascular injury [33, 34]. This risk factor is reason enough to take regular cardiac vitals to monitor modifiable risk factors. However, no suggestions or guidelines exist regarding cardiovascular risk screening and testing [35].

The link between obesity and primary headaches is well-established. A large case-controlled study indicated that the relative odds of CDH were five times higher with a body mass index (BMI) of at least 30 and three times higher with a BMI from 25 to 29 [36]. The increased inflammatory mediators found in obese individuals are important in headache pathophysiology, including interleukins and calcitonin gene-related peptide [37, 38].

Physical Examination

Physical and emotional sensitivity of patients with CDH make it difficult to assess and examine them; however, the physical exam is a crucial part of adequate monitoring. Besides a thorough neurological exam, we recommend tailoring the physical exam toward CDH mimics, and therefore ophthalmological, otolaryngologic, and musculoskeletal systems should always be assessed.

Assessment by a headache specialist or neurologist is often the only time outside of optometry and ophthalmology visits where patients have their eyes evaluated. Ophthalmological assessment begins with examination of fundi for evidence of papilledema, abnormal cup-to-disk ratios, loss of venous pulsation, and retinal changes. The evaluation of papilledema is essen-

tial as it is often the only sign of intracranial hypotension, whether idiopathic or secondary to mass lesion or tumor. Visual fields should also be assessed at each encounter as should acuity with best-corrected vision. These quick and cheap tests can often lead to identification of easily treated issues such as glaucoma, hyperopia, or myopia. Examination of extraocular muscles, eyelids, and pupils can also reveal cranial nerve palsy indicating a compressing mass or an aneurysm. Additionally, appreciation of ptosis or Horner's syndrome could be a sign of a cluster headache or in some cases a more menacing entity.

Otolaryngologic assessment should focus more so on the sinuses and throat. The tympanic membrane should be evaluated for pathology as this could be an aggravating factor toward headache. Additionally, the clinical exam should assess the vestibulocochlear nerve, which if pathologic could indicate a compressing mass. The sinuses should be palpated to assess for a chronic or acute sinusitis as this is often an undertreated cause of chronic headaches. On the other hand, a chronic primary headache disorder can be mislabeled and mistreated as a sinus issue. Assessment of the oral cavity should focus on the anatomy. An underdiagnosed secondary cause of CDH is obstructive sleep apnea (OSA); furthermore, studies of CDH patients have indicated that they are more likely to be habitual snorers. While a Mallampati score (grade of oropharyngeal appearance) should not be used exclusively to predict OSA, but with a corroborating history, it can prompt further evaluation [39]. The relationship between obstructive sleep apnea and CDH is not fully understood but may involve intracranial and arterial pressure fluctuations during snoring. This may occur particularly in individuals susceptible to pain progression, hypoxia, hypercapnia, sleep fragmentation, and disruptions with increased muscle activation during awakenings [40].

Musculoskeletal pathology is dynamic, and assessment should always include a thorough evaluation. Patients with tenderness involving pericranial and paravertebral muscles are likely to benefit from physical or osteopathic evaluation. Similarly, evaluation of the range of motion of the cervical spine could also indicate structural deficits or alert concern for meningitis. In older adults, the temporal arteries should be assessed for pulse, elevation, and tenderness as this is often the first clinical sign of giant cell arteritis. The temporomandibular joints (TMJ) should be palpated and assessed for mobility in all patients regardless of baseline complaints. A TMJ disorder can coincide with dysfunction of the upper cervical spine as well as with chronic headaches. One also assesses trigger point evaluation of the cervicoscapular musculature as a potential pain-generating source. The presence of active trigger points in the cervicoscapular musculature has been identified in patients with primary headache disorders when compared to age-matched controls, and these points correlate with longer duration and increased intensity of headaches [41].

While a tailored exam for CDH does not need to always include assessment of cardiac, pulmonary, hepatic, endocrine, and dermatological systems, all of these should be at least addressed once in the care of the CDH patient. Of note, while the clinical exam can often reveal pathology, a normal examination without focal signs does not rule out serious etiologies for CDH.

Laboratory Assessment

Similar to vitals, laboratory assessments serve as indicators of medication side effects as well as have the potential to reveal various pathologies that may be the cause of exacerbating CDH. Please see Chap. 12 for an in-depth review of this topic. The ease and multitude of laboratory tests have prompted some clinicians to use a shotgun approach particularly in cases of refractory patients. This shotgun method is, in fact, disadvantageous as a false negative can lead providers and patients down a dangerous path.

There is little clinical utility in continuously monitoring laboratory data outside of drug levels or screening for medication side effects, but a complete blood count with differential as well as comprehensive metabolic needs to be assessed at least once during the evaluation of CDH patient. Laboratory tests should be considered on a case-

by-case basis in the CDH patient. For example, if a patient has history of intracranial thrombosis, a hypercoagulability panel must be pursued. At-risk populations should be screened for human immunodeficiency virus as it is a common cause of primary and secondary headaches. In areas of endemic Lyme disease, a screening enzyme-linked immunosorbent to assess for antibodies to *Borrelia burgdorferi* should be considered or done if meningismus is present. If temporal arteritis is of concern, obtain inflammatory markers such as sedimentation rate and C-reactive protein. These are just a few examples for which laboratory and other workups may be different or unique to one specific headache disorder.

Monitoring of drug levels can serve to identify noncompliant individuals as well as those who engage in medication over usage. We do not discuss the specifics of monitoring individual levels of pharmaceuticals in this section. Due to predisposition to pain sensitivity, CDH patients often are wary of engaging in blood testing. Additionally, serum levels are more of a snapshot rather than reliable marker of intake over time. A new but not commercially available tool is, however, addressing both of these issues. Researchers have shown that you can reliably measure via hair analysis, intake of amitriptyline, citalopram, delorazepam, duloxetine, lorazepam, and venlafaxine over previous months [42].

Radiological Monitoring

While neuroimaging is not always a regular part of monitoring a patient with CDH, it may be an essential part of the initial evaluation. Just like other monitoring tools, consider neuroimaging on a case-by-case basis. Plain head computed tomography (CT) is a good screening test in a patient, but an enhanced CT often provides more information with little risk. Clinicians do need to avoid enhanced CT in cases where concern for hemorrhage is present. General limitations in CT scan include the exposure to radiation and an overall lack of sensitivity; however, the latter helps avoid nonspecific and nondiagnostic white matter changes that are particularly common on magnetic resonance imaging (MRI). Nevertheless, an MRI with gadolinium enhancement is considered the best testing method for overall evaluation of CDH patients. The limitations of MRI may be the missed cases of cerebral venous thrombosis or arterial dissection, but overall it is more sensitive than CT scan mainly for evaluation of posterior fossa, leptomeninges, and dura.

Specialized Testing

The lumbar puncture (LP) is an invasive and painful test but can provide information that no other test can ascertain and considered in patients with suspected cerebral spinal hypotension, idiopathic intracranial hypertension (IIH), or chronic meningitis. Due to the invasive nature of the test, an opening and closing pressure should always be obtained as well as basic labs (cell count, protein, glucose, and Gram stain) to avoid repeating the test. The opening pressure is of particular importance during lumbar puncture as this could be the only indicator of IIH as papilledema is often not present. It is also imperative to delay the LP until checking the head imaging for an intracranial lesion and subsequent mass effect as this could put the patient at risk for brain herniation and demise.

In 1995 the American Academy of Neurology published their practice parameter regarding electroencephalogram (EEG) utility in evaluation of headache. The overall recommendation was that EEG is not useful in the routine assessment of patients with headache. While this statement is undoubtedly accurate, this does not preclude the use of EEG. CDH presentations that have symptoms of a seizure disorder such as complicated migraines or episodic loss of awareness should include an evaluation via EEG [43].

Headache Diaries

Headache diaries have been the standard part of most clinicians' armamentarium in the assessment of headaches for decades [44]. Traditionally, paper diaries have been used to investigate headache frequency, intensity, duration, and medication compliance/usage as well as trigger exposure and other patterns, just to name a few data points. However, the paper diary method has led to a lot of criticism because diaries are bulky and require a lot of effort by the participants and not to mention they can be lost or forgotten. Furthermore, compliance with paper diaries can be a problem; individuals may be completing multiple diary entries concurrently at a later date which raises reliability concerns. Due to the lack of alternatives, for many years the paper-based diaries were the standard for behavior assessment of CDH; however, limitations of paper diaries, along with recent advances in mobile technology, have led to the increasing adoption of electronic diaries (e-diaries).

E-diaries use a computer-based system to record what would be in a paper diary. Overall several studies have indicated that e-diaries may be superior to paper diaries in that they offer advantages such as a reduction of recall bias, easy accessibility for physicians and patients, and improved compliance [45, 46]. The e-diary for many years had its limitations due to lack of access to the Internet and overall computer illiteracy. However, this situation has changed dramatically over last decade with the advent of handheld computers and smartphones. These devices have allowed the creation of easy-to-use applications (apps) that collect and sort patients' headache data. Today's clinicians face the challenge of identifying and recommending the best "e-diary." Clinicians often express concern regarding the quality of e-diaries due to lack of oversight in the mobile health app market. One recent comprehensive analysis of e-diary apps allowed identification of the most clinically relevant apps.

Published in 2014, Hundert and colleagues analyzed 38 applications in Apple iTunes and Google Play store [47]. To assess the applications, the researchers set seven criteria that defined an ideal headache app, and quality of the apps was determined by the number of app criteria met. Criteria were as follows: apps created with headache expertise, formal psychometric and feasibility testing, clinically relevant headache variables measured, usable apps, customizable answer options and reports, reports linking multiple variables, and ability to export headache data from the app. The three highest scoring apps (iHeadache, ecoHeadache, and Headache Diary Pro) only met five of these seven criteria. Of concern is that none of the apps in this study including the three highest scoring had undergone formal feasibility or psychometric property testing. The iHeadache app is appealing in that it is the only one of the three applications created by a physician with headache medicine expertise. Additionally, it provides succinct information in that it records all clinically relevant variables without requiring nonessential information. EcoHeadache, on the other hand, provides significantly more information and can generate a variety of chart reports and customizable reports. The third option Headache Diary Pro is overall rated less usable compared to the apps mentioned above but is the highest scoring Android application as the prior apps are only available on iOS or Apple systems.

Conclusion

Chronic daily headache's wide prevalence in society as well its tremendous cost burden has made efficacious treatment of this disorder of utmost importance. Ineffective headache diagnosis and treatment has led to repeated consultations of different disciplines, expenditure on alternative therapies, and unnecessary hospitalizations. Certainly, this has led to frustrated and suffering patients. It is abundantly clear that to manage CDH patients effectively, clinicians need to monitor their patients adequately. Utilizing the information in this chapter, clinicians should be able to comprehensively monitor their CDH patients which can lead to better outcomes overall.

References

1. Silberstein SD, Lipton RB, Sliwinski M. Classification of daily and near-daily headaches: field trial of revised IHS criteria. Neurology. 1996;47(4):871–5.
2. Headache Classification Committee of the International Headache, S. The international classifi-

cation of headache disorders, 3rd edition (beta version). Cephalalgia. 2013;33(9):629–808.
3. Dodick DW. Clinical practice. Chronic daily headache. N Engl J Med. 2006;354(2):158–65.
4. Lanteri-Minet M, et al. Prevalence and description of chronic daily headache in the general population in France. Pain. 2003;102(1–2):143–9.
5. Lu SR, et al. Chronic daily headache in Taipei, Taiwan: prevalence, follow-up and outcome predictors. Cephalalgia. 2001;21(10):980–6.
6. Scher AI, et al. Prevalence of frequent headache in a population sample. Headache. 1998;38(7):497–506.
7. Stovner L, et al. The global burden of headache: a documentation of headache prevalence and disability worldwide. Cephalalgia. 2007;27(3):193–210.
8. Wiendels NJ, et al. Chronic frequent headache in the general population: prevalence and associated factors. Cephalalgia. 2006;26(12):1434–42.
9. Lanteri-Minet M, et al. Quality of life impairment, disability and economic burden associated with chronic daily headache, focusing on chronic migraine with or without medication overuse: a systematic review. Cephalalgia. 2011;31(7):837–50.
10. Hu XH, et al. Burden of migraine in the United States: disability and economic costs. Arch Intern Med. 1999;159(8):813–8.
11. Abu Bakar N, et al. Quality of life in primary headache disorders: a review. Cephalalgia. 2016;36(1):67–91.
12. Gunreben-Stempfle B, et al. Effectiveness of an intensive multidisciplinary headache treatment program. Headache. 2009;49(7):990–1000.
13. Lemstra M, Stewart B, Olszynski WP. Effectiveness of multidisciplinary intervention in the treatment of migraine: a randomized clinical trial. Headache. 2002;42(9):845–54.
14. Maizels M, Saenz V, Wirjo J. Impact of a group-based model of disease management for headache. Headache. 2003;43(6):621–7.
15. Saper JR, et al. Comprehensive/tertiary care for headache: a 6-month outcome study. Headache. 1999;39(4):249–63.
16. Wallasch TM, Kropp P. Multidisciplinary integrated headache care: a prospective 12-month follow-up observational study. J Headache Pain. 2012;13(7):521–9.
17. Harpole LH, et al. Headache management program improves outcome for chronic headache. Headache. 2003;43(7):715–24.
18. Gaul C, et al. Clinical outcome of a headache-specific multidisciplinary treatment program and adherence to treatment recommendations in a tertiary headache center: an observational study. J Headache Pain. 2011;12(4):475–83.
19. Gaul C, et al. Team players against headache: multidisciplinary treatment of primary headaches and medication overuse headache. J Headache Pain. 2011;12(5):511–9.
20. Sahai-Srivastava S, et al. Multidisciplinary team treatment approaches to chronic daily headaches. Headache. 2017;57(9):1482–91.

21. Butcher, J. N., Dahlstrom, W. G., Graham, J. R., Tellegen, A., & Kaemmer, B. Minnesota Multiphasic Personality Inventory–2 (MMPI-2): Manual for administration and scoring. Minneapolis, MN: University of Minnesota Press. 1989.

22. Amoils S, et al. The positive impact of integrative medicine in the treatment of recalcitrant chronic daily headache: a series of case reports. Glob Adv Health Med. 2014;3(4):45–54.

23. Juang KD, et al. Comorbidity of depressive and anxiety disorders in chronic daily headache and its subtypes. Headache. 2000;40(10):818–23.

24. Couch JR. Update on chronic daily headache. Curr Treat Options Neurol. 2011;13(1):41–55.

25. Verri AP, et al. Psychiatric comorbidity in chronic daily headache. Cephalalgia. 1998;18(Suppl 21):45–9.

26. Grisanzio KA, et al. Transdiagnostic symptom clusters and associations with brain, behavior, and daily function in mood, anxiety and trauma disorders. JAMA Psychiat. 2017;75(2):201–9.

27. Spitzer RL, et al. Utility of a new procedure for diagnosing mental disorders in primary care. The PRIME-MD 1000 study. JAMA. 1994;272(22):1749–56.

28. Beck, A.T., Steer, R.A., & Brown, G.K. Manual for the Beck Depression Inventory-II. San Antonio, TX: Psychological Corporation. 1996.

29. Steer RA, et al. Use of the beck depression inventory for primary care to screen for major depression disorders. Gen Hosp Psychiatry. 1999;21(2):106–11.

30. Kroenke K, Spitzer RL, Williams JB. The PHQ-9: validity of a brief depression severity measure. J Gen Intern Med. 2001;16(9):606–13.

31. Leyfer OT, Ruberg JL, Woodruff-Borden J. Examination of the utility of the Beck anxiety inventory and its factors as a screener for anxiety disorders. J Anxiety Disord. 2006;20(4):444–58.

32. Spitzer RL, et al. A brief measure for assessing generalized anxiety disorder: the GAD-7. Arch Intern Med. 2006;166(10):1092–7.

33. Schurks M, et al. Migraine and cardiovascular disease: systematic review and meta-analysis. BMJ. 2009;339:b3914.

34. Scher AI, et al. Cardiovascular risk factors and migraine: the GEM population-based study. Neurology. 2005;64(4):614–20.

35. Kirkham KE, Colon RJ, Solomon GD. The role of cardiovascular screening in headache patients. Headache. 2011;51(2):331–7.

36. Scher AI, et al. Factors associated with the onset and remission of chronic daily headache in a population-based study. Pain. 2003;106(1–2):81–9.

37. Bigal ME, Lipton RB. Putative mechanisms of the relationship between obesity and migraine progression. Curr Pain Headache Rep. 2008;12(3):207–12.

38. Bigal ME, et al. Obesity, migraine, and chronic migraine: possible mechanisms of interaction. Neurology. 2007;68(21):1851–61.

39. Friedman M, et al. Diagnostic value of the Friedman tongue position and Mallampati classification for obstructive sleep apnea: a meta-analysis. Otolaryngol Head Neck Surg. 2013;148(4):540–7.

40. Scher AI, Lipton RB, Stewart WF. Habitual snoring as a risk factor for chronic daily headache. Neurology. 2003;60(8):1366–8.

41. Giamberardino MA, et al. Contribution of myofascial trigger points to migraine symptoms. J Pain. 2007;8(11):869–78.

42. Ferrari A, et al. Monitoring of adherence to headache treatments by means of hair analysis. Eur J Clin Pharmacol. 2017;73(2):197–203.

43. Practice parameter: the electroencephalogram in the evaluation of headache (summary statement). Report of the quality standards subcommittee of the American Academy of Neurology. Neurology. 1995;45(7):1411–3.

44. Russell MB, et al. Presentation of a new instrument: the diagnostic headache diary. Cephalalgia. 1992;12(6):369–74.

45. Goldberg J, et al. Evaluation of an electronic diary as a diagnostic tool to study headache and premenstrual symptoms in migraineurs. Headache. 2007;47(3):384–96.

46. Nappi G, et al. Diaries and calendars for migraine. A review. Cephalalgia. 2006;26(8):905–16.

47. Hundert AS, et al. Commercially available mobile phone headache diary apps: a systematic review. JMIR Mhealth Uhealth. 2014;2(3):e36.

Medication Overuse in Chronic Daily Headache

14

Hans-Christoph Diener, Dagny Holle-Lee, and Frederick G. Freitag

Introduction

The frequent or regular intake of medication to treat acute headache episodes can lead to an increase in headache frequency and finally to a transition from episodic to chronic headache. Many patients with chronic headache take abortive medication on a daily basis. Medication overuse headache (MOH) is defined by the International Classification of Headache Disorders as a headache in patients with a pre-existing primary headache disorder (e.g., migraine or tension-type headache) occurring on ≥15 days per month for >3 months. Also, these primary headache disorders occur in association with overuse of medication for acute or symptomatic headache treatment. The prevalence of MOH in the general population is around 1%. MOH is more common in people with chronic migraine and chronic daily headache than in patients with episodic migraine. The phenotype of the headache in MOH depends on the initial primary headache and the type of overused acute medication. Treatment of MOH occurs in three stages. First, we educate patients about the relationship between frequent intake of acute headache medication and MOH to reduce intake of acute medication. In a second step migraine prevention should be initiated in chronic migraine (topiramate or onabotulinumtoxinA in migraine) or amitriptyline in chronic tension-type headache. In patients who fail to cease overuse of overused medication with preventive therapy, then detoxification occurs on an outpatient basis or in a day hospital or inpatient setting, depending on severity and comorbidities. The success rate of treatment is around 50–70%, with higher relapse rates in patients with opioid overuse. Patient education and continuity of care in the follow-up period reduce relapse rates. This chapter is based on a recently published review on MOH in *Nature Reviews Neurology* [1].

Definitions

Medication overuse headache MOH (8.2 IHS Classification 3rd edition) [2] is defined as headache occurring on 15 or more days per month developing as a consequence of regular overuse of acute or symptomatic headache medication (on 10 or more or 15 or more days per month, depending on the medication) for more than 3 months. It usually, but not invariably, resolves after the overuse stops.

H.-C. Diener (✉)
Clinical Neurosciences, Department of Neurology, University Duisburg-Essen, Essen, Germany
e-mail: hans.diener@uk-essen.de

D. Holle-Lee
Department of Neurology and Headache Center, University Hospital Essen, Essen, Germany

F. G. Freitag
Department of Neurology, Medical College of Wisconsin, Milwaukee, WI, USA

© Springer International Publishing AG, part of Springer Nature 2019
M. W. Green et al. (eds.), *Chronic Headache*, https://doi.org/10.1007/978-3-319-91491-6_14

Diagnostic Criteria

A. Headache occurring on ≥15 days per month in a patient with a pre-existing headache disorder.
B. Regular overuse for >3 months of one or more drugs that can be taken for acute and/or symptomatic treatment of headache.
   Simple analgesics on >15 days per month.
   Combination analgesics, triptans, ergots, or opioids >10 days per month.
C. Not better accounted for by another ICHD-3 diagnosis.

Chronic daily headaches (CDHs) occur 15 days or more a month, for at least 3 months. Primary chronic daily headaches were another condition that does not imply causation. There are short-lasting and long-lasting chronic daily headaches. Long-lasting headache last more than 4 h. They include chronic migraine, chronic tension-type headache, new daily persistent headache, and hemicrania continua.

The overuse of any medication to treat acute headache episodes can lead to MOH. These medications include simple analgesics, combination analgesics, ergots, triptans, opioids, and barbiturates [3–8]. Whether NSAIDs belong in this group is still controversial. The causal relationship between the frequent or daily headache of abortive medication and MOH can only be established when the headache frequency improves with the less frequent or termination of intake of the assumed drug or drugs supposed to cause MOH. Frequent intake of acute medication does not necessarily lead to MOH. Some patients might use triptans on 15–20 days per month for many years without developing a daily headache and without the more frequent intake of triptans per month. This condition is called "medication overuse" [9].

Epidemiology

Medication overuse headache affects 1–2% of the general population [10, 11]. The prevalence, however, depends on the definition of MOH [12]. Patients with MOH constitute 25–50% of all patients with chronic headache [13] and 40–50% of all patients seen in tertiary headache centers. Prospective studies in headache centers observed that up to 14% of patients with an episodic headache develop a chronic headache per year. The majority of these patients overuse acute medication [14].

Diagnosis and Clinical Features

The characteristics of headache in MOH depend on the primary headache [15]. Migraine patients who overuse triptans report a migraine-like daily headache or a marked increase in migraine frequency. In some of the patients, the phenotype of migraine attacks changes with increasing attack frequency with fewer and less pronounced autonomic features. Patients with chronic tension-type headache overusing acute medication report an increase in headache days with features of tension-type headache [15]. The evolution toward MOH is substance-specific and is faster in patients who overuse triptans, opioids, and combination analgesics compared with those who overuse simple analgesics [15]. This evolution was confirmed by a French study with 82 patients overusing triptans [16]. In a population-based study in the USA [17], including 24,000 headache patients, opioids and barbiturates increased the risk for chronification of headache. This risk was not observed for triptans [18]. A systematic literature review of 29 studies [19] confirmed a similar increased risk of MOH related to opioid intake [19].

The diagnosis of MOH is based on the patient's history and documentation of drug intake. Patients who develop a chronic headache at age >60 years or focal neurological symptoms or psychopathological features require imaging with CT or MRI. In women with a high BMI, measurement of the CSF pressure might be indicated to rule out idiopathic intracranial hypertension [20]. Similarly, patients with certain comorbidities (e.g., positional orthostatic tachycardia, Marfan's syndrome, Ehlers-Danlos syndrome) and long-standing CDH resistant to treatment should be considered for a spontaneous intracranial hypotension evaluation.

Most patients with MOH originally suffer from a primary headache disorder like migraine or tension-type headache [6, 21]. Some patients with cluster headache may develop MOH in particular if they also suffer from migraine or have a family history of migraine [22]. Patients with other chronic pain syndromes like chronic low back pain or arthrosis will not develop MOH if they take NSAIDs on a daily basis [23, 24].

Pathophysiology

The pathophysiological mechanisms leading to MOH are still enigmatic. One clinical observation is that patients with migraine and TTH are at higher risk to develop MOH compared to patients without any primary headache disorder [25].

Therefore, one hypothesis is that the migrainous/TTH headache brain itself may be prone to develop MOH when it is exposed to increased amount of acute medication over a longer period. In contrast, patients who suffer from cluster headache usually do not develop MOH except for the patients who additionally suffer from migraine or have a family history of migraine [26]. Specific genetic profiles might be involved, including angiotensin-converting enzyme (ACE) I/D polymorphism [27], brain-derived neurotrophic factor Val66Met polymorphism [28], and polymorphism in COMT and SLC6A4 genes [29].

Although prolonged exposure to all classes of pain medication can lead to MOH, some drugs will more often and faster lead to MOH than others. For example, triptan intake is associated with a higher risk for developing MOH than overuse of simple analgesics. Alteration of neurotransmitter metabolism might be one pathophysiological correlate especially regarding the serotonergic [30–32] and endocannabinoid systems [33, 34]. Electrophysiological investigations (e.g., sensory-evoked potentials [35] and laser-evoked potentials [36]) have shown neuronal hyperexcitability of the MOH brain in terms of increased stimulus response and habituation deficits. These observations can be made not only regarding cephalic but also extra-cephalic stimulation [35]. After stopping medication overuse, most of the electrophysiological changes were reversible [35, 36].

Imaging studies in MOH show different kinds of structural, functional, and metabolic changes. Mainly alterations of the central pain network can be observed picturing the multidimensional properties of pain disorders and MOH (sensory discrimination, cognitive, attentional, and emotional dimensions). Results from migraine/pain/depression questionnaires correlate positively with gray matter changes detected via Voxel-based morphometry (VBM) [37]. Structural changes may also resolve after cessation of medication overuse [38–40]. However, all observed pathological changes are not specific for MOH, and similar changes can be observed in other headache/pain or affective disorders.

Risk Factors

Risk factors for development of MOH include primary headache disorders (migraine, tension-type headache), female sex, >10 headache days/month, lower social class, other chronic pain conditions, stress, physical inactivity, obesity, smoking, dependency behavior, and comorbid psychiatric disorders [41, 42]. In a large population-based study in Norway with 51,383 participants and an 11-year follow-up, the incidence of MOH was 0.72 per 1000 person-years. In the multivariate analyses, a fivefold risk for developing MOH occurred among certain individuals. Those individuals who at baseline reported regular use of tranquilizers [odds ratio 5.2 (3.0–9.0)] or who had a combination of chronic musculoskeletal complaints, gastrointestinal complaints, and hospital anxiety and depression scale score >/ = 11 [odds ratio 4.7 (2.4–9.0)] had the highest risk. Smoking and physical inactivity more than doubled the risk of MOH [43].

Patients at high risk of MOH should be identified via prescriptions for excessive amounts of specific migraine drugs and followed up. In a multicenter study, educational strategies applied in a cognitive-behavioral minimal contact program, with either group sessions or written material provided for the patient, showed success in reducing the rate of MOH occurrence in patients at risk without institution of other medication treatments [44].

A commonly held concept of medication overuse headache and chronic daily headache disorders is that they are truly daily headache disorders. However, a variety of studies for treatment of chronic migraine show this not to be the case. A recent study of chronic headaches associated with medication overuse suggests that patients with daily headache are not the same as those with near daily headache [45]. The patients who had migraine or chronic migraine as well as medication overuse entered a program of treatment. Only 8 had daily headache, whereas the other 69 had near daily headache with a mean of almost 19 headache days per month. The daily headache group was more likely to adhere to treatment, not relapse back to overuse, while both groups demonstrated a significant reduction in their headache frequency back to the range of episodic migraine.

Treatment

The treatment of MOH is based on four consecutive approaches:

1. Firstly, informing the patient about the mechanism of MOH with the aim to reduce the intake of acute medication for headache (below the threshold of 10 days/previous month for specific drugs and opioids and combination analgesics and below 15 days for simple analgesics).
2. Next, begin medical and nonmedical preventive therapy.
3. Thirdly, detoxification from the overused acute medication occurs by either abrupt withdrawal of drugs by itself or done in conjunction with "bridge therapies" to aid in the transition.
4. Lastly, these steps are followed by immediate or delayed preventative therapy.

Most of the randomized studies investigating these approaches were small and underpowered. A study in Italy compared the effectiveness of advice with either outpatient or inpatient withdrawal in patients with MOH. The study performed in a tertiary headache center and included 120 patients with MOH [46]. Advice alone was as effective as the other two interventions, with a success rate after 2 months of >70%. A second study compared the effectiveness of an educational strategy (advice to withdraw the overused medication or medications) with that of two structured pharmacological detoxification pro-

grams in patients with MOH and migraine as the primary headache in 137 patients [47]. One group of 46 patients received intensive advice to reduce the intake of the overused medication(s). The second group of 46 patients underwent a standard detoxification program as outpatients (advice + steroids + preventive treatment). The third group of 45 patients underwent a standard inpatient withdrawal program (advice + steroids + fluid replacement and antiemetics plus preventive treatment). The success rate was 60% of the patients in the first two groups and 89% of those in the third group. A meta-analysis which compared outpatient withdrawal with inpatient treatment found no difference in responder rates or the reduction in headache days [48]. A prospective cohort study in Norway was comprised of 109 participants with chronic headache (mostly tension-type headache) and MOH who received short written information about the possible role of medication overuse in headache chronification [49]. Patients were followed for 18 months. At baseline, the mean duration of chronic headaches was 8–18 years, and the mean duration of medication overuse was between 5 and 10 years. At follow-up, the mean medication days went from 22 days to 6 days per month. Seventy-six percent of patients no longer overused medication [49]. The approach of providing advice can also be applied in the general practice [50].

Krause and colleagues examined the impact of a 3-week outpatient interdisciplinary program which included medical interventions addressing long-term preventative medications, intravenous bridge therapies such as intravenous dihydroergotamine, and optimization of acute migraine and headache management strategies [51]. Outcome parameters were physical functioning and psychological impairment in chronic headache patients. Three hundred seventy-nine patients admitted to an outpatient chronic headache treatment program agreed to provide assessment. Assessments of headache severity, psychological status, and functional impairment were completed by 371 (97.8%) of these at the time of admission. At discharge, 340 subjects (89.7%) provided assessment data, and 152 (40.1%) provided data at 1-year follow-up. At entry subjects' mean headache pain was 6.1, declining at discharge of 3.5

and at follow-up of 3.3. A measure of functional impairment, the HIT-6 score improved following treatment from 66.1 on admission to 55.4 at discharge and 51.9 at 1-year follow-up. Depression and anxiety also showed marked improvement although depression scores lapsed back toward admission levels at the 1 year follow-up.

In conclusion, advice alone might be an appropriate approach in patients who overuse triptans or simple analgesics and who do not have major psychiatric comorbidity. Advice alone can be provided by GPs, neurologists in private practice, and headache nurses. However, advice alone might not be enough for patients who overuse opioids tranquilizers or barbiturates or who have had repeated episodes of overuse. These patients need referral to a headache specialist or a headache center.

Preventive Migraine Therapy in MOH

Most patients with MOH who are referred to headache centers have already failed preventive therapy with beta blockers, flunarizine, valproic acid, or amitriptyline. At present scientific evidence for effective preventive therapy in patients with MOH from randomized trials exists for topiramate and onabotulinumtoxinA and some of the monoclonal CGRP-antibodies.

Topiramate was investigated in a European study and included patients with chronic migraine who were randomized to topiramate or placebo for a 16-week double-blind trial. Topiramate was titrated from 25 mg weekly to a target dose of 100 mg/day, allowing dosing flexibility from 50 to 200 mg/day. Thirty-two patients in the intention-to-treat population received topiramate, and 27 patients received placebo. Seventy-eight percent of patients met the criteria for medication overuse at baseline. Topiramate significantly reduced the mean number of monthly migraine days by 3.5 compared with placebo (−0.2 days) [52]. This trial showed that topiramate was effective and reasonably well tolerated when used for the preventive treatment of chronic migraine with medication overuse. A second trial conducted in the USA compared topiramate with placebo for the prevention of chronic migraine [53]. A subgroup analysis of the patients with MOH at baseline showed a nonsignificant reduction in mean monthly migraine/migrainous days compared with placebo [54]. The trials differed from the European trial in inclusion criteria and the classes of overused medications [53, 55, 56].

About 65% of patients fulfilled the criteria for MOH in the two pivotal trials comparing onabotulinumtoxinA with placebo injections in patients with chronic migraine, [57–59]. Excluded patients from the trials were those with opioid overuse. At week 24, statistically significant results favoring onabotulinumtoxinA versus placebo were observed for headache days (primary endpoint, −8.2 versus −6.2, $p < 0.001$). Significant result occurred as well for secondary endpoints such as frequencies of migraine days ($p < 0.001$), moderate/severe headache days ($p < 0.001$), cumulative headache hours on headache days ($p < 0.001$), headache episodes ($p = 0.028$), and migraine episodes ($p = 0.018$) [60].

Observational and underpowered randomized trials investigated valproic acid, cannabinoids, pregabalin, occipital nerve stimulation, and acupuncture for the treatment of MOH (summarized by [61]). Due to the methodological shortcomings, the results of these studies have no impact on the practical treatment of patients with MOH.

Management of Symptoms During Detoxification

Most studies in patients with MOH investigated drug withdrawal or detoxification. After discontinuation of migraine drugs or analgesics, most patients experience a transient deterioration of the underlying headache with autonomic disturbances, anxiety, and sleep problems [6]. These symptoms last 2–7 days depending on the overused medication [62]. The shortest duration of withdrawal symptoms is in patients overusing triptans and the longest in patients overusing ergots, barbiturate compounds, or opioids.

A systematic review identified 27 studies reporting the treatment response to discontinuation or withdrawal, 19 of them with preventive medication [61]. In the studies included in the review, the withdrawal program was either performed in an outpatient setting, in a day hospital or inpatient setting. Therapies included fluid replacement (if necessary) and some drug treatments, including corticosteroids, neuroleptic drugs, tranquilizers, ergots, and simple analgesics. Adding preventive medication to early discontinuation led to a better outcome than early discontinuation alone. For patients with chronic migraine and medication overuse, randomized controlled trials supported the use of onabotulinumtoxinA and topiramate without early discontinuation of overuse (see above).

Two placebo-controlled trials investigating the use of corticosteroids versus placebo for the treatment of withdrawal symptoms, one in Norway and one in Germany [63, 64]. Both studies found no benefit of prednisone or prednisolone versus placebo.

The majority of the studies of withdrawal-associated symptoms in MOH conducted to date have been observational. A large multinational study with centers from Europe and South America (COMOESTAS) recruited 376 patients with MOH [65]. Patients went through detoxification followed by the initiation of preventive therapy. The choice of preventive medication was dependent on comorbid disorders. The post-detoxification follow-up lasted 6 months. At the final evaluation, two-thirds of the participants were no longer overusing acute medication, and in 46.5% of participants, the headache had reverted to an episodic pattern of headache. When comparing the participants who underwent outpatient detoxification with those treated with inpatient detoxification, both regimens proved effective. The dropout rate was higher in the outpatient approach [65]. The number of patients with depression and/or anxiety decreased over time, and the disability improved [66].

The use of bridging therapies has been advocated to ease the severity of the withdrawal headaches and associated symptoms. Steroids used as a bridging therapy during the first week of treatment did not offer any long-term advantages to standard therapy of changes in preventative medications coupled with use of a triptan and a NSAID for acute headache treatment to a maximum of twice a week [67]. Bridging therapy with avoidance of all other acute medications for migraine and pain and replacement of them with naproxen sodium alone during the withdrawal

period was associated with a significant reduction in headache frequency without institution of new preventative treatments [68]. This may be the result of the action of naproxen on P2X3 receptors on sensitized trigeminal neurons in addition to effects on cyclooxygenase [69]. The combined use of a tizanidine, an alpha agonist, coupled with a once daily COX-2 inhibitor led to marked reduction in additional acute medication use over a several month trial period [70].

Dihydroergotamine mesylate is used in the USA in the management of chronic migraine with and without medication overuse headache [71]. By comparison to ergotamine tartrate and the triptan class of medication, medication overuse headache has not been reported, but rather it may be a useful adjunct as part of a comprehensive management strategy [72]. In chronic migraine without medication overuse, it produces a robust reduction in migraine during the infusion for most patients and coupled with symptom management [73] may afford early relief to these patients and potentially improve the long-term outcome for reduction of headaches.

Historically, in the USA, as well as elsewhere, the use of an inpatient environment to initiate treatment has been used [74]. This allows for aggressive medical management of the headache and associated symptoms, especially during medication overuse withdrawal. It permits early intervention with non-pharmacological strategies and behavioral medicine assessments in a controlled environment. Despite insurance attempts to reduce this type of treatment for cost concerns, it remains an important method of addressing the patient's needs [75] when outpatient services have not proven effective. Moreover, an inpatient program may be associated with containment of long-term healthcare costs as well [76]. While outpatient treatment of chronic migraine with medication overuse produced a 4% reduction in healthcare expenditure, this was compared to nearly 33% reduction in long-term costs among those treated initially on an inpatient basis. Both groups had about a 75% reduction in MIDAS scores, although those treated in inpatient hospital had roughly twice the number of day's reduction of headache over 6 months (Table 14.1).

Table 14.1 Outcome parameters comparing outpatient and inpatient treatment of MOH

Parameter	Chronic migraine *without* medication overuse						Chronic migraine *with* medication overuse					
	Outpatient treatment			Inpatient treatment			Outpatient treatment			Inpatient treatment		
	Pre-treatment	Post-treatment	% change	Pre-treatment	Post-treatment	% change	Pre-treatment	Post-treatment	% change	Pre-treatment	Post-treatment	% change
Number of patients	27			46			57			23		
Age (years)	48			50			52			50		
Comorbid medical disorders	2.8			2.8			2.7			2.8		
Disease duration	14			14			15.9			18		
Cost/6 months	2724	2646	−2.8%	3677	3518	−0.4%	7859	7529	−4.2%	6671	4502	−32.5%
Headache days/3 months	54.4	48.1	−11.5%	59.2	53.3	−9.9%	75.5	49	−35.1%	65	23	−64.6%
MIDAS	55.1	27.6	−49.9%	83	39.6	−53.4%	123.9	25.4	−79.5%	91	21.5	−76.4%
MD visits/6 months	5.18	0.56	−89.2%	6.8	1.27	−81.3%	10	1.88	−81.2%	7.9	2.8	−64.5%
ED visits/6 months	1.27	0.38	−70.3%	1.41	0.63	−55.3%	1.79	0.95	−46.9%	1.38	0.4	−71%
Inpatient admisssions/6 months	0.42	0.18	−57.1%	0.26	0.81	+211%	0.51	0.72	+41%	0.48	0.2	−58.3%

Reprinted from [76], courtesy of Baylor University Medical Center at Dallas

Long-term benefits associated with the use of intravenous DHE during the initiation of treatment revealed significant benefit. The authors found that >90% of patient were headache-free within 3 days [71]. In a study examining long-term outcomes, 78% of 278 patients had at least moderate reduction in their headache pain parameters [77].

Another potential bridge treatment that has been effective has been the use of daily 25 mg three times per day dosing of sumatriptan given steadily until the patient has headache freedom for more than 24 h. In the study by Tepper et al., 58% of 26 patients had reverted to an episodic pattern with this treatment in addition to new preventative medications [78].

One randomized trial compared three treatment approaches for MOH. This 1-year open-labelled, multicenter study included 56 patients who were randomly assigned to receive prophylactic treatment from the start without detoxification, undergo a standard outpatient detoxification program without prophylactic treatment from the start, or to have no specific treatment (5-month follow-up). The primary outcome measure, change in headache days per month, did not differ significantly between groups. However, the prophylaxis group had the greatest decrease in headache days compared with baseline and also a significantly greater reduction in total headache index (headache days/month x headache intensity x headache hours) at months 3 ($P = 0.003$) and 12 ($P = 0.017$) compared with the withdrawal group. At month 12, 53% of patients in the prophylaxis group had $\geq 50\%$ reduction in monthly headache days compared with 25% in the withdrawal group ($P = 0.081$) [79].

A Danish study investigated the effects of a 2-month medication period in 337 patients with probable MOH [80]. Only two-thirds of the patients completed the study. Forty-five percent of the patients improved, 48% had no change in headache, and 7% experienced an increase in headache days. Patients with migraine showed a higher rate of improvement than patients with tension-type headache. Patients overusing triptans improved the most.

Relapse of MOH

Chiang et al. summarized the remission and relapse rates after discontinuation from 22 studies [61] with a follow-up of 2 and 60 months (most studies 12 months). The relapse rate varied between 0% and 45%, with most studies showing a relapse rate between 25% and 35%. Predictors of relapses were chronic tension-type headache versus migraine as the primary headache, overuse of opioids versus triptans, and comorbid psychiatric disorders. Depression is an important predictor of relapse [81].

The most important recommendations for the management of MOH are:

- Patients with MOH should be managed by a multidisciplinary team of neurologists or pain specialists and behavioral psychologists.
- Patient education is of significant importance.
- Patients with MOH should undergo drug withdrawal. One can abruptly terminate in patients overusing simple analgesic, ergot, or triptan medication. In patients with long-lasting abuse of opioids, barbiturates, or tranquilizers, slow tapering of these drugs can be an option.
- Detoxification can be performed on an outpatient basis, in a day-care setting or an inpatient setting. All settings have a similar success rate because of the different complexities suited to each setting. Headache history may help to assign patients to a given setting (Table 14.2).
- Patients who do not want to undergo detoxification can initiate migraine preventive therapy with either topiramate or onabotulinumtoxinA.

Table 14.2 Treatment strategies in MOH

Outpatient withdrawal	Inpatient treatment
• No opioid, barbiturates, or tranquilizer	• Long-lasting MOH (>5 years)
• Motivated patient	• Overuse of opioids or barbiturates
• Support by family or friends	• Overuse of psychotropic medication (hypnotics, anxiolytics, tranquilizers
Day-care setting	
• Comorbidity with depression or anxiety	• Failed outpatient withdrawal
• Comorbidity with other chronic pain syndromes (low back pain, fibromyalgia)	• Psychiatric comorbidity

Disclosures H. C. Diener received honoraria for his participation in clinical trials, contribution to advisory boards, or oral presentations from Addex Pharma, Alder, Allergan, Almirall, Amgen, Autonomic Technology, AstraZeneca, Bayer Vital, Berlin Chemie, Böhringer Ingelheim, Bristol-Myers Squibb, Chordate, Coherex, CoLucid, Electrocore, GlaxoSmithKline, Grünenthal, Janssen-Cilag, Labrys Biologics, Lilly, La Roche, 3 M Medica, Medtronic, Menerini, Minster, MSD, Neuroscore, Novartis, Johnson & Johnson, Pierre Fabre, Pfizer, Schaper and Brümmer, Sanofi, St. Jude, Teva, and Weber & Weber. Financial support for research projects was provided by Allergan, Almirall, AstraZeneca, Bayer, Electrocore, GSK, Janssen-Cilag, MSD and Pfizer. Headache research at the Department of Neurology in Essen is supported by the German Research Council (DFG), the German Ministry of Education and Research (BMBF), and the European Union. H.C. Diener has no ownership interest and does not own stocks of any pharmaceutical company. HCD serves on the editorial boards of *Cephalalgia* and Lancet Neurology. HCD chairs the Clinical Guidelines Committee of the German Society of Neurology.

D. Holle-Lee has received financial support for research projects from Allergan, Grünenthal, and Lilly and research support from EFIC.

F. Freitag is an advisor to the Migraine Research Foundation and BioHealthonomics. He has received financial support for clinical research, consulting, and educational presentations from Alder, Allergan, Amgen, Avanir, Depomed, Mayo Clinic Phoenix, Dr. Reddy, Teva, and Weber & Weber.

References

1. Diener HC, Holle D, Solbach K, Gaul C. Medication-overuse headache: risk factors, pathophysiology and management. Nat Rev Neurol. 2016;12(10):575–83.
2. Headache Classification Committee of the International Headache Society. The international classification of headache disorders, 3rd edition (beta version). Cephalalgia. 2013;33(9):629–808.
3. Dichgans J, Diener HC, Gerber WD, Verspohl EJ, Kukiolka H, Kluck M. Analgetika-induzierter Dauerkopfschmerz. Dtsch med Wschr. 1984;109:369–73.
4. Horton BT, Peters GA. Clinical manifestations of excessive use of ergotamine preparations and management of withdrawal effect: report of 52 cases. Headache. 1963;3:214–26.
5. Kaube H, May A, Diener HC, Pfaffenrath V. Sumatriptan misuse in daily chronic headache. BMJ. 1994;308:1573.
6. Diener HC, Limmroth V. Medication-overuse headache: a worldwide problem. Lancet Neurol. 2004;3:475–83.
7. Diener HC, Katsarava Z, Limmroth V. Headache attributed to a substance or its withdrawal. Handb Clin Neurol. 2010;97:589–99.
8. Abrams BM. Medication overuse headaches. Med Clin North Am. 2013;97(2):337–52.
9. Kristoffersen ES, Lundqvist C. Medication-overuse headache: epidemiology, diagnosis and treatment. Ther Adv Drug Saf. 2014;5(2):87–99.
10. Stovner LJ, Andree C. Prevalence of headache in Europe: a review for the Eurolight project. J Headache Pain. 2010;11(4):289–99.
11. Straube A, Pfaffenrath V, Ladwig KH, Meisinger C, Hoffmann W, Fendrich K, et al. Prevalence of chronic migraine and medication overuse headache in Germany–the German DMKG headache study. Cephalalgia. 2010;30(2):207–13.
12. Westergaard ML, Hansen EH, Glumer C, Olesen J, Jensen RH. Definitions of medication-overuse headache in population-based studies and their implications on prevalence estimates: a systematic review. Cephalalgia. 2014;34(6):409–25.
13. Stovner L, Hagen K, Jensen R, Katsarava Z, Lipton R, Scher A, et al. The global burden of headache: a documentation of headache prevalence and disability worldwide. Cephalalgia. 2007;27(3):193–210.
14. Katsarava Z, Schneeweiss S, Kurth T, Kroener U, Fritsche G, Eikermann A, et al. Incidence and predictors for chronicity of headache in patients with episodic migraine. Neurology. 2004;62(5):788–90.
15. Limmroth V, Katsarava Z, Fritsche G, Przywara S, Diener H. Features of medication overuse headache following overuse of different acute headache drugs. Neurology. 2002;59:1011–4.
16. Creac'h C, Radat F, Mick G, Guegan-Massardier E, Giraud P, Guy N, et al. One or several types of triptan overuse headaches? Headache. 2009;49(4):519–28.
17. Bigal ME, Borucho S, Serrano D, Lipton RB. The acute treatment of episodic and chronic migraine in the USA. Cephalalgia. 2009;29(8):891–7.
18. Bigal ME, Lipton RB. Excessive acute migraine medication use and migraine progression. Neurology. 2008;71(22):1821–8.
19. Thorlund K, Sun-Edelstein C, Druyts E, Kanters S, Ebrahim S, Bhambri R, et al. Risk of medication overuse headache across classes of treatments for acute migraine. J Headache Pain. 2016;17(1):107.
20. Chai NC, Scher AI, Moghekar A, Bond DS, Peterlin BL. Obesity and headache: part I–a systematic review of the epidemiology of obesity and headache. Headache. 2014;54(2):219–34.
21. Zeeberg P, Olesen J, Jensen R. Discontinuation of medication overuse in headache patients: recovery of therapeutic responsiveness. Cephalalgia. 2006;26(10):1192–8.
22. Paemeleire K, Evers S, Goadsby PJ. Medication-overuse headache in patients with cluster headache. Curr Pain Headache Rep. 2008;12(2):122–7.
23. Lance F, Parkes C, Wilkinson M. Does analgesic abuse cause headache de novo? Headache. 1988;38:61–2.
24. Bahra A, Walsh M, Menon S, Goadsby PJ. Does chronic daily headache arise de novo in association with regular use of analgesics? Headache. 2003;43:179–90.

25. Lance F, Parkes C, Wilkinson M. Does analgesic abuse cause headaches de novo? Headache. 1988;28(1):61–2.

26. Paemeleire K, Bahra A, Evers S, Matharu MS, Goadsby PJ. Medication-overuse headache in patients with cluster headache. Neurology. 2006;67(1):109–13.

27. Di Lorenzo C, Coppola G, Curra A, Grieco G, Santorelli FM, Lepre C, et al. Cortical response to somatosensory stimulation in medication overuse headache patients is influenced by angiotensin converting enzyme (ACE) I/D genetic polymorphism. Cephalalgia. 2012;32(16):1189–97.

28. Di Lorenzo C, Di Lorenzo G, Sances G, Ghiotto N, Guaschino E, Grieco GS, et al. Drug consumption in medication overuse headache is influenced by brain-derived neurotrophic factor Val66Met polymorphism. J Headache Pain. 2009;10(5):349–55.

29. Cargnin S, Viana M, Ghiotto N, Bianchi M, Sances G, Tassorelli C, et al. Functional polymorphisms in COMT and SLC6A4 genes influence the prognosis of patients with medication overuse headache after withdrawal therapy. Eur J Neurol. 2014;21(7):989–95.

30. Srikiatkhachorn A, Anthony M. Serotonin receptor adaptation in patients with analgesic-induced headache. Cephalalgia. 1996;16(6):419–22.

31. Srikiatkhachorn A, Anthony M. Platelet serotonin in patients with analgesic-induced headache. Cephalalgia. 1996;16(6):423–6.

32. Srikiatkhachorn A, Puangniyom S, Govitrapong P. Plasticity of 5-HT serotonin receptor in patients with analgesic-induced transformed migraine. Headache. 1998;38(7):534–9.

33. Rossi C, Pini LA, Cupini ML, Calabresi P, Sarchielli P. Endocannabinoids in platelets of chronic migraine patients and medication-overuse headache patients: relation with serotonin levels. Eur J Clin Pharmacol. 2008;64(1):1–8.

34. Cupini LM, Costa C, Sarchielli P, Bari M, Battista N, Eusebi P, et al. Degradation of endocannabinoids in chronic migraine and medication overuse headache. Neurobiol Dis. 2008;30(2):186–9.

35. Ayzenberg I, Obermann M, Nyhuis P, Gastpar M, Limmroth V, Diener HC, et al. Central sensitization of the trigeminal and somatic nociceptive systems in medication overuse headache mainly involves cerebral supraspinal structures. Cephalalgia. 2006;26(9):1106–14.

36. Ferraro D, Vollono C, Miliucci R, Virdis D, De Armas L, Pazzaglia C, et al. Habituation to pain in "medication overuse headache": a CO2 laser-evoked potential study. Headache. 2012;52(5):792–807.

37. Riederer F, Marti M, Luechinger R, Lanzenberger R, von Meyenburg J, Gantenbein AR, et al. Grey matter changes associated with medication-overuse headache: correlations with disease related disability and anxiety. World J Biol Psychiatry. 2012;13(7):517–25.

38. Riederer F, Gantenbein AR, Marti M, Luechinger R, Kollias S, Sandor PS. Decrease of gray matter volume in the midbrain is associated with treatment response in medication-overuse headache: possible influence of orbitofrontal cortex. J Neurosci. 2013;33(39):15343–9.

39. Grazzi L, Chiapparini L, Ferraro S, Usai S, Andrasik F, Mandelli ML, et al. Chronic migraine with medication overuse pre-post withdrawal of symptomatic medication: clinical results and FMRI correlations. Headache. 2010;50(6):998–1004.

40. Ferraro S, Grazzi L, Mandelli ML, Aquino D, Di Fiore D, Usai S, et al. Pain processing in medication overuse headache: a functional magnetic resonance imaging (fMRI) study. Pain Med. 2012;13(2):255–62.

41. Sarchielli P, Corbelli I, Messina P, Cupini LM, Bernardi G, Bono G, et al. Psychopathological comorbidities in medication-overuse headache: a multicentre clinical study. Eur J Neurol. 2015;23(1):85–91.

42. Westergaard ML, Glumer C, Hansen EH, Jensen RH. Medication overuse, healthy lifestyle behaviour and stress in chronic headache: results from a population-based representative survey. Cephalalgia. 2016;36(1):15–28.

43. Hagen K, Linde M, Steiner TJ, Stovner LJ, Zwart JA. Risk factors for medication-overuse headache: an 11-year follow-up study. The Nord-Trondelag health studies. Pain. 2012;153(1):56–61.

44. Fritsche G, Frettloh J, Huppe M, Dlugaj M, Matatko N, Gaul C, et al. Prevention of medication overuse in patients with migraine. Pain. 2010;151(2):404–13.

45. Krymchantowski AV, Tepper SJ, Jevoux C, Valenca MM. Medication-overuse headache: differences between daily and near-daily headache patients. Brain Sci. 2016;6:3.

46. Rossi P, Di Lorenzo C, Faroni J, Cesarino F, Nappi G. Advice alone vs. structured detoxification programmes for medication overuse headache: a prospective, randomized, open-label trial in transformed migraine patients with low medical needs. Cephalalgia. 2006;26(9):1097–105.

47. Rossi P, Faroni JV, Tassorelli C, Nappi G. Advice alone versus structured detoxification programmes for complicated medication overuse headache (MOH): a prospective, randomized, open-label trial. J Headache Pain. 2013;14:10.

48. de Goffau MJ, Klaver AR, Willemsen MG, Bindels PJ, Verhagen AP. The effectiveness of treatments for patients with medication overuse headache; a systematic review and meta-analysis. J Pain. 2016;18(6):615–27.

49. Grande RB, Aaseth K, Benth JS, Lundqvist C, Russell MB. Reduction in medication-overuse headache after short information. The Akershus study of chronic headache. Eur J Neurol. 2011;18(1):129–37.

50. Kristoffersen ES, Straand J, Russell MB, Lundqvist C. Disability, anxiety and depression in patients with medication-overuse headache in primary care–the BIMOH study. Eur J Neurol. 2016;23(Suppl 1):28–35.

51. Krause SJ, Stillman MJ, Tepper DE, Zajac D. A prospective cohort study of outpatient interdisciplinary rehabilitation of chronic headache patients. Headache. 2017;57(3):428–40.

52. Diener HC, Bussone G, Van Oene JC, Lahaye M, Schwalen S, Goadsby PJ. Topiramate reduces headache days in chronic migraine: a randomized, double-blind, placebo-controlled study. Cephalalgia. 2007;27(7):814–23.

53. Silberstein SD, Lipton RB, Dodick DW, Freitag FG, Ramadan N, Mathew N, et al. Efficacy and safety of topiramate for the treatment of chronic migraine: a randomized, double-blind, placebo-controlled trial. Headache. 2007;47(2):170–80.

54. Silberstein S, Lipton R, Dodick D, Freitag F, Mathew N, Brandes J, et al. Topiramate treatment of chronic migraine: a randomized, placebo-controlled trial of quality of life and other efficacy measures. Headache. 2009;49(8):1153–62.

55. Diener HC, Dodick DW, Goadsby PJ, Bigal ME, Bussone G, Silberstein SD, et al. Utility of topiramate for the treatment of patients with chronic migraine in the presence or absence of acute medication overuse. Cephalalgia. 2009;29(10):1021–7.

56. Silberstein SD. Topiramate in migraine prevention: a 2016 perspective. Headache. 2017;57(1):165–78.

57. Aurora SK, Dodick DW, Turkel CC, DeGryse RE, Silberstein SD, Lipton RB, et al. OnabotulinumtoxinA for treatment of chronic migraine: results from the double-blind, randomized, placebo-controlled phase of the PREEMPT 1 trial. Cephalalgia. 2010;30(7):793–803.

58. Diener HC, Dodick DW, Aurora SK, Turkel CC, DeGryse RE, Lipton RB, et al. OnabotulinumtoxinA for treatment of chronic migraine: results from the double-blind, randomized, placebo-controlled phase of the PREEMPT 2 trial. Cephalalgia. 2010;30(7):804–14.

59. Dodick DW, Turkel CC, DeGryse RE, Aurora SK, Silberstein SD, Lipton RB, et al. OnabotulinumtoxinA for treatment of chronic migraine: pooled results from the double-blind, randomized, placebo-controlled phases of the PREEMPT clinical program. Headache. 2010;50(6):921–36.

60. Silberstein SD, Blumenfeld AM, Cady RK, Turner IM, Lipton RB, Diener HC, et al. OnabotulinumtoxinA for treatment of chronic migraine: PREEMPT 24-week pooled subgroup analysis of patients who had acute headache medication overuse at baseline. J Neurol Sci. 2013;331(1–2):48–56.

61. Chiang CC, Schwedt TJ, Wang SJ, Dodick DW. Treatment of medication-overuse headache: a systematic review. Cephalalgia. 2015;36(4):371–86.

62. Katsarava Z, Fritsche G, Muessig M, Diener HC, Limmroth V. Clinical features of withdrawal headache following overuse of triptans and other headache drugs. Neurology. 2001;57:1694–8.

63. Rabe K, Pageler L, Gaul C, Lampl C, Kraya T, Foerderreuther S, et al. Prednisone for the treatment of withdrawal headache in patients with medication overuse headache: a randomized, double-blind, placebo-controlled study. Cephalalgia. 2013;33(3):202–7.

64. Boe MG, Mygland A, Salvesen R. Prednisolone does not reduce withdrawal headache: a randomized, double-blind study. Neurology. 2007;69(1):26–31.

65. Tassorelli C, Jensen R, Allena M, De Icco R, Sances G, Katsarava Z, et al. A consensus protocol for the management of medication-overuse headache: evaluation in a multicentric, multinational study. Cephalalgia. 2014;34(9):645–55.

66. Bendtsen L, Munksgaard S, Tassorelli C, Nappi G, Katsarava Z, Lainez M, et al. Disability, anxiety and depression associated with medication-overuse headache can be considerably reduced by detoxification and prophylactic treatment. Results from a multicentre, multinational study (COMOESTAS project). Cephalalgia. 2014;34(6):426–33.

67. Krymchantowski AV, Tepper SJ, Jevoux C, Valenca M. Medication-overuse headache: protocols and outcomes in 149 consecutive patients in a tertiary Brazilian headache center. Headache. 2017;57(1):87–96.

68. Cady R, Nett R, Dexter K, Freitag F, Beach ME, Manley HR. Treatment of chronic migraine: a 3-month comparator study of naproxen sodium vs SumaRT/nap. Headache. 2014;54(1):80–93.

69. Hautaniemi T, Petrenko N, Skorinkin A, Giniatullin R. The inhibitory action of the antimigraine nonsteroidal anti-inflammatory drug naproxen on P2X3 receptor-mediated responses in rat trigeminal neurons. Neuroscience. 2012;209:32–8.

70. Smith TR. Low-dose Tizanidine with nonsteroidal anti-inflammatory drugs for detoxification from analgesic rebound headache. Headache. 2002;42:175–7.

71. Silberstein SD, Schulman EA, McFaden HM. Repetitive intravenous DHE in the treatment of refractory headache. Headache. 1990;30:334–9.

72. Saper JR, Silberstein S, Dodick D, Rapoport A. DHE in the pharmacotherapy of migraine: potential for a larger role. Headache. 2006;46(Suppl 4):S212–20.

73. Eller M, Gelfand AA, Riggins NY, Shiboski S, Schankin C, Goadsby PJ. Exacerbation of headache during dihydroergotamine for chronic migraine does not alter outcome. Neurology. 2016;86(9):856–9.

74. Freitag FG, Lake A 3rd, Lipton R, Cady R, Diamond S, Silberstein S, et al. Inpatient treatment of headache: an evidence-based assessment. Headache. 2004;44(4):342–60.

75. Relja G, Granato A, Bratina A, Antonello RM, Zorzon M. Outcome of medication overuse headache after abrupt in-patient withdrawal. Cephalalgia. 2006;26(5):589–95.

76. Freitag FG, Lyss H, Nissan GR. Migraine disability, healthcare utilization, and expenditures following treatment in a tertiary headache center. Proc (Bayl Univ Med Cent). 2013;26(4):363–7.

77. Lake AE III, Saper JR, Hamel RL. Comprehensive inpatient treatment of refractory chronic daily headache. Headache. 2009;49(4):555–62.

78. Drucker P, Tepper S. Daily sumatriptan for detoxification from rebound. Headache. 1998;38:687–90.

79. Hagen K, Albretsen C, Vilming ST, Salvesen R, Gronning M, Helde G, et al. Management of medication overuse headache: 1-year randomized multicentre open-label trial. Cephalalgia. 2009;29(2):221–32.

80. Zeeberg P, Olesen J, Jensen R. Probable medication-overuse headache: the effect of a 2-month drug-free period. Neurology. 2006;66(12):1894–8.

81. Raggi A, Giovannetti AM, Leonardi M, Sansone E, Schiavolin S, Curone M, et al. Predictors of 12-months relapse after withdrawal treatment in hospitalized patients with chronic migraine associated with medication overuse: a longitudinal observational study. Headache. 2017;57(1):60–70.

Optimizing Acute Headache Treatment in the Setting of Chronic Migraine

Amanda Tinsley and John Farr Rothrock

Successful reduction of headache burden in patients with chronic migraine (CM) most often will require an integrated management strategy that involves much more than simply the prescription of an oral prophylactic agent or administration of onabotulinumtoxinA. In most cases, pharmacologic prophylactic therapy represents the final, albeit critical, component of any management plan designed to suppress CM. An example of a rational, multidimensional plan is outlined below.

Management Plan for the Suppression of Chronic Migraine
- Intensive patient education
- Avoidance of acute migraine "triggers"/chronic migraine aggravators
- Elimination/avoidance of symptomatic medication overuse
- Aggressive and appropriate treatment of acute "breakthrough" headaches
- "Customized"* aerobic conditioning program
- Treatment of coexisting sleep or mood disorder
- Use of a headache diary
- Ongoing follow-up with provider
- Appropriate pharmacologic prophylactic therapy

*i.e., appropriate to the patient's baseline level cardiovascular fitness

A. Tinsley (✉) · J. F. Rothrock
Department of Neurology, GW-MFA Headache Center, George Washington University School of Medicine and Health Sciences, Washington, DC, USA
e-mail: ammichael@mfa.gwu.edu

The Therapeutic Paradox

For the patient with CM and daily or near-daily headache, two components of this management

© Springer International Publishing AG, part of Springer Nature 2019
M. W. Green et al. (eds.), *Chronic Headache*, https://doi.org/10.1007/978-3-319-91491-6_15

plan—*aggressive treatment of acute headache* and *avoidance of symptomatic medication overuse*—may seem contradictory. Especially in the early weeks of treatment, when any prophylactic treatment prescribed or administered has yet to exert a therapeutic effect, how does one manage to treat effectively each headache that occurs without straying into the self-defeating realm of symptomatic medication overuse and medication overuse headache (MOH)?

Consequences of Inadequately Treated Acute Migraine

There are both short- and long-term consequences that result from inadequate acute headache treatment. Aside from the misery, inconvenience, and cost that attend an untreated or incompletely treated acute migraine attack, such attacks may negatively influence the afflicted individual's subsequent headache pattern. Increasing headache attack frequency is a potent risk factor for "transformation" of episodic migraine (EM) into its chronic variant, and congruent with this is the observation that prolonged attacks of severe migraine headache appear to amplify sensitization of the anatomical pathways that signal migrainous head pain [1, 2]. In the setting of CM, wherein those pathways already have become persistently sensitized, such amplification will serve to render the patient yet more headache-prone and further complicate the task of achieving a significant reduction in headache burden.

Medication Overuse Headache

If frequent migraine headaches predispose to and reinforce CM, why burden the patient with any limit on the use/frequency of symptomatic medication? Issues of side effects, abuse/addiction, and habituation aside, unrestricted acute headache treatment unfortunately may result in MOH. While some persuasively have argued that the frequency and clinical influence of MOH have been overstated, it remains the prevailing

opinion in the field of headache medicine that frequent use of virtually any of the over-the-counter or prescription medications commonly used to treat acute migraine headache will lead to an increase in overall headache burden [3–6]. Although the propensity for the development of MOH well may vary from one migraineur to another, current International Headache Society guidelines indicate that use of "simple" analgesics (e.g., acetaminophen) more than 14 days per month for at least 3 consecutive months or use of an opiate/opioid, butalbital, ergotamine, or triptan more than 9 days per month will add to the migraineur's primary headache disorder a component of MOH [7].

Symptomatic medication overuse is prevalent [8]. Among patients presenting to a subspecialty headache clinic, as many as two-thirds report overusing symptomatic medication [8]. At least in this clinic population, both the frequency of MOH and the type of medication overused may vary significantly according to geographic region. In one study, patients at a university-affiliated headache clinic in the District of Columbia were significantly less likely to report or exhibit overuse of symptomatic medication than patients at a university-affiliated clinic in Nevada, and among those in the former group, the prevalence of overuse of an opiate/opioid or butalbital was also significantly lower [9, 10].

Patients often use "rebound headache" as a term they consider to be synonymous with MOH. The authors have found that when patients who report "rebound" caused by a given medication are questioned more closely, what the patient often is describing is an acute migraine headache that responded to treatment with a given symptomatic agent but then soon recurred, frequently with a vengeance. In short, they are describing precisely what one would expect from an incompletely treated acute migraine episode wherein early headache recurrence will occur once the initially effective symptomatic medication is metabolized and eliminated. For example, the half-life of subcutaneously administered sumatriptan is only 1–2 h. While the therapy's swift Tmax may lead to a rapid and dramatic reduction in acute headache, its short half-life ensures that many patients will experience early headache recurrence (especially if treatment has been delayed and the initial headache is reduced but not eliminated).

Medication overuse headache is often far less vivid and much more insidious than the term "rebound" would imply. Although there are patients overusing symptomatic medication who exhibit an obvious temporal relationship between administration of drug and development of headache (e.g., a consistent pattern of being awakened from sleep by recurrent, severe headache), MOH more often blends seamlessly with the afflicted patient's primary headache disorder. Medication overuse headache takes time to develop. In isolation, a "bad week" wherein a patient uses a triptan 4 or 5 days is unlikely to generate MOH. Instead, the months pass, the medication—say, acetaminophen—is taken on what amounts to a scheduled basis, the CM patient simply continues to suffer from pervasive headache, and aside from the potential development of drug tolerance or side effects, the headache disorder's clinical characteristics remain more or less unchanged.

Thus MOH may be obscured by the CM itself. If the potential for developing MOH varies according to the class of symptomatic medication involved and, even more problematic, the physiology of the given individual, how, then, can the clinician know when a patient's CM has become complicated by MOH? While elegant preclinical and clinical studies have established an objective scientific basis for the existences of MOH, at this point there is no easily available laboratory test or imaging study available to confirm the clinical suspicion of MOH [11]. The best the provider can do is attempt to prevent overuse from the start, assume MOH is present if persistent overuse is known to be occurring, and then work with the patient to curtail overuse.

The individual with CM who substantially reduces his or her use of the offending symptomatic medication(s) may not be immediately rewarded for that effort by any meaningful reduction in headache burden. Just as it may take months of overuse for MOH to develop, a similarly extended period may be required for the biologic process that generates MOH to dissipate and clinical improvement to begin. The rapidity with which improvement occurs appears to vary according to the class of symptomatic medication involved. With the triptans and ergotamines, cessation of overuse tends to produce clinical improvement within days to a few weeks, but with virtually all other symptomatic medications—from acetaminophen to oxycodone—such improvement may be much slower in coming. An absence of any early positive reinforcement obviously can be discouraging for the patient, and on a more general level, it calls into question the utility of short-term hospitalization or use of outpatient infusion centers for the primary purpose of treating MOH via acute "detoxification."

Rational Pharmacologic Management of Acute Migraine in the CM Patient

The individual with CM typically is more familiar and experienced with acute therapies than the average migraineur. Often times, CM patients have tried numerous symptomatic medications and experienced disappointing results, leading to increased direct and indirect costs and patient frustration. In this patient population, it is especially important to obtain detailed information regarding what has constituted treatment "failure." In many cases, suboptimal doses, poorly timed administration of a given medication, or an inappropriate formulation may have been employed. Ascertain whether the patient has tried combination therapies and/or non-oral formulations. Simply adjusting the dose or matching drug and formulation to headache intensity and associated symptoms may improve the patient's ability to control acute attacks. Perhaps of greatest importance, whenever possible ensure the patient treats the acute headache attack early, while pain intensity is still mild.

As implied earlier, the major difference in treating acute migraine attacks for CM patients compared to episodic migraine (EM) patients is that aggressive treatment of all attacks places CM patient at risk for developing MOH. About the best the provider can do is educate the patient as to that risk, provide parameters for how often a given medication or class of medications should be utilized, and prescribe multiple abortive therapies intended to "fit" the individual headache's level of intensity without overuse of one particular medication or class.

The patient-provider alliance is of utmost value when developing a regimen for acute management of CM. A discussion on realistic expectations of acute therapy in the office can lead to improved patient education and satisfaction.

Although the goals of acute therapy (pain freedom, rapid and complete restoration of function, and absence of early headache recurrence) are ideal, this will not be possible in all cases. In many cases of CM, simply achieving the goals of pain reduction, decreased utilization of urgent care centers or emergency rooms (ERs), and reduced migraine-related disability may have to suffice.

Patients should be encouraged to keep a headache "diary" to monitor headache frequency and severity and acute medication use, and this record should be reviewed at follow-up visits to track the progress of the patient's headache burden and its change (or lack of change) subsequent to implementation of a management plan. While the authors have not found elaborate hour-by-hour journals detailing food and beverage intake, weather, physical and social activity, etc. to be especially helpful in managing CM, for cycling female patients, the inclusion of menstrual flow onset and cessation in the diary may provide another avenue for achieving a reduction in headache burden.

There is an a priori reason why the development of an *evidence-based* plan for acute treatment in the setting of CM can be difficult: to date, the great majority of clinical trials evaluating therapies for acute migraine have systematically excluded patients with CM. Navigating the acute management of the CM patient population consequently requires a blend of "art" and extrapolation from clinical trials data relevant to the EM population. At present, there can be no scientifically derived consensus regarding the pharmacologic specifics of acute therapy in CM patients.

Selecting a Therapy

Acute treatment regimens necessarily are often dynamic, changing based on the patient's response to a given medication and other circumstances (e.g., financial considerations). Interactions with other medications the patient is taking and comorbidities such as hypertension, vascular disease, and gastrointestinal disorders must be considered when selecting an acute treatment. Many patients with CM do not respond well to acute monotherapy, and so combination therapies with drugs possessing different mechanisms of action may be needed.

Acute therapies can be either nonspecific or specific, with the latter intended to target receptors or other mechanisms of electrochemical transmission known to be integral to the generation of migrainous head pain.

Major Categories of Acute Migraine Treatments
  Nonspecific Acute Migraine Therapies
  • Nonsteroidal anti-inflammatory drugs (NSAIDs)
  • Acetaminophen
  • Opioids
  • Benzodiazepines
  • Corticosteroids
  • Propofol (IV only)
  • Ketamine (IV only)
  Specific Acute Migraine Therapies
  • Triptans
  • Ergots
  • Dopamine antagonists
  • Diphenhydramine
  • Calcitonin gene-related peptide (CGRP) antagonists (currently under study)
  Therapies with Uncertain Mechanisms
  • Valproic acid (IV)
  • Magnesium sulfate (IV)
  • Occipital nerve blocks

Nonspecific Migraine Therapies

The most commonly used acute medications for migraine are the nonsteroidal anti-inflammatory drugs (NSAIDs). NSAIDs exert their effect by inhibiting cyclooxygenase, decreasing prostaglandin synthesis in the central nervous system and systemically. Given that migraine is classified as a *neuro-inflammatory disorder*, it's hardly surprising that many drugs in this class have performed well in trials involving acute migraine. The NSAIDs with the most consistently positive clinical trials evidence of efficacy in the setting of acute migraine treatment are aspirin, diclofenac potassium/sodium, flurbiprofen, ibuprofen, naproxen sodium, and tolfenamic acid.

Especially when the headache is moderate to severe in intensity, an oral NSAID may fail to abort an acute migraine attack. Parenteral ketorolac can be helpful in these cases and is the only NSAID available in intravenous (IV) or intramuscular (IM) formulations in the United States. In the ER or urgent care setting, ketorolac 15–30 mg IV or 30–60 mg IV is used as a first-line treatment; in clinical trials, the IV route has yielded a higher response rate. Theoretically, the high concentration of NSAID that reaches the CNS with the parenteral administration of the medication accounts for the increase in efficacy relative to the oral formulation. Patients can also self-administer ketorolac intramuscularly with prefilled syringes, eliminating the need for utilization of an ER or urgent care center.

Gastrointestinal (GI) intolerance and bleeding is the major potential complication associated with NSAID use. Oral celecoxib (100–400 mg), a selective cyclooxygenase-2 (COX-2) inhibitor, can be considered if NSAIDs are contraindicated secondary to gastrointestinal bleeding but may convey an increased risk for cardiovascular events. For patients who fail to respond to an oral NSAID, exhibit extreme GI intolerance, and cannot/will not self-inject ketorolac, indomethacin 50 mg is available as compounded suppository.

Acetaminophen, like aspirin often referred to as a "simple analgesic," may not be as effective for acute migraine treatment as the NSAIDs but has been consistently superior to placebo in clinical trials. Excedrin, a patented over-the-counter combination medication containing aspirin, acetaminophen, and caffeine, has been shown to be effective and has received US Food and Drug Administration approval for acute migraine treatment [12].

Opiate/opioid treatment of acute migraine is controversial, and such treatment is typically best avoided or minimized whenever possible. In select cases of acute, severe migraine headache wherein all other medication options have failed, are contraindicated, or are not tolerated, opiate/opioid therapy may be considered as an option, but the frequency of use should be kept to a minimum so as to reduce the complications of MOH, dependence/addiction, decreased responsiveness to prophylactic therapy, or tardive development of CM.

Benzodiazepines provide sedation but little analgesic benefit. They are not ideal first-line abortive agents due to their side effect profile (drowsiness, confusion), association with dependence/addiction, and risk of overdose. Even so, benzodiazepines may be particularly helpful in promoting sleep in a patient with a prolonged migraine attack, and sleep itself may terminate a migraine attack. Oral diazepam 5 mg tablets can be used in the outpatient setting, and multiple IV formulations exist for urgent care settings.

Steroids may suppress the inflammatory processes thought to be involved in migraine. In the absence of little supportive evidence from research trials, clinicians often prescribe a short course (3–10 days) of oral steroids to "break" status migrainosus and/or reduce the risk of headache recurrence following treatment of that condition. Because chronic steroid use can lead to a host of long-term sequelae (e.g., osteoporosis, aseptic necrosis, cataracts, diabetes, weight gain, skin thinning, immunosuppression), their use must be limited, and even brief courses of oral steroids should be restricted to ~8 times per year. There is currently no evidence available regarding which steroid and dosing paradigm is most effective in the outpatient setting, and current prescribing patterns are based primarily on provider preference. Common regimens include dexamethasone 4 mg tid for 3 days, prednisone 60 mg in the morning with food for 3–5 days, or prepackaged tapering regimen of methylprednisolone (i.e., a "dosepak"). In the ER setting, corticosteroids (10–25 mg IM/IV) have been shown to be effective in decreasing the risk of headache recurrence when used as an adjunctive therapy with other abortive agents.

The administration of sub-anesthetic doses (1 mg/kg or less) of propofol IV for acute treatment of refractory migraine has been shown to be efficacious and safe in several case studies, but practical considerations have limited its use in the setting of acute migraine headache [13–16]. In a recently published retrospective analysis, sub-anesthetic doses of IV ketamine were reported to be helpful in treating patients with CM and new daily persistent headache who had failed traditional therapies [17].

"Specific" Migraine Therapies

Relatively more migraine-specific acute treatments include the triptans and ergotamine derivatives, which act as 5-hydroxytryptamine (5-HT) agonists at serotonin receptors inhibitory to head pain transmission. While a more central action cannot be excluded, these drugs may exert their therapeutic effect by blocking the extravasation of pro-inflammatory plasma proteins from dural blood vessels and by constricting dilated extracerebral cranial blood vessels.

For now, subcutaneously injected sumatriptan (3.4, or 6 mg) must be considered the most effective self-administered therapy for "rescue" from migraine headache of moderate to severe intensity. It's often astounding efficacy may be attributed to the drug's rapid Tmax and relatively high Cmax, pharmacokinetic variables which unfortunately also tend to produce the familiar array of triptan side effects more frequently and at a higher level of intensity than other triptan formulations.

The intranasal formulation of sumatriptan appears to offer little advantage over the oral and is less effective than the injectable. Intranasal zolmitriptan, however, may represent an attractive option for patients who are reluctant to self-inject but do not respond consistently to the oral formulations of this or the other triptans. Of the "fast-onset" oral triptans—sumatriptan, zolmitriptan, rizatriptan, almotriptan, eletriptan—patient response tends to be highly idiosyncratic; some patients prefer one over the others, some respond well to all, and some respond to none. While the oral triptans clearly are more effective if taken early in a migraine attack, when pain intensity is mild to moderate, their FDA indications were derived from registration trials involving headache of moderate to severe intensity, and at this writing we lack data to indicate they are any more effective for early migraine than the NSAIDs or other cheaper, more accessible treatment options. As for the "slow-onset" oral triptans—naratriptan and frovatriptan—their relatively slow onset of therapeutic action is such that their use is largely restricted to patients intolerant of faster-onset triptans or those requiring triptan "miniprophylaxis" (e.g., as for menstrually related migraine).

Relative to the triptans, the ergotamines have the advantage of longer half-lives, a longer duration of therapeutic effect, and a lower rate of early headache recurrence. As for their negative attributes, the oral ergotamines are poorly absorbed, subcutaneously administered dihydroergotamine (DHE) is less rapidly effective than injectable sumatriptan, and the ergotamines as a group are more likely than the triptans to cause nausea. Intranasally administered DHE appeared in phase 3 trials to offer an intriguing alternative to the oral and intranasal triptans or to subcutaneous therapy, but its expense and tendency to promote nasal congestion have limited its use.

As for the dopamine antagonists, with the exception of oral metoclopramide, self-administration of these agents is most commonly reserved to treat migraine-associated nausea rather than the headache itself. Their efficacy in treating headache increases dramatically when they are administered via the intravenous route (see below).

Status Migrainosus

Aggressive treatment of acute migraine may be beneficial for many reasons, but such treatment is especially appropriate for patients with prolonged attacks that exceed 3 days or more ("status migrainosus"). In the setting of acute migraine, once a certain level of biologic sensitization has been reached, medications typically effective when administered earlier in the attack may lose their therapeutic benefit [18]. In addition, there is much clinical and biological evidence to support the adage that "headache begets headache," and prolonged attacks of severe migrainous head pain may be particularly inclined to enhance sensitization of the central and peripheral pathways integral to signaling of head pain. As for the worst case scenario, any clinician who sees a high volume of migraine has encountered patients whose status migrainosus progressed from being atypically prolonged into the pervasive headache of chronic migraine.

Provider-administered "rescue therapy" ideally should be delivered in a setting absent of stimuli which aggravate acute migraine (e.g., light, noise), wherein the patient can be treated rapidly by providers familiar with acute migraine management and, better yet, familiar with the individual patient's history and particular needs. Unfortunately, such is rarely the case in emergency rooms and urgent care centers. Confronted with the option of suffering in silence at home and facing the long wait time and bright neon lights of the ER, many patients with acute migraine understandably choose the former. The attack persists untreated until it finally runs its course, and at its conclusion the migraineur is left with a yet more sensitized biologic system primed to generate more headaches.

A third option for provider-administered acute migraine treatment is beginning to gain traction. "Headache rescue rooms" which are embedded in subspecialty headache centers may provide an excellent alternative to an ER, urgent care center, or simple endurance in a dark, silent room. "Rescue room" utilization is associated with high rates of headache relief, low rates of early headache recurrence, high patient satisfaction, and a significant reduction in direct medical costs [19].

In the ER and elsewhere, the use of nonspecific parenteral opiates and opioids to treat acute migraine headache remains discouragingly high. Despite their frequency of use and the potential for abuse, little evidence exists to suggest that these traditional nostrums convey much in the way of meaningful efficacy.

Among the more specific medications which have been used to treat status migrainosus, droperidol administered intramuscularly became widely utilized by ER physicians for the treatment of acute migraine headache [20]. In 2001, however, the drugs' controversial acquisition of a "boxed warning" related to QTc prolongation led to an abrupt

decline in its use and, eventually, its availability. Although there is little evidence to suggest that other dopamine antagonists commonly administered for the treatment of acute migraine have more or less potential for producing QTc prolongation or significant cardiac arrhythmia, the FDA warning and the corresponding need to obtain and evaluate an electrocardiogram prior to administration of droperidol and maintain cardiac monitoring over the subsequent hours have served to effectively eliminate its role in migraine treatment.

As for the other dopamine antagonists often used to treat acute migraine headache—metoclopramide, prochlorperazine, promethazine, chlorpromazine, and haloperidol—there are few data to suggest that anyone is better suited for that purpose than another. By virtue of its consistently positive performance in ER-based clinical trials involving migraine headache and relatively high tolerability, intravenously administered metoclopramide is considered by many to be the dopamine antagonist of first choice for migraine therapy.

Early headache recurrence following transiently successful termination of status migrainosus is not uncommon, and to assist in avoiding that complication, it may be helpful to add intravenous steroid to whatever other else is administered and to prescribe a short course of high-dose oral steroid to be taken over the days immediately ensuing.

Pharmacologic intervention aside, optimal management of status migrainosus requires that the provider ensure the patient is adequately hydrated and that the blood pressure is maintained at an appropriate level. Patients with prolonged migraine frequently have reduced intravascular volume due to decreased oral intake and migraine-associated vomiting, and dehydration reinforces the migraine process. Even typically normotensive patients with acute, severe migraine headache may exhibit a considerable elevation of systemic blood pressure during attacks, and if the elevated pressure fails to decrease following treatment directed at reduction of headache intensity, then more specific antihypertensive therapy is indicated.

An evidence-based algorithm for provider-administered treatment of acute migraine is presented in Fig. 15.1. Interestingly, in one scholarly meta-analysis involving ER-based trials that

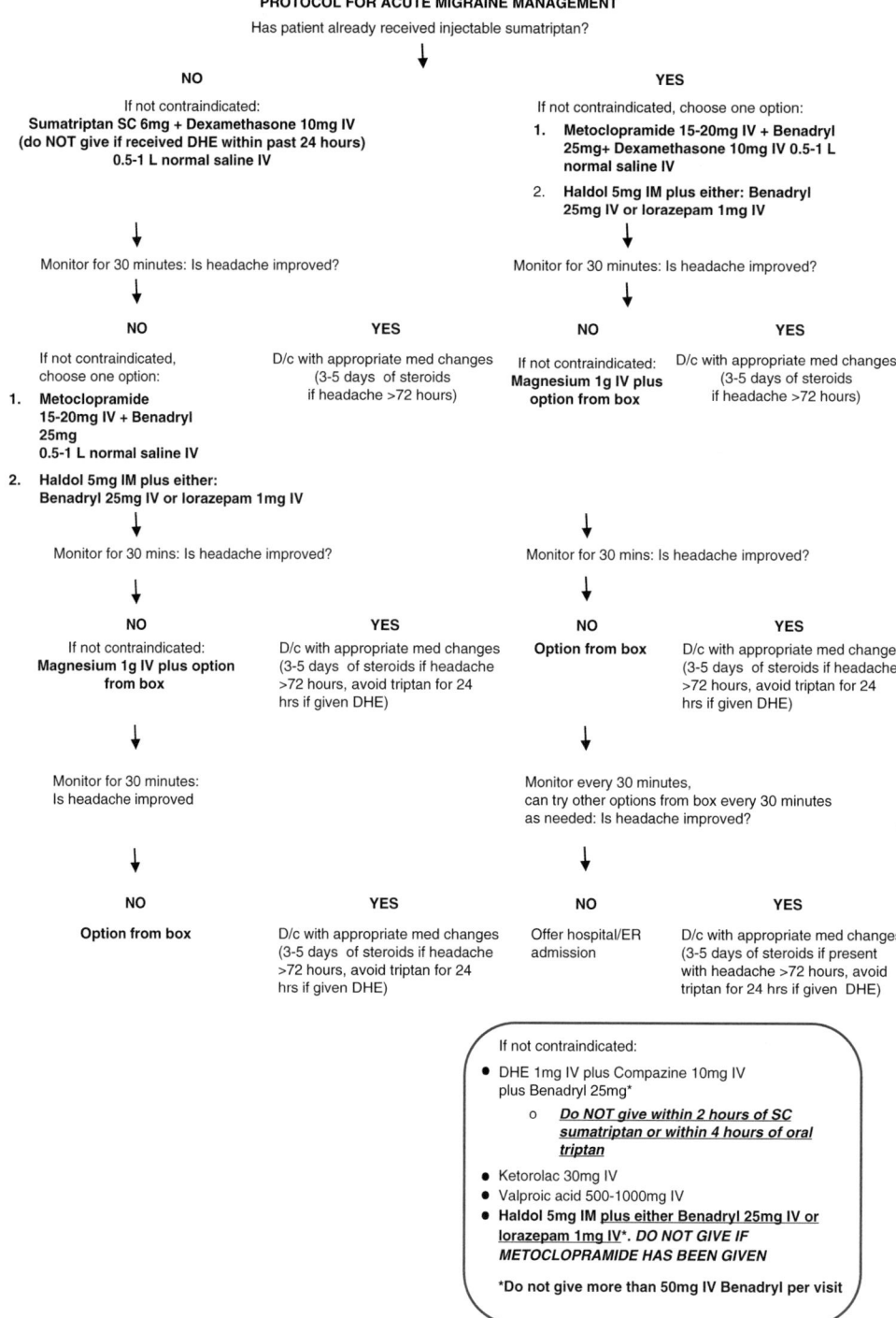

Fig. 15.1 Protocol for acute migraine management

examined various medications used for treatment of acute migraine headache, the authors found that subcutaneously injected sumatriptan possessed the strongest evidence base of all the therapies evaluated [21]. As injectable sumatriptan is the only therapy among those listed in Fig. 15.1 which routinely may be self-administered, it would make sense that positively responding patients for whom this treatment is not contraindicated should receive a prescription for the medication/formulation so as to preclude the need for provider-initiated "rescue" when future attacks occur.

References

1. Burstein R. Deconstructing migraine headache into peripheral and central sensitization. Pain. 2001;89:107.
2. Scher A, Stewart W, Ricci J, Lipton R. Factors associated with the onset and remission of chronic daily headache in a population-based study. Pain. 2003;106:81.
3. Dodick D, Freitag F. Evidence-based understanding of medication-overuse headache: clinical implications. Headache. 2006;46((suppl) 4):S202.
4. Katsavara Z, Jensen R. Medication-overuse headache: where are we now? Curr Opin Neurol. 2007;20:326.
5. Abrams B. Medication overuse headache. Med Clin North Am. 2013;97:337.
6. Scher A, Rizzoli P, Loder E. Medication overuse headache. An entrenched idea in need of scrutiny. Neurology. 2017;89(12):1296–304.
7. Headache Classification Committee of the International Headache Society (HIS). The international classification of headache disorders, 3rd edition (beta version). Cephalalgia. 2013;33:629.
8. Katsavara Z, Muessig M, Dzagnidze A, et al. Medication overuse headache: rates and predictors for relapse in a 4-year prospective study. Cephalalgia. 2005;25:12.
9. Choi J, Michael A, Andress-Rothrock D, Rothrock J. A regional comparison of headache clinic populations: demography, diagnoses, and frequencies/types of symptomatic medication overuse. Headache. 2016;56(suppl 1):45.
10. Mendizabal J, Rothrock J. An inter-regional comparative study of headache clinic populations. Cephalalgia. 1998;18:57.
11. Srikiatkhachorn A, le Grand S, Supornsilpchai W, Storer J. Pathophysiology of medication overuse headache-an update. Headache. 2014;54:204.
12. Stewart WF, Ryan RE Jr, et al. Efficacy and safety of acetaminophen, aspirin, and caffeine in alleviating migraine headache pain: three double-blind, randomized, placebo-controlled trial. Arch Neurol. 1998;55:210.
13. Sato K, Hida A, Arai N, et al. Low-dose intravenous propofol as a possible therapeutic option for acute confusional migraine. Am J Emerg Med. 2017;35:195.e5.
14. Krusz JC, Scott V, Belaner J. Intravenous propofol: unique effectiveness in treating intractable migraine. Headache. 2000;49:224.
15. Mendes PM, Silberstein SD, Young WB, Rozen TD, et al. Intravenous propofol in the treatment of refractory headache. Headache. 2002;42:638.
16. Mosier J, Roper G, Hays D, et al. Sedative dosing of propofol for treatment of migraine headache in the emergency department: a case series. West J Emerg Med. 2013;14:646.
17. Pomery JL, Marmua MJ, Nahas SJ, Viscusi ER. Ketamin infusions for treatment refractory headache. Headache. 2017;57(2):276.
18. Burstein R, Collins B, Jakubowski M. Defeating migraine pain with triptans: a race against the development of cutaneous allodynia. Ann Neurol. 2004;55:19–26.
19. Morey V, Rothrock J. Examining the utility of in-clinic "rescue" therapy for acute migraine. Headache. 2008;48:939.
20. Silberstein S, Young W, Mendizabal J, Rothrock J, Alam A. Efficacy of intramuscular droperidol for migraine treatment: a dose response study. Neurology. 2003;60:315.
21. Orr S, Friedman B, Christie S, et al. Management of adults with acute migraine in the emergency department: the American headache society evidence assessment of parenteral pharmacotherapies. Headache. 2016;56:911.

Pharmacologic Approaches to CDH: Evidence and Outcomes

16

Miguel J. A. Láinez and Ane Mínguez-Olaondo

Introduction

Chronic daily headache (CDH) is a frequent condition in headache referral center; most patients with CDH have chronic migraine (CM). Because most of the recent pharmacologic studies targeted CM, therefore, the primary focus of this chapter will be the pharmacologic treatment of CM. CM has a prevalence of at least 1–2% and CDH 4–5% in the general population [1]. The treatment of these patients is complex and includes patient education, lifestyle modifications, strict control of the predisposing factors, management of the comorbidities, and pharmacological treatment. Behavioral therapies are also important and discussed in another chapter.

In migraine, the most frequently used drugs for acute attacks are triptans, NSAIDs, antiemetics, and analgesics combinations. A patient with headaches most days of the month needs acute treatment for pain management. Principles of acute treatment in CDH are similar to those for episodic headache, and the goals are headache

freedom at 2 h with good tolerability and without recurrence. But in CDH, the need to alleviate the pain should be balanced with the efforts to avoid medication-overuse headache and medication side effects. The choice of acute treatment should be individualized, depending on patient needs. There are no specific studies regarding efficacy of different acute treatments in patients with CDH or CM; triptans and NSAIDs are the most commonly used. Opiates and opioid combinations should be avoided to prevent pharmacological dependency. If possible, acute treatment should be reserved for the exacerbations, trying to reduce the number of days with acute medication.

Preventive treatment is the most important pharmacological approach in patients with CDH. In the standard preventive treatments of migraine, several drugs have shown a superiority compared to placebo, but only a few have been specifically investigated for their effectiveness in CDH and CM [2]. The objective of this chapter is to review the published data on the preventive pharmacological treatment of CDH and CM.

M. J. A. Láinez (✉)
Department of Neurology, Neurology Service, University Clinical Hospital, Catholic University of Valencia, Valencia, Spain
e-mail: miguel.lainez@sen.es

A. Mínguez-Olaondo
Neurology Service, University Clinical Hospital, Catholic University of Valencia, Valencia, Spain

Preventative Treatment

CDH is a condition in which the threshold for developing headache attacks is lower, and therefore these attacks occur with higher frequency. The main objective of treatment is to increase the

© Springer International Publishing AG, part of Springer Nature 2019
M. W. Green et al. (eds.), *Chronic Headache*, https://doi.org/10.1007/978-3-319-91491-6_16

threshold for headache and thereby reduce the number of attacks. Additionally the aim of the preventive treatment beyond reducing headache frequency is to reduce the severity and associated disability of the attacks and reduce the need for acute care medications which contribute to medication-overuse headache [3]. For all these reasons, prophylactic treatment should be considered in all patients with CDH.

Medication overuse contributes to an increase in headache frequency, which facilitates migraine progression [4–7]. In a patient who fulfills criteria for medication-overuse headache, early discontinuation of acute medication produces a substantial alleviation of headache in a significant proportion of patients, although the overuse is not always the driver of the chronification [5]. In this group of patients with overuse, there is a debate about the ideal time to initiate preventive medication. Some authors advocate for initial withdrawal of the overused medication alone, but there is more data in favor of combining withdrawal with early prophylaxis.

Together with prophylactic medication for migraine, it is important to recognize that many patients with CDH have other conditions that can exacerbate their headaches: depression, anxiety, other pain syndromes like fibromyalgia, or sleep disorders. These comorbidities also need management, and there are some drugs that can help both conditions.

For episodic migraine, multiple drugs have proven efficacy in randomized controlled studies, but in CM the randomized controlled trials are scarce. OnabotulinumtoxinA is the only FDA-approved drug for the prevention of CM. The use of topiramate is supported by two double-blind controlled studies, but is not FDA-approved for this indication.

There are other medications that have shown some benefit in single randomized or open-label studies in CDH or CM. These medications may be considered for patients with CM, particularly when comorbid conditions such as hypertension or mood disorders might benefit or when use of the more proven therapies is not feasible [8].

Oral Preventive Treatment: Drugs

Antiepileptics (Table 16.1)

In episodic migraine, the American Academy of Neurology and the American Headache Society classify topiramate and valproate sodium as level A medications and recommend offering them to patients for prophylaxis. Gabapentin, pregabalin, levetiracetam, zonisamide, and even carbamazepine can be useful in selected patients, despite a lack of clear scientific evidence [9]. A recent meta-analysis suggests that topiramate and divalproex (and propranolol) are more efficacious than other prophylactic medications [10].

Topiramate
Topiramate is the only oral drug with a level of evidence I, grade of recommendation A used as a preventive treatment in CM [11]. There are two main studies, one American [12] and the other

Table 16.1 Antiepileptics

Drug	Studies	Scientific evidence	Adverse events
Topiramate	>1 RCT	Strong	Paresthesia, cognitive impairment
Valproate sodium	1RCT for CM	Weak	Weight gain, hair loss, and tremor. Notice it is teratogenic
Gabapentin	1RCT for CM	Weak	Sleepiness, dizziness, ataxia, tiredness, nystagmus
Pregabalin	1 open-label design	Weak	Dizziness, somnolence, and thought disturbance
Zonisamide	2 open-label multicenter design	Weak	Anorexia, nervousness, irritability, irritabilidad, confusion, depression, ataxia, dizziness, amnesia, somnolence
Levetiracetam	1 placebo-controlled trial	Weak	Somnolence, headaches, rhinopharyngitis

European [13], in which the efficacy was demonstrated comparing placebo with a dose of topiramate between 50 and 200 mg/day. In those studies and others [13], the target dose proposed was 100 mg/day; however, doses as low as 50 mg/day can also be effective [2]. The use of topiramate can prevent the evolution of episodic migraine to CM [14] and can induce a change from chronic to episodic migraine [15]. This is not guaranteed, as shown in the INTREPID trial. In that study, topiramate intervention to prevent transformation of episodic migraine was analyzed for 26 weeks. Progression from high-frequency episodic migraine to CDH could not be completely prevented by 100 mg topiramate per day, although the proportion of transformed patients was low [16].

Topiramate reduces headache days effectively from the first month of treatment [17], which is significant for patients. Even though migraineurs are often more sensitive to topiramate-associated side effects compared to patients with epilepsy [18], it is well tolerated [19]. Possible side effects include behavioral and cognitive disturbances, impaired vision (due to increased intraocular pressure), weight loss, renal stone formation, and a tingling or prickling sensation in the hands and feet. Most adverse events are minimized by titrating the dose upward by 15–25 mg per week to reach the target dose [20], and those symptoms usually resolve over time. The cognitive complaints can be managed similarly [2, 12, 21]. Since it favors the development of metabolic acidosis and renal stones, which are an increased risk in migraineurs, patients should maintain hydration [18]. Topiramate improves quality of life [2, 22] and reduces frequency of migraine-accompanying photophobia, phonophobia, and vomiting [23]. The European study results differed from previous studies in the treatment of CM associated with medication overuse; CM patients with acute medication overuse improved significantly with topiramate [13] without first having withdrawal of the overused medication.

It is not recommended in women of childbearing age planning pregnancy as cleft palate has occurred in newborns whose mothers used the drug during the first trimester of pregnancy (Pregnancy Category D) [18, 20].

Valproate Sodium

Valproate sodium at doses of 500–1000 mg per day shows good efficacy and tolerability [20, 24, 25]. In the extended release formulation, it can be used as a once-a-day prophylactic antimigraine medication [26]. There is one prospective, double-blind, randomized, placebo-controlled trial study published on the efficacy of sodium valproate in patients with CDH. Of the 70 patients included in the study, 29 had CM. Visual analog scale (VAS) and pain frequency (PF) were evaluated. Sodium valproate 500 mg twice a day, compared with placebo, decreased the maximum pain VAS levels (MaxVAS) and PF at the end of the study, but did not change general pain VAS (GnVAS) levels. It was more effective in the group of patients with CM (level of evidence III, grade of recommendation C) [27]. In the other study, sodium valproate (800 mg/day) was superior to placebo in the treatment of medication-overuse headache with history of migraine after detoxification [28]. The most common adverse events are weight gain, hair loss, and tremor. Valproate is a severely teratogenic drug, which is why it should not be used as first-line migraine prophylaxis in women of childbearing age [20]. Other contraindications include thrombocytopenia, pancytopenia, and bleeding disorders [29].

Gabapentin

Gabapentin has been studied against placebo for the prophylaxis of CDH in a multicenter randomized placebo-controlled crossover study. The target dose was 2400 mg per day, a total of 133 patients were enrolled, and 95 were evaluated for efficacy. There was a 9.1% difference in headache-free rates favoring gabapentin over placebo. This is the only study with gabapentin. Unlike other preventive drugs in episodic migraine, the efficacy data of gabapentin is questionable. Gabapentin (1800 mg per day to 2400 mg per day) showed efficacy in a placebo-controlled double-blind trial only when a modified intent-to-treat analysis was used [30]. Thus, in several trials, gabapentin was not superior to placebo [31]. Recent reviews [32], including a Cochrane review [33], conclude that further evaluation of gabapentin in migraine prophylaxis is warranted.

Pregabalin

In an open-label study in CM patients, pregabalin, dosed at 75 mg/day, with an increase depending on the clinical response and the tolerability, was associated with significant decreases in headache frequency and severity and the use of rescue medication. Side effects including dizziness, somnolence, and thought disturbance were frequent [34]. There are no controlled studies on pregabalin in CDH or CM or episodic migraine [33]. Due to its anxiolytic effect, its efficacy in other chronic pain conditions, and possible reduction of central sensitization, it could be a potential therapy in CM, but more evidence is necessary.

Zonisamide

There is some data about the efficacy of zonisamide in patients with CM who are refractory to other preventives or are responsive to, but unable to, tolerate topiramate. The studies are open-label, but multicenter and with an adequate number of patients, although retrospective [35, 36]. These results, obtained in a large sample of patients refractory or intolerant to topiramate and other preventives, indicate that zonisamide, at low doses, is an option for the preventive treatment of patients with frequent migraine [36]. It represents a well-tolerated and effective alternative in case of intolerable side effects to topiramate [37, 38]. Patients should be informed that there is insufficient scientific support for their use in migraine [9]. The recommended dose is between 100 and 200 mg/day.

Levetiracetam

The only placebo-controlled trial published with levetiracetam (3000 mg/day) in patients with CDH (most of them having CM) was negative [39].

β-Blockers (Table 16.2)

Beta-blockers were introduced in migraine prevention by serendipity but can be first-line drugs in migraine prophylaxis. Metoprolol, timolol, and propranolol, in many studies, have proved their efficacy in preventing episodic migraine and are recommended at level A in the majority of guidelines. Others like atenolol, nadolol, nebivolol, and pindolol are recommended as grade B or C. There are however few studies with beta-blockers in the prevention of CDH or CM.

Propranolol

There is one study in which propranolol slow-release 160 mg has been compared to candesartan 16 mg and placebo in a randomized, triple-blind, double crossover study, in patients with episodic or CM [40]. Both drugs have a similar effect size against placebo but, although they include patients with a high number of headache days (8.21 per 4 weeks), only 1 in 72 patients was affected by CM. In open-label studies, beta-blockers (propranolol or nadolol) combined with sodium valproate [41] and topiramate showed better efficacy and good tolerability in patients refractory to both treatments alone. This strategy was studied in a double-blind, placebo-controlled, randomized clinical trial conducted through the National Institute of Neurological Disorders and Stroke Clinical Research Collaboration [43]. In CM subjects inadequately controlled ($\geq$10 headaches/month) with topiramate (50–100 mg/day) alone were treated with either propranolol long acting or placebo. The study was terminated because the ability to complete the trial was not possible. However there may be other combinations that are effective [42].

Atenolol

In an open-label study, atenolol, used at 50 per day, was safe and effective in reducing the number of headache days and intensity, in a small population of CM patients [43]. Controlled trials have not confirmed this. Two old and small trials in migraine patients were negative, which included some patients with more than 16 headache days a month and using atenolol and atenolol versus propranolol [31, 44].

Tricyclic Antidepressants

Tricyclic antidepressants are used for migraine prevention; however, only one tricyclic antidepressant (amitriptyline) has proven clear efficacy [7, 45].

Table 16.2 Other drugs

Drug		Studies	Scientific evidence	Adverse events
β-blockers	Propranolol	Randomized, triple-blind, double crossover study in EM and CM against candesartan and placebo	Weak	Tiredness, vomits, diarrhea, sleep disorder, bronchitis
	Atenolol	Open-label study	Weak	Tiredness
Tricyclic antidepressant	Amitriptyline	>1 RCT (but for EM)	Weak	Dry mouth, a metallic taste, epigastric distress, constipation, dizziness, mental confusion, tachycardia, palpitations, blurred vision, and urinary retention
Selective serotonin reuptake inhibitors and serotonin-norepinephrine reuptake inhibitors	Fluoxetine	RCT	Weak	Nausea, dry mouth, headaches, insomnia, anxiety
	Venlafaxine	Randomized double-blind crossover study where effect of amitriptyline and venlafaxine was compared	Weak	Insomnia, nervousness, mydriasis, and seizures
	Duloxetine	Open-label trial	Weak	Nausea, headaches, dry mouth, dizziness
Calcium channel blockers	Flunarizine	Prospective, randomized, open-label, blinded-endpoint	Weak	Weight gain and depression
Angiotensin II receptor blockers	Candesartan	RCT but no specific data in CM	Weak	Dizziness, vertigo, headaches, abdominal pain, dyspepsia, nausea, vomits, diarrhea
Alpha-blockers	Tizanidine	RCT but no specific for CM, single-blind, placebo-controlled trial	Weak	Somnolence, dizziness, dry mouth, and asthenia
Others	Memantine	Small, partly open-label studies	Weak	Vertigo, headaches, somnolence, constipation, high blood pressure
	Ketamine	Small case series	Weak	Anorexia, nausea, vomits, somnolence, hallucination

Amitriptyline

The use of amitriptyline is common in clinical practice in patients with chronic headaches. Approximately 50% of patients with migraine are improved by more than 50%, results comparable to the use of propranolol and sodium valproate. However, the evidence as treatment for CM is scarce. There is a strong evidence for its use in preventing episodic migraine. It has been studied in four placebo-controlled trials, all with positive results, using doses of 10–150 mg per day [46, 47]. Use of low-dosage amitriptyline may also improve medication compliance, which is an important clinical consideration in the management of this common and chronic condition. This has been an issue in studies for amitriptyline use in headaches, but not only for CM [46]. In a meta-analysis, amitriptyline outperformed candesartan, fluoxetine, propranolol, topiramate, and valproate and was equivalent to atenolol, flunarizine, clomipramine, or metoprolol. This was not confirmed in head-to-head studies [31]. In a randomized clinical trial with two groups of patients with CDH, one group was treated with 25 or 50 mg/day of amitriptyline and the other with 250 U of onabotulinumtoxinA. Amitriptyline was as effective as onabotulinumtoxinA for the prophylactic treatment of chronic daily migraines both reduced by 70% the number of headache days, more than 50% the intensity, and more than 70% the use of acute medications; the distribution of the injection sites was different from PREEMPT [47]. In other study about the efficacy of amitriptyline in episodic migraine, a small group of patients fulfilling criteria of CDH were included; in this subgroup there was a trend for amitriptyline to be superior to placebo [48].

Although there is little evidence supporting amitriptyline, this drug and other antidepressants, which may treat some comorbidities, are frequently used in CM. Prophylactic medication should be tailored according to patient preferences, characteristics, and side effect profiles [31].

Adverse events are common with tricyclic antidepressant use; antimuscarinic effects include dry mouth, a metallic taste, epigastric distress, constipation, dizziness, mental confusion, tachycardia, palpitations, blurred vision, and urinary retention. Other adverse events include weight gain (rarely seen with protriptyline), orthostatic hypotension, reflex tachycardia, palpitations, QT interval prolongation, decreased seizure threshold, and sedation [30]. If the tricyclic antidepressant being used for migraine prevention is too sedating, a switch from a tertiary tricyclic antidepressant (e.g., amitriptyline, doxepin) to a secondary tricyclic antidepressant (e.g., nortriptyline, protriptyline) is suggested [30].

Selective Serotonin Reuptake Inhibitors and Serotonin-Norepinephrine Reuptake Inhibitors

Fluoxetine

Fluoxetine, in doses from 10 to 40 mg per day, may be effective in the management of episodic migraine [49]. In a RCT trial of fluoxetine titrated to 40 mg daily, depending upon patient response, and in a group of patients with migraine and CDH, fluoxetine was moderately effective (improvement of 50% in overall headache status in the fluoxetine group and 11% in placebo) in CDH, but not in migraine [50, 51]. Other SSRIs, femoxitine and sertraline, were not more effective than placebo [31].

Venlafaxine

Venlafaxine has been used (dose, 75–150 mg) in the preventive treatment of episodic migraine found superior to placebo [49] and could be useful in some patients with migraine and mood disorders. It is recommended at B level in most guidelines [52]. A randomized double-blind crossover study, where amitriptyline and venlafaxine were compared, it was suggested that venlafaxine may be considered for the prophylaxis of migraine because of its tolerable side effect profile [53]. In another study which compared the efficacy of venlafaxine to escitalopram, both were found to be effective in the prophylaxis of migraine headache without depression and anxiety [54]. Adverse events include insomnia, nervousness, mydriasis, and seizures [30].

Venlafaxine may be a good alternative in patients with CM and depression; the efficacy is similar to amitriptyline and better tolerated.

Duloxetine

The efficacy of duloxetine can be explained by its multilevel modulatory influence which includes the activity of antinociceptive systems of the brainstem and of brain nociceptive systems, through the decrease of central sensitization [31, 55]. In patients with chronic headache and major depressive disorders, duloxetine 60 mg/day was effective, fast acting, and well tolerated [56].

Nefazodone

It is an atypical antidepressant which was first marketed in 1994, but even if efficacy of nefazodone in the prophylaxis of chronic daily headache was seen [57], it was discontinued because of the rare incidence of severe liver damage.

Calcium Channel Blockers

Flunarizine

Flunarizine is effective in migraine prophylaxis at doses of 5–10 mg per day [46]. In a case series including a study of 348 patients with CM and medication overuse, flunarizine was compared with topiramate; flunarizine was more effective in reducing the number of days with headaches and had minor side effects compared to topiramate [58]. In a prospective, randomized, open-label, blinded-endpoint 8-week trial, 10 mg/d flunarizine was more effective than 50 mg/d topiramate for CM prophylaxis [59]. Possible side effects include weight gain and depression [58]. This drug is not available in the USA, but it is commonly used in some European countries, Canada, and South America [49].

Angiotensin II Receptor Blockers

Candesartan

It provided effective prophylaxis in episodic migraine, with a tolerability profile comparable to that of placebo [60]. Current evidence supports the use of candesartan for long-term migraine preven-

tion and blood pressure control [61]. There is no specific data in CM, only that mentioned above, in the comparative study with propranolol.

Alpha-Blockers

Tizanidine

Tizanidine is an alpha2-adrenergic agonist, with antinociceptive effects. In a single-blind, placebo-controlled trial in patients with chronic migrainous headache or chronic tension-type headache, tizanidine was shown to be superior to placebo in reducing the overall headache index and other measures. There was no statistically significant difference in outcome for patients with CM compared to those with migrainous or tension-type headache. Adverse effects included somnolence dizziness, dry mouth, and asthenia [62].

Other Drugs

There are small open-label studies which support the effectiveness of memantine in refractory migraine (episodic migraine with 8–14 days of headache per month or transformed migraine) [63]. Intravenous ketamine has been reported as a subacute treatment with improvement in a small number of patients with CM [64].

Many patients with CM do not experience substantial improvement with the mentioned oral preventive drugs. For them, there are other options such as blockades or injections with onabotulinumtoxinA. Neuromodulation techniques are another alternative and are emerging therapies such as antibodies and analogs targeting CGRP or its receptors.

Anaesthetic Blocks

Sphenopalatine Ganglion Blockade

Some nonsurgical interventions targeting the sphenopalatine ganglion have demonstrated a potential in the management of CM. In a double-blind study, the instillation of local anaesthetic using a small device led to a decrease in the intensity of pain in patients with CM. The administration of bupivacaine for 6 consecutive weeks was successful as acute treatment and the Headache Impact Test-6 scores were statistically significantly decreased [65].

In a prospective, open-label, uncontrolled study after 1-month baseline, bilateral injections of 25 IU onabotulinumtoxinA (total dose 50 IU) in the sphenopalatine ganglion in a single outpatient session were administered to 10 patients with intractable migraine. At 12 weeks follow-up, eight out of ten patients experienced at least 50% reduction of moderate and severe headache days compared to baseline [66].

Anaesthetic Occipital Nerve Blockade

Occipital blockade is a well-tolerated treatment [67], but the results of the trials are inconclusive. In a controlled trial, blockade with local anaesthetic and methylprednisolone was not superior to placebo in a group of patients with either episodic or CM [68]. In another blind trial, blockade of the occipital with bupivacaine nerve during 4 consecutive weeks significantly decreased the number of days with headache in a group of patients with CM [69]. A recent study from 2016 has suggested that occipital nerve blockade with bupivacaine is superior to placebo, has longer-lasting effect than placebo, and is found to be effective for the treatment of CM [70]. In a recent trial, anaesthetic blocks appear to be effective in the short term in CM, as measured by a reduction in the number of days with moderate-to-severe headache or any headache during the week following injection [71]. Occipital blockade has shown superiority to placebo in patients with triptan-overuse headache [70].

This procedure could be an alternative short-term treatment in some patients with CM to avoid medication overuse and as a transitional therapy in combination with other treatments.

Preventive Treatment with OnabotulinumtoxinA

OnabotulinumtoxinA is recommended for patients with lack of response or intolerance to beta-blockers, topiramate, or other preventive medications. Those treatments should be used with an adequate dose and for at least for 3 months [72, 73].

OnabotulinumtoxinA is indicated for CM (level of evidence I, grade of recommendation A), after the publication of two large-scale phase III randomized controlled trials called Phase III Research Evaluating Migraine Prophylaxis Therapy (PREEMPT) 1 and 2. OnabotulinumtoxinA, at a minimum dose of 155 U, was shown to effectively reduce total headache days in CM patients with or without acute medication overuse [74–76] when injected every 12 weeks in frontal, temporal, occipital, and neck muscles in a standardized scheme. Treatment effects were observed at 24 weeks [74–76] and 56 weeks. These results have been replicated in many clinical studies [77–79].

The fact that onabotulinumtoxinA is useful in the subgroup of patients with CM with an excessive use of acute drugs was especially significant. The difference in the decrease of headache days was notable (−8,2 compared to −6,2 in the placebo group) [80]. In another randomized controlled trial, onabotulinumtoxinA as a prophylactic treatment in medication-overuse headache, without withdrawal of the overused medicine, failed to reduce headache days [81]. There are studies in which the discontinuation of acute medication overuse was achieved with long-term use of onabotulinumtoxinA [81]. The prolonged use of the toxin also reduced depressive symptoms in patients with CM and comorbid depression [82, 83].

In a sub-analysis of the PREEMPT study, 49.3% of the patients responded for the first time during the first cycle (decrease of at least 50% in the number of days of headache). 11.3% responded for the first time during the second cycle and 10.3% responded for the first time during at least two cycles [84]. It is necessary to wait until completion of the third cycle to know whether the patient is responsive [73].

In the meta-analysis, conducted by the US Agency for Research and Quality of Health, which compiled information from 20 randomized trials with onabotulinumtoxinA, involving 4237 patients, it was more effective than placebo in patients with CDH and CM. Only 26/1000 (95%

CI 10–43) abandoned the treatment because of side effects [85].

In double-blind comparative studies, onabotulinumtoxinA compared to other prophylactic standard medication (topiramate and amitriptyline), the toxin demonstrated similar efficacy for subjects with CM [47, 86].

There is controversy about the ideal timing of administration. In a Spanish study with 69 patients, onabotulinumtoxinA provided greater benefits in patients with shorter history of CM [87].

It is common knowledge that allodynia is more frequent in chronic migraine [88, 89]. There have been several studies on this symptom; as an extensive study on this aspect and its relationship with the chronification of migration, it seems that allodynia could improve with the administration of botulinum toxin [90], even if no clear clinical or demographic markers have been found to predict the response to onabotulinumtoxinA [91]. Pretreatment CGRP levels measured outside a migraine attack can predict the response of patients with CM [92].

OnabotulinumtoxinA not only reduces the number of headache days and the use of rescue medication, it improves other parameters. Besides the clinical trials, there are also many studies done in a clinical practice. One with 254 patients showed a decrease in work absenteeism and an improvement in the quality of life [78]. There are studies indicating that the efficacy of onabotulinumtoxinA increases after the second injection [93] with a significant decrease in emergency room visits and the use of triptans as a symptomatic treatment, specifically subcutaneous sumatriptan [94].

With long-term use, according to a study carried out in a typical clinical setting of a headache unit, a positive response to onabotulinumtoxinA was observed in more than 100 patients for whom treatment lasted for more than 1 year. 74.2% of these patients continued to respond in the second year of treatment. In 10% the treatment was temporarily suspended due to lack of attacks, and in 43.9% it was possible to extend the time between injections from 3 to 4 months. Long-term treatment led to additive adverse effects in two cases with more than 5 years of therapy, in which well-tolerated frontal and temporal atrophy occurred [95].

The clinical trials and the clinical practice results strongly support the use of onabotulinumtoxinA for the prophylaxis of CM. This intervention has proven to be effective, safe, and well tolerated in patients [96]. The safety and efficacy of onabotulinumtoxinA for CM prophylaxis have been demonstrated for up to nine treatment cycles [97]. Currently an ongoing study named Chronic migraine OnabotulinumtoxinA Prolonged Efficacy open-label (COMPEL) study, aims to investigate the long-term safety, efficacy, and tolerability of nine cycles of repetitive injections administered every 12 weeks [98]. The preliminary results of this study (716 patients followed during 108 weeks) confirm the progressive efficacy and tolerability of the toxin. The side effects described in the PREEMPT trials arose from the injection sites and the involvement of the trapezius muscles in the neck. Specifically, 6.7% of the patients had cervical pain, compared to 2.2% of the placebo group, and muscle weakness in 5.3% in the treated group compared to 0.3% in the placebo group. Ptosis appeared in 3.2% of the treated group, compared to 0.3% in the placebo group [74, 99].

How to Use it

A dilution of 5 U is required for each inoculum of 0.1 ml. To do this, dilute the product in 2 ml of saline, if the vial is 100 U, and in 1 ml if it is 50 U. The corresponding quantities (5 U per injection point) will be applied at key points where sensory nerve terminals are responsible for painful conduction [100]. Table 16.3 shows the toxin distribution in each muscle until completing 155 U.

The PREEMPT protocol allows the use of 40 U in additional areas to follow the pain (2 additional points at a temporary level, 2 additional occipital points and 4 extra points at the trapezoid level). If bruxism is present, injection of masseters could be helpful [97].

A recent dose comparison study with onabotulinumtoxinA in a clinical setting demonstrated the superior efficacy of onabotulinumtoxinA 195 U compared to 155 U in CM patients with medication-overuse headache during a 2-year treatment period with similar safety and tolerability profile [101].

In summary, onabotulinumtoxinA is a good choice in the management of patients with CM. The efficacy in short and long term is well documented in clinical trials and in clinical practice, and it is well tolerated.

Table 16.3 OnabotulinumtoxinA units distribution according to the protocol PREEMPT [100]

OnabotulinumtoxinA units according to the protocol PREEMPT	
Muscle	Units (U)
Corrugator	10 (5 in each side)
Prócer	5
Frontal	20 (10 in each side)
Temporal	40 (20 in each side)
Occipital	30 (15 in each side)
Cervical paraspinal	20 (10 in each side)
Trapezoid	30 (15 in each side)
	155

How to Manage Preventive Treatment in CM

A paradigm to manage CM is shown in Fig. 16.1.

Topiramate is recommended as primary treatment, and if this fails or is not well tolerated, change to another neuromodulator, e.g., zonisamide. If the response is insufficient, add amitriptyline or other SNRI (the effects are independent of depression). A combination with propranolol or flunarizine may be helpful. If there is an insufficient response with two or more preventives (or because of poor tolerability), onabotulinumtoxinA is recommended. An initial dose of 155 IU could be administered; in case of partial or no response or short duration of improvement (less than 3 months), a higher dose (195) is recommended [72].

Future

There are a number of promising molecules in the pipeline with potential impact on chronic

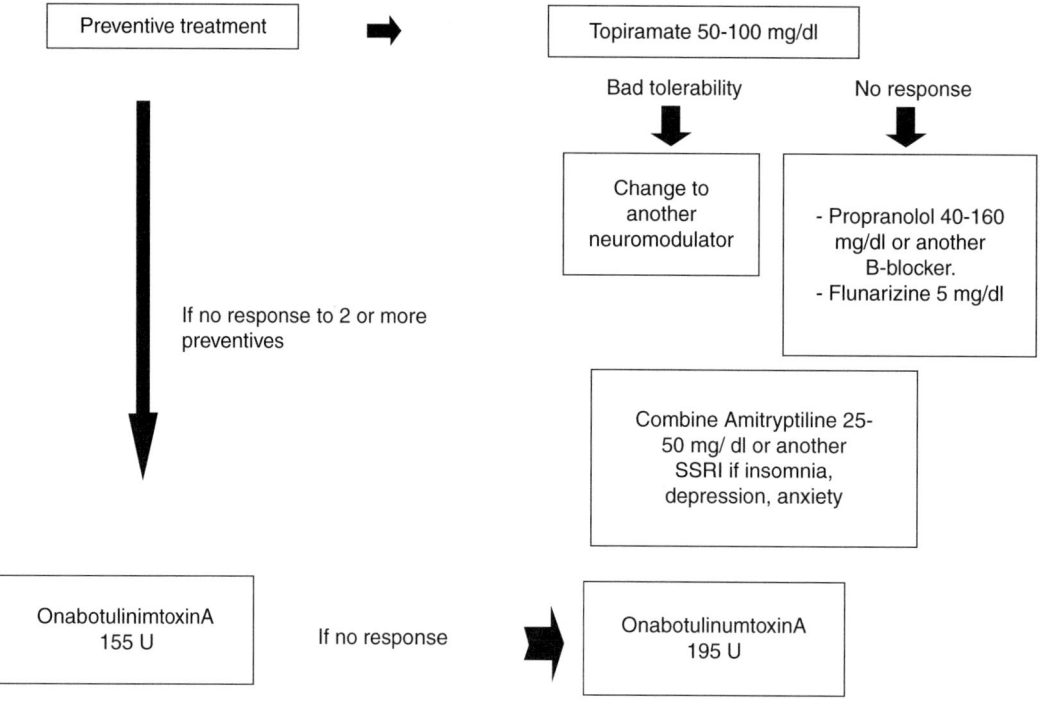

Fig. 16.1 Practical management of CM

daily headache. The first novel agent likely to come to market will be agents that block calcitonin gene-related peptide (CGRP). CGRP is a potent vasodilator and pain-signaling neuropeptide, and it has shown to be a useful therapeutic target for migraine [102]. This represents the first specific, mechanism-based, migraine prophylactic treatment and appears to be without significant adverse events such as cardiovascular effects [103]. Four different antibodies from four different companies are in development, as well as at least two small-molecule CGRP antagonists. A recent review of the five completed trials published at the time of this writing concludes that CGRP: mAbsMAbs are effective as antimigraine therapy with few side effects [104, 105]. In addition to demonstrating efficacy that is roughly equivalent to that seen in the PREEMPT trials, it is noteworthy that the side effect profile is excellent and there appear to be subpopulations within the studies that show dramatic and early onset of benefits [106]. If these results are confirmed in ongoing studies, the anti-CGRP mAbs could make an important contribution to the therapeutic arsenal.

References

1. Natoli JL, Manack A, Dean B, Butler Q, Turkel CC, Stovner L, et al. Global prevalence of chronic migraine: a systematic review. Cephalalgia. 2010;30(5):599–609.
2. Silvestrini M, Bartolini M, Coccia M, Baruffaldi R, Taffi R, Provinciali L. Topiramate in the treatment of chronic migraine. Cephalalgia. 2003;23(8):820–4.
3. Sun-Edelstein C, Rapoport AM. Update on the pharmacological treatment of chronic migraine. Curr Pain Headache Rep. 2016;20(1):6.
4. Scher AI, Stewart WF, Ricci JA, Lipton RB. Factors associated with the onset and remission of chronic daily headache in a population-based study. Pain. 2003;106(1–2):81–9.
5. Mathew NT, Kurman R, Perez F. Drug induced refractory headache--clinical features and management. Headache. 1990;30(10):634–8.
6. Zwart JA, Dyb G, Hagen K, Svebak S, Holmen J. Analgesic use: a predictor of chronic pain and medication overuse headache: the head-HUNT study. Neurology. 2003;61(2):160–4.
7. Dodick DW, Silberstein SD. Migraine prevention. Pract Neurol. 2007;7(6):383–93.
8. Becker WJ. The diagnosis and management of chronic migraine in primary care. Headache. 2017;57(9):1471–81.
9. Bagnato F, Good J. The use of antiepileptics in migraine prophylaxis. Headache. 2016;56(3):603–15.
10. He A, Song D, Zhang L, Li C. Unveiling the relative efficacy, safety and tolerability of prophylactic medications for migraine: pairwise and network-meta analysis. J Headache Pain. 2017;18(1):26.
11. Aurora SK, Brin MF. Chronic migraine: an update on physiology, imaging, and the mechanism of action of two available pharmacologic therapies. Headache. 2017;57(1):109–25.
12. Silberstein SD, Lipton RB, Dodick DW, Freitag FG, Ramadan N, Mathew N, et al. Efficacy and safety of topiramate for the treatment of chronic migraine: a randomized, double-blind, placebo-controlled trial. Headache. 2007;47(2):170–80.
13. Diener HC, Bussone G, Van Oene JC, Lahaye M, Schwalen S, Goadsby PJ, et al. Topiramate reduces headache days in chronic migraine: a randomized, double-blind, placebo-controlled study. Cephalalgia. 2007;27(7):814–23.
14. Limmroth V, Biondi D, Pfeil J, Schwalen S. Topiramate in patients with episodic migraine: reducing the risk for chronic forms of headache. Headache. 2007;47(1):13–21.
15. Mei D, Ferraro D, Zelano G, Capuano A, Vollono C, Gabriele C, et al. Topiramate and triptans revert chronic migraine with medication overuse to episodic migraine. Clin Neuropharmacol. 2006;29(5):269–75.
16. Lipton RB, Silberstein S, Dodick D, Cady R, Freitag F, Mathew N, et al. Topiramate intervention to prevent transformation of episodic migraine: the topiramate INTREPID study. Cephalalgia. 2011;31(1):18–30.
17. Brandes JL, Saper JR, Diamond M, Couch JR, Lewis DW, Schmitt J, et al. Topiramate for migraine prevention: a randomized controlled trial. JAMA. 2004;291(8):965–73.
18. Silberstein SD. Topiramate in migraine prevention: a 2016 perspective. Headache. 2017;57(1):165–78.
19. May A, Schulte LH. Chronic migraine: risk factors, mechanisms and treatment. Nat Rev Neurol. 2016;12(8):455–64.
20. Antonaci F, Ghiotto N, Wu S, Pucci E, Costa A. Recent advances in migraine therapy. Springerplus. 2016;5:637.
21. Diener HC, Tfelt-Hansen P, Dahlof C, Lainez MJ, Sandrini G, Wang SJ, et al. Topiramate in migraine prophylaxis–results from a placebo-controlled trial with propranolol as an active control. J Neurol. 2004;251(8):943–50.
22. Dodick DW, Silberstein S, Saper J, Freitag FG, Cady RK, Rapoport AM, et al. The impact of topiramate on health-related quality of life indicators in chronic migraine. Headache. 2007;47(10):1398–408.
23. Silberstein S, Lipton R, Dodick D, Freitag F, Mathew N, Brandes J, et al. Topiramate treatment of chronic migraine: a randomized, placebo-controlled trial of quality of life and other efficacy measures. Headache. 2009;49(8):1153–62.
24. Klapper J. Divalproex sodium in migraine prophylaxis: a dose-controlled study. Cephalalgia. 1997;17(2):103–8.

25. Mathew NT, Saper JR, Silberstein SD, Rankin L, Markley HG, Solomon S, et al. Migraine prophylaxis with divalproex. Arch Neurol. 1995;52(3):281–6.

26. Freitag FG, Collins SD, Carlson HA, Goldstein J, Saper J, Silberstein S, et al. A randomized trial of divalproex sodium extended-release tablets in migraine prophylaxis. Neurology. 2002;58(11):1652–9.

27. Yurekli VA, Akhan G, Kutluhan S, Uzar E, Koyuncuoglu HR, Gultekin F. The effect of sodium valproate on chronic daily headache and its subgroups. J Headache Pain. 2008;9(1):37–41.

28. Sarchielli P, Messina P, Cupini LM, Tedeschi G, Di Piero V, Livrea P, et al. Sodium valproate in migraine without aura and medication overuse headache: a randomized controlled trial. Eur Neuropsychopharmacol. 2014;24(8):1289–97.

29. Gursoy AE, Ertas M. Prophylactic treatment of migraine. Noro Psikiyatr Ars. 2013;50(Suppl 1):S30–S5.

30. Silberstein SD. Preventive migraine treatment. Continuum (Minneap Minn). 2015;21(4 Headache):973–89.

31. Jackson JL, Cogbill E, Santana-Davila R, Eldredge C, Collier W, Gradall A, et al. A comparative effectiveness meta-analysis of drugs for the prophylaxis of migraine headache. PLoS One. 2015;10(7):e0130733.

32. Perloff MD, Berlin RK, Gillette M, Petersile MJ, Kurowski D. Gabapentin in headache disorders: what is the evidence? Pain Med. 2016;17(1):162–71.

33. Mulleners WM, Chronicle EP. Anticonvulsants in migraine prophylaxis: a Cochrane review. Cephalalgia. 2008;28(6):585–97.

34. Calandre EP, Garcia-Leiva JM, Rico-Villademoros F, Vilchez JS, Rodriguez-Lopez CM. Pregabalin in the treatment of chronic migraine: an open-label study. Clin Neuropharmacol. 2010;33(1):35–9.

35. Pascual-Gomez J, Alana-Garcia M, Oterino A, Leira R, Lainez-Andres JM. Preventive treatment of chronic migraine with zonisamide: a study in patients who are refractory or intolerant to topiramate. Rev Neurol. 2008;47(9):449–51.

36. Pascual-Gomez J, Gracia-Naya M, Leira R, Mateos V, Alvaro-Gonzalez LC, Hernando I, et al. Zonisamide in the preventive treatment of refractory migraine. Rev Neurol. 2010;50(3):129–32.

37. Villani V, Ciuffoli A, Prosperini L, Sette G. Zonisamide for migraine prophylaxis in topiramate-intolerant patients: an observational study. Headache. 2011;51(2):287–91.

38. Mohammadianinejad SE, Abbasi V, Sajedi SA, Majdinasab N, Abdollahi F, Hajmanouchehri R, et al. Zonisamide versus topiramate in migraine prophylaxis: a double-blind randomized clinical trial. Clin Neuropharmacol. 2011;34(4):174–7.

39. Beran RG, Spira PJ. Levetiracetam in chronic daily headache: a double-blind, randomised placebo-controlled study. (the Australian KEPPRA headache trial [AUS-KHT]). Cephalalgia. 2011;31(5):530–6.

40. Stovner LJ, Linde M, Gravdahl GB, Tronvik E, Aamodt AH, Sand T, et al. A comparative study of candesartan versus propranolol for migraine prophylaxis: a randomised, triple-blind, placebo-controlled, double cross-over study. Cephalalgia. 2014;34(7):523–32.

41. Pascual J, Leira R, Lainez JM. Combined therapy for migraine prevention? Clinical experience with a beta-blocker plus sodium valproate in 52 resistant migraine patients. Cephalalgia. 2003;23(10):961–2.

42. Pascual J. Combination therapy for chronic migraine: bad news but not the last word. Neurology. 2012;78(13):940–1.

43. Edvardsson B. Atenolol in the prophylaxis of chronic migraine: a 3-month open-label study. Springerplus. 2013;2:479.

44. Punay NC, Couch JR. Antidepressants in the treatment of migraine headache. Curr Pain Headache Rep. 2003;7(1):51–4.

45. Freitag FG, Lake A 3rd, Lipton R, Cady R, Diamond S, Silberstein S, et al. Inpatient treatment of headache: an evidence-based assessment. Headache. 2004;44(4):342–60.

46. Doyle Strauss L, Weizenbaum E, Loder EW, Rizzoli PB. Amitriptyline dose and treatment outcomes in specialty headache practice: a retrospective cohort study. Headache. 2016;56(10):1626–34.

47. Magalhaes E, Menezes C, Cardeal M, Melo A. Botulinum toxin type a versus amitriptyline for the treatment of chronic daily migraine. Clin Neurol Neurosurg. 2010;112(6):463–6.

48. Couch JR. Amitriptyline versus placebo study G. Amitriptyline in the prophylactic treatment of migraine and chronic daily headache. Headache. 2011;51(1):33–51.

49. Evers S, Afra J, Frese A, Goadsby PJ, Linde M, May A, et al. EFNS guideline on the drug treatment of migraine--revised report of an EFNS task force. Eur J Neurol. 2009;16(9):968–81.

50. Evans RW. A rational approach to the management of chronic migraine. Headache. 2013;53(1):168–76.

51. Saper JR, Silberstein SD, Lake AE 3rd, Winters ME. Double-blind trial of fluoxetine: chronic daily headache and migraine. Headache. 1994;34(9):497–502.

52. Silberstein SD, Holland S, Freitag F, Dodick DW, Argoff C, Ashman E, et al. Evidence-based guideline update: pharmacologic treatment for episodic migraine prevention in adults: report of the quality standards subcommittee of the American academy of neurology and the American headache society. Neurology. 2012;78(17):1337–45.

53. Bulut S, Berilgen MS, Baran A, Tekatas A, Atmaca M, Mungen B. Venlafaxine versus amitriptyline in the prophylactic treatment of migraine: randomized, double-blind, crossover study. Clin Neurol Neurosurg. 2004;107(1):44–8.

54. Tarlaci S. Escitalopram and venlafaxine for the prophylaxis of migraine headache without mood disorders. Clin Neuropharmacol. 2009;32(5):254–8.

55. Artemenko AR, Kurenkov AL, Nikitin SS, Filatova EG. Duloxetine in the treatment of chronic

migraine. Zh Nevrol Psikhiatr Im S S Korsakova. 2010;110(1):49–54.

56. Volpe FM. An 8-week, open-label trial of duloxetine for comorbid major depressive disorder and chronic headache. J Clin Psychiatry. 2008;69(9):1449–54.

57. Saper JR, Lake AE, Tepper SJ. Nefazodone for chronic daily headache prophylaxis: an open-label study. Headache. 2001;41(5):465–74.

58. Gracia-Naya M, Rios C, Garcia-Gomara MJ, Sanchez-Valiente S, Mauri-Llerda JA, Santos-Lasaosa S, et al. A comparative study of the effectiveness of topiramate and flunarizine in independent series of chronic migraine patients without medication abuse. Rev Neurol. 2013;57(8):347–53.

59. Lai KL, Niddam DM, Fuh JL, Chen SP, Wang YF, Chen WT, et al. Flunarizine versus topiramate for chronic migraine prophylaxis: a randomized trial. Acta Neurol Scand. 2017;135(4):476–83.

60. Tronvik E, Stovner LJ, Helde G, Sand T, Bovim G. Prophylactic treatment of migraine with an angiotensin II receptor blocker: a randomized controlled trial. JAMA. 2003;289(1):65–9.

61. Feher G, Pusch G. Role of antihypertensive drugs in the treatment of migraine. Orv Hetil. 2015;156(5):179–85.

62. Saper JR, Lake AE 3rd, Cantrell DT, Winner PK, White JR. Chronic daily headache prophylaxis with tizanidine: a double-blind, placebo-controlled, multicenter outcome study. Headache. 2002;42(6):470–82.

63. Bigal M, Rapoport A, Sheftell F, Tepper D, Tepper S. Memantine in the preventive treatment of refractory migraine. Headache. 2008;48(9):1337–42.

64. Lauritsen C, Mazuera S, Lipton RB, Ashina S. Intravenous ketamine for subacute treatment of refractory chronic migraine: a case series. J Headache Pain. 2016;17(1):106.

65. Cady RK, Saper J, Dexter K, Cady RJ, Manley HR. Long-term efficacy of a double-blind, placebo-controlled, randomized study for repetitive sphenopalatine blockade with bupivacaine vs. saline with the Tx360 device for treatment of chronic migraine. Headache. 2015;55(4):529–42.

66. Bratbak DF, Nordgard S, Stovner LJ, Linde M, Dodick DW, Aschehoug I, et al. Pilot study of sphenopalatine injection of onabotulinumtoxinA for the treatment of intractable chronic migraine. Cephalalgia. 2017;37(4):356–64.

67. Saracco MG, Valfre W, Cavallini M, Aguggia M. Greater occipital nerve block in chronic migraine. Neurol Sci. 2010;31(Suppl 1):S179–80.

68. Dilli E, Halker R, Vargas B, Hentz J, Radam T, Rogers R, et al. Occipital nerve block for the short-term preventive treatment of migraine: a randomized, double-blinded, placebo-controlled study. Cephalalgia. 2015;35(11):959–68.

69. Inan LE, Inan N, Karadas O, Gul HL, Erdemoglu AK, Turkel Y, et al. Greater occipital nerve blockade for the treatment of chronic migraine: a randomized, multicenter, double-blind, and placebo-controlled study. Acta Neurol Scand. 2015;132(4):270–7.

70. Gul HL, Ozon AO, Karadas O, Koc G, Inan LE. The efficacy of greater occipital nerve blockade in chronic migraine: a placebo-controlled study. Acta Neurol Scand. 2016;136(2):138–44.

71. Cuadrado ML, Aledo-Serrano A, Navarro P, Lopez-Ruiz P, Fernandez-de-Las-Penas C, Gonzalez-Suarez I, et al. Short-term effects of greater occipital nerve blocks in chronic migraine: a double-blind, randomised, placebo-controlled clinical trial. Cephalalgia. 2016;37(9):864–72.

72. Cernuda-Morollon E, Pascual J. Something's moving in chronic migraine. Rev Neurol. 2014;58(1):1–3.

73. D. Ezpeleta PPR. Guías diagnósticas y terpeútica de la Sociedad Española de Neurología 2015. 3. Guía oficial de práctica clínica en cefaleas2015 2015.

74. Aurora SK, Dodick DW, Turkel CC, DeGryse RE, Silberstein SD, Lipton RB, et al. OnabotulinumtoxinA for treatment of chronic migraine: results from the double-blind, randomized, placebo-controlled phase of the PREEMPT 1 trial. Cephalalgia. 2010;30(7):793–803.

75. Diener HC, Dodick DW, Aurora SK, Turkel CC, DeGryse RE, Lipton RB, et al. OnabotulinumtoxinA for treatment of chronic migraine: results from the double-blind, randomized, placebo-controlled phase of the PREEMPT 2 trial. Cephalalgia. 2010;30(7):804–14.

76. Dodick DW, Turkel CC, DeGryse RE, Aurora SK, Silberstein SD, Lipton RB, et al. OnabotulinumtoxinA for treatment of chronic migraine: pooled results from the double-blind, randomized, placebo-controlled phases of the PREEMPT clinical program. Headache. 2010;50(6):921–36.

77. Lia C, Tosi P, Giardini G, Caligiana L, Bottacchi E. Onabotulinumtoxin a for prophylaxis in chronic migraine: preliminary data from headache regional Centre of Aosta valley. Neurol Sci. 2014;35(Suppl 1):175–6.

78. Khalil M, Zafar HW, Quarshie V, Ahmed F. Prospective analysis of the use of OnabotulinumtoxinA (BOTOX) in the treatment of chronic migraine; real-life data in 254 patients from hull, U.K. J Headache Pain. 2014;15:54.

79. Grazzi L, Usai S. Onabotulinum toxin a (Botox) for chronic migraine treatment: an Italian experience. Neurol Sci. 2015;36(Suppl 1):33–5.

80. Silberstein SD, Blumenfeld AM, Cady RK, Turner IM, Lipton RB, Diener HC, et al. OnabotulinumtoxinA for treatment of chronic migraine: PREEMPT 24-week pooled subgroup analysis of patients who had acute headache medication overuse at baseline. J Neurol Sci. 2013;331(1–2):48–56.

81. Sandrini G, Perrotta A, Tassorelli C, Torelli P, Brighina F, Sances G, et al. Botulinum toxin type-a in the prophylactic treatment of medication-overuse headache: a multicenter, double-blind, randomized, placebo-controlled, parallel group study. J Headache Pain. 2011;12(4):427–33.

82. Boudreau GP, Grosberg BM, McAllister PJ, Lipton RB, Buse DC. Prophylactic onabotulinumtoxinA

in patients with chronic migraine and comorbid depression: an open-label, multicenter, pilot study of efficacy, safety and effect on headache-related disability, depression, and anxiety. Int J Gen Med. 2015;8:79–86.

83. Maasumi K, Thompson NR, Kriegler JS, Tepper SJ. Effect of OnabotulinumtoxinA injection on depression in chronic migraine. Headache. 2015; 55(9):1218–24.

84. Silberstein SD, Dodick DW, Aurora SK, Diener HC, DeGryse RE, Lipton RB, et al. Per cent of patients with chronic migraine who responded per onabotulinumtoxinA treatment cycle: PREEMPT. J Neurol Neurosurg Psychiatry. 2015;86(9):996–1001.

85. Jackson JL, Kuriyama A, Hayashino Y. Botulinum toxin a for prophylactic treatment of migraine and tension headaches in adults: a meta-analysis. JAMA. 2012;307(16):1736–45.

86. Cady RK, Schreiber CP, Porter JA, Blumenfeld AM, Farmer KU. A multi-center double-blind pilot comparison of onabotulinumtoxinA and topiramate for the prophylactic treatment of chronic migraine. Headache. 2011;51(1):21–32.

87. Castrillo Sanz A, Morollon Sanchez-Mateos N, Simonet Hernandez C, Fernandez Rodriguez B, Cerdan Santacruz D, Mendoza Rodriguez A, et al. Experience with botulinum toxin in chronic migraine. Neurologia. 2016;S0213-4853(16):30209-2.

88. Benatto MT, Florencio LL, Carvalho GF, Dach F, Bigal ME, Chaves TC, et al. Cutaneous allodynia is more frequent in chronic migraine, and its presence and severity seems to be more associated with the duration of the disease. Arq Neuropsiquiatr. 2017;75(3):153–9.

89. Louter MA, Bosker JE, van Oosterhout WP, van Zwet EW, Zitman FG, Ferrari MD, et al. Cutaneous allodynia as a predictor of migraine chronification. Brain. 2013;136(Pt 11):3489–96.

90. Burstein R, Jakubowski M, Garcia-Nicas E, Kainz V, Bajwa Z, Hargreaves R, et al. Thalamic sensitization transforms localized pain into widespread allodynia. Ann Neurol. 2010;68(1):81–91.

91. Pagola I, Esteve-Belloch P, Palma JA, Luquin MR, Riverol M, Martinez-Vila E, et al. Predictive factors of the response to treatment with onabotulinumtoxinA in refractory migraine. Rev Neurol. 2014;58(6):241–6.

92. Cernuda-Morollon E, Ramon C, Martinez-Camblor P, Serrano-Pertierra E, Larrosa D, Pascual J. OnabotulinumtoxinA decreases interictal CGRP plasma levels in patients with chronic migraine. Pain. 2015;156(5):820–4.

93. Pedraza MI, de la Cruz C, Ruiz M, Lopez-Mesonero L, Martinez E, de Lera M, et al. OnabotulinumtoxinA treatment for chronic migraine: experience in 52 patients treated with the PREEMPT paradigm. Springerplus. 2015;4:176.

94. Oterino A, Ramon C, Pascual J. Experience with onabotulinumtoxinA (BOTOX) in chronic refractory migraine: focus on severe attacks. J Headache Pain. 2011;12(2):235–8.

95. Cernuda-Morollon E, Ramon C, Larrosa D, Alvarez R, Riesco N, Pascual J. Long-term experience with onabotulinumtoxinA in the treatment of chronic migraine: what happens after one year? Cephalalgia. 2015;35(10):864–8.

96. Vikelis M, Argyriou AA, Dermitzakis EV, Spingos KC, Mitsikostas DD. Onabotulinumtoxin-a treatment in Greek patients with chronic migraine. J Headache Pain. 2016;17(1):84.

97. Diener HC, Dodick DW, Turkel CC, Demos G, Degryse RE, Earl NL, et al. Pooled analysis of the safety and tolerability of onabotulinumtoxinA in the treatment of chronic migraine. Eur J Neurol. 2014;21(6):851–9.

98. Blumenfeld AM, Aurora SK, Laranjo K, Papapetropoulos S. Unmet clinical needs in chronic migraine: rationale for study and design of COMPEL, an open-label, multicenter study of the long-term efficacy, safety, and tolerability of onabotulinumtoxinA for headache prophylaxis in adults with chronic migraine. BMC Neurol. 2015;15:100.

99. Aicua-Rapun I, Martinez-Velasco E, Rojo A, Hernando A, Ruiz M, Carreres A, et al. Real-life data in 115 chronic migraine patients treated with Onabotulinumtoxin a during more than one year. J Headache Pain. 2016;17(1):112.

100. Blumenfeld A, Silberstein SD, Dodick DW, Aurora SK, Turkel CC, Binder WJ. Method of injection of onabotulinumtoxinA for chronic migraine: a safe, well-tolerated, and effective treatment paradigm based on the PREEMPT clinical program. Headache. 2010;50(9):1406–18.

101. Negro A, Curto M, Lionetto L, Martelletti P. A two years open-label prospective study of OnabotulinumtoxinA 195 U in medication overuse headache: a real-world experience. J Headache Pain. 2015;17:1.

102. Barbanti P, Aurilia C, Fofi L, Egeo G, Ferroni P. The role of anti-CGRP antibodies in the pathophysiology of primary headaches. Neurol Sci. 2017;38(Suppl 1):31–5.

103. Bigal ME, Walter S, Rapoport AM. Therapeutic antibodies against CGRP or its receptor. Br J Clin Pharmacol. 2015;79(6):886–95.

104. Pellesi L, Guerzoni S, Pini LA. Spotlight on anti-CGRP monoclonal antibodies in migraine: the clinical evidence to date. Clin Pharmacol Drug Dev. 2017;6(6):534–47. https://doi.org/10.1002/cpdd.345.

105. Hou M, Xing H, Cai Y, Li B, Wang X, Li P, et al. The effect and safety of monoclonal antibodies to calcitonin gene-related peptide and its receptor on migraine: a systematic review and meta-analysis. J Headache Pain. 2017;18(1):42.

106. Bigal ME, Dodick DW, Krymchantowski AV, VanderPluym JH, Tepper SJ, Aycardi E, et al. TEV-48125 for the preventive treatment of chronic migraine: efficacy at early time points. Neurology. 2016;87(1):41–8.

Shalonda S. Slater and Hope L. O'Brien

Non-pharmacological treatments are often used in conjunction with or in place of pharmacological treatments for chronic daily headache. These non-pharmacological treatments include behavioral approaches such as cognitive behavioral therapy, relaxation training, biofeedback, acceptance and mindfulness treatments, and a focus on healthy lifestyle recommendations. Behavioral approaches to headache care may be preferred for patients with a poor response to medications, actual or planned pregnancy, history of overuse of acute headache medication, a preference for non-pharmacological treatments, significant stress, poor coping, or comorbid medical or psychological disorders [1, 2]. Relaxation training, thermal biofeedback combined with relaxation training, electromyographic biofeedback, and cognitive behavioral therapy are treatment options supported as Grade A by the American Academy of Neurology [3]. Behavioral treatments aim to reduce functional disability, improve coping, and decrease pain intensity.

S. S. Slater (✉)
Division of Behavioral Medicine and Clinical Psychology, Department of Pediatrics, Cincinnati Children's Hospital Medical Center, University of Cincinnati College of Medicine, Cincinnati, OH, USA
e-mail: Shalonda.Slater@cchmc.org

H. L. O'Brien
Division of Neurology, Department of Pediatrics, Cincinnati Children's Hospital Medical Center, University of Cincinnati College of Medicine, Cincinnati, OH, USA

Psychological Interventions

Cognitive behavioral therapy (CBT) is a behavioral approach widely supported as an efficacious treatment for many chronic pain conditions including chronic daily headaches. CBT is often a part of a multidisciplinary treatment plan, which often includes medication, physical therapy, and complementary and alternative medicine (CAM) in the management of headache symptoms. Given the advanced knowledge of psychological principles and intense clinical training required, this behavioral treatment should be conducted by a psychologist or other trained mental health professional.

CBT is a psychological treatment that teaches a patient to cope with pain and stress by identifying and challenging negative thoughts and problematic beliefs that generate stress and worsen headaches and by identifying and changing behaviors that may trigger or increase pain episodes. CBT, based on the biobehavioral model of chronic pain, asserts that physical symptoms such as pain are influenced by emotional, behavioral, and social factors [4]. CBT for pain is typically a time-limited course of 6–10 weekly to bi-weekly sessions. The length of a course of treatment depends on the patient's pain severity, the level of disability, and comorbid psychological issues. Also, CBT describes a structured intervention that follows a course of treatment involving instruction in specific strategies for coping with chronic pain. Each treatment session includes a focus on instruction in coping skills, self-monitoring, homework review, and a homework plan for the practice of skills outside of the session. Self-monitoring refers to the patient keeping track, often with a pain diary, of environmental and internal factors that may be contributing to headaches. Identifying factors that may be triggering or worsening headaches is important to progress in treatment.

Components of CBT

CBT typically includes biobehavioral treatment components of cognitive training (e.g., cognitive modification, problem-solving, and distraction) and behavioral strategies (e.g., relaxation training with or without biofeedback, activity pacing, and adherence).

- An example of skills taught in each week of treatment.
    - Week 1: Rationale for treatment and explanation of gate control theory of pain.
    - Week 2: Relaxation instruction (diaphragmatic breathing).
    - Week 3: Progressive muscle relaxation and imagery.
    - Week 4: Cognitive strategies.
    - Week 5: Behavioral activation, pleasant activities, and distraction.
    - Week 6: Activity pacing.
    - Week 7: Problem-solving.
    - Week 8: Summary of coping strategies.

Psychological Education

At the start of treatment, one provides education about the connection between thoughts, feelings, and pain. Information is provided about the gate control theory of pain. This theory of pain processing explains how psychological factors can change a person's experience of pain [5]. According to this theory, there is a process of communication between the spinal cord and the brain that functions like a gate opening and closing, and pain signals must pass through the gate to reach the brain. If the gate is open, many pain signals pass through, and a person feels a great deal of pain. However, if the gate is closed, the pain signals do not pass through, and although pain signals are present in the body, they do not carry their message to the brain, and the person does not feel pain. Factors such as emotions, cognitions, or focus on pain can affect the position of the gate and change the pain experience, even when the pain stimulus remains the same. An understanding of this pain process can help a patient recognize how cognitive and behavioral strategies impact the experience of chronic pain.

Cognitive Strategies

Another core component of CBT is the focus on identifying cognitions that trigger or worsen chronic headaches. Cognitive strategies help the patient change thoughts and interpretations of events. These cognitive changes can lead to an adjustment in behavior and improve the patient's ability to cope with pain and distress effectively. In CBT, patients with negative thought patterns are taught skills to alter these patterns by using strategies such as thought stopping, cognitive restructuring, and positive self-talk.

Behavioral Strategies

Activity pacing is an intervention often included in CBT for chronic pain conditions. This strategy involves teaching a patient to structure daily activities in a way that prevents over- or under-exertion and a worsening of chronic pain. Behavioral activation or pleasant activities are another core skill included in CBT. Chronic headaches can often result in a patient restricting participation in activities due to fear that the activity will worsen pain. Scheduling regular physical activity, or an enjoyable activity, can be beneficial in improving mood and activity level by increasing opportunities for positive experiences.

Relaxation Techniques

Relaxation strategies are a core component in behavioral treatments for chronic headaches.

These behavioral strategies have been studied extensively for the treatment of primary headache and migraine [6]. Patients are taught skills to reduce muscle tension and stress to prevent or reduce distressing physical symptoms. These strategies include deep breathing, progressive muscle relaxation, imagery, and hypnosis.

Diaphragmatic or abdominal breathing is a technique of taking slow, deep breaths from the diaphragm instead of short, shallow breaths from the chest. Progressive muscle relaxation (PMR) involves systematically tensing and relaxing various muscle groups to increase awareness of distinctions between tension and relaxation, ultimately increasing feelings of relaxation over time. Imagery refers to a strategy in which relaxation is induced by instructing the patient to think about a peaceful and calming scene. Hypnosis describes the use of three components (induction, deepening, suggestions) to help the patient achieve a deep state of relaxation. Note that hypnosis requires special training, provided through several professional organizations. Though relaxation strategies are often included as a component in studies evaluating the effectiveness of treatments such as CBT and biofeedback, no randomized controlled trials (RCTs) have been conducted with relaxation skills alone [7].

Biofeedback and Neurofeedback

Relaxation therapies have been examined in connection with biofeedback training. In addition, biofeedback without relaxation has been used as a treatment for chronic pain. Biofeedback, a self-regulation technique, involves monitoring and voluntary control of physiological processes such as muscle activity, skin temperature, respiration, and blood flow to reduce sympathetic arousal. Patients are attached to specific devices and receive feedback on selected parameters to learn ways to control or refine their physiological response [6].

Peripheral skin temperature feedback (TEMP), blood-volume-pulse feedback (BVP), and electromyographic feedback (EMG) are the most commonly used biofeedback techniques for migraine treatment. Many systematic reviews have found that biofeedback is an effective treatment for migraine and tension-type headaches. In a recent review, these three biofeedback methods showed effectiveness in preventing migraine [8].

Few studies have evaluated the use of biofeedback for treatment of chronic daily headaches. A recent review described two studies, which supported the use of biofeedback in the preventive treatment of chronic headaches [7]. A study comparing a biofeedback group to a control group in a sample of patients with MOH found that the biofeedback group reported a lower number of headache days and a lower risk of MOH relapse relative to the control group at the 3-year follow-up, though not at the 1-year follow-up [9]. Another study found that EMG biofeedback reduced headache frequency from chronic to episodic at 8 weeks and 1 year [10].

Evidence and Outcomes for CBT

CBT is well established as a treatment of migraine in adults though efficacy varies widely from 20 to 67%, as described in a systematic review by Sullivan [11]. This review showed that CBT, relaxation therapy, and biofeedback resulted in significant improvements in headache, psychological disability, and quality of life outcomes when combined with pharmacological treatment. Many studies that were reviewed utilized CBT plus relaxation therapy and had a minimal contact study design, though higher contact therapies had a larger effect. The authors noted that minimal contact designs had been used more often in recent studies because of concerns about cost effectiveness. In addition, a review of treatments for chronic migraine concluded that cognitive behavioral therapy, biofeedback, and relaxation techniques were associated with a significant improvement in headache symptoms and are recommended treatments for chronic migraine [7].

Another recent review of CBT for migraine found that the treatment reduced the physical symptoms of migraine in adults but concluded that other benefits are unclear [12]. Harris et al. noted that differences in treatment outcomes might have been due to variations in the components of CBT employed in these studies or differences in the way the therapy was implemented. Ten RCTs evaluating the use of CBT for the treatment of chronic migraine/headache met criteria for review, indicating that a small number of studies have been conducted with this patient population.

A large study assessing the use of CBT was conducted by Holroyd and colleagues [13]. The researchers evaluated the use of CBT and preventive medication treatment in a randomized placebo-controlled trial. Patients with frequent migraine headaches were randomized to one of the four preventative treatment groups: β-blocker, matched placebo, behavioral migraine management plus placebo, or behavioral migraine management plus a β-blocker. Behavioral treatment was a structured, manually guided treatment and included four monthly migraine management sessions and learning with the application of skills through a behavioral migraine management and workbook and accompanying ten audio lessons. Skills included deep breathing, progressive muscle relaxation, imagery, thermal biofeedback, cognitive behavioral stress management, and medication adherence. Results suggested that the addition of combined β-blocker and behavioral migraine management, but not the addition of β-blocker alone or behavioral migraine management alone, improved outcomes of optimized acute treatment.

In addition, an RCT evaluated the benefit of CBT in pediatric patients with chronic daily headache prescribed amitriptyline as a preventative headache medication [14, 15]. Participants were randomized to receive CBT plus amitriptyline or headache education plus amitriptyline. Participants attended ten psychotherapy sessions for 20 weeks and less frequent follow-up sessions for 1 year. The CBT group received instruction in relaxation skills, activity pacing, cognitive skills, and problem-solving, and the headache education group received information about headache management. Results of the study showed that participants in the CBT plus amitriptyline group had greater reductions in days with headache and migraine-related disability compared to the headache education plus amitriptyline group.

Acceptance-Based Interventions

Mindfulness-based therapy approaches emphasize developing cognitive distance from facing expectations that cannot or need not be changed. As a result, the goal of therapy is learning how to accept life's uncontrollable events. Acceptance and commitment therapy (ACT), mindfulness-based stress reduction (MBSR), and mindfulness-based cognitive therapy (MBCT) are therapy approaches that are emerging as treatment options. Acceptance and commitment therapy (ACT) is a mindfulness-based approach that has been used with patients with chronic pain, including headaches. ACT emphasizes the necessity of pain acceptance to improve functioning. Exposure strategies aim to guide the patient to engage in functional behaviors, which result in valued actions.

In a review of mindfulness-based therapies for headaches, the researchers suggest that mindfulness alone may be comparable to pharmacological treatment alone for chronic migraine accompanied by medication overuse [16]. However, the review noted that additional research is needed to more fully document the role and long-term value of mindfulness for specific headache types.

Healthy Habits

This section reviews the evidence to support daily activities or lifestyle practices that promote healthy living and well-being for those with chronic daily headaches. It is important to educate patients on ways to modify their lifestyle and to encourage taking an active role in managing their headaches that may not involve taking medication. Adhering to regular daily exercise, eating a well-balanced diet that includes vegetables and protein, limiting caffeine intake, staying hydrated, and maintaining good sleep hygiene are common recommendations among those who treat headache disorders. Unlike conventional treatment options, lifestyle modification may take longer to show benefit compared to traditional therapies [17]. Research determining whether physical and behavioral changes are linked to improvement of headaches has been difficult to study for many reasons. Determining measures for obtaining headache diagnosis, preconceived biases, and subjective responses are just a few of obstacles toward deter-

Nutrition

Traditionally, diet has played an important role in headache management. Few studies have shown that vitamins, contained in food, can help reduce headache frequency and severity, and foods that contain nutrients and vitamins are essential in headache control [18, 19]. Vitamins in the form of nutraceuticals that have been most studied include coenzyme Q10, magnesium, and riboflavin. Coenzyme Q 10 is a cofactor involved in energy metabolism within the cell mitochondria, and studies have shown that increasing levels may be linked to improving headache outcomes [20, 21]. Foods that contain coenzyme Q10 include meat and oily fish such as salmon, mackerel, and peanuts [19]. Magnesium is a chemical element, endogenous to the body, and essential for hormone regulation, neurotransmitter function, and anti-inflammatory properties. Low levels of magnesium have been associated with cortical spreading depression, vasoconstriction, and neuro-inflammatory release linked to the onset of headache [22–24]. Although there are conflicting studies on the benefits of magnesium in reducing migraine frequency, there may be a benefit in those with migraine aura [25–28]. Foods rich in magnesium include almonds, spinach, potatoes, sunflower seeds, whole grains, and dairy products [19]. Riboflavin, also known as vitamin B2, is also a cofactor involved in energy metabolism and is derived from a reduced sugar and a structure that when oxidized, forms a bright yellow appearance in urine. Studies of patients taking riboflavin show improvement in headache frequency, although the proper dosing required remains unclear [29–31]. Patients are encouraged to consume foods rich in riboflavin and magnesium such as dairy products, almonds, fortified grains, and dark green vegetables. When recommending dietary supplementation, keep in mind that the doses studied are higher than ordinarily ingested in one meal and results may be delayed. Checking vitamin levels may be reasonable to provide guidance about which supplements and amounts are needed to increase levels to normal values [32]. However encouraging patients to incorporate such foods in their diet may help improve levels and may be an alternative than having to oral medication.

Avoiding potential food triggers is a common practice among migraineurs, despite limited scientific evidence supporting the relationship between headache and certain foods. A low-fat diet resulting in weight loss may improve headaches over time especially as obesity is a known risk factor associated with worsening headache outcomes [33–35]. Individuals with food sensitivities and those adhering to a ketogenic or modified Atkins's diet may benefit from eliminating foods that result in antibodies against certain food antigens [36–39]. Avoiding fasting states and hypoglycemic episodes and increasing the intake of omega-3 fatty acids may offer reduction in headache frequency [18, 40, 41]. Other triggers identified by patients believed to cause or worsen headache include the following: stress, bright lights, odors, loud noises, physical activity, chocolate, nitrates, monosodium glutamate, artificial sweeteners, nuts, cheese, nicotine, menstruation, and atmospheric changes [42]. An individual may have more than one trigger, and once identified, patients are instructed to avoid potential triggers that are under their control. Avoidance and implementing behavioral medicine interventions such as cognitive behavioral therapy may help in coping and managing pain if triggers have been identified. In general, recommendations regarding trigger avoidance are based on small studies that are limited in quality, and further research is needed to determine whether this is effective in improving migraine outcomes. It can be helpful to remind patients that triggers are often partial and additive in their effect on headache and that absolute triggers are much less common.

Hydration

Dehydration has been described as a headache trigger [43]. The underlying mechanism is unclear but thought to be due to low vascular fluid volume resulting in a decrease of oxygen flow to the brain, triggering head pain response. Increasing the intake of fluids that contain salts and electrolytes can improve vascular tone and hydration and help "dizziness" commonly described in migraine patients [44]. Drinking 200–1500 ml of water may provide headache relief in as early as 30 min [45]. The consensus among headache providers regarding fluid intake is for patients to stay well hydrated and avoid or limit alcohol and caffeine intake, which have been shown to be potential triggers for migraine [46–48].

Exercise

Patients who present with the complaint of frequent headache are often told to exercise as part of their treatment regimen [49]. Outside of observational reports, there is limited evidence to support that exercise can decrease headache frequency and severity, especially among patients with migraine. Busch and Gaul [50] did a literature review and reported that studies on patients with migraine and the influence of exercise were small with poorly defined methods used in determining headache diagnosis, frequency, and intensity of attacks, type, length, and adherence to exercise program. One study suggested regular exercise averaging 8 h per month may reduce headache pain intensity, and there were conflicting studies that did not show any change in headache outcomes [51, 52]. There is no dispute that regular exercise is important to improving and maintaining good physical health overall and has been incorporated in multidisciplinary programs focused on improving function in patients with chronic pain disorders [53]. The combination of a healthy diet and regular exercise can help prevent obesity which is a known risk factor for developing chronic migraine [33].

Sleep

Sleep disorders are common in patients with primary headache, and there is limited data that poor sleep quality, lack or excess of sleep, may precipitate headaches [54, 55]. The causal relationship between sleep and headaches is unclear. One study with primary headaches showed that insufficient and poor quality sleep was associated with increased headache frequency and intensity [56]. In another study, improvement of sleep hygiene through cognitive behavioral therapy led to a reduction in migraine frequency [57]. Recommendations to improve good sleep hygiene could have a positive impact on headache control.

Conclusion

There are options for treating chronic daily headache aside from traditional pharmaceutical therapy. Behavioral management interventions such as CBT offer the most evidence, particularly among adolescent patients. Although there is limited evidence on the impact of lifestyle modification, developing the habit of eating foods that contain key vitamins and nutrients, staying hydrated, and optimizing restful sleep and regular exercise can have a positive impact on physical health, which can improve overall function and lessen disability caused by chronic daily headache. The causal relationship between triggers and headache remains unclear; avoidance of potential triggers should be individualized to the patient. Non-pharmacological options for managing chronic daily headache have been used in combination or conjunction with pharmacotherapy; however, based on this review, further research is needed regarding outcomes and to further guide recommendations.

References

1. Penzien DB, Irby MB, Smitherman TA, Rains JC, Houle TT. Well established and empirically supported behavioral treatments for migraine. Curr Pain Headache Rep. 2015;19:34.
2. Faedda N, Cerutti R, Verdecchia P, Migliorini D, Arruda M, Guidetti V. Behavioral management of headache in children and adolescents. J Head Pain. 2016;17:80.
3. Silberstein SD. Practice parameter: evidence-based guidelines for migraine headache (an evidence-based review): report of the quality standards Subcommittee

of the American Academy of neurology. Neurology. 2000;55(6):754–62.

4. Drossman DA. Gastrointestinal illness and the biopsychosocial model. Psychosom Med. 1998;60:258–67.

5. Melzack R, Wall PD. Pain mechanisms: a new theory. Surv Anesthesiol. 1967;11(2):89–90.

6. Fraser F, Matsuzawa Y, Lee YSC, Minen M. Behavioral treatments for post-traumatic headache. Curr Pain Headache Rep. 2017;21(5):22.

7. Cho SJ, Song TJ, Chu MK. Treatment update of chronic migraine. Curr Pain Headache Rep. 2017;21(6):26.

8. Nestoriuc Y, Rief W, Andrasik F. Biofeedback treatment for headache disorders: a comprehensive efficacy review. Appl Psychophysiol Biofeedback. 2008;33(3):125–40.

9. Grazzi L, Andrasik F, D'Amico D, Leone M, Usai S, Kass SJ, et al. Behavioral and pharmacologic treatment of transformed migraine with analgesic overuse: outcome at 3 years. Headache. 2002;42(6):483–90.

10. Rausa M, Palomba D, Cevoli S, Lazzerini L, Sancisi E, Cortelli P, et al. Biofeedback in the prophylactic treatment of medication overuse headache: a pilot randomized controlled trial. J Headache Pain. 2016;17(1):87.

11. Sullivan A, Cousins S, Ridsdale L. Psychological interventions for migraine: a systematic review. J Neurol. 2016;263(12):2369–77.

12. Harris P, Loveman E, Clegg A, Easton S, Berry N. Systematic review of cognitive behavioural therapy for the management of headaches and migraines in adults. Br J Pain. 2015;9:213–24.

13. Holroyd KA, Cottrell CK, O'Donnell FJ, et al. Effect of preventive (beta blocker) treatment, behavioural migraine management, or their combination on outcomes of optimised acute treatment in frequent migraine: randomised controlled trial. BMJ. 2010;341:c4871.

14. Powers SW, Kashikar-Zuck SM, Allen JR, LeCates SL, Slater SK, Zafar M, et al. Cognitive behavioral therapy plus amitriptyline for chronic migraine in children and adolescents: a randomized clinical trial. JAMA. 2013;310(24):2622–30.

15. Kroner JW, Hershey AD, Kashikar-Zuck SM, LeCates SL, Allen JR, Slater SK, et al. Cognitive behavioral therapy plus amitriptyline for children and adolescents with chronic migraine reduces headache days to ≤ 4 per month. Headache. 2016;56(4):711–6.

16. Andrasik F, Grazzi L, D'Amico D, Sansone E, Leonardi M, Raggi A, et al. Mindfulness and headache: a "new"old treatment, with new findings. Cephalalgia. 2016;36(12):1192–205.

17. Tepper SJ. Nutraceutical and other modalities for the treatment of headache. Continuum (Minneap Minn). 2015;21(4):1018–31.

18. Orr SL. Diet and nutraceutical interventions for headache management: a review of the evidence. Cephalalgia. 2016;36(12):1112–33.

19. Murray KA, O'Neal KS, Weisz M. Dietary suggestions for migraine preventions. Am J Health Sys Pharm. 2015;72(7):519–21.

20. Sandor PS, Di Clemente L, Coppola G, et al. Efficacy of coenzyme Q10 in migraine prophylaxis: a randomized controlled trial. Neurology. 2005;64:713–5.

21. Hershey AD, Powers SW, Vockell A-LB, et al. Coenzyme Q10 deficiency and response to supplementation in pediatric and adolescent migraine. Headache. 2007;47:73–80.

22. Mody I, Lambert JD, Heinemann U. Low extracellular magnesium induces epileptiform activity and spreading depression in rat hippocampal slices. J Neurophysiol. 1987;57(3):869–88.

23. Altura BT, Altura BM. Withdrawal of magnesium causes vasospasm while elevated magnesium produces relaxation of tone in cerebral arteries. Neurosci Lett. 1980;20(3):323–7.

24. Weglicki WB, Phillips TM. Pathobiology of magnesium deficiency: a cytokine/neurogenic inflammation hypothesis. Am J Phys. 1992;263(3 pt 2):R734–7.

25. Peikert A, Wilimzig C, Kohne-Volland R. Prophylaxis of migraine with oral magnesium: results from a prospective, multi-center, placebo-controlled and double-blind randomized study. Cephalalgia. 1996;16(4):257–63.

26. Pfaffenrath V, WEsseley P, Meyer C, Isler HR, Evers S, Grotemeyer KH, et al. Magnesium in the prophylaxis of migraine-a double=blind placebo-controlled study. Cephalalgia. 1996;16(6):436–40.

27. Bianchi A, Salomone S, Caraci F, Pizza V, Bernardina R, D'Amato CC. Role of magnesium, coenzyme Q10, riboflavin, and vitamin B12 in migraine prophylaxis. Vitam Horm. 2004;69:297–312.

28. Bigal ME, Bordini CA, Tepper SJ, Speciali JG. Intervenous magnesium sulphate in the acute treatment of migraine without aura and migraine with aura. A randomized, double-blind, placebo-controlled study. Cephalalgia. 2002;22(5):345–53.

29. O'Brien HL, Hershey AD. Vitamin s and paediatric migraine: riboflavin as a preventative medication. Cephalalgia. 2010;30(12):1417–8.

30. Schoenen J, Jacquy J, Lenaerts M. Effectiveness of high-dose riboflavin in migraine prophylaxis. A randomized controlled trial. Neurology. 1998;50:466–70.

31. Maizels M, Blumenfeld A, Burchette R. A combination of riboflavin, magnesium, and feverfew for migraine prophylaxis: a randomized trial. Headache. 2004;44:885–90.

32. Rajapakse R, Pringsheim T. Nutraceuticals in migraine: a summary of existing guidelines for use. Headache. 2016;56(4):808–16.

33. Bigal ME, Lipton RB. Obesity is a risk factor for transformed migraine but not chronic tension-type headache. Neurology. 2006;67(2):252–7.

34. Bic Z, Blix G, Hopp H, et al. The influence of a low-fat diet on incidence and severity of migraine headaches. J Womens Health Gend Based Med. 1999;8:623–30.

35. Bunner AE, Agarwal U, Gonzales JF, et al. Nutrition intervention for migraine: a randomized crossover trial. J Headache Pain. 2014;15:1–9.

36. Arroyave Hernandez C, Echavarria Pinto M, Hernandez Montiel HL. Food allergy mediated by

IgG antibodies associated with migraine in adults. Rev Alerg Mex. 2007;54:162–8.

37. Alpay K, Ertax M, Orhan EH, et al. Diet restriction in migraine, based on IgG against foods: a clinical double-blind, randomized, cross-over trial. Cephalalgia. 2010;30:829–37.

38. Barborka CJ. Migraine: results of treatment by ketogenic diet in fifty cases. JAMA. 1930;95:1825–8.

39. Kossoff EH, Huffman J, Turner Z, et al. Use of the modified Atkins diet for adolescents with chronic daily headache. Cephalalgia. 2010;30:1014–6.

40. Dexter J, Roerts J, Byer J. The five hour glucose tolerance test and effect of low sucrose diet in migraine. Headache. 1978;18:91–4.

41. Ramsden C, Faurot K, Zamora D, Suchindran CM, Macintosh BA, Gaylord S, et al. Targeted alteration of dietary n-3 and n-6 fatty acids for the treatment of chronic headaches: a randomized trial. Pain. 2013;154:1–22.

42. Peris F, Donoghue S, Torres F, Mian A, Wober C. Towards improved migraine management: determining potential trigger factors in individual patients. Cephalalgia. 2016;37(5):452–63.

43. Martins IP, Gouveia RG. More on water and migraine. Cephalalgia. 2007;27:372–4.

44. Carvalho GF, Chaves TC, Dach F, Pinheiro CF, Goncalves MC, Florencio LL, Ferreira KS, Bigal ME, Bevilaqua-Grossi D. Influence of migraine and migraine aura on balance and mobility - a controlled study. Headache. 2013;53:1116–22.

45. Blau JN, Kell CA, Sperling JM. Water-deprivation headache: a new headache with two variants. Headache. 2004;44:79–83.

46. Sun-Edelstein C, Mauskop A. Foods and supplements in the management of migraine headaches. Clin J Pain. 2009;25(5):446–52.

47. Kelman L. The triggers or precipitants of the acute migraine attack. Cephalalgia. 2007;27:394–402.

48. Ravishankar K, Evans RW, Wang S-J. Modern day management of headache questions and answers. New Delhi: The Health Sciences Publishers; 2017.

49. Matthew N, Tfelt-Hansen P. General and pharmacologic approach to migraine management. In: Olesen J, Tfelt-Hansen P, Welch KMA, editors. The headaches. Philadelphia, PA: Lippincott Williams & Wilkins; 2006. p. 433–40.

50. Busch W, Gaul C. Exercise in migraine therapy-is there any evidence for efficacy? A critical review. Headache. 2008;48:890–9.

51. Lockett DM, Campbell JF. The effects of aerobic exercise on migraine. Headache. 1992;32:50–4.

52. Nordlander E, Cider A, Carlsson J, Linde M. Improvement of exercise capacity in patients with migraine–methodological considerations. Cephalalgia. 2007;27:575–9.

53. Zheng Y, Tepper SJ, Covington EC, Mathews M, Scheman J. Retrospective outcome analysis for headache in a pain rehabilitation interdisciplinary program. Headache. 2014;54:520–7.

54. Sahota PK, Dexter JD. Sleep and headache syndromes: a clinical review. Headache. 1990;30:80–4.

55. Jennum P, Jensen R. Sleep and headache. Sleep Med Rev. 2002;6:471–9.

56. Gilman DK, Palermo TM, Kabbouche MA, Hershey AD, Powers SW. Primary headache and sleep disturbances in adolescents. Headache. 2007;47:1189–94.

57. Calhoun AH, Ford S. Behavioral sleep modification may revert transformed migraine to episodic migraine. Headache. 2007;47:1178–83.

Complementary and Alternative Approaches to Chronic Daily Headache: Part I—Mind/Body

Rebecca Erwin Wells, Laura Granetzke, and Brielle Paolini

Introduction to Parts I, II, and III: Complementary and Alternative Approaches for Chronic Daily Headache

The refractory nature of chronic daily headache makes it challenging to treat. Both patients and providers become frustrated with the often-poor treatment responses and persistent symptoms, and as a result many patients turn to complementary and alternative medicine (CAM) for relief. CAM therapies include diverse medical and healthcare systems, practices, and products not presently considered as part of conventional medicine [1]. These options can be used as alternatives or complements to traditional western medical options. Many CAM therapies address and target other factors (e.g., stress) that may be involved in development or persistence of medical symptoms. Typical pharmacologic options are often limited by side effects, poor tolerance, limited efficacy, patient noncompliance or non-adherence, medication contraindications, and comorbidities or coexisting conditions (e.g., pregnancy/nursing). Overuse of medications can become a critical problem, especially with chronic daily headache and the potential development of medication-overuse headache.

Some CAM therapies may be appealing because of their minimal cost, as well as patients' views that such products are more aligned with their personal health and wellness beliefs. Since they can be used concurrently with medications, many patients may use them without discussing them with their providers. However, these therapies may have side effects, and their costs may not be negligible. Understanding the benefits and risks of these therapies is critical for patients, who should seek appropriate provider counseling about CAM treatment options for headache [2].

Headache is among the most common neurological conditions associated with CAM use [3–5]. The prevalence of CAM use in patients with headaches ranges from 29 to 74% [3, 6–13]. This may even be an underestimate; one study ($n = 484$) determined prevalence based on initial admittance of use to be 17%, but follow-up questioning determined actual use to be 42% [3]. In an analysis of the 2007 National Health Interview Survey (NHIS, $n = 23,393$), 49.5% of adults with self-reported migraines/severe headache reported using CAM therapies versus 33.9% of those without migraines/severe headaches ($p < 0.001$) [6]. Therapies reported included mind/body therapies (30.2%), biologically based therapies such as herbs/supplements (23.7%), manipulation-based therapies such as chiropractic and massage (20.6%), and alternative systems such as acu-

R. E. Wells (✉) · L. Granetzke
Neurology, Wake Forest School of Medicine,
Winston-Salem, NC, USA
e-mail: rewells@wakehealth.edu

B. Paolini
Wake Forest School of Medicine,
Winston-Salem, NC, USA

© Springer International Publishing AG, part of Springer Nature 2019
M. W. Green et al. (eds.), *Chronic Headache*, https://doi.org/10.1007/978-3-319-91491-6_18

puncture and homeopathy (5.2%). This study was limited because patients did not report using the CAM therapy specifically for their headaches. An analysis of the 2012 NHIS data reports similar prevalence of CAM for adults with migraines/severe headaches (44%) but with manipulation-based therapies most commonly used (23.7%), followed by biologically based therapies (22.2%), and then mind/body therapies (19.0%) [13]. Differences in rates from the 2007 to the 2012 analyses may be due to actual changes in use or different definitions of the CAM modalities in the analyses [6, 13]. A smaller survey from a Turkish headache clinic reported massage (51%) as most frequently used [7]. Since pediatric patients and their parents and providers often wish to avoid pharmacologic options due to risks of side effects and fear for long-term use, CAM is often used in children and adolescents [10]. In a survey of 124 pediatric headache patients from Italy, 76% reported using CAM, most often herbal preparations (64%). Eighty percent of respondents used CAM as a preventive treatment option [10].

If patients decide to use CAM, most report using three or more types of therapies [8, 14]. In addition, if used for headache, patients will often use CAM for other medical conditions. Headache patients most commonly use CAM based on provider recommendation, cost or ineffectiveness of conventional treatments [6], the wish of avoiding chronic use of drugs with their related side effects, the desire for an integrated approach, inefficacy of conventional medicine [10], the hope for a potential improvement of headache [9], or as a last resort after trying all conventional therapies [15]. The most common source of CAM referral is usually a friend or relative [8, 9]. For those who report using CAM, up to 42–62% do not discuss their use with their provider [6, 8, 9], although many say this is because the provider did not ask about their use, rather than fear of discouragement or lack of understanding [8]. In headache patients, predictors or correlates of CAM use include headache disability (e.g., headache impact test-6 [HIT-6] scores) [8], higher income, more frequent headaches [9], anxiety, joint or low back pain, alcohol use, higher education, and living in the western USA [6]. Using

CAM therapies does not exclude the use of conventional therapies, and some research suggests the contrary. For example, youth with headaches who used CAM, compared to nonusers, had higher expenditures while using most types of conventional care [11].

Many of the surveys assessing CAM use have also questioned perceived efficacy. A survey from a UK headache clinic ($n = 92$, with 32% reporting CAM use) demonstrated that 60% of CAM users perceived the therapy as beneficial in helping reduce headache frequency or intensity, 58% reported being satisfied or very satisfied with the treatment, and none felt the CAM therapy worsened their headaches [8]. However, several surveys report less than half of patients experiencing satisfaction from their CAM therapy. A Norwegian survey with 62% prevalence of CAM use in those with primary chronic headaches found a range of 0–43% perceived efficacy, without significant differences between gender, headache diagnoses, medication use, physician contact, and co-occurrence of migraine [12]. Another survey, based out of a Turkish headache clinic, found that out of all CAM modalities, only those using massage reported benefit and in only 33% of those patients [7]. Only 23% of 2477 chronic migraineurs reported satisfaction with their CAM treatment [14]. The type of headache treated may also affect perceived efficacy, as a survey of CAM use in cluster patients reported that only 8% perceived benefit and 28% had partial effectiveness [9].

Compared to those not using CAM, those who use CAM are more likely to have comorbid mental health issues, have more intense headaches, and experience more negative life impact from migraines [14]. Interestingly, CAM treatment satisfaction was inversely related to the number of psychiatric comorbidities, the frequency of migraines, and the number of migraine symptoms, although CAM treatment satisfaction was more strongly correlated with migraine outcomes than psychiatric comorbidities. Disability associated with chronic headaches may make it difficult to use extensive non-home-based CAM treatments, although for the same reasons chronic migraineurs may be more amenable to home options such as meditation. The 2012 NHIS analysis of CAM use in adults with migraines found that women are more likely to use CAM than men and that CAM use was associated with decreased odds of moderate mental distress only in women [13]. The authors argue that women with migraines/severe headaches may have benefited from CAM for their mental distress.

Providers have also been surveyed to assess their opinion on CAM efficacy. A survey was administered to 223 different UK CAM organizations, and headaches/migraine was the second most commonly cited condition that would benefit by CAM (behind stress/anxiety) [16]. The recommended treatment options for headache/migraines included massage, yoga, reflexology, aromatherapy, and chiropractic treatments, along with other options not discussed in this chapter (Bowen technique, hypnotherapy, nutrition, Reiki). A survey completed by 1247 healthcare professionals in Switzerland reports that they would most likely refer patients for acupuncture for migraine (75%) or tension headaches (71%), although over half had never referred a patient to a CAM provider, and 84% felt they lacked the knowledge to inform their patients on CAM [17].

This review focuses on the evidence and outcomes to date for CAM therapies of mind/body therapies, Part I (e.g., meditation, yoga, tai chi, deep breathing); manipulation-based therapies, Part II (e.g., acupuncture, acupressure, dry needling, chiropractic manipulation, massage, craniosacral therapy, reflexology); and other CAM options (aromatherapy, homeopathy, hydrotherapy, daith piercing, and hyperbaric oxygen therapy) for headache. Part III summarizes this evidence for nutraceutical options for headache, specifically feverfew, riboflavin, magnesium, coenzyme Q10, melatonin, vitamin D, and ginkgo. Most of these therapies have very little research supporting their use, and the research that has been conducted is limited by critical methodologic concerns (e.g., small sample sizes, no active control groups, etc.). By the very nature of being "CAM," these therapies do not yet have the research evidence base to be accepted into mainstream medicine. Further, research on these therapies for headache, and specifically chronic daily headache, is limited. The goal of this review is to describe the research on CAM therapies for headache and, when available, chronic daily headache. If not available, the research presented for headache can be extrapolated for consideration in the treatment of chronic daily headache.

Mind/Body and Chronic Daily Headache

Mind/body practices are based on the awareness of the mind and body connection, to enhance the mind's positive influence on the body's physical functioning and thus promote health. Mind/body therapies are often considered treatments that target stress. Since stress is the most cited trigger for migraine attacks [18] and has a complex relationship with headaches [19], headaches may be particularly amenable to mind/body therapies. Many mind/body therapies are also considered "behavioral treatments." Currently, "behavioral treatments" for headache include cognitive behavioral therapy, biofeedback, and relaxation training (Table 18.1) [20], with the goal of training patients in these "headache management skills." These therapies have been researched within the context of headache medicine for many years; the first study evaluating biofeedback for headaches appeared in 1969. Based on a large systematic review evaluating behavioral treatments for headache [21], the US Headache Consortium gave Grade A evidence for the use of relaxation train-

Table 18.1 Behavioral and mind/body treatment options

Behavioral	Mind/body
• Cognitive behavioral therapy	• Meditation
– Stress management	• Yoga
– Coping skills	• Guided imagery
• Biofeedback	• Biofeedback
• Relaxation training	• Hypnosis
	• Tai chi
	• Qi gong
	• Deep breathing exercises
	• Progressive muscular relaxation

Reproduced with permission from John Wiley & Sons, Inc. from the journal *Headache* [19]

ing, thermal biofeedback with relaxation, electromyographic (EMG) biofeedback, and cognitive behavioral therapy [22]. Because of their increasing acceptance into mainstream headache medicine, these therapies may not be considered "CAM" anymore.

However, many typical "mind/body" approaches have been used in Eastern medicine for many years and are only now gaining attention in Western medicine, with limited research evidence for their use. Many mind/body therapies incorporate components of evidence-based behavioral treatments, such as relaxation, deep breathing, and guided imagery. Although clearly there is overlap between the two categories, Table 18.1 delineates the differences between behavioral treatments and mind/body treatments. For this chapter, the evidence and potential mechanisms for the mind/body approaches of meditation, yoga, tai chi, and deep breathing will be discussed. Few studies have been conducted evaluating these approaches in general and even fewer that are specific to chronic daily headache. Therefore, much of the evidence described will focus on these approaches to any type of headache, with the consideration of extrapolating the information to chronic daily headache.

Meditation

Meditation has long historical roots in religious and spiritual traditions, with goals of reaching heightened levels of spiritual awareness. In the last several decades, meditation has been researched for its physiological benefits. Benson published early investigations of meditation and its ability to elicit the "relaxation response" [23]. His research on the effects of the relaxation response through mantra-based transcendental meditation for cluster, migraine, and tension headaches demonstrated that twice-daily, 20-min sessions for 4–14 months resulted in significant clinical improvements for 6 of 17 headache patients [24, 25].

Kabat-Zinn's research further developed this line of inquiry through a program to teach "mindfulness meditation," defined as "paying attention

in a particular way: on purpose, in the present moment, and non-judgmentally" [26]. Through the daily practice of mindfulness meditation, participants are encouraged to apply mindfulness in daily activities. The practice of mindfulness promotes an attitude of acceptance, curiosity, and openness. His original research focused on those with "chronic pain," including headache. Participants had improvements in pain symptoms, anxiety, depression, and drug utilization, with most effects maintained at 15 months follow-up [27, 28]. This program blossomed into the "mindfulness-based stress reduction (MBSR)" program, a standardized program of 8 weekly 2.5 h classes that has been taught to over 22,000 individuals, with referrals from over 6000 providers.

As a standardized intervention, MBSR has been helpful for a multitude of different medical conditions [29], with chronic pain being one of the most commonly studied conditions. A systematic review evaluated the benefits of MBSR or a variation of the program for chronic pain in 38 randomized clinical trials (RCTs) [30]. The authors reported that mindfulness meditation improves pain, depression, and quality of life, although they argued that larger, more well-designed and rigorous RCTs are needed to provide better estimates of efficacy [30]. Five of the RCTs included in this review evaluated mindfulness for headache; all are limited by lack of an active control [31–35].

We conducted the first RCT of MBSR in adults with episodic migraine ($n = 19$), one of the studies included in the systematic review. Both groups received usual care, and the active group also received MBSR. Most participants (89%) were taking migraine prophylactics daily and had an average of ten headaches/month. We observed statistically significant improvements in headache duration (captured with daily headache logs), disability (HIT-6 and Migraine Disability Assessment [MIDAS]), self-efficacy, and mindfulness. Adherence and study participation were excellent, with no adverse events. Although our small sample size limited the study's power to detect statistically significant differences in headache frequency or severity, a strength of this study (standard for strong headache studies but unusual in the CAM literature) was use of daily headache logs for assessment of headache outcomes, with baseline data completed prior to randomization. The major limitation was the lack of an active control group.

Additional studies included in this review [30] evaluated MBSR or variations for different types of headaches. Two studies were conducted in Iran. One evaluated MBSR for "chronic headache" (primary chronic migraine or tension-type headache) versus usual care ($n = 40$), with pain and quality of life (SF-36) questionnaires at baseline and follow-up [35]. MBSR improved pain intensity and quality of life vs. the control group. However, the study was considered of "poor" quality in the systematic review because of weak statistical analyses, no active control group, and how headache outcomes were assessed. Rather than daily headache logs, headache outcomes were limited to a perceived pain intensity of headache at each time point, with a cumulative assessment and score for pain ratings, duration, and frequency of headaches in the prior month (not a typical headache outcome). Another RCT conducted in Iran of MBSR for tension headache (uncertain if episodic or chronic, $n = 60$) demonstrated improvements in headache severity (measured by daily headache logs) and mindfulness (mindfulness attention awareness scale) [34] and reported separately perceived stress and general mental health (Brief Symptom inventory) [36]. Although this study had a 3-month follow-up, it was also limited by lack of an active control group.

An RCT in Australia evaluated a briefer version of MBSR (classes twice weekly for 3 weeks) vs. wait-list control ($n = 58$) for ICHD-II defined chronic tension-type headache, with headache outcomes captured with 2-week headache diaries before/after the intervention and mindfulness assessed before/after with the Five-Factor Mindfulness Questionnaire. Headache frequency decreased in the intervention group compared to the control group; headache duration and intensity did not show improvements with MBSR. The intervention group had better scores on the observe scale from the Five-Factor Mindfulness

Scale compared to the control group. The study was limited by significant dropouts (58 randomized but only 42 analyzed), no active control group, and a novel intervention with unknown reliability and validity. Another RCT evaluated a variant of MBSR, mindfulness-based cognitive therapy (that incorporates facets of both MBSR and CBT), for adults with "headache pain" (3+ days/month of any primary headache disorder) compared to delayed treatment control ($n = 36$) [33]. Compared to the control group, intervention participants reported better pain acceptance and self-efficacy, with additional improvements seen in pain interference and pain catastrophizing among those who completed the study ($n = 24$). Improvements in headache outcomes were not seen. Limitations included lack of an active control and limited headache log data (only 1-week baseline data, no posttreatment data); these weaknesses may have affected outcome assessments of headache. In a follow-up analysis to evaluate responders versus nonresponders, the authors reported pain acceptance and pain catastrophizing were key factors underlying treatment response [33].

After the systematic review [30] was conducted, a unique clinic-based "effectiveness" trial compared a mindfulness-based training group (6 weekly 45-min sessions, an MBSR variant) and prophylactic medication group in 44 adults with chronic migraine and medication-overuse headache [37]. Participants first completed a withdrawal program in a day hospital and then were given the option of which group to join; participants were not randomized. Both groups had statistically significant decreases in monthly headache days, monthly use of abortive medications intake, headache disability, and depression after the intervention compared to baseline, without differences between groups, with effects persisting to 12-month follow-up. Although limited by its non-randomized approach, this study provides evidence that a mindfulness program may be as effective as standard of care for patients with chronic migraine and medication-overuse headache.

A few other meditation studies for headache, not specifically of mindfulness meditation, were not included in the mindfulness for chronic pain systematic review [30]. A study from India in chronic tension-type headaches compared two groups of 70 patients [38]. Both received twice-daily abortive medications; one group also received eight additional lessons in a form of spiritual meditation known as "Rajyoga meditation," which incorporates visualization of meaningful images with a focus on positive thoughts of a universal force. Within-group analyses showed that both groups had improvements in headache severity, frequency, and duration, although significant relief in headache severity, duration, and frequency was much higher in the meditation group (94/91/97% vs. 36/36/49%). This study was limited by within-group analyses and high participant dropout (only 50 participants completed).

Several studies have compared "spiritual meditation" (spiritually inspired mantras) to "secular meditation" (secular mantras) to "relaxation" (progressive muscular relaxation) [39–43]. The first study [39] in 68 healthy college students showed that "spiritual meditation" (20 min/day for 2 weeks) appeared to have the most benefits on anxiety, mood, spiritual health, and pain tolerance compared to "secular meditation" and "relaxation" [39]. Two follow-up studies in adults ($n = 83$ and $n = 92$) with two or more migraines per month also showed improvements with "spiritual meditation" compared to "secular meditation" and "relaxation" on measures of headache frequency, anxiety, negative affect, pain tolerance, headache related, and self-efficacy [40, 41]. A third study reported that a 20-minute meditation intervention improved immediate pain and emotional tension scores in 27 adults who had 2–10 migraines/month [42]. A more recent study ($n = 107$ randomized, 74 analyzed) showed that mindfulness meditation improved pain-related stress compared to simple relaxation and the mindfulness meditation intervention provided similar outcomes to spiritual mindfulness in pain-related outcomes [43]. Unfortunately, since participants in these studies were generally healthy, non-treatment seeking young adults, the results may not generalize to other populations. Further, many participants dropped out after

being randomized (from 84 to 68 in one study and from 107 to 74 in another study) [39, 43].

A small non-randomized study [44] of a mindfulness-based intervention in 20 adolescents with "recurrent headaches" (4 or more per month) showed safety (no adverse events), feasibility (median class attendance 7 out of 8), and improvements in depression, quality of life, and acceptance of pain; no changes in headache frequency or severity were seen. This was a pilot study and was not powered for headache outcomes but shows the possibility of using mindfulness interventions in adolescents with headaches.

In a study that tracked outcomes after an MBSR course in patients with a variety of chronic pain conditions, those with chronic headache/migraine experienced the smallest improvements in pain and quality of life compared to the other chronic pain conditions [45]. However, this study was limited by its observational nature and lacked a control group and direct measures of pain. The small sample sizes for each specific chronic pain condition limited statistical power and reliability of effect sizes (e.g., only 34 of 133 participants had headaches).

Potential Mechanisms of Meditation

Proposed mechanisms to explain the potential impact of meditation on pain (including headaches) include neurobiological changes in pain processing, stress reduction, changes in relevant psychological constructs, effects on other behaviors, and/or placebo [46]. The strongest evidence comes from the neuroscientific research that has demonstrated the specific neural pathways involved in meditation and pain relief. Mind/body therapies may be effective because they target the cognitive and affective control of pain [47]. Meditation may attenuate pain by improving its emotional and cognitive modulation at the cortical level [48]. In studies assessing the impact of meditation on experimentally induced heat pain in healthy controls, meditation-induced decreases in pain intensity were associated with increases in anterior insula and anterior cingulate activity detected on MRI—key regions for cognitive modulation of pain processing [49]. Meditation-induced decreases in pain unpleasantness were associated with orbitofrontal activation (that could explain the cognitive reframing of sensory events with meditation) and thalamic deactivation (suggesting that meditation may downregulate the thalamus, the key relay station for pain transmission from sensory receptors to the brain). Additional research has shown that meditation-based pain relief does not require or use endogenous opioids [50] and has a distinct neurobiological signature from placebo analgesia [51].

Further research on the neuroscientific underpinnings of meditation has indicated that meditation may enhance frontal attentional control, increase cortical thickness, and activate areas of the brain important for pain modulation (hippocampus, insula, cingulate cortex, prefrontal cortex, and parietal cortex), thereby helping to decouple sensory-discriminative and cognitive-evaluative brain networks [52–54].

Meditation also fosters a calm state of focused attention that may better balance the parasympathetic and sympathetic systems. Meditation lowers stress levels [55], the most frequently cited trigger for migraine [18]. Further, the presence of migraine may impact stress-related dysregulation of the autonomic nervous system [56–58]. In a study that assessed heart rate variability in headache patients (randomized to either a mindfulness intervention or a control group) after a cognitive stress induction test [59], headache patients were more likely to have dysregulated stress recovery compared to controls. These data suggest that mindfulness practice may promote effective heart rate regulation, especially after a stressful event.

Other research has suggested the important role cognitive and psychological factors play in the relationship between meditation and migraines. In a cross-sectional study that compared stress-coping styles among migraineurs, meditators, and healthy controls, migraineurs used negative stress-coping strategies significantly more than the other groups, especially "rumination" [60]. In secondary analyses of the previously described RCT of MBCT for headache by Day and colleagues [33], pain acceptance was a significant mediator underlying improve-

ment in pain after MBCT [61]. Additional secondary analyses also demonstrated the importance of pretreatment expectations, patient motivation, and the development of strong rapport with the therapist as critical components to improving pain outcomes [62]. Day and colleagues developed a theoretical model to explain mindfulness-based pain relief, organized into the overarching factors of environment, brain state, cognitive content and coping/processes, behavior, and emotion and affect [54]. The cognitive factors not already discussed that they included in this model include increased self-efficacy, emotion regulation, positive affect, and decreased pain catastrophizing and negative affect.

In mindfulness meditation, participants are taught to notice sensations distinct from the thoughts related to the sensation; this detachment may alter pain perception. Participants may continue to have headaches but are able to better cope with the pain [28]. This flexible attentional capacity may help relieve the suffering of pain and improve quality of life.

Finally, mindfulness meditation, like all mind/body therapies, may work by helping to improve other behaviors that result in improvement of headaches. For example, meditation may improve sleep, and this effect could improve headaches. Meditation may also enhance a person's ability to engage in other healthy behaviors, such as improved diet and more exercise, which also could improve headaches.

Summary: Meditation and Chronic Daily Headache

The research on meditation for headaches is limited by the lack of active control groups, small sample sizes, and lack of long-term follow-up. However, the evidence suggests that meditation could benefit headache patients as a complement to standard of care. Meditative practices can be practiced anywhere, increasing adherence. Once the technique is learned, it requires little financial investment, so it may be applicable to a broader audience than typical psychological resources such as biofeedback. It does require active participation and self-responsibility, which may be critical ingredients for its success. Although such active involvement may improve self-efficacy, it does require significant time, energy, and a commitment to regular practice. In a case report of a migraineur ultimately benefiting from mindfulness training, it took years of encouragement from a provider before the patient was ready to adopt a mind-body practice [63]. Another case report suggested that mindfulness meditation initially induced headaches in one patient but then became a powerful treatment option [64]. If helpful, research suggests that benefits may persist for up to 4 years [65]. Most research to date has focused on mindfulness meditation, although spiritual meditative techniques and transcendental meditation have also been explored. Future research needs to include active control groups and larger studies of appropriate design and longer follow-up periods.

Yoga

Yoga is a mind/body treatment that combines the physical exercise of postures ("asanas") with breathing ("pranayama") and deep relaxation ("shavasana") to create a meditative experience. Evidence suggests yoga may be beneficial for many health conditions and their associated symptoms (cancer, hypertension, diabetes mellitus type 2, multiple sclerosis, Parkinson's, depression, anxiety, pregnancy, pre−/postpartum depression, etc.) [66]. Although yoga has long been used to treat many different chronic pain conditions [67], a systematic review looking for RCTs of yoga specifically for headache [68] found only one publication from a headache clinic in India [69]. This study compared 12 weeks of yoga to a headache education group in 72 migraineurs without aura (uncertain if episodic or chronic). The yoga group practiced 5 days/week for 60 min, and participants were also instructed to practice as an abortive migraine treatment but only during the prodromal phase of a migraine. The intervention involved yoga postures, breathing practices, yoga breathing, relaxation practices, and meditation. Headache education group participants received headache education once/month for 3 months plus handouts on self-care.

Those in the yoga group had significant decreases in headache intensity, frequency, pain rating index, affective pain rating index, total pain rating index, anxiety, depression, and symptomatic medication use. Unfortunately, analyses did not compare baseline and end-of-study results; it only compared post-study results between groups. The study lacked matching on time and attention between the two groups, and the participants were not blinded. There was no long-term follow-up to assess treatment durability, and no adverse events were mentioned.

A few smaller studies provide additional insight on the impact and potential mechanisms of yoga on headache. As tension-type headache has long been viewed as a condition of muscular tension, many have felt yoga may be particularly applicable. A different study from India ($n = 16$) compared EMG biofeedback with yogic shavasana relaxation (both practiced twice per week in 30-min sessions for 10 weeks); the two groups had equally improved tension headaches (occurring at least twice per week for over a year) [70]. Interestingly, "complete remission" was achieved after only 13 sessions with the yoga group, compared to 16 sessions with the biofeedback group. Although small, this study suggests yoga may have similar benefits to EMG biofeedback. Another small study ($n = 15$ headache patients) compared NSAID treatment (undefined dosage/frequency), botulinum toxin (undefined frequency), and an intense yoga program (3 h/day for 2 weeks) for treatment of chronic tension-type headache [71] and found that subjective pain scores improved in all three groups. In another study, 32 women with migraines (uncertain if episodic or chronic) were randomized to either 12 weeks of medication treatment under a neurologist's supervision (undefined medication type, dosage, frequency) or medical treatment plus yoga [72]. Metabolites of nitric oxide, hypothesized as having a role in the mechanism of yoga on headache, were measured in both groups. Those in the yoga group (75-min guided sessions three times per week) had significant reductions in headache frequency and severity, but plasma nitric oxide levels were not different between groups before and after the study.

A more recent study assessed changes in endothelial function after yoga (three 75-min sessions per week for 12 weeks) compared to medication (undefined drug/dose/frequency) in 42 migraineurs (unclear if episodic or chronic) [73]. The study focused on plasma concentrations of intercellular adhesion molecule (ICAM) and vascular cell adhesion molecule (VCAM) as possible mechanisms for triggering vascular inflammatory responses; no headache measures were assessed. After treatment, plasma concentrations of ICAM decreased in the yoga group compared to the control group, with no differences detected in VCAM concentrations. Although the authors concluded that the intervention might improve vascular function in migraineurs, the methodologic concerns (only data from 32 participants were reported), lack of headache measures/outcomes, and inconsistent results between ICAM and VCAM limit such a conclusion.

In a recent pilot study of 8 weeks of 75-min yoga classes for pediatric patients with headache [74], 19 of 57 patients approached agreed to participate, but only 7 actually attended classes, with the weekly no-show rate ranging from 1 to 3 participants. This study demonstrates the challenges of adherence to interventions that involve significant time, although children may have more scheduling limitations than adults.

Summary: Yoga and Headache

Yoga may be a valuable treatment option for adults with headaches, but most studies are limited by serious methodologic concerns. In addition, the interventions studied to date have been intense programs, requiring significant time and motivation, limiting feasibility for many patients. Several studies have attempted to assess pathophysiologic mechanisms of yoga on migraine, with unclear results. Additional research is needed to assess other potential hypothesized mechanisms, such as the improvement in parasympathetic tone and calming of the stress response through active yoga postures, deep breathing, and deep relaxation states. However, yoga is now widely available, and among some settings, illiteracy and poverty make some behavioral treatments (like biofeedback) more challenging; yoga could be a more easily accessible and inexpensive treatment option [70].

Tai Chi

Tai chi is a form of traditional Chinese medicine that incorporates physical, cognitive, social, and meditative components into this mind/body activity [75]. As a "moving meditation," the goal is to rebalance the body's own healing capacity. Evidence suggests it can prevent falls and improve balance and is helpful for many chronic musculoskeletal pain conditions [76]. Since tai chi overlaps with both mind/body interventions and other traditional Chinese medicine treatments like acupuncture, and both may help headaches, tai chi has been hypothesized to improve headaches. However, only one RCT has assessed tai chi for headache [77]. This study compared biweekly 60-min tai chi sessions for 15 weeks to a wait-list control group using the classical Yang style of tai chi with 24 standardized movements. Those in the intervention group demonstrated improvements in pain, energy/fatigue, social functioning, emotional well-being, and mental health summary scores on the HIT-6 and SF-36 instruments. Although 47 were randomized, only 30 completed the study; outcomes did not assess headache measures but rather only quality of life measures. Nonetheless, while this study suggests tai chi may be helpful for tension-type headaches, larger, more rigorous studies are needed for further recommendations.

Deep Breathing

In the National Health Interview Survey, "deep breathing" is assessed as a mind/body CAM medical treatment option. Of adults with a history of severe headaches/migraines, 24% report using deep breathing exercises, the highest prevalence of all mind/body therapies [6]. Unfortunately, what "deep breathing" entails is not defined in the survey or by participants. Although most proponents of mind/body therapies would argue that breathing is a critical component of the intervention, no specific studies evaluate the sole benefit of deep breathing for headache. Many patients in pain often hold their breath or in moments of anxiety take shorter, more shallow, and frequent breaths; thus, deep breathing may help ease pain, anxiety, or panic. Despite the lack of research for this modality for headache, many providers may recommend it, with specific instructions on how to achieve ideal "deep breathing" [78]. Some argue that patients may be more receptive to this technique than less familiar interventions such as meditation. A survey of adolescents with headache demonstrated that 72% were interested in learning deep breathing, while only 21% wanted to learn the relaxation response or biofeedback, and none were interested in meditation [11]. Deep breathing for pain is not a new concept—e.g., in the Lamaze technique, deep breathing is taught to help ease the pain of childbirth. Migraine involves dysfunction of the autonomic nervous system [56–59], so targeting this dysfunction through deep breathing may provide headache benefit. Additional research into this modality for headaches is needed, especially evaluating its role in all mind/body therapies.

Summary: Mind Body and Chronic Daily Headache

Chronic daily headache is often refractory to conventional treatment options, and CAM treatments may provide relief. However, research of CAM treatments for chronic daily headache is limited, so research evidence is reviewed for CAM to treat headache. The mechanisms of mind/body approaches such as meditation, yoga, tai chi, and deep breathing suggest they should be helpful for headaches, especially considering their overlap with well-researched behavioral treatments, but research is just now emerging regarding true efficacy. Mindfulness meditation has the most research to date of all mind/body therapies for headaches. The evidence is promising but limited by methodologic concerns such as lack of active control groups, small sample sizes, and lack of

long-term follow-up. The one RCT of yoga for migraine suggests a benefit, but additional studies are needed. Other yoga studies for headache have been limited by significant methodologic concerns, and the yoga interventions have been time-intensive. Tai chi has minimal evidence to suggest benefit for tension-type headache. Research needs to be conducted to assess "deep breathing" as an independent modality for headache.

Part II summarizes manipulation-based treatment options (acupuncture, chiropractic, and massage) and other CAM treatments. Part III reviews the evidence regarding nutraceuticals and homeopathy for chronic daily headache and final conclusions from Parts I, II, and III.

Acknowledgments Dr. Wells is supported by the National Center for Complementary and Integrative Health of the National Institutes of Health under Award Number K23AT008406. The content is solely the responsibility of the authors and does not necessarily represent the official views of the National Institutes of Health. We gratefully acknowledge the editorial assistance of Karen Klein, MA, in the Wake Forest Clinical and Translational Science Institute, funded by the National Center for Advancing Translational Sciences (NCATS), National Institutes of Health, through Grant Award Number UL1TR001420. We also thank Mark McKone, Librarian at Carpenter Library, Wake Forest School of Medicine, for his help with the use of Zotero. We are appreciative of the help from Nakiea Choate from the Department of Neurology at Wake Forest Baptist for her administrative support.

References

1. Complementary and Alternative Medicine [Internet]. [cited 2017 May 15]. Available from: https://www.nlm.nih.gov/tsd/acquisitions/cdm/subjects24.html
2. Wells RE, Baute V, Wahbeh H. Complementary and integrative medicine for neurologic conditions. Med Clin N Am. 2017;101(5):881–9.
3. Kenney D, Jenkins S, Youssef P, Kotagal S. Patient use of complementary and alternative medicines in an outpatient pediatric neurology clinic. Pediatr Neurol. 2016;58:48–52.e7.
4. Morone NE, Moore CG, Greco CM. Characteristics of adults who used mindfulness meditation: United States, 2012. J Altern Complement Med. 2017;23(7):545–50.
5. Wells RE, Phillips RS, Schachter SC, McCarthy EP. Complementary and alternative medicine use among US adults with common neurological conditions. J Neurol. 2010;257(11):1822–31.

6. Wells RE, Bertisch SM, Buettner C, Phillips RS, McCarthy EP. Complementary and alternative medicine use among adults with migraines/severe headaches. Headache. 2011;51(7):1087–97.

7. Karakurum Göksel B, Coşkun Ö, Ucler S, Karatas M, Ozge A, Ozkan S. Use of complementary and alternative medicine by a sample of Turkish primary headache patients. Agri. 2014;26(1):1–7.

8. Lambert TD, Morrison KE, Edwards J, Clarke CE. The use of complementary and alternative medicine by patients attending a UK headache clinic. Complement Ther Med. 2010;18(3–4):128–34.

9. Rossi P, Torelli P, Di Lorenzo C, Sances G, Manzoni GC, Tassorelli C, et al. Use of complementary and alternative medicine by patients with cluster headache: results of a multi-Centre headache clinic survey. Complement Ther Med. 2008;16(4):220–7.

10. Dalla Libera D, Colombo B, Pavan G, Comi G. Complementary and alternative medicine (CAM) use in an Italian cohort of pediatric headache patients: the tip of the iceberg. Neurol Sci. 2014;35(Suppl 1):145–8.

11. Bethell C, Kemper KJ, Gombojav N, Koch TK. Complementary and conventional medicine use among youth with recurrent headaches. Pediatrics. 2013;132(5):e1173–83.

12. Kristoffersen ES, Aaseth K, Grande RB, Lundqvist C, Russell MB. Self-reported efficacy of complementary and alternative medicine: the Akershus study of chronic headache. J Headache Pain. 2013;14:36.

13. Rhee TG, Harris IM. Gender differences in the use of complementary and alternative medicine and their association with moderate mental distress in U.S. adults with migraines/severe headaches. Headache. 2017;57(1):97–108.

14. Lee J, Bhowmick A, Wachholtz A. Does complementary and alternative medicine (CAM) use reduce negative life impact of headaches for chronic migraineurs? A national survey. Springerplus. 2016;5(1):1006.

15. Gaul C, Schmidt T, Czaja E, Eismann R, Zierz S. Attitudes towards complementary and alternative medicine in chronic pain syndromes: a questionnaire-based comparison between primary headache and low back pain. BMC Complement Altern Med. 2011;11:89.

16. Long L, Huntley A, Ernst E. Which complementary and alternative therapies benefit which conditions? A survey of the opinions of 223 professional organizations. Complement Ther Med. 2001;9(3):178–85.

17. Aveni E, Bauer B, Ramelet A-S, Kottelat Y, Decosterd I, Finti G, et al. The attitudes of physicians, nurses, physical therapists, and midwives toward complementary medicine for chronic pain: a survey at an academic hospital. Explore NY. 2016;12(5):341–6.

18. Peroutka SJ. What turns on a migraine? A systematic review of migraine precipitating factors. Curr Pain Headache Rep. 2014;18(10):454.

19. Martin PR. Stress and primary headache: review of the research and clinical management. Curr Pain Headache Rep. 2016;20(7):45.

20. Wells RE, Loder E. Mind/body and behavioral treatments: the evidence and approach. Headache. 2012;52(Suppl 2):70–5.

21. Goslin RE, Gray RN, McCrory DC, Penzien D, Rains J, Hasselblad V. Behavioral and physical treatments for migraine headache [Internet]. Rockville (MD): Agency for Health Care Policy and Research (US); 1999 [cited 2017 Feb 5]. (AHRQ Technical Reviews). Available from: http://www.ncbi.nlm.nih.gov/books/NBK45267/

22. Campbell J, Penzien D, Wall E. Evidence-based guidelines for migraine headache: Behavioral and physical treatments. US Headache Consortium; 2000.

23. Benson H, Klipper MZ. The relaxation response. New York, NY: William Morrow and Company, Inc.; 1975.

24. Benson H, Malvea BP, Graham JR. Physiologic correlates of meditation and their clinical effects in headache: an ongoing investigation. Headache. 1973;13(1):23–4.

25. Benson H, Klemchuk HP, Graham JR. The usefulness of the relaxation response in the therapy of headache. Headache. 1974;14(1):49–52.

26. Kabat-Zinn J. Wherever you go, there you are. New York, NY: Hyperion books; 1994.

27. Kabat-Zinn J. An outpatient program in behavioral medicine for chronic pain patients based on the practice of mindfulness meditation: theoretical considerations and preliminary results. Gen Hosp Psychiatry. 1982;4(1):33–47.

28. Kabat-Zinn J, Lipworth L, Burney R. The clinical use of mindfulness meditation for the self-regulation of chronic pain. J Behav Med. 1985;8(2):163–90.

29. Grossman P, Niemann L, Schmidt S, Walach H. Mindfulness-based stress reduction and health benefits. A meta-analysis. J Psychosom Res. 2004;57(1):35–43.

30. Hilton L, Hempel S, Ewing BA, Apaydin E, Xenakis L, Newberry S, et al. Mindfulness meditation for chronic pain: systematic review and meta-analysis. Ann Behav Med. 2017;51(2):199–213.

31. Wells RE, Burch R, Paulsen RH, Wayne PM, Houle TT, Loder E. Meditation for migraines: a pilot randomized controlled trial. Headache. 2014;54(9):1484–95.

32. Cathcart S, Galatis N, Immink M, Proeve M, Petkov J. Brief mindfulness-based therapy for chronic tension-type headache: a randomized controlled pilot study. Behav Cogn Psychother. 2014;42(1):1–15.

33. Day MA, Thorn BE, Rubin NJ. Mindfulness-based cognitive therapy for the treatment of headache pain: a mixed-methods analysis comparing treatment responders and treatment non-responders. Complement Ther Med. 2014;22(2):278–85.

34. Omidi A, Zargar F. Effect of mindfulness-based stress reduction on pain severity and mindful awareness in patients with tension headache: a randomized controlled clinical trial. Nurs Midwifery Stud. 2014;3(3):e21136. [cited 2017 Apr 25]; Available from: http://www.ncbi.nlm.nih.gov/pmc/articles/PMC4332994/

35. Bakhshani NM, Amirani A, Amirifard H, Shahrakipoor M. The effectiveness of mindfulness-based stress reduction on perceived pain intensity and quality of life in patients with chronic headache. Glob J Health Sci. 2015;8(4):142–51.
36. Omidi A, Zargar F. Effects of mindfulness-based stress reduction on perceived stress and psychological health in patients with tension headache. J Res Med Sci. 2015;20(11):1058–63.
37. Grazzi L, Sansone E, Raggi A, D'Amico D, De Giorgio A, Leonardi M, et al. Mindfulness and pharmacological prophylaxis after withdrawal from medication overuse in patients with chronic migraine: an effectiveness trial with a one-year follow-up. J Headache Pain. 2017;18(1):15.
38. Kiran, Girgla KK, Chalana H, Singh H. Effect of rajyoga meditation on chronic tension headache. Indian J Physiol Pharmacol. 2014;58(2):157–61.
39. Wachholtz AB, Pargament KI. Is spirituality a critical ingredient of meditation? Comparing the effects of spiritual meditation, secular meditation, and relaxation on spiritual, psychological, cardiac, and pain outcomes. J Behav Med. 2005;28(4):369–84.
40. Wachholtz AB, Pargament KI. Migraines and meditation: does spirituality matter? J Behav Med. 2008;31(4):351–66.
41. Wachholtz AB, Malone CD, Pargament KI. Effect of different meditation types on migraine headache medication use. Behav Med. 2015;11:1–8.
42. Tonelli ME, Wachholtz AB. Meditation-based treatment yielding immediate relief for meditation-naïve migraineurs. Pain Manag Nurs. 2014;15(1):36–40.
43. Feuille M, Pargament K. Pain, mindfulness, and spirituality: a randomized controlled trial comparing effects of mindfulness and relaxation on pain-related outcomes in migraineurs. J Health Psychol. 2015;20(8):1090–106.
44. Hesse T, Holmes LG, Kennedy-Overfelt V, Kerr LM, Giles LL. Mindfulness-based intervention for adolescents with recurrent headaches: a pilot feasibility study. Evid Based Complement Alternat Med. 2015;2015:e508958.
45. Rosenzweig S, Greeson JM, Reibel DK, Green JS, Jasser SA, Beasley D. Mindfulness-based stress reduction for chronic pain conditions: variation in treatment outcomes and role of home meditation practice. J Psychosom Res. 2010;68(1):29–36.
46. Wells RE, Smitherman TA, Seng EK, Houle TT, Loder EW. Behavioral and mind/body interventions in headache: unanswered questions and future research directions. Headache. 2014;54(6):1107–13.
47. Bushnell MC, Ceko M, Low LA. Cognitive and emotional control of pain and its disruption in chronic pain. Nat Rev Neurosci. 2013;14(7):502–11.
48. Zeidan F, Martucci KT, Kraft RA, Gordon NS, McHaffie JG, Coghill RC. Brain mechanisms supporting the modulation of pain by mindfulness meditation. J Neurosci. 2011;31(14):5540–8.
49. Zeidan F, Grant JA, Brown CA, McHaffie JG, Coghill RC. Mindfulness meditation-related pain relief: evidence for unique brain mechanisms in the regulation of pain. Neurosci Lett. 2012;520(2):165–73.
50. Zeidan F, Adler-Neal AL, Wells RE, Stagnaro E, May LM, Eisenach JC, et al. Mindfulness-meditation-based pain relief is not mediated by endogenous opioids. J Neurosci. 2016;36(11):3391–7.
51. Zeidan F, Emerson NM, Farris SR, Ray JN, Jung Y, McHaffie JG, et al. Mindfulness meditation-based pain relief employs different neural mechanisms than placebo and sham mindfulness meditation-induced analgesia. J Neurosci. 2015;35(46):15307–25.
52. Tang Y-Y, Hölzel BK, Posner MI. The neuroscience of mindfulness meditation. Nat Rev Neurosci. 2015;16(4):213–25.
53. Creswell JD. Mindfulness interventions. Annu Rev Psychol. 2017;68:491–516.
54. Day MA, Jensen MP, Ehde DM, Thorn BE. Toward a theoretical model for mindfulness-based pain management. J Pain. 2014;15(7):691–703.
55. Chiesa A, Serretti A. A systematic review of neurobiological and clinical features of mindfulness meditations. Psychol Med. 2010;40(8):1239–52.
56. Shechter A, Stewart WF, Silberstein SD, Lipton RB. Migraine and autonomic nervous system function: a population-based, case-control study. Neurology. 2002;58(3):422–7.
57. Koenig J, Williams DP, Kemp AH, Thayer JF. Vagally mediated heart rate variability in headache patients– a systematic review and meta-analysis. Cephalalgia. 2016;36(3):265–78.
58. Mamontov OV, Babayan L, Amelin AV, Giniatullin R, Kamshilin AA. Autonomic control of cardiovascular reactivity in patients with episodic and chronic forms of migraine. J Headache Pain. 2016;17:52.
59. Azam MA, Katz J, Mohabir V, Ritvo P. Individuals with tension and migraine headaches exhibit increased heart rate variability during post-stress mindfulness meditation practice but a decrease during a post-stress control condition–a randomized, controlled experiment. Int J Psychophysiol. 2016;110:66–74.
60. Keller A, Meyer B, Wöhlbier H-G, Overath CH, Kropp P. Migraine and meditation: characteristics of cortical activity and stress coping in migraine patients, meditators and healthy controls—an exploratory cross-sectional study. Appl Psychophysiol Biofeedback. 2016;41(3):307–13.
61. Day MA, Thorn BE. The mediating role of pain acceptance during mindfulness-based cognitive therapy for headache. Complement Ther Med. 2016;25:51–4.
62. Day MA, Halpin J, Thorn BE. An empirical examination of the role of common factors of therapy during a mindfulness-based cognitive therapy intervention for headache pain. Clin J Pain. 2016;32(5):420–7.
63. Oberg EB, Rempe M, Bradley R. Self-directed mindfulness training and improvement in blood pressure, migraine frequency, and quality of life. Glob Adv Health Med. 2013;2(2):20–5.
64. Sun T-F, Kuo C-C, Chiu N-M. Mindfulness meditation in the control of severe headache. Chang Gung Med J. 2002;25(8):538–41.

65. Kabat-Zinn J, Lipworth L, Burney R, Sellers W, Brew M. Reproducibility and four year follow-up of a training program in mindfulness meditation for the self-regulation of chronic pain. Pain. 1984;18:S303.

66. Field T. Yoga research review. Complement Ther Clin Pract. 2016;24:145–61.

67. Büssing A, Ostermann T, Lüdtke R, Michalsen A. Effects of yoga interventions on pain and pain-associated disability: a meta-analysis. J Pain. 2012;13(1):1–9.

68. Kim S-D. Effects of yoga exercises for headaches: a systematic review of randomized controlled trials. J Phys Ther Sci. 2015;27(7):2377–80.

69. John PJ, Sharma N, Sharma CM, Kankane A. Effectiveness of yoga therapy in the treatment of migraine without aura: a randomized controlled trial. Headache. 2007;47(5):654–61.

70. Sethi BB, Trivedi JK, Anand R. A comparative study of relative effectiveness of biofeedback and shav-asana (yoga) in tension headache. Indian J Psychiatry. 1981;23(2):109–14.

71. Bhatia R, Dureja GP, Tripathi M, Bhattacharjee M, Bijlani RL, Mathur R. Role of temporalis muscle over activity in chronic tension type headache: effect of yoga based management. Indian J Physiol Pharmacol. 2007;51(4):333–44.

72. Boroujeni MZ, Marandi SM, Esfarjani F, Sattar M, Shaygannejad V, Javanmard SH. Yoga intervention on blood NO in female migraineurs. Adv Biomed Res. 2015;4:259.

73. Naji-Esfahani H, Zamani M, Marandi SM, Shaygannejad V, Javanmard SH. Preventive effects of a three-month yoga intervention on endothelial function in patients with migraine. Int J Prev Med. 2014;5(4):424–9.

74. Hainsworth KR, Salamon KS, Khan KA, Mascarenhas B, Davies WH, Weisman SJ. A pilot study of yoga for chronic headaches in youth: promise amidst challenges. Pain Manag Nurs. 2014;15(2):490–8.

75. Wayne PM, Walsh JN, Taylor-Piliae RE, Wells RE, Papp KV, Donovan NJ, et al. Effect of tai chi on cognitive performance in older adults: systematic review and meta-analysis. J Am Geriatr Soc. 2014;62(1):25–39.

76. Hall A, Copsey B, Richmond H, Thompson J, Ferreira M, Latimer J, et al. Effectiveness of tai chi for chronic musculoskeletal pain conditions: updated systematic review and meta-analysis. Phys Ther. 2017;97(2):227–38.

77. Abbott RB, Hui K-K, Hays RD, Li M-D, Pan T. A randomized controlled trial of tai chi for tension headaches. Evid Based Complement Alternat Med. 2007;4(1):107–13.

78. Gerik SM. Pain management in children: developmental considerations and mind-body therapies. South Med J. 2005;98(3):295–302.

Complementary and Alternative Approaches to Chronic Daily Headache: Part II—Manipulation-Based Therapies and Other CAM Therapies

Brielle Paolini, Laura Granetzke, and Rebecca Erwin Wells

Manipulation-Based Therapies: Overview

The manipulation-based complementary and alternative medicine (CAM) therapies assessed in this chapter for headache include acupuncture, acupressure, dry needling, chiropractic manipulation (spinal manipulative and mobilization therapy), massage, craniosacral therapy, and reflexology. Only a few have evidence specific for chronic daily headache (acupuncture and chiropractic); for the other therapies, we review the evidence for other headache types with intent to extrapolate findings for chronic daily headache. Notably, in most studies, manipulation-based techniques are used as preventive therapies rather than abortive treatment.

Acupuncture

Acupuncture dates back to 200 BC [1, 2] and involves the placement of needles at specific

B. Paolini
Wake Forest School of Medicine,
Winston-Salem, NC, USA

L. Granetzke · R. E. Wells (✉)
Neurology, Wake Forest School of Medicine,
Winston-Salem, NC, USA
e-mail: rewells@wakehealth.edu

points throughout the body based on meridians (i.e., channels in the body). These needles are thought to help balance the traditional Chinese medicine concept of *Qi*, or "life force," resulting in improved imbalances and illnesses. Acupuncture is one of the most widely used CAM therapies [3–5]. Its effects are believed to be due to a combination of local effects, spinal and supraspinal mechanisms, and other cortical (i.e., psychological or placebo) responses.

Although acupuncture is extensively used clinically, research into acupuncture has challenges, especially complete blinding of the control group. Sham control is traditionally considered the ideal strategy. The most common sham methods are touching needles to acupuncture points, touching non-acupuncture points without penetration, or superficial needling at non-acupuncture points. No technique is perfect; touching needles to acupuncture points may affect meridians, and physiologic effects of superficial needling may resemble those of true acupuncture. Ideal studies would include a non-active control group and a sham control group, to fully elucidate treatment effects of placebo responses.

Acupuncture and Chronic Daily Headache

Many acupuncture studies use "chronic headache" as an umbrella term, while others differentiate the type as either "chronic migraine" or "chronic tension-type headache" or "chronic mixed type." Also, several studies use the term "chronic headache" to imply the headache has been present for a certain period of time, rather than using ICHD diagnostic criteria of "chronic" defined as meeting a threshold of headache frequency/month (e.g., >15 days/month for migraine and tension-type) for at least 3 months.

The most comprehensive assessment of acupuncture for chronic daily headache was a systematic review published in 2008 that summarized results of 31 clinical trials with 3916 participants—17 trials for migraine, 10 for tension-type headache, and 4 for mixed chronic headache [6]. Only 19 trials used ICHD criteria to diagnose chronic headache. Three trials used ad hoc information, two trials used resistance to traditional therapy, and seven trials used no formal criteria for diagnosis. Using the modified Oxford scale to assess quality (maximum score of 7; 4+ was considered high quality), 14 trials scored more than 4 points, and 5 studies scored a maximum score of 7. The duration of treatment varied (average 10 sessions, range 6–16) over a mean of 8 weeks (range 4–24 weeks). The sham designs were heterogeneous. Randomization was sufficiently addressed in only nine trials, and the longest follow-up period was 2 years (used in five trials).

In the 14 studies comparing acupuncture vs. sham with reported follow-up data, the true acupuncture group had a significantly higher response rate, defined as at least a 33% improvement in headaches (measured by the headache index or headache frequency) than sham (53% vs. 45% response rate, respectively) [6]. Subgroup analyses revealed similar outcomes for tension-type but not migraine headache. No differences were found in headache intensity, frequency, or health-related quality of life when data for the two groups were pooled for each follow-up period. Of the eight studies of acupuncture compared to medication treatment, headache intensity and frequency were reduced in the acupuncture group. Three of the four trials that compared acupuncture to other non-pharmacological treatments found that the other therapy (e.g., massage or physiotherapy) was more effective than acupuncture.

Twelve studies reported acupuncture side effects and 11 provided details. Common acupuncture side effects reported included minor bleeding, bruising, or local paresthesias at needle insertion sites, or triggering of a headache by needle insertion. There were fewer side effects compared to medication treatment trials. The heterogeneity of the studies (in treatment protocol and headache type and the frequent lack of proper control groups) makes it difficult to fully elucidate the placebo response in the reported results. When compared to sham or medication, the results favor acupuncture, suggesting it may have a specific effect beyond placebo for chronic headache; however, the evidence is still quite limited.

Since publication of this systematic review in 2008, a few other studies have investigated acupuncture for chronic headache. A large study compared acupuncture to routine care for primary headache (defined as more than 12 months of having 2 or more headaches per month) in 11,874 non-randomized participants and 3,182 randomized participants [7]. In both groups acupuncture decreased headache days and intensity of pain and persistently improved quality of life through the 6-month follow-up period. One small study ($n = 26$) showed within-group improvements (i.e., no control group) on frequency, duration, and intensity of chronic daily headache diagnosed with IHS criteria after acupuncture (30-min sessions twice a week for 4 weeks, followed by once a week for 4 weeks) [8]. Acupuncture point injection (API) involves the injection of a small amount of medicine or vitamin to enhance the stimulation of acupuncture points. One randomized, double-blinded study of 40 participants with chronic daily headache (minimum of 15 headaches per month) demonstrated that Carthami-Semen (safflower seed) extract API compared to normal saline API resulted in improved quality of life and headache-free days after biweekly injections for 4 weeks [9]. No adverse events were reported.

In summary, acupuncture appears to have beneficial effects on chronic daily headache compared to sham acupuncture and medication treatment, with minimal side effects. The data suggest that acupuncture may have a potential role in management of chronic daily headache. To better assess acupuncture's clinical efficacy and significance regarding chronic daily headache, further studies with more rigorous blinded-controlled designs, longer follow-up periods, and more standardized treatment interventions are needed.

Acupuncture and Migraine

In 2011, a randomized controlled trial (RCT) was published comparing effects of acupuncture and topiramate in 66 patients with chronic migraine [10]. Both the acupuncture (24 sessions over 12 weeks) and the topiramate groups (25 mg daily, titrating weekly to 100 mg/day for 8 weeks) demonstrated improved headache frequency after treatment; however, acupuncture's improvement was larger (20.2 days to 9.8 days vs. 19.8 days to 12.0 days, $p < 0.01$). Differences persisted even in participants with medication overuse. Adverse events were 66% in the topiramate group and only 6% in the acupuncture group. This study lacked a sham acupuncture control group, limiting the interpretation since active procedures such as acupuncture consistently have higher placebo response rates than those with oral medication. Additionally, the acupuncture group had significantly more provider time than the topiramate group (24 versus 6 visits), and patients were unblinded. Despite these limitations, this study demonstrates acupuncture may be of similar benefit for chronic migraine as a daily prophylactic medication such as topiramate, without the frequent side effects. Future work should focus on whether acupuncture as an add-on therapy to topiramate or other prophylactic medication has additive or synergistic effects on chronic migraine [11].

A Cochrane database review in 2016 investigating acupuncture for episodic migraine prophylaxis (22 trials with 4,985 participants) found a small but statistically significant reduction in headache frequency over sham, usual care and drug prophylaxis at 2 months; however, the findings were statistically heterogeneous [12]. A recent study ($n = 249$) demonstrated that 30-minute sessions of acupuncture (5 days/week for 4 weeks) with electrical stimulation decreased migraine frequency and intensity after 16 weeks compared to sham acupuncture [13].

Acupuncture and Tension Headache

A number of studies have evaluated acupuncture specifically for chronic tension-type headaches and are well summarized in a Cochrane systematic review (initially published in 2009, updated in 2016 including only one new trial) [14]. The review analyzed 12 RCTs of at least 8-week duration, which included 2,349 patients with either episodic or chronic tension-type headache. Treatments varied (6–15 weekly sessions and follow-up periods of 8–24 weeks). Acupuncture point selection also varied across studies. Quality assessment of all studies was low to moderate due to a high risk of bias, lack of blinding and variable effect sizes in diverse trials. Seven studies compared acupuncture to sham acupuncture; of the five studies with data for meta-analyses, acupuncture had benefit over sham acupuncture (51% vs. 43% with at least 50% reduction in headache frequency), with effects lasting 6 months. Only three of the seven trials reported an adverse event (17% with acupuncture and 12% with sham). In the two trials that compared acupuncture to routine care, those who received acupuncture had a greater likelihood of a 50% reduction in headache frequency. Four trials compared acupuncture to physiotherapy, massage, or exercise; acupuncture was not superior to the other interventions, and some outcomes demonstrated better results for the other treatment option. The review concluded that the quality of evidence is moderate or low and that acupuncture is effective for treating frequent episodic or chronic tension-type headaches.

It is unclear whether patients with tension-type headaches respond differently to acupuncture compared to migraine patients and whether the presence of more than one headache type influences outcome. A study of self-reported CAM efficacy reported that acupuncture was effective in 38% of participants with chronic tension-type headache and co-occurrence of migraine, compared to only 11% without the co-occurrence [15].

Considering its low risk, acupuncture may be a worthwhile option for patients suffering from chronic tension-type headache, especially those unwilling or unable to tolerate long-term medication management [16]. Future work should include comparing acupuncture with other treatment options [14, 17].

Acupuncture and Cluster Headache

Limited evidence exists for CAM therapies and cluster headache [18–20]. In one small case report, four patients with cluster headaches (three with episodic and one with chronic) reported reduction or elimination of attacks with acupuncture treatment (twice/week for 2 weeks, then once/week for 8 weeks, and then once/alternate weeks for 2 weeks) combined with verapamil or alone [21]. Such a report is encouraging, but further research is needed to evaluate acupuncture for cluster.

Acupuncture and Pediatric Headache

Only a few studies have evaluated acupuncture in pediatric headache patients and none specifically for chronic headache. One RCT of 43 patients under 18 years old with episodic migraine (n = 22) or tension-type headache (n = 21) showed that 4 weekly treatments of laser acupuncture was more effective in decreasing headache frequency, severity, and duration than placebo laser acupuncture [22]. This research suggests that laser acupuncture, which uses a low-energy laser to stimulate headache-related acupuncture points [23], could be a useful non-traumatic, non-painful treatment for children (considered safe as long as the proper energy dosage is used with eye protection), especially those who are afraid of needles or intolerant of medications. A study of 19 pediatric patients who received auricular acupuncture (where acupuncture needles are applied to the ear) demonstrated it might be an option for abortive treatment in the emergency department [24]. However, this study did not have a control group.

Acupuncture and Cost Analysis

Lack of affordability is one of the most frequently cited reasons for not having acupuncture. Two RCTs investigated the cost-effectiveness of acupuncture for headache. In 1 study of 401 patients with "chronic headache" (defined as at least 2 headaches/month) in Wales and England, participants were randomized to acupuncture (12 sessions over 3 months) or usual care alone. Acupuncture was more expensive (~$768 vs. $413/year), but the mean health gain from acupuncture was 0.021 quality-adjusted life years (QALYs), and the cost difference for acupuncture was substantially lower when evaluated per QALY. The authors conclude that since "acupuncture for chronic headache improves health-related quality of life at a small additional cost, it is relatively cost-effective [25]." A similar RCT involving 3,182 patients in Germany found similar increased costs with acupuncture, but it still met the international thresholds for cost-effectiveness [26]. Nonetheless, insurance companies rarely cover acupuncture. In addition, the time and energy to complete a course of acupuncture treatment must be considered. To be compliant, one needs lifestyle flexibility to attend treatment without negative impact on missed partial days of work or school [27]. Future studies should consider these additional factors in assessing cost benefit for acupuncture with long-term follow-up.

Acupuncture Summary of Evidence and Recommendations

Acupuncture research is challenging to evaluate because of the variability of protocols (e.g., frequency and duration of treatment, location of acupuncture points), the heterogeneity of control groups and blinding, and the resulting high risk of bias. Despite these limitations, the evidence for acupuncture for headache is promising. Some moderate evidence supports the use of acupuncture in chronic daily headache, and weak evidence supports the use of acupuncture point injection (API) therapy in the treatment of chronic daily headache. Acupuncture may be as efficacious for chronic migraine as topiramate and has many fewer side effects [10]. There is only weak or moderate evidence for acupuncture in treating episodic or chronic tension-type headaches. The limited data on acupuncture for cluster headaches preclude any recommendations. Although acupuncture costs more than usual care alone, its improvements in health-related quality of life might be worth the small additional cost. In a participant with the financial means and time availability, acupuncture may be an effective treatment for chronic daily headache, chronic migraine, and possibly chronic tension-type headache. Considering the overall low risks, acupuncture is an important headache treatment consideration, especially in those unwilling or unable to tolerate long-term medication management [16].

Acupressure

Acupressure uses fingers instead of needles at acupuncture points and is a low-cost, noninvasive technique with very limited side effects [28]. A small ($n = 28$) RCT in "chronic headache" (defined as over 6 months of headaches, with four or more per month) demonstrated the benefit of acupressure plus "placebo" (15 mg/day of riboflavin/vitamin B2) over the muscle relaxant mephenoxalone, based on self-appraised pain scores at 1 and 6 months of follow-up. Unfortunately, this study did not include headache frequency or duration effects, and the "placebo" pill of vitamin B2 may have benefited headache, limiting its clinical usefulness [28]. The acupressure wristband Sea-Band®, used to stimulate a distinct acupoint that helps nausea, showed benefit in aborting migraine-associated nausea in a study of 40 participants [29].

Limited research and methodologic concerns of acupressure for headache prevents the recommendation of its use. If an individual has chronic migraine and cannot tolerate an antiemetic, acupressure may be a non-drug option. Future RCTs should include active placebo groups as well as a non-active control to tease out placebo responses and include metrics of headache frequency, duration, and medication use.

Dry Needling

Dry needling has becoming increasingly popular over the last decade to treat headaches [30, 31]. It is defined by the American Physical Therapy Association (APTA) as a "skilled intervention using a thin filiform needle to penetrate the skin and stimulate trigger points, muscles, and connective tissues for the treatment of musculoskeletal disorder [32]." Unlike acupuncture, dry needling is not based in the theoretical concept of *Qi*, and it is not administered along meridians. Instead, the practitioner identifies tender taut bands within a muscle that are thought to be hyperalgesic [33]. The most common technique is the "fast-in and fast-out" technique [34] where a needle is inserted into a trigger point until a quick twitch is observed (a sudden contraction of the muscle fibers in the taut band). Once the twitch is obtained, the needle is then moved up and down around 3–5 mm at a frequency of 1 Hz. The duration of treatment depends on the irritation of the trigger point [31]. The pathophysiology and mechanism of action of dry needling is under debate but is thought to decrease concentrations of pro-inflammatory substances locally [31, 35] and to induce ischemia and hypoxia resulting in vasodilation, potential angiogenesis and altered glucose metabolism [30]. Additionally, dry needling is thought to decrease peripheral sensitization and mitigate central sensitization [30, 31] by diminishing the prolonged cause of peripheral nociceptive input modulating the dorsal horn's response and activating central inhibitory pain pathways [36].

Despite its increasing use, the evidence supporting dry needling therapy for headache is limited. A recent systematic review on dry needling for cervicogenic or tension-type headache [37] resulted in the analysis of 3 studies, two RCTS (with n's of 45 and 30 participants with tension-type and/or migraine headaches) and a third case report ($n = 1$) on cervicogenic headache. All three studies showed significant improvement with dry needling over 4–5 weeks of treatment; however, they did not show greater effectiveness than other techniques (e.g., lidocaine injections, lidocaine plus corticosteroid injections, or superficial dry needling). The case report supported the addition of dry needling to conventional physiotherapy versus dry needling alone in cervicogenic headache. Adverse effects were not sufficiently reported or described. The three studies used different needling methodologies and had very heterogeneous samples with varying control groups, limiting the power of their evidence [31]. One prospective study investigating adverse events found that out of 7,629 treatments, only 1,463 (9%) reported mild adverse events (e.g., bruising, bleeding, or pain), and no physiotherapists reported serious adverse events [38]. In summary, there is insufficient evidence to strongly support the use of dry needling to treat chronic daily headache or other types of headache. Further research should be done with greater methodologic rigor and with attention to potential side effects.

Chiropractic Manipulation

Chiropractic manipulation includes spinal manipulation (more commonly used) and spinal mobilization. Spinal manipulation uses high-velocity, low-amplitude forces to move a joint slightly beyond its passive range [39]. Through spinal mobilization, the application of low-velocity, variable amplitude force is intended to cause movement of the joint within its natural passive range [39]. Spinal manipulation and mobilization are thought to exert benefit in two ways—by decreasing nociceptive input from the cervical spine structure and by modulating pain centrally through spinal and supraspinal mechanisms [40–47]. However, other cortical modulators also may play a role, such as expectancy, placebo, and other nonspecific effects [39].

Chiropractic Manipulation and "Chronic Daily Headache"

A 2001 systematic review of spinal manipulation for "chronic headache" (tension, migraine, and cervicogenic) included 9 RCTs with nearly 683 patients [48]. Spinal manipulation was considered superior to massage for cervicogenic headache and may have an effect similar to first-line prophylactic medications for tension-type and migraine headaches. Importantly, the review included studies with episodic headache (one study of episodic tension, one study with both episodic and chronic tension), and four were spe-

cific to chronic headache (including migraine, cervicogenic, and muscle-tension headache). Many studies had very poor to adequate methodologic quality and heterogeneous methodologies which prevented pooled analyses, greatly limiting the review's conclusions. In addition to the evidence described, the Cochrane database plans to release a review on manual treatments for prevention of migraine, tension-type headache, and cervicogenic headache that will provide additional understanding of the evidence to date [49].

Chiropractic Manipulation and Cervicogenic Headache

A 2015 Cochrane review of chiropractic manipulation for neck pain [50] included 51 trials but only 2 trials [51, 52] for treatment of cervicogenic headache (total $n = 125$ participants). Both studies had low methodologic quality; the authors concluded that multiple sessions of spinal manipulative therapy were superior to light massage in improving pain and function of chronic cervicogenic headache at short-term and immediate-term follow-up [50, 53]. Of the 51 studies, less than half reported adverse events; of those, only temporary and benign side effects were reported [50]. The needed frequency and duration of treatment for effect remain unclear. Although 12 sessions appear better than 3 sessions [51], no differences were seen between 12 to 16 and 3 to 8 treatments [51, 52]. A recent review of 10 RCTs ($n = 685$) investigated chiropractic manipulation for cervicogenic headache [47], and all studies had an active control group (physical therapy) or placebo [36, 41, 51, 53–58]. Many of the studies in this review have already been discussed. One study determined that manipulation was more effective than mobilization in decreasing cervicogenic headache duration, frequency, and associated disability [47]. A dose-response study of spinal manipulation for cervicogenic headache [59] with pending results per clinicaltrials.gov [60] may provide additional insight on the effect of cervical manipulation for cervicogenic headache. In addition, a single-blinded, placebo-controlled RCT investigating spinal manipulative therapy for cervicogenic headache [61] also has pending results [62].

Chiropractic Manipulation and Tension Headache

Currently, two RCTs have investigated spinal manipulative therapy for chronic tension-type headaches. Some studies evaluating the effectiveness of spinal manipulative therapy tend to group it with massage and physical therapy, under the umbrella term "manual therapies." For instance, one partially blinded, multicenter RCT ($n = 82$) found that manual therapy (mobilization of the cervical and thoracic spine, exercises, and postural correction; maximum of nine treatments over 8 weeks) reduced headache frequency, improved disability and cervical function, and decreased medication use more than usual care for chronic tension-type headaches [63]. Since this study included multiple modalities, the findings are not specific for spinal manipulation. Adverse events were not reported.

A well-designed older RCT ($n = 150$; included in the review above with chronic headaches) showed that 6 weeks of amitriptyline was more effective in reducing pain than spinal manipulative therapy (twice weekly for 6 weeks at 20 min/session) to treat chronic tension-type headache (1 headache/week for at least 3 months). Those receiving amitriptyline had more side effects (82% vs. 4%); as expected, effects disappeared once amitriptyline was stopped. However, 4 weeks after treatment, those who underwent spinal manipulative therapy had statistically significant improvement in headache frequency, intensity, medication use, and functional health status (on the SF-36 instrument) compared to baseline [64]. Of the participants who completed the study, 43 (82.1%) in the amitriptyline group reported side effects (drowsiness, dry mouth, and weight gain), and three (4.3%) in the spinal manipulative group reported side effects (neck soreness and stiffness).

Both of these studies lacked blinding, increasing their risk of bias. The preliminary data are somewhat promising for spinal manipulative therapy for chronic tension-type headache, but currently there are not enough strong data to support its use. A Cochrane database protocol was published assessing manual treatment for the prevention of tension-type headache, but results are pending [49, 65]. A 2006 review of six studies included a variety of manual therapies, limiting its specificity for spinal manipulative therapies; this review concluded that there was no evidence that manual therapies are effective for tension-type headache [66].

A 2012 systematic review of five ($n = 348$), mostly high-quality RCTs (Jada scores between 2 and 4, scale is from 1 to 5) investigated spinal manipulative therapy for tension-type headache [67]. Two of the studies were mentioned above and found a benefit of spinal manipulative therapy for chronic tension-type headache [64, 68]. Of the three other studies, one found no significant difference between spinal manipulative therapy and control groups in daily headache hours, headache intensity, or medication use in individuals with tension-type headache (IHS criteria) [69]. There were no adverse events. Another study ($n = 22$) found improved subjective ratings of pain relief after osteopathic spinal manipulative therapy versus palpatory examination or no intervention for muscle contraction headache; however, the limited outcome measures and lack of randomization limit its clinical usefulness [70]. Adverse events were not reported. The final study ($n = 19$) compared cervical spinal manipulative therapy plus amitriptyline to cervical spinal manipulative therapy + placebo vs. sham cervical spinal manipulation plus amitriptyline vs. sham cervical spinal manipulation plus placebo (three times/week for 6 weeks, one time/week for 4 weeks). The only group that had a statistically significant reduction in headache frequency was the combined treatment (spinal manipulative therapy and amitriptyline) [71]. The small sample size and wide confidence intervals limit the clinical usefulness of the findings. Four subjects experienced AEs after spinal manipulative therapy (e.g., minor aggravations of neck pain or headaches) and five after amitriptyline (e.g., nausea, fatigue, sleep disturbance, dry mouth, and constipation).

Since these reviews appeared, two additional RCTs were published investigating spinal manipulative therapy and tension-type headache. One study randomized participants ($n = 84$, episodic tension-type headache 57.1%, chronic tension-type headache 42.9%) into manual therapy, manipulative therapy, a combination of manual or manipulative therapy (4 treatments over 4 weeks for all previous groups), or a control group. All treatment groups had statistically significant improvements in pain perception, frequency, and intensity; however, the manipulative treatment was most effective, showing statistically significant improvement in all pain dimensions at post-treatment and 4-week follow-up. Importantly, the control group also had significant differences in three of five dimensions of pain (sensory, evaluative, and intensity) on the McGill Pain Questionnaire. Headache frequency was significantly lower at follow-up in the combination treatment group [72]. No adverse events were reported. The second RCT ($n = 105$) published in 2016 found that manipulation treatment plus massage (4 treatments over 4 weeks) decreased headache frequency compared to massage only in patients with tension-type headache. Headache disability inventory (HDI) scores improved in both groups. This study lacks a true control group, so it is impossible to differentiate the results from a placebo response, providing limited evidence for massage alone or combined with manipulative therapy for tension-type headache [73].

One study assessed the benefit of using a self-acupressure pillow daily versus chiropractic care alone for patients with both tension-type and cervicogenic headache ($n = 34$). Both groups improved, but no difference between groups was found [74].

Chiropractic Manipulation and Migraine

In 2011, a systematic review summarized three RCTs that investigated spinal manipulative therapy for migraine [75]. The RCTs had mostly poor methodologic quality (1–3 on Jadad scale that ranges from 1 to 5) [76–78]. Two were described above in the chronic headache review and suggested no effect of spinal manipulation on the headache index or migraine duration and disability compared to drug therapy, spinal manipulation plus drug therapy, or mobilization [76, 77]. One RCT showed significantly reduced migraine frequency, intensity, duration, and disability

compared with a control group that underwent detuned interferential therapy (electrodes without current) [78]. However, this study lacked appropriate randomization, blinding, and intention-to-treat analysis and included selective reporting (Jadad scale 1). One observational study and one recent RCT have been published subsequently. The first study ($n = 11$, $n = 6$ chronic migraine) found a statistically and clinically significant reduction in headache days and headache disability after atlas vertebra realignment compared to baseline; however, there was no control or placebo group. Studies of pharmacologic interventions indicate that the placebo response is high in migraineurs [79]. Future studies should include a proper control.

A recent, well-designed, single-blinded, prospective RCT ($n = 104$) investigated spinal manipulative therapy for migraine (at least one attack/month) [80]. The study had three groups including spinal manipulative therapy, a placebo group (i.e., sham maneuvers to the scapula and/or gluteal region), and a control group of usual care. The treatment period was 3 months, and follow-up occurred at 3, 6, and 12 months. The study used a newly validated sham placebo for manual therapy [81], and this is the first manual-therapy RCT to document successful blinding [80]. Migraine days were significantly reduced for all three groups compared to baseline, and this effect remained at follow-up for the spinal manipulative and placebo groups at all time points. The control group (usual care) did return to baseline posttreatment. The authors concluded that improvements in migraine with chiropractic spinal manipulation were likely only due to placebo response.

Chiropractic Manipulation and Pediatrics

One prospective, randomized, single-blind multicenter study ($n = 52$) found that both spinal manipulative therapy and placebo (i.e., light touch in a specific cervical segment without manipulation) decreased the frequency of headaches posttreatment compared to baseline in children and adolescents with cervicogenic headache; however, no difference existed between treatment and placebo [55]. Neither placebo nor spinal manipulation decreased the duration or intensity of the headaches or use of medication from baseline to posttreatment.

Chiropractic Manipulation and Cost Analysis

Little data are available on cost-benefit analysis of spinal manipulative and mobilization therapy for headache. One Cochrane review published in 2004 concluded, "there is moderate evidence for an economic advantage in using multidisciplinary care, defined as mobilization and manipulation plus exercise, for mechanical neck disorders" [82]. In addition to the financial cost of treatment, participants need flexible schedules to attend treatments regularly. Lack of insurance coverage also impacts availability and access to care. Future studies should be conducted on the cost-benefit ratio for spinal manipulative and mobilization therapy with long-term follow-up.

Chiropractic Manipulation and Adverse Events

A recent review found that out of 118 reviews, 54 concluded that manipulation was safe, 15 concluded that it was harmful, and the remainder were neutral or unclear [83]. The most common adverse events were stroke, headache, and vertebral artery dissection, with incidence estimates for such serious adverse events ranging from 1 in 20,000 to 1 in 250,000,000 manipulations. A 2017 literature review assessing the risk of adverse events after cervical spinal manipulation found that although women had a slightly increased risk compared to men, the authors could not delineate a clear patient profile related to risk [84]. The recent well-designed RCT with three arms evaluating chiropractic spinal manipulation in migraineurs (with the sham maneuver control group) [80] closely monitored for side effects prospectively in the 70 participants and found that of the 703 sessions, local tenderness (7–11%) and fatigue (1–9%) were the most common side effects, with no severe or serious AEs reported [85]. A few case-control studies have also suggested a link between spinal manipulative therapy and stroke from cervical artery dissection [86–88], and in one large nested case-control study ($n = 457$), spinal manipulative therapy was independently associated with vertebral arterial dissection, even after controlling for neck pain [89]. However a case-control and case-crossover study using 100 million person-years of data found no excess risk of stroke in those who had chiropractic care versus medical care [90]. The authors argue that the association arises from individuals seeking treatment for neck pain and headache, symptoms that precede 80% of vertebrobasilar strokes. However, as we recently concluded, "[arterial dissection or stroke post spinal manipulative therapy] are catastrophic events which, however rare, must weigh heavily in any assessment of this approach" [91].

Chiropractic Manipulation: Summary of Recommendations

There is no specific evidence for the use of spinal manipulative therapy for chronic daily headache. There is some evidence supporting its use in chronic cervicogenic headache based on two RCTs. The data for episodic cervicogenic headache are heterogeneous, limiting their clinical usefulness. One well-designed RCT suggested that spinal manipulative therapy was helpful for the long-term treatment of chronic tension-type headaches. Amitriptyline outperformed spinal manipulative therapy in the short term, but it was associated with more adverse events. The other study on chronic tension-type headache used a number of modalities, limiting specificity for spinal manipulative therapy treatment. The data for chiropractic treatment and episodic tension-type headache are weak. Most studies investigating spinal manipulative therapy and migraine are of poor methodologic quality. A recent well-designed RCT concluded that the benefit of spinal manipulative therapy for migraine is likely due to the placebo response [80]. No evidence supports the use of spinal manipulative therapy in children or adolescents. While the studies presented reported only minor adverse events, the risk of a cervical dissection or stroke, however unlikely, is serious and must be weighed into any clinical decision. At this time, the lack of strong data supporting the use of spinal manipulation therapy combined with the lack of good data investigating its potential serious risk precludes a recommendation for treatment of chronic daily headache.

Massage

Massage is defined as the manipulation of muscles and other soft tissues. There are many specific types (e.g., trigger point therapy, Swedish, structural, relaxation, Thai massage, traditional, traditional court-type Thai, connective tissue release, and cross-friction massage) [39]. The mechanism of action is considered to be similar to spinal manipulative therapy and dry needling (see above) by decreasing nociceptive input from the cervical spine and by modulating pain centrally.

Massage and "Chronic Headache"

Currently, no studies directly investigate massage therapy for chronic daily headache. A few exist for chronic tension-type headache, and one study included both chronic tension-type headache and chronic migraine patients. Many studies are small and do not include headache frequency or duration measures, significantly limiting their clinical relevance. The study of both migraine and tension-type chronic headache patients ($n = 72$) randomized individuals to receive traditional Thai massage or sham ultrasound (both groups received nine sessions over 3 weeks) and found no statistically significant difference in headache intensity [92].

Massage and Tension Headache

The first systematic review of manual therapy for primary chronic headache was published in 2014 and included six RCTs; however, only one study addressed massage therapy [93]. It was a prospective crossover RCT of 11 participants with chronic tension-type headache; headache intensity decreased 24 h after a massage (2 treatments within 1 week) compared to the control group (which received detuned ultrasound and electrodes without current) [94].

A RCT ($n = 60$) published in 2015 reported that individuals with chronic tension-type headache randomized to receive court-type traditional

Thai massage (45-min Thai massage twice per week for 4 weeks) had lower pain intensity (VAS scores) at 2, 4, and 6 weeks compared to medication treatment (25 mg of amitriptyline daily for 4 weeks). The court-type traditional Thai massage group also had decreased tissue hardness and increased heart rate variability suggesting that this treatment is a modulator of parasympathetic activity [95]. However, the study lacked relevant metrics for headache parameters, limiting its clinical significance.

Three additional small studies were done on chronic tension-type headache and massage. The first ($n = 11$) found a single session of massage was associated with significant increases in heart rate variability, decreases in head pain at 24 h, and decreased negative mood states (tension-anxiety and anger-hostility subscales of the profile of mood states) after treatment; the placebo group (detuned ultrasound) did not have these changes [94]. This study also lacked relevant headache parameters. The second study ($n = 11$) found a significant decrease in headache frequency 1 week after massage treatment (4 weeks of biweekly 30-min massage treatments) that lasted until the end of the study [96]. There was no change in headache intensity after treatment compared to the 8-week baseline, but a trend existed for a shorter duration of headaches. This study had a high dropout rate (6/10), and it did not have an adequate control or placebo group, limiting its conclusions. The third study ($n = 21$) included only women and found that upper body massage (ten sessions) significantly decreased pain intensity (VAS scale), the number of days with neck pain, and scores on the Finnish Pain Questionnaire while increasing range of motion [97]. This study lacked a control or placebo group, as well as measurements of relevant headache parameters.

Two RCTs [98, 99], one previously mentioned study [73] and one pilot study [100], have examined massage therapy for tension-type headache. The first recent RCT [98] ($n = 97$) included individuals with both chronic and episodic tension-type headache diagnosed by ICHD criteria. Its four-arm design included placebo superficial massage, soft tissue techniques, neural mobilization techniques, or a combination of soft tissue and neural mobilization techniques (each arm included 6 15-min treatments). The soft tissue, neural mobilization, and the combination group all reported increased pain pressure thresholds, fewer headaches, less maximal intensity of headaches, and improved quality of life (HIT-6) compared to baseline and the placebo group. The combination group had the highest pain pressure threshold and the lowest headache frequency and HIT-6 values after intervention.

In one study described above in the chiropractic section, Espi-Lopez et al. found that massage treatment improved Headache Disability Index (HDI) scores and cervical range of motion in 105 patients with tension-type headache; however, the effect was enhanced when combined with spinal manipulative therapy [73]. This study lacks a true control group limiting evidence for massage alone or combined with manipulative therapy for tension-type headache.

Another RCT conducted in 2015 found myofascial trigger point massage (12 45-min treatments over 6 weeks) decreased headache frequency significantly from baseline for recurrent tension-type headache in 56 participants; however, the placebo group (detuned ultrasound) also had statistically significant decreases in headache frequency from baseline, and no differences were found between groups [99]. This study likely only captured a placebo response, underscoring the importance of including both active placebo and control groups in a well-designed trial [99].

In 2008, a pilot study with tension-type headache (2004 IHS guidelines and physician confirmation, 13 = chronic, 3 = episodic) found massage therapy (45-min biweekly massages for 6 weeks) significantly reduced headache frequency, intensity, and duration and improved HDI scores compared to baseline [100]. Future work should include a larger sample size, a placebo group, and proper controls.

Massage and Migraine

Only one RCT has addressed chronic migraine and massage [101]. In this study of 26 individuals, migraine was diagnosed by questionnaire.

The study reported that massage therapy (30 min/week for 5 weeks) reduced pain intensity by 71% compared to a control group (unchanged from baseline). It is unknown what questionnaire criteria were used to diagnose chronic migraine, and the study did not track migraine frequency or duration, limiting the clinical significance of its findings.

Two RCTs [102, 103] and one small study [104] have also been conducted on massage and migraine. The first RCT (n = 64) randomized individuals with migraine (with and without aura, diagnosed by IHS criteria) to lymphatic drainage (a gentle pressure technique thought to improve lymphatic flow), traditional massage, or a waiting group [102]. After a 4-week baseline, the treatment period was 8 weeks followed by a 4-week observation period. At the end of the observation period, both treatment groups had significantly fewer migraine attacks and migraine days than the waiting group. The lymphatic drainage group also had significantly less medication use during the intervention than the other two groups. The second RCT [103] recruited 47 individuals with migraine (51% had more than one attack/month, with 48-h mean duration) diagnosed by questionnaire. The massage group (weekly massage sessions for 5 weeks) had greater improvements in migraine frequency and sleep quality during the intervention and in the 3 follow-up weeks compared to the control group. There was no difference in the intensity of the attacks between groups or medication use, but a trend existed for perceived stress and coping efficacy for the massage group. Migraine duration changes were not reported. The final study investigated the use of massage and spinal manipulation during an acute migraine attack in ten men [104]. After treatment, the participants had a statistically significant decrease in pain intensity. No adverse events were reported, but other headache parameters were not investigated.

Massage and Cervicogenic Headache

Three studies have been conducted on massage for the treatment of cervicogenic headache, including one pilot RCT and two small studies.

One randomized study ($n = 136$) published in 2015 found a specific form of micro-regulating massage (described as "micro-regulating with vertical cross press lying on one side") was associated with lower headache intensity and decreased headache frequency, compared to traditional massage. It is unknown what criteria were used to diagnose cervicogenic headache, and the study did not have a control group, seriously limiting its clinical interpretation [105].

A pilot RCT ($n = 20$) found that trigger point therapy (manual therapy on active trigger points in the sternocleidomastoid muscle) decreased headache and neck pain intensity and improved motor performance more than a control treatment (simulated trigger point therapy without pressure application) in individuals with a known diagnosis of cervicogenic headache, using the criteria of Sjaastad and Fredricksen [106]. This study demonstrated feasibility of study design; however, it did not include measures of headache duration or frequency, limiting its clinical utility [107].

A single-group, pre-post test pilot study found that soft tissue cervical massage (three treatments of 8 min over 1 week) improved range of motion in eight individuals with cervicogenic headache; however, headache intensity, duration, and frequency were not studied [108].

It is unknown how much range of motion clinically relates to these important headache variables.

Massage and Pediatric Headaches

One small pilot study ($n = 9$, all girls) found that trigger point-specific physical therapy (twice weekly over 4 weeks) reduced headache frequency by 67.7%, intensity by 74.3%, and duration by 77.3% [109]. This study lacked a control group, making it impossible to detect placebo effects.

Massage and Cost Analysis

Few data are available on cost-benefit analysis of massage therapy for headache. In addition to the financial cost of treatment, participants need to have flexible schedules to attend treatment regularly. Lack of insurance coverage also impacts availability and access to care. Future studies should be conducted on cost benefit for massage therapy with long-term follow-up, including quality -of -life metrics.

Massage and Adverse Events

Many massage studies do not report on adverse events. A systematic review of adverse events due to "pain-related massage" from case reports published between 2003 and 2013 (clinical trials were excluded) found 43 case reports, with only 7 containing reports of 95 adverse events [110]. From the seven reports, massage was only reported in one of the cases as the manual therapy utilized, and cervical disc herniation was reported. The other treatment modalities were actually spinal manipulative therapies.

Massage: Summary of Recommendations

Currently, no studies have examined the use of massage therapy for chronic daily headache. Those that have investigated massage and chronic headache are severely limited by their exclusion of standard headache metrics. Many studies were small and lacked proper control groups. There are some preliminary data from two RCTs supporting massage for episodic migraine treatment; however, the optimal mode of treatment, intervals, and frequency are still unknown. The long-term impact of massage therapy on disease process should also be studied in larger patient groups. The three studies investigating massage for episodic cervicogenic headache were too poorly designed to provide any evidence for the use of massage for cervicogenic headache. There is some preliminary evidence supporting massage therapy for episodic tension headache, based on the findings of one well-designed RCT [98]. The efficacy of massage therapy for pediatric patients is currently unknown.

The current evidence on massage and chronic daily headache is inconclusive. There is some weak evidence for massage for episodic migraine and tension-type headache. The studies reviewed used a variety of manual therapy techniques and study designs, making global clinical inferences challenging. At this time evidence is lacking to recommend massage for treatment of chronic daily headache. It may be a useful adjunct for medication-resistant or medication-intolerant individuals, as massage is typically considered safe; however, additional research into adverse events is needed. The biggest barrier for most patients' use of massage therapy is cost, as it is rarely covered by insurance. Some patients report using a pretax health savings or flex spending account to help cover the costs.

Craniosacral Manipulation

Craniosacral therapy is based on the idea that a craniosacral fluid rhythm exists and, if restricted, can be released by a practitioner who is manually identifying restrictions in the craniosacral system and using gentle hand adjustments to release and restore these rhythms [111]. One small study ($n = 20$) of CST vs. wait-list control demonstrated improvements in HIT-6 scores after 6 craniosacral treatments over 4 weeks for treatment of migraine (via ICHD criteria; at least 5–15 headaches per month for at least 2 years) [111]. The lack of a control group limits the interpretation of these findings. The lack of high-quality evidence limits the recommendation of craniosacral therapy for chronic daily headache.

Reflexology

Reflexology is a type of foot massage based on the theory that various reflex zones on the feet correspond to a particular organ of the body and its associated energy level. Reflexologists believe that circulation improves when the reflex zones are stimulated with pressure [112]. No specific studies have investigated reflexology for chronic daily headache. One prospective, exploratory study without a control group assessed the impact of 6 months of reflexology treatments on 220 migraine or tension-type patients in Denmark; 81% reported improvements in their headaches. Due to the lack of high-quality evidence, reflexology is not recommended for the treatment of chronic daily headache.

Other Complementary and Alternative Treatment Approaches

Several other complementary therapies discussed include aromatherapy, hydrotherapy, daith piercing, and oxygen administration.

Aromatherapy

Aromatherapy and oils have been used as early as 800–900 AD [113]. Peppermint, eucalyptus, chamomile, and lavender are examples of oils commonly used by patients. Inhaler lavender significantly reduced headache severity in control (3.6 ± 2.8) compared to placebo (1.6 ± 1.6) groups in one clinical trial ($n = 47$). Another study analyzed neurophysiologic and analgesic effects of peppermint and/or eucalyptus and/or ethanol when topically applied to the forehead and temples ($n = 32$) [114]. Although no combinations were associated with reduced experimental pain sensitivity, sensitivity to head stimulus was significantly reduced in the peppermint plus ethanol group. Further research is needed to further elucidate the potential benefits of aromatherapy for headache.

Hydrotherapy

Hydrotherapy, the use of water for pain relief, is a very old treatment reported to help many chronic pain and arthritis conditions. There are many different techniques, but most either submerge the body or part of the body in hot or cold water and/or apply hot or cold compresses to the body. Due to the hypothesized pathophysiology of local vasoconstriction followed by reflexive vasodilation, it has been theorized to be beneficial for migraine [115]. One small study ($n = 40$) evaluated hydrotherapy (45 days of hot arm and foot bath of 103–110 °F and 20 min of daily head ice massage) plus conventional medication therapy or conventional medication therapy alone for chronic migraine [115]. Both groups had improved headache outcomes and HIT-6 scores, although more so in the hydrotherapy group. Better heart rate variability in the hydrotherapy group led to the assessment of "improved vagal tone." However, the paucity of data limits our ability to recommend hydrotherapy for chronic daily headache at this time.

Daith Piercing

Daith piercing, a piercing located in the innermost cartilage fold of the ear, has become increasingly popular for the treatment of headaches due to individual reports via social media and a website that reports 40 anecdotal cases of benefit after receiving the piercing [116]. The piercing does not coincide with any known acupuncture point for headache treatment [117]. There are no systematic studies investigating its effectiveness, and experts believe that the relief is often temporary (1–2 weeks). The cost is usually minimal; however, extreme care must be taken up to 6 months after the piercing to avoid infection [117]. Given the potential risk of infection and the lack of evidence supporting benefit, daith piercing is not recommended for chronic daily headache.

Oxygen Administration

Oxygen administration therapies take two forms. One administers oxygen at high percentage of normal atmospheric pressure (normobaric oxygen therapy), and the other administers 100% oxygen at pressures above one atmosphere (hyperbaric oxygen therapy). Normobaric oxygen therapy has Grade A evidence for its use as an abortive treatment option for cluster headache [118] and is thus not considered a CAM therapy for cluster treatment. Interestingly, one recent 2016 pilot study ($n = 22$) demonstrated potential efficacy for the use of normobaric oxygen treatment for migraine [119]. While the primary endpoint was negative (mean decrease in pain score at 30 min), overall relief of pain, nausea, and

visual symptoms at 60 min were better in oxygen group compared to air group, without any significant adverse events. Hyperbaric oxygen therapy has limited evidence yet many purport its benefits, with the hypothesized mechanism of oxygen as a serotonergic agonist, an immuno-modulator of substance P and neuropeptides, and a modulator of inflammatory pathways [120–125]. The remainder of this section will discuss evidence for hyperbaric oxygen use for headache treatment. There is currently no specific data on oxygen administration for chronic daily headache.

A 2015 Cochrane review (11 studies and 209 participants) had 2 new studies to update the prior 2008 review [126] investigating the effectiveness and safety of oxygen administration for migraine and cluster headache [124]. For prevention of migraine, one study failed to show a difference between hyperbaric oxygen ($n = 20$) and sham ($n = 20$) for mean number of headache days, proportion of participants with nausea/vomiting, or the use of rescue medicine compared to sham therapy [127]. Three of the five studies were pooled ($n = 58$) and found hyperbaric oxygen to be more effective in treating acute migraine headaches compared to sham. One study ($n = 56$) found a significant reduction in pain intensity (VAS scores) after 1 h of normobaric oxygen administration compared to sham for acute migraine treatment. Only two small ($n = 16$ and $n = 16$) studies have evaluated hyperbaric oxygen for abortive [128] and prophylactic [129] cluster treatment (respectively), and both were negative.

While oxygen administration has major risks, such as fire (especially for smokers—and most cluster patients smoke), respiratory arrest (which can occur in chronically hypercarbic patients relying on hypoxic drive for respiration), pulmonary barotraumas, worsening of shortsightedness (reversible), claustrophobia, and oxygen poisoning, only two trials specifically mentioned adverse events [127, 130], and only four very minor adverse events (claustrophobia and running out of trial gas) were reported [124].

In summary, there is minimal evidence for the use of hyperbaric oxygen for abortive migraine treatment and no evidence for its use for preventive migraine treatment or chronic daily headache. Hyperbaric oxygen has failed to show any benefit for abortive or prophylactic cluster treatment and has the potential for major risks.

Summary: Manipulation-Based and Other Therapies for Chronic Daily Headache

Manipulation-based therapies have been reported more extensively than mind/body options, although many studies have similar methodologic concerns. Heterogeneous interventions add challenges to interpretation and generalizability of such interventions. The strongest evidence for acupuncture is for chronic migraine, and cost analyses suggest it may have overall cost benefit. There is some evidence for spinal manipulative therapy for chronic cervicogenic headache or chronic tension-type headache, but most chiropractic studies also have major methodologic limitations. The potential for major adverse events, such as cervical dissection, limit more widespread recommendation for use. There are no data supporting the use of massage for any chronic headache conditions. Other complementary therapies (aromatherapy, homeopathy, daith piercing, and hyperbaric oxygen administration) have minimal evidence to support their use for chronic daily headache.

Part III reviews the evidence regarding nutraceuticals and homeopathy for chronic daily headache and final conclusions from Parts I, II, and III.

Acknowledgments Dr. Wells is supported by the National Center for Complementary and Integrative Health of the National Institutes of Health under Award Number K23AT008406. The content is solely the responsibility of the authors and does not necessarily represent the official views of the National Institutes of Health. We gratefully acknowledge the editorial assistance of Karen Klein, MA, in the Wake Forest Clinical and Translational Science Institute, funded by the National Center for Advancing Translational Sciences (NCATS), National Institutes of Health, through Grant Award Number UL1TR001420. We also thank Mark McKone, Librarian at Carpenter Library, Wake Forest School of Medicine, for his help with the use of Zotero. We are appreciative of the help from Nakiea Choate from the Department of Neurology at Wake Forest Baptist for her administrative support.

References

1. Kaptchuk TJ. Acupuncture: theory, efficacy, and practice. Ann Intern Med. 2002;136(5):374–83.
2. Cady RK, Farmer K. Acupuncture in the treatment of headache: a traditional explanation of an ancient art. Headache. 2015;55(3):457–64.
3. Endres HG, Diener H-C, Molsberger A. Role of acupuncture in the treatment of migraine. Expert Rev Neurother. 2007;7(9):1121–34.
4. Kristoffersen ES, Grande RB, Aaseth K, Lundqvist C, Russell MB. Management of primary chronic headache in the general population: the Akershus study of chronic headache. J Headache Pain. 2012;13(2):113–20.
5. Wells RE, Bertisch SM, Buettner C, Phillips RS, McCarthy EP. Complementary and alternative medicine use among adults with migraines/severe headaches. Headache. 2011;51(7):1087–97.
6. Sun Y, Gan TJ. Acupuncture for the management of chronic headache: a systematic review. Anesth Analg. 2008;107(6):2038–47.
7. Jena S, Witt CM, Brinkhaus B, Wegscheider K, Willich SN. Acupuncture in patients with headache. Cephalalgia. 2008;28(9):969–79.
8. Plank S, Goodard J. The effectiveness of acupuncture for chronic daily headache: an outcomes study. Mil Med. 2009;174(12):1276–81.
9. Park J-M, Park S-U, Jung W-S, Moon S-K. Carthami-semen acupuncture point injection for chronic daily headache: a pilot, randomised, double-blind, controlled trial. Complement Ther Med. 2011;19(Suppl 1):S19–25.
10. Yang C-P, Chang M-H, Liu P-E, Li T-C, Hsieh C-L, Hwang K-L, et al. Acupuncture versus topiramate in chronic migraine prophylaxis: a randomized clinical trial. Cephalalgia. 2011;31(15):1510–21.
11. Wang S-J, Young WB. Needling the pain and comforting the brain: acupuncture in the treatment of chronic migraine. Cephalalgia. 2011;31(15):1507–9.
12. Linde K, Allais G, Brinkhaus B, Fei Y, Mehring M, Vertosick EA, et al. Acupuncture for the prevention of episodic migraine. Cochrane Database Syst Rev. 2016;6:CD001218.
13. Zhao L, Chen J, Li Y, Sun X, Chang X, Zheng H, et al. The long-term effect of acupuncture for migraine prophylaxis: a randomized clinical trial. JAMA Intern Med. 2017;177(4):508–15.
14. Linde K, Allais G, Brinkhaus B, Fei Y, Mehring M, Shin B-C, et al. Acupuncture for the prevention of tension-type headache. Cochrane Database Syst Rev. 2016;4:CD007587.

15. Kristoffersen ES, Aaseth K, Grande RB, Lundqvist C, Russell MB. Self-reported efficacy of complementary and alternative medicine: the Akershus study of chronic headache. J Headache Pain. 2013;14:36.

16. Glickman-Simon R. Acupuncture may be effective for prevention of tension-type headache, but magnitude of improvement may be small compared to sham. Explore NY. 2016;13(2):145–6.

17. Coeytaux RR, Befus D. Role of acupuncture in the treatment or prevention of migraine, tension-type headache, or chronic headache disorders. Headache. 2016;56(7):1238–40.

18. Cheng AC. The treatment of headaches employing acupuncture. Am J Chin Med. 1975;3(2):181–5.

19. Thoresen A. Alternative therapy of cluster headache. Tidsskr Den Nor Laegeforening Tidsskr Prakt Med Ny Raekke. 1998;118(22):3508.

20. Gwan KH. Treatment of cluster headache by acupuncture. Am J Chin Med. 1977;5(1):91–4.

21. Fofi L, Allais G, Quirico PE, Rolando S, Borgogno P, Barbanti P, et al. Acupuncture in cluster headache: four cases and review of the literature. Neurol Sci. 2014;35(Suppl 1):195–8.

22. Gottschling S, Meyer S, Gribova I, Distler L, Berrang J, Gortner L, et al. Laser acupuncture in children with headache: a double-blind, randomized, bicenter, placebo-controlled trial. Pain. 2008;137(2):405–12.

23. Ebneshahidi NS, Heshmatipour M, Moghaddami A, Eghtesadi-Araghi P. The effects of laser acupuncture on chronic tension headache–a randomised controlled trial. Acupunct Med. 2005;23(1):13–8.

24. Graff DM, McDonald MJ. Auricular acupuncture for the treatment of pediatric migraines in the emergency department. Pediatr Emerg Care. 2016;34(4):258–62.

25. Wonderling D, Vickers AJ, Grieve R, McCarney R. Cost effectiveness analysis of a randomised trial of acupuncture for chronic headache in primary care. BMJ. 2004;328(7442):747.

26. Witt CM, Reinhold T, Jena S, Brinkhaus B, Willich SN. Cost-effectiveness of acupuncture treatment in patients with headache. Cephalalgia. 2008;28(4):334–45.

27. Solomon S. Acupuncture for headache. It's still all placebo. Headache. 2017;57(1):143–6.

28. Hsieh LL-C, Liou H-H, Lee L-H, Chen TH-H, Yen AM-F. Effect of acupressure and trigger points in treating headache: a randomized controlled trial. Am J Chin Med. 2010;38:1):1–14.

29. Allais G, Rolando S, Castagnoli Gabellari I, Burzio C, Airola G, Borgogno P, et al. Acupressure in the control of migraine-associated nausea. Neurol Sci. 2012;33(Suppl 1):S207–10.

30. Kietrys DM, Palombaro KM, Mannheimer JS. Dry needling for management of pain in the upper quarter and craniofacial region. Curr Pain Headache Rep. 2014;18(8):437.

31. Fernández-De-Las-Peñas C, Cuadrado ML. Dry needling for headaches presenting active trigger points. Expert Rev Neurother. 2016;16(4):365–6.

32. Gardner K. Dry needling in physical therapy [Internet]. [cited 2017 Mar 8]. Available from: http://www.apta.org/StateIssues/DryNeedling/.

33. Cagnie B, Dewitte V, Barbe T, Timmermans F, Delrue N, Meeus M. Physiologic effects of dry needling. Curr Pain Headache Rep. 2013;17(8):348.

34. Hong CZ. Lidocaine injection versus dry needling to myofascial trigger point. The importance of the local twitch response. Am J Phys Med Rehabil. 1994;73(4):256–63.

35. Shah JP, Phillips TM, Danoff JV, Gerber LH. An in vivo microanalytical technique for measuring the local biochemical milieu of human skeletal muscle. J Appl Physiol. 2005;99(5):1977–84.

36. Dunning JR, Butts R, Mourad F, Young I, Fernandez-de-Las Peñas C, Hagins M, et al. Upper cervical and upper thoracic manipulation versus mobilization and exercise in patients with cervicogenic headache: a multi-center randomized clinical trial. BMC Musculoskelet Disord. 2016;17:64.

37. France S, Bown J, Nowosilskyj M, Mott M, Rand S, Walters J. Evidence for the use of dry needling and physiotherapy in the management of cervicogenic or tension-type headache: a systematic review. Cephalalgia. 2014;34(12):994–1003.

38. Brady S, McEvoy J, Dommerholt J, Doody C. Adverse events following trigger point dry needling: a prospective survey of chartered physiotherapists. J Man Manip Ther. 2014;22(3):134–40.

39. Haas M, Brønfort G, Evans RL, Leininger B, Schmitt J, Levin M, et al. Spinal rehabilitative exercise or manual treatment for the prevention of cervicogenic headache in adults. Cochrane Database Syst Rev. 2016;5:CD012205.

40. Coronado RA, Gay CW, Bialosky JE, Carnaby GD, Bishop MD, George SZ. Changes in pain sensitivity following spinal manipulation: a systematic review and meta-analysis. J Electromyogr Kinesiol. 2012;22(5):752–67.

41. Jull G, Trott P, Potter H, Zito G, Niere K, Shirley D, et al. A randomized controlled trial of exercise and manipulative therapy for cervicogenic headache. Spine. 2002;27(17):1835–43. discussion 1843

42. O'Leary S, Falla D, Jull G. Recent advances in therapeutic exercise for the neck: implications for patients with head and neck pain. Aust Endod J. 2003;29(3):138–42.

43. Bialosky JE, Bishop MD, Price DD, Robinson ME, George SZ. The mechanisms of manual therapy in the treatment of musculoskeletal pain: a comprehensive model. Man Ther. 2009;14(5):531–8.

44. Bialosky JE, George SZ, Horn ME, Price DD, Staud R, Robinson ME. Spinal manipulative therapy-specific changes in pain sensitivity in individuals with low back pain (NCT01168999). J Pain. 2014;15(2):136–48.

45. Pickar JG, Bolton PS. Spinal manipulative therapy and somatosensory activation. J Electromyogr Kinesiol. 2012;22(5):785–94.

46. Zhou L, Hud-Shakoor Z, Hennessey C, Ashkenazi A. Upper cervical facet joint and spinal rami

blocks for the treatment of cervicogenic headache. Headache. 2010;50(4):657–63.

47. Garcia JD, Arnold S, Tetley K, Voight K, Frank RA. Mobilization and manipulation of the cervical spine in patients with cervicogenic headache: any scientific evidence? Front Neurol. 2016;7:40.

48. Bronfort G, Assendelft WJ, Evans R, Haas M, Bouter L. Efficacy of spinal manipulation for chronic headache: a systematic review. J Manip Physiol Ther. 2001;24(7):457–66.

49. Brønfort G, Haas M, Evans RL, Goldsmith CH, Assendelft WJJ, Bouter LM. WITHDRAWN: non-invasive physical treatments for chronic/recurrent headache. Cochrane Database Syst Rev. 2014;8:CD001878.

50. Gross A, Langevin P, Burnie SJ, Bédard-Brochu M-S, Empey B, Dugas E, et al. Manipulation and mobilisation for neck pain contrasted against an inactive control or another active treatment. Cochrane Database Syst Rev. 2015;9:CD004249.

51. Haas M, Groupp E, Aickin M, Fairweather A, Ganger B, Attwood M, et al. Dose response for chiropractic care of chronic cervicogenic headache and associated neck pain: a randomized pilot study. J Manip Physiol Ther. 2004;27(9):547–53.

52. Haas M, Spegman A, Peterson D, Aickin M, Vavrek D. Dose response and efficacy of spinal manipulation for chronic cervicogenic headache: a pilot randomized controlled trial. Spine J. 2010;10(2):117–28.

53. Youssef EF, Shanb A-SA. Mobilization versus massage therapy in the treatment of cervicogenic headache: a clinical study. J Back Musculoskelet Rehabil. 2013;26(1):17–24.

54. Haas M, Schneider M, Vavrek D. Illustrating risk difference and number needed to treat from a randomized controlled trial of spinal manipulation for cervicogenic headache. Chiropr Osteopat. 2010;18:9.

55. Borusiak P, Biedermann H, Bosserhoff S, Opp J. Lack of efficacy of manual therapy in children and adolescents with suspected cervicogenic headache: results of a prospective, randomized, placebo-controlled, and blinded trial. Headache. 2010;50(2):224–30.

56. Shin E-J, Lee B-H. The effect of sustained natural apophyseal glides on headache, duration and cervical function in women with cervicogenic headache. J Exerc Rehabil. 2014;10(2):131–5.

57. Nilsson N, Christensen HW, Hartvigsen J. The effect of spinal manipulation in the treatment of cervicogenic headache. J Manip Physiol Ther. 1997;20(5):326–30.

58. Hall T, Chan HT, Christensen L, Odenthal B, Wells C, Robinson K. Efficacy of a C1-C2 self-sustained natural apophyseal glide (SNAG) in the management of cervicogenic headache. J Orthop Sports Phys Ther. 2007;37(3):100–7.

59. Hanson L, Haas M, Bronfort G, Vavrek D, Schulz C, Leininger B, et al. Dose-response of spinal manipulation for cervicogenic headache: study protocol for a randomized controlled trial. Chiropr Man Therap. 2016;24:23.

60. Haas M. Cervicogenic headache dose-response [Internet]. clinicaltrials.gov. [cited 2017 Jun 30]. Available from: https://clinicaltrials.gov/show/NCT01530321.

61. Chaibi A, Benth JŠ, Tuchin PJ, Russell MB. Chiropractic spinal manipulative therapy for cervicogenic headache: a study protocol of a single-blinded placebo-controlled randomized clinical trial. Springerplus. 2015;4:779.

62. Chaibi A. Is chiropractic spinal manipulative therapy an efficient treatment option in cervicogenic headache [Internet]. clinicaltrials.gov. [cited 2017 Jun 30]. Available from: https://clinicaltrials.gov/show/NCT01687881.

63. Castien RF, van der Windt DAWM, Grooten A, Dekker J. Effectiveness of manual therapy for chronic tension-type headache: a pragmatic, randomised, clinical trial. Cephalalgia. 2011;31(2):133–43.

64. Boline PD, Kassak K, Bronfort G, Nelson C, Anderson AV. Spinal manipulation vs. amitriptyline for the treatment of chronic tension-type headaches: a randomized clinical trial. J Manip Physiol Ther. 1995;18(3):148–54.

65. Leininger B, Brønfort G, Haas M, Schmitt J, Evans RL, Levin M, et al. Spinal rehabilitative exercise or manual treatment for the prevention of tension-type headache in adults. Cochrane Database Syst Rev. 2016;2016(4):CD012139.

66. Fernández-de-Las-Peñas C, Alonso-Blanco C, Cuadrado ML, Miangolarra JC, Barriga FJ, Pareja JA. Are manual therapies effective in reducing pain from tension-type headache?: a systematic review. Clin J Pain. 2006;22(3):278–85.

67. Posadzki P, Ernst E. Spinal manipulations for tension-type headaches: a systematic review of randomized controlled trials. Complement Ther Med. 2012;20(4):232–9.

68. Castien RF, van der Windt DAWM, Dekker J, Mutsaers B, Grooten A. Effectiveness of manual therapy compared to usual care by the general practitioner for chronic tension-type headache: design of a randomised clinical trial. BMC Musculoskelet Disord. 2009;10:21.

69. Bove G, Nilsson N. Spinal manipulation in the treatment of episodic tension-type headache: a randomized controlled trial. JAMA. 1998;280(18):1576–9.

70. Hoyt WH, Shaffer F, Bard DA, Benesler JS, Blankenhorn GD, Gray JH, et al. Osteopathic manipulation in the treatment of muscle-contraction headache. J Am Osteopath Assoc. 1979;78(5):322–5.

71. Vernon H, Jansz G, Goldsmith CH, McDermaid C. A randomized, placebo-controlled clinical trial of chiropractic and medical prophylactic treatment of adults with tension-type headache: results from a stopped trial. J Manip Physiol Ther. 2009;32(5):344–51.

72. Espí-López GV, Gómez-Conesa A. Efficacy of manual and manipulative therapy in the perception

of pain and cervical motion in patients with tension-type headache: a randomized, controlled clinical trial. J Chiropr Med. 2014;13(1):4–13.

73. Espí-López GV, Zurriaga-Llorens R, Monzani L, Falla D. The effect of manipulation plus massage therapy versus massage therapy alone in people with tension-type headache. A randomized controlled clinical trial. Eur J Phys Rehabil Med. 2016;52(5):606–17.

74. Vernon H, Borody C, Harris G, Muir B, Goldin J, Dinulos M. A randomized pragmatic clinical trial of chiropractic care for headaches with and without a self-acupressure pillow. J Manip Physiol Ther. 2015;38(9):637–43.

75. Posadzki P, Ernst E. Spinal manipulations for the treatment of migraine: a systematic review of randomized clinical trials. Cephalalgia. 2011;31(8):964–70.

76. Nelson CF, Bronfort G, Evans R, Boline P, Goldsmith C, Anderson AV. The efficacy of spinal manipulation, amitriptyline and the combination of both therapies for the prophylaxis of migraine headache. J Manip Physiol Ther. 1998;21(8):511–9.

77. Parker GB, Tupling H, Pryor DS. A controlled trial of cervical manipulation of migraine. Aust NZ J Med. 1978;8(6):589–93.

78. Tuchin PJ, Pollard H, Bonello R. A randomized controlled trial of chiropractic spinal manipulative therapy for migraine. J Manip Physiol Ther. 2000;23(2):91–5.

79. Hróbjartsson A, Gøtzsche PC. Placebo interventions for all clinical conditions. Cochrane Database Syst Rev. 2010;1:CD003974.

80. Chaibi A, Benth JŠ, Tuchin PJ, Russell MB. Chiropractic spinal manipulative therapy for migraine: a three-armed, single-blinded, placebo, randomized controlled trial. Eur J Neurol. 2017;24(1):143–53.

81. Chaibi A, Šaltytė Benth J, Bjørn Russell M. Validation of placebo in a manual therapy randomized controlled trial. Sci Rep. 2015;5:11774.

82. Gross AR, Hoving JL, Haines TA, Goldsmith CH, Kay T, Aker P, et al. A Cochrane review of manipulation and mobilization for mechanical neck disorders. Spine. 2004;29(14):1541–8.

83. Nielsen SM, Tarp S, Christensen R, Bliddal H, Klokker L, Henriksen M. The risk associated with spinal manipulation: an overview of reviews. Syst Rev. 2017;6(1):64.

84. Kranenburg HA, Schmitt MA, Puentedura EJ, Luijckx GJ, van der Schans CP. Adverse events associated with the use of cervical spine manipulation or mobilization and patient characteristics: a systematic review. Musculoskelet Sci Pract. 2017;28:32–8.

85. Chaibi A, Benth JŠ, Tuchin PJ, Russell MB. Adverse events in a chiropractic spinal manipulative therapy single-blinded, placebo, randomized controlled trial for migraineurs. Musculoskelet Sci Pract. 2017;29:66–71.

86. Kawchuk GN, Jhangri GS, Hurwitz EL, Wynd S, Haldeman S, Hill MD. The relation between the spatial distribution of vertebral artery compromise and exposure to cervical manipulation. J Neurol. 2008;255(3):371–7.

87. Biller J, Sacco RL, Albuquerque FC, Demaerschalk BM, Fayad P, Long PH, et al. Cervical arterial dissections and association with cervical manipulative therapy: a statement for healthcare professionals from the american heart association/american stroke association. Stroke. 2014;45(10):3155–74.

88. Church EW, Sieg EP, Zalatimo O, Hussain NS, Glantz M, Harbaugh RE. Systematic review and meta-analysis of chiropractic care and cervical artery dissection: no evidence for causation. Cureus. 2016;8(2):e498.

89. Smith WS, Johnston SC, Skalabrin EJ, Weaver M, Azari P, Albers GW, et al. Spinal manipulative therapy is an independent risk factor for vertebral artery dissection. Neurology. 2003;60(9):1424–8.

90. Cassidy JD, Boyle E, Côté P, He Y, Hogg-Johnson S, Silver FL, et al. Risk of vertebrobasilar stroke and chiropractic care: results of a population-based case-control and case-crossover study. J Manip Physiol Ther. 2009;32(2 Suppl):S201–8.

91. Wells RE. Spinal manipulation for headaches: will better quality trials do the trick? Headache. 2011;51(7):1149–51.

92. Chatchawan U, Eungpinichpong W, Sooktho S, Tiamkao S, Yamauchi J. Effects of Thai traditional massage on pressure pain threshold and headache intensity in patients with chronic tension-type and migraine headaches. J Altern Complement Med. 2014;20(6):486–92.

93. Chaibi A, Russell MB. Manual therapies for primary chronic headaches: a systematic review of randomized controlled trials. J Headache Pain. 2014;15:67.

94. Toro-Velasco C, Arroyo-Morales M, Fernández-de-Las-Peñas C, Cleland JA, Barrero-Hernández FJ. Short-term effects of manual therapy on heart rate variability, mood state, and pressure pain sensitivity in patients with chronic tension-type headache: a pilot study. J Manip Physiol Ther. 2009;32(7):527–35.

95. Damapong P, Kanchanakhan N, Eungpinichpong W, Putthapitak P, Damapong P. A randomized controlled trial on the effectiveness of court-type traditional thai massage versus amitriptyline in patients with chronic tension-type headache. Evid Based Complement Altern Med. 2015;2015:930175.

96. Quinn C, Chandler C, Moraska A. Massage therapy and frequency of chronic tension headaches. Am J Public Health. 2002;92(10):1657–61.

97. Puustjärvi K, Airaksinen O, Pöntinen PJ. The effects of massage in patients with chronic tension headache. Acupunct Electrother Res. 1990;15(2):159–62.

98. Ferragut-Garcías A, Plaza-Manzano G, Rodríguez-Blanco C, Velasco-Roldán O, Pecos-Martín D, Oliva-Pascual-Vaca J, et al. Effectiveness of a treatment involving soft tissue techniques and/or neural mobilization techniques in the management of tension-type headache: a randomized controlled

trial. Arch Phys Med Rehabil. 2017;98(2):211–219. e2.

99. Moraska AF, Stenerson L, Butryn N, Krutsch JP, Schmiege SJ, Mann JD. Myofascial trigger point-focused head and neck massage for recurrent tension-type headache: a randomized, placebo-controlled clinical trial. Clin J Pain. 2015;31(2):159–68.

100. Moraska A, Chandler C. Changes in clinical parameters in patients with tension-type headache following massage therapy: a pilot study. J Man Manip Ther. 2008;16(2):106–12.

101. Hernandez-reif M, Dieter J, Field T, Swerdlow B, Diego M. Migraine headaches are reduced by massage therapy. Int J Neurosci. 1998;96(1–2):1–11.

102. Happe S, Peikert A, Siegert R, Evers S. The efficacy of lymphatic drainage and traditional massage in the prophylaxis of migraine: a randomized, controlled parallel group study. Neurol Sci. 2016;37(10):1627–32.

103. Lawler SP, Cameron LD. A randomized, controlled trial of massage therapy as a treatment for migraine. Ann Behav Med. 2006;32(1):50–9.

104. Noudeh YJ, Vatankhah N, Baradaran HR. Reduction of current migraine headache pain following neck massage and spinal manipulation. Int J Ther Massage Bodywork. 2012;5(1):5–13.

105. Ding H, Tang X. Study on the clinical effect of the massage method of micro-regulating with vertical cross pressing lying on one side in treating cervicogenic headache. Zhongguo Gu Shang. 2015;28(8):722–6.

106. Sjaastad O, Fredriksen TA. Cervicogenic headache: criteria, classification and epidemiology. Clin Exp Rheumatol. 2000;18(2 Suppl 19):S3–6.

107. Bodes-Pardo G, Pecos-Martín D, Gallego-Izquierdo T, Salom-Moreno J, Fernández-de-Las-Peñas C, Ortega-Santiago R. Manual treatment for cervicogenic headache and active trigger point in the sternocleidomastoid muscle: a pilot randomized clinical trial. J Manip Physiol Ther. 2013;36(7):403–11.

108. Hopper D, Bajaj Y, Kei Choi C, Jan O, Hall T, Robinson K, et al. A pilot study to investigate the short-term effects of specific soft tissue massage on upper cervical movement impairment in patients with cervicogenic headache. J Man Manip Ther. 2013;21(1):18–23.

109. von Stülpnagel C, Reilich P, Straube A, Schäfer J, Blaschek A, Lee S-H, et al. Myofascial trigger points in children with tension-type headache: a new diagnostic and therapeutic option. J Child Neurol. 2009;24(4):406–9.

110. Yin P, Gao N, Wu J, Litscher G, Xu S. Adverse events of massage therapy in pain-related conditions: a systematic review. Evid Based Complement Altern Med. 2014;2014:480956.

111. Mann JD, Faurot KR, Wilkinson L, Curtis P, Coeytaux RR, Suchindran C, et al. Craniosacral therapy for migraine: protocol development for an exploratory controlled clinical trial. BMC Complement Altern Med. 2008;8:28.

112. Launsø L, Brendstrup E, Arnberg S. An exploratory study of reflexological treatment for headache. Altern Ther Health Med. 1999;5(3):57–65.

113. Zargaran A, Borhani-Haghighi A, Faridi P, Daneshamouz S, Kordafshari G, Mohagheghzadeh A. Potential effect and mechanism of action of topical chamomile (Matricaria chammomila L.) oil on migraine headache: a medical hypothesis. Med Hypotheses. 2014;83(5):566–9.

114. Göbel H, Schmidt G, Soyka D. Effect of peppermint and eucalyptus oil preparations on neurophysiological and experimental algesimetric headache parameters. Cephalalgia. 1994;14(3):228–34. discussion 182.

115. Sujan MU, Rao MR, Kisan R, Abhishekh HA, Nalini A, Raju TR, et al. Influence of hydrotherapy on clinical and cardiac autonomic function in migraine patients. J Neurosci Rural Pract. 2016;7(1):109–13.

116. Does daith piercing really work?: First anecdotal study of its kind [Internet]. The daily migraine. [cited 2017 Feb 4]. Available from: http://www.the-dailymigraine.com/blog/2016/3/1/does-daith-piercing-really-work-first-anecdotal-study-of-its-kind.

117. Does daith ear piercing help with migraines? [Internet]. [cited 2017 Mar 6]. Available from: http://www.acupuncture.org.uk/public-content/public-ask-an-expert/ask-an-expert-neuro-and-psycho-logical/ask-an-expert-headache/4974-does-daith-ear-piercing-help-with-migraines.html.

118. Francis GJ, Becker WJ, Pringsheim TM. Acute and preventive pharmacologic treatment of cluster headache. Neurology. 2010;75(5):463–73.

119. Singhal AB, Maas MB, Goldstein JN, Mills BB, Chen DW, Ayata C, et al. High-flow oxygen therapy for treatment of acute migraine: a randomized cross-over trial. Cephalalgia. 2016;37(8):730–6.

120. Di Sabato F, Giacovazzo M, Cristalli G, Rocco M, Fusco BM. Effect of hyperbaric oxygen on the immunoreactivity to substance P in the nasal mucosa of cluster headache patients. Headache. 1996;36(4):221–3.

121. Di Sabato F, Rocco M, Martelletti P, Giacovazzo M. Hyperbaric oxygen in chronic cluster headaches: influence on serotonergic pathways. Undersea Hyperb Med. 1997;24(2):117–22.

122. Slotman GJ. Hyperbaric oxygen in systemic inflammation … HBO is not just a movie channel anymore. Crit Care Med. 1998;26(12):1932–3.

123. Sümen G, Cimşit M, Eroglu L. Hyperbaric oxygen treatment reduces carrageenan-induced acute inflammation in rats. Eur J Pharmacol. 2001;431(2):265–8.

124. Bennett MH, French C, Schnabel A, Wasiak J, Kranke P, Weibel S. Normobaric and hyperbaric oxygen therapy for the treatment and prevention of migraine and cluster headache. Cochrane Database Syst Rev. 2015;12:CD005219.

125. Rozen TD. Inhaled oxygen for cluster headache: efficacy, mechanism of action, utilization, and economics. Curr Pain Headache Rep. 2012;16:175–9.

126. Bennett MH, French C, Schnabel A, Wasiak J, Kranke P. Normobaric and hyperbaric oxygen ther-

apy for migraine and cluster headache. Cochrane Database Syst Rev. 2008;3:CD005219.

127. Eftedal OS, Lydersen S, Helde G, White L, Brubakk AO, Stovner LJ. A randomized, double blind study of the prophylactic effect of hyperbaric oxygen therapy on migraine. Cephalalgia. 2004;24(8):639–44.

128. Di Sabato F, Fusco BM, Pelaia P, Giacovazzo M. Hyperbaric oxygen therapy in cluster headache. Pain. 1993;52(2):243–5.

129. Nilsson Remahl AIM, Ansjön R, Lind F, Waldenlind E. Hyperbaric oxygen treatment of active cluster headache: a double-blind placebo-controlled cross-over study. Cephalalgia. 2002;22(9):730–9.

130. Cohen AS, Burns B, Goadsby PJ. High-flow oxygen for treatment of cluster headache: a randomized trial. JAMA. 2009;302(22):2451–7.

Complementary and Alternative Approaches to Chronic Daily Headache: Part III—Nutraceuticals

20

Laura Granetzke, Brielle Paolini, and Rebecca Erwin Wells

Nutraceuticals

The term "nutraceutical" was coined by Dr. Stephen DeFelice in 1989 as a combination of "nutrition" and "pharmaceutical" and was defined as "a food, or part of a food, that provides medical or health benefits, including the prevention and/or treatment of a disease" [1]. Currently, this term is used loosely and has no regulatory definition. The Dietary Supplement Health and Education Act (DSHEA) of 1994 defined the US Food and Drug Administration's (FDA) statutory authority over dietary supplements [2]. A dietary supplement is "a product that is intended to supplement the diet and may contain one or more dietary ingredients. A dietary ingredient may be any of the following: a vitamin or mineral; an herb or other botanical; amino acid; a dietary substance for use by humans to supplement the diet by increasing the total dietary intake; a concentrate, metabolite, constituent, extract, or combination of the preceding ingredients."

Dietary supplements are used by nearly half of the US population [3]. Unlike pharmaceutical products, the FDA expects the manufacturer to maintain quality and safety standards. Thus, dietary supplements are not required to pass safety and efficacy studies in humans before production and sale. Voluntary adverse event reporting exists, and if the FDA has scientific proof and determines a product to be unsafe, the FDA can issue a warning or require that it be removed [4]. Past products have required numerous years to assemble sufficient data and prove harm prior to market removal [3]. The FDA also oversees the health claims that are used for dietary supplements. Specifically, supplements are allowed to make claims of health benefit, nutrient content, and structure/function, but not of specific disease treatment or prevention [5].

The supplement market has grown from 4000 products in 1994 to over 85,000 by 2014, and the ability to purchase them online has increased their accessibility [3]. In addition, the high cost of prescription drugs, disparities in prescription coverage, and the public's perception that all "natural" medicines are good are cited as reasons for the explosion of this market [1]. Many patients report using supplements to avoid side effects associated with some prescription medications (70%) or because they have an integrated approach to their health (52%) or are generally dissatisfied with conventional medicine (32%) [6]. However, since the FDA allows companies control over the manufacturing process, the accuracy of labeling and purity of some supplements have come into question. Investigations of supplements are ongoing for (1) claims of potential

20

L. Granetzke (✉) · R. E. Wells
Neurology, Wake Forest School of Medicine,
Winston-Salem, NC, USA
e-mail: rewells@wakehealth.edu

B. Paolini
Wake Forest School of Medicine,
Winston-Salem, NC, USA

© Springer International Publishing AG, part of Springer Nature 2019
M. W. Green et al. (eds.), *Chronic Headache*, https://doi.org/10.1007/978-3-319-91491-6_20

contaminants [7] and (2) poor quality (lack of advertised ingredient or different dosage from claim) [8]. Supplement companies can pay for third-party testing to confirm content and accuracy. Consumers can use this "stamp of approval" on bottles to confirm accuracy and quality of the product.

In the 2007 National Health Interview Survey (n = 23,393), 26.7% of adults with self-reported migraines/severe headaches reported using herbal/other supplements (even without including multivitamins in this category); usage was split across 44 different supplements [9]. Children also frequently use supplements. In an Italian survey of 124 4- to 16-year-old children with a primary headache diagnosis by IHS criteria, 64% reported use of herbal remedies (such as *Valeriana*, *Ginkgo biloba*, *Boswellia serrata*, *Vitex agnus-castus*, passionflower, linden tree), and 40% reported use of vitamins/mineral supplements (such as magnesium, 5-hydroxytryptophan, vitamin B6 or B12, multivitamin compounds); baseline CAM use in this group was 76% [6]. A larger, multicenter Italian study (n = 706 children/adolescents with a primary headache disorder using ICHD-IIIβ criteria) found a lower, but still meaningful, prevalence of nutraceutical use (32%) and melatonin use (10%) [10]. Of note, perceived efficacy of melatonin and nutraceuticals was similar to prophylactic drugs (75% vs. 68% vs. 75%, respectively). Despite such frequent use, it is estimated that 60% of patients do not report CAM use to their providers [9, 11].

Few studies have evaluated the benefit of nutraceuticals specifically for chronic daily headache. Therefore, the research evidence conducted for headache will be described, with the hope that this information can help inform use in those with chronic daily headache. Based on evidence and efficacy for headache, nutraceuticals included in this review are *Tanacetum parthenium* (feverfew), riboflavin, magnesium, CoQ10, melatonin, vitamin D, and ginkgolide B (*Ginkgo biloba*). The evidence for homeopathy is also discussed.

Although Level A evidence exists for *Petasites* (butterbur), it is not currently recommended secondary to potential for liver toxicity [4, 12, 13].

Feverfew

The herb *Tanacetum parthenium* (feverfew) is a perennial plant that belongs to the family Asteraceae (daisy). Its Latin origin *febrifugia* means "fever reducer" [4]. Although native to the Balkan Peninsula, it can now be seen growing along roadsides, field, and wooded areas in the USA, Africa, Australia, China, Japan, and Europe [14]. It is used for numerous medical conditions [14] and comes in a variety of formulations, but its mechanism of action is not fully understood. It is thought that parthenolide, a sesquiterpene lactone, is the principle active ingredient [4, 12, 15]. Parthenium may inhibit the release of serotonin and potentially serve as an anti-inflammatory agent by inhibiting prostaglandin and phospholipase A production, thus improving vascular contraction and relaxation [4, 12, 15]. It may also inhibit platelet secretion and histamine release [14]. Parthenolide may not be the only active ingredient; some varieties of feverfew also contain a high concentration of melatonin [15], which is also thought to be helpful in many headache types (see below).

Evidence of Feverfew for Headache

Feverfew is one of the most thoroughly studied nutraceuticals for headache prevention, and two Cochrane reviews have evaluated its efficacy [15, 16]. The first review in 2004 concluded that insufficient evidence exists to suggest an effect of feverfew over placebo in preventing migraine. The publication of a larger (n = 218) and more rigorous study [17] with a stable feverfew extract (MIG-99) resulted in a new Cochrane review in 2015. This new review evaluated all randomized, placebo-controlled, double-blind trials assessing feverfew mono-preparations for preventing migraines in all ages, resulting in an analysis of 6 studies with 561 participants. Pooled analyses were not possible due to study and dose heterogeneity; participant inclusion criteria, feverfew preparation/dosage, and length of treatment varied considerably. Of the 4 studies that found some benefit [17–20], 3 had small sample sizes (between 17 and 60 participants). Two more rigorous studies (n = 50 and 147 participants, respectively) found no significant effects [21, 22]. The newest study [17] had the largest sample size of all studies to date ($n = 218$) and found that feverfew may reduce migraine by 0.6 headaches per month compared to placebo [17] (from 4.8 to 2.9 attacks/month vs. 4.8–3.5, respectively, $P = 0.0456$). Adverse events were mild and not significantly different from placebo, with gastrointestinal complaints the most common side effect. A "post feverfew syndrome" was reported when the substance was withdrawn in long-term users. Symptoms included joint/muscle aches and stiffness, nervousness, anxiety, and poor sleep [18]. The new study added positive evidence to the prior mixed and inconclusive findings, but the overall quality evidence is still low and not conclusive.

While the Cochrane reviews evaluated the evidence for feverfew as a prophylactic migraine treatment, a recent study evaluated feverfew plus ginger given sublingually (1 unit dose applicator; exact dose was not listed) as first-line abortive for mild headache [23]. After 2 h, 32% of patients who received active medication were pain-free versus 16% who received placebo ($P = 0.02$). However, the two groups were not randomized with respect to baseline average severity of headache (1.41 in active group, on a scale 0–3, versus 1.67 placebo group). In summary, although robust data may be lacking in support of feverfew for migraine, its side effect profile is favorable. Care must be taken to obtain a high-quality product, as the amount of parthenolide may vary among brands. Feverfew should be avoided during pregnancy because it may stimulate contractions. Thus, it should be recommended with caution for women of childbearing age.

Feverfew Guideline Recommendations
The evidence for efficacy of feverfew (studied dose, 50–300 mg bid; 2.08–18.75 tid of MIG-99) is considered Level B (probably effective) per the 2012 American Headache Society (AHS) and the American Academy of Neurology (AAN) guidelines [24]. The recent Canadian Headache Society guidelines recommend against its use [25], citing insufficient evidence of benefit. The European Federation of Neurological Societies (EFNS) considers the evidence for efficacy of feverfew as Level C [26].

Riboflavin

Riboflavin, or vitamin B2, is a water-soluble vitamin that is a cofactor in the mitochondrial electron transport chain. The name originates from "ribitol" (sugar whose reduced form provides part of the chemical structure) and "flavin" (functional group which gives patient's urine the characteristic yellow color upon oxidization) [4]. It has a 1 h half-life, so absorption is poor unless taken with food [27]. Riboflavin plays a role in the Krebs cycle, production of ATP, and mitochondrial energy metabolism and generation [12, 28]. There may be a relationship between migraine and mitochondrial dysfunction which leads to "decreased ATP production and energy metabolism, imbalance in calcium ions, increased neuronal information processing, decreased migraine threshold, and ultimately cortical spreading depression" [27].

Evidence of Riboflavin for Headache
Dating back to 1946, a case series was published in which 19 patients with migraine reported positive results from using riboflavin for variable lengths of time [29]. In a randomized clinical trial (RCT) in 1998, 3 months of 400 mg daily riboflavin resulted in statistically significant reductions in migraine headache days ($P = 0.012$) and frequency ($P = 0.005$) compared to placebo. Treatment effect was seen at 1 month but was highest after 3 months of treatment [30]. Another study comparing 4 months of preventive use of beta-blockers ($n = 11$) to riboflavin ($n = 15$) for migraine found that treatment response (patients with ≥50% decrease in attack frequency) was similar in both groups (beta-blocker 55% and riboflavin 53%), but auditory evoked cortical responses tended to normalize only after beta-blocker use, suggesting different pathophysiological mechanisms of action [31]. A small ($n = 23$) open-label study showed that 400 mg daily riboflavin decreased migraine frequency (from 4 to 2 days/month at 3 and 6 month follow-ups,

$P < 0.05$) and use of acute medications, but not headache duration or intensity [32]. Minor side effects (diarrhea, abdominal pain, facial erythema, and polyuria) were reported by a few patients.

The few studies of riboflavin for headache in pediatric patients have yielded conflicting results. A double-blind RCT showed that 200 mg daily riboflavin did not improve headaches more than placebo in 48 children. The placebo rate was high (66.6%) and the dose used for this study was lower than typical [33]. Another double-blind, crossover RCT in 42 children with migraines also found no benefit of riboflavin (at 50 mg/day) vs. placebo, although they did find a reduction in frequency of tension-type headaches [34]. No adverse reactions were noted in this study. In a retrospective chart analysis of 41 pediatric/adolescent patients with various headache subtypes, those receiving either 200 mg or 400 mg of riboflavin daily for 3, 4, or 6 months had fewer headaches (68.4% of patients) and less intense pain (21% of patients). Full benefit was seen after 4 months of treatment. A few patients reported decreased or resolution of aura. One patient stopped due to vomiting, and another complained of increased appetite, otherwise few side effects were reported [35]. Results of this study need to be interpreted with caution, as it was retrospective and lacked a placebo group and blinding. A case study of three children reported that riboflavin significantly improved ICHD-diagnosed cyclic vomiting syndrome, a condition hypothesized to be related to deficient mitochondrial energy supplies [36].

Riboflavin Guideline Recommendations

Evidence for efficacy of riboflavin (studied dose: 400 mg daily) was categorized as Level B in the 2012 AHS and the AAN guidelines. The Canadian Headache Society guidelines report strong but low-quality evidence. The EFNS considered the evidence for riboflavin as Level C and classified it as a third-line option.

Magnesium

The essential mineral nutrient magnesium (Mg^{2+}) exists in every cell type and plays a major role in energy metabolism. Nearly half of US adults have poor dietary intake of magnesium [37]. Diets low in magnesium have been associated with type 2 diabetes, premenstrual syndrome symptoms, asthma, osteoporosis, elevated plasma levels of C-reactive protein, hypertension, cardiovascular disease, and sudden death [37, 38]. Magnesium deficiency may play a role in many factors associated with migraine pathophysiology, including cortical spreading depression, substance P release, serotonin-related vasoconstriction, N-methyl-D-aspartate (NMDA) glutamate transmission, and nitric oxide production [39]. Magnesium deficiency may be present in up to half of patients with migraine [38]. However, conflicting evidence exists regarding serum magnesium levels in migraineurs. In one study using a magnesium load test (3000 mg of magnesium lactate), 24 h urinary magnesium excretion was lower in the migraine group versus controls, suggesting magnesium retention occurred in the migraineurs because of systemic underlying deficiency, but baseline serum levels were similar between groups [40]. In a case control study (50 migraineurs and 50 healthy controls), serum magnesium levels were lower in migraineurs vs. controls at baseline, although there were no differences in serum magnesium during or between migraine headache events [41]. In a separate matched case-control study (40 migraineurs, 40 healthy controls), serum ionized magnesium levels were lower between attacks and during acute attacks in cases compared to controls, with odds of acute migraine significantly increasing when serum levels of magnesium were low (OR 35.3, 95% CI 12.4–95.2, $p = 0.001$) [42]. Low ionized magnesium levels have been reported during acute menstrual migraine attacks [43].

Factors limit simple magnesium blood level testing to assess for magnesium deficiency [38]. Of total body magnesium stores, 31% are intracellular, 67% in the bone, and only 2% in the extracellular space, where it could be accurately measured with a blood draw; thus, blood magnesium levels do not reflect true body stores [38]. As magnesium is depleted from the blood, it is pulled from the cells in attempts to maintain adequate levels. A magnesium test in red blood cells may be more accurate, but it is not available at all institutions and can be costly.

Evidence for Treatment of Headache with Magnesium

In one study, 81 patients with migraines used 600 mg of trimagnesium dicitrate daily for 12 weeks versus placebo. Migraine attack frequency was reduced in 41.6% in the magnesium group versus 15.8% in the placebo group ($p < 0.05$). Diarrhea and gastric complaints were reported in about a quarter of participants [44].

A recent meta-analysis reviewed 21 studies of magnesium for migraine using Cochrane review criteria. In 11 studies, magnesium was given intravenously for acute treatment; in 10 studies, oral magnesium was used as a preventive [45]. The 10 studies of oral magnesium included 789 participants (6 studies in China) and used 6 different forms of the salt and/or combinations, for periods of 4–12 weeks. Overall findings were positive. Oral magnesium decreased frequency and intensity of migraine (odds ratios [ORs] 0.20 and 0.27). Intravenous magnesium aborted acute migraine within 14–45 min, 120 min, and 24 h after infusion, respectively (ORs of 1.23, 1.20, and 1.25, respectively). Only one study [46] used blinding of participants, personnel, and outcome assessments. However, the results are difficult to interpret because the treatment group received a combination of riboflavin, magnesium, and feverfew; the "placebo" group received a smaller dose of riboflavin [46].

In 1996, Pfaffenrath et al. reported the results of a randomized, double-blind, multicenter placebo-controlled phase III study of 10 mmol magnesium twice daily in patients with 2–6 migraines without aura per month. The study was stopped early due to lack of an effect (goal $n = 150$, stopped after interim analysis of 69 patients) [47]. Response rates were equivocal in the two groups (28.6% with magnesium, 29.4% with placebo). No difference was seen in numbers of migraine days or migraine attacks. Adverse events were noted in 45% of the magnesium group including diarrhea or soft stools ($n = 10$) and palpitations ($n = 3$), thus suggestive that the form of magnesium may have been poorly absorbed and patients may not have received full benefit. In addition, more than 50% of participants in both groups had previously failed one or more prophylactic agents; thus, they may have been more refractory to treatment.

Two studies have evaluated oral magnesium in children with migraine. A randomized, double-blind, placebo-controlled study tested oral magnesium oxide (9 mg/kg/day divided tid with food) versus placebo for 16 weeks among children with migraine [48]. The magnesium group reported fewer headaches of lower severity ($p = 0.0037$ and $p = 0.0029$, respectively). There was also a placebo response in headache frequency that waned after 6 weeks. In a second study of 45 children given 2.25 g of magnesium pidolate twice/daily for 3 months (in an unblinded, open-label design), treatment improved MIDAS scores, headache days (decreased by 69.9%), and use of analgesics (65.4% lower) [49]. However, only 22 participants completed the full 12-month follow-up period. Unpleasant taste was the only adverse effect noted.

Magnesium was recently reclassified from category A to D during pregnancy based on evidence that intravenous magnesium sulfate injections may have teratogenic effects on fetal bone growth. Evidence is limited on the safety of daily oral magnesium in pregnancy; given this new potential risk and categorization, precaution is advised for use in pregnancy [50].

Magnesium Guideline Recommendations

Evidence for efficacy of magnesium (studied dose: 600 mg trimagnesium dicitrate daily) is considered Level B by the AHS and AAN guidelines. The Canadian Headache Society guidelines made a strong recommendation for its use, whereas the EFNS considered the evidence as a Level C, denoting a third-line option. According to the 2015 American Headache Society Evidence Assessment, 1–2 g of magnesium given intravenously as abortive relief of migraine with aura has Level B evidence. There is no evidence of significant adverse reactions with oral magnesium in those without pre-existing severe renal disease.

Coenzyme Q10 (CoQ10)

Coenzyme Q10 (ubiquinone) is a hydrophobic substance found in all cell membranes that serves critical roles in the electron transport chain [39] and in mitochondrial function [39, 51] by helping convert fats and sugar into energy. As a free radical scavenger, it is an antioxidant with numerous anti-inflammatory properties [39, 52]. CoQ10 has long been studied for its cardiovascular benefits, such as blood pressure reduction, hypothesized to be secondary to improved endothelial function. Severe CoQ10 deficiencies are found in mitochondrial diseases (neonatal encephalopathy with nephropathy, Leigh syndrome, lactic acidosis, infantile nephropathy, recessive ataxia, cerebellar atrophy ± retardation) [53], and CoQ10 supplementation can significantly reduce symptoms. Ubiquinol was recently approved by the FDA as an orphan drug to treat primary CoQ10 deficiencies. Some hypothesize that migraine may be a disorder of mitochondrial energy deficiency [54] and that inflammation present during a migraine leads to depletion of CoQ10 [55].

Evidence for CoQ10 for Headache

In a double-blind, randomized, placebo-controlled study published in Neurology, CoQ10 100 mg tid improved attack frequency ($p = 0.05$) and days with nausea after 3 months of treatment ($p = 0.02$) in 42 participants with episodic migraine with and without aura, compared to placebo. The 50% responder rate for attack frequency was greater for those receiving CoQ10 than placebo (47.6% CoQ10 vs. 14.4%; $p = 0.05$). Mean duration, severity, and abortive medication use did not differ between groups. One patient reported cutaneous allergy, but otherwise no other adverse reactions were noted [56].

A randomized, double-blind, placebo-controlled, crossover study (in addition to a multidisciplinary clinic approach) of 100 mg CoQ10 was conducted in 6- to 17-year-old participants with episodic or chronic migraine with and without aura. Both groups improved from baseline, without a difference between coenzyme Q10 and placebo [57]. Chronic migraine patients taking CoQ10 did have a greater initial reduction in headache frequency from baseline to week 1–4 compared to placebo. Similarly, episodic migraineurs who crossed over from placebo to CoQ10 improved after the first 4 weeks (but declined with the opposite crossover). There was a high dropout rate; the authors suggest that after

rapid improvement, patients may not have felt a need for continued therapy. The study was also limited because baseline headache frequency was based on report, whereas treatment headache frequency was based on headache diaries. The dose used in this study was lower than in the adult studies (only 100 mg daily rather than 100 mg tid) and was an add-on to an already effective multidisciplinary clinic approach; CoQ10 as monotherapy was not evaluated. Based on evidence from an open-label study in 32 adults [58], 150 mg daily of CoQ10 reduced average number of days with migraine from 7.34 to 2.95 in the last 60 days of treatment ($P < 0.0001$). These findings are supported by a recent study done by Shoeibi et al. [59]. No adverse effects were reported in either study [58, 59].

Some authors suggest testing coenzyme Q10 levels in patients prior to supplementation [4]. One-third of 1550 patients aged 3 to 22 with diagnoses of migraine with and without aura, probable migraine, and chronic migraine had CoQ10 deficiency [52]. Once diagnosed, they were then started on 1–3 mg/kg/day of CoQ10. Although there was no control group for comparison, at follow-up evaluation (mean 97 + _56 days later), headache frequency (46.3% with 50% reduction; $p < 0.001$) and headache disability scores both improved significantly (from 47.4 ± 50.6 to 22.8 ± 30.6; $p < 0.001$).

CoQ10 Guideline Recommendations

Coenzyme Q10 (studied dose 100 mg tid) was given Level C evidence and judged as possibly effective by the AHS and AAN guidelines. The Canadian Headache Society guidelines strongly encouraged offering it based on low-quality evidence but low adverse effects. The EFNS considered the evidence for efficacy of coQ10 as Level C, denoting a third-line option.

Melatonin

Melatonin is a hormone produced by the pineal gland associated with regulation of the circadian rhythm. Melatonin is thought to have anti-inflammatory properties, inhibits both nitric oxide synthesis and dopamine, and may have a role in glutamate transmission. Its safety profile for short-term use has been established in both human and animal studies, but data are lacking during pregnancy and lactation. Melatonin may enhance opioid efficacy; thus, caution should be used in prescribing melatonin to patients using opioids. Supplements produced in a lab may be safer than products made from animal sources, which may contain contaminants. Lower doses are proposed to have a greater phase-shifting effect on human circadian rhythms [60, 61].

Evidence for Melatonin for Headache

Studies evaluating melatonin for headache are challenging to summarize given the variety of headache diagnoses, melatonin dosages, forms (immediate versus extended release), and duration of treatments. In a randomized, double-blind, placebo-controlled trial of amitriptyline 25 mg, melatonin 3 mg, and placebo for 12 weeks in 196 participants with episodic migraine with and without aura [62], the amitriptyline and melatonin groups had fewer migraine headache days per month compared to placebo. Compared to baseline, after 12 weeks, headache frequency was reduced by 2.7 days in the melatonin group, 2.2 days in the amitriptyline group, and 1.1 days in the placebo group. Melatonin reduced headache frequency compared to placebo ($p = 0.009$) but not compared to amitriptyline ($p = 0.19$). As a secondary end point, more patients taking melatonin had >50% reduction in headache frequency versus amitriptyline ($p < 0.05$) and placebo ($p < 0.01$). Those receiving both melatonin and amitriptyline had reductions in migraine duration and intensity and less analgesic use compared to placebo. Adverse effects were similar in the melatonin and placebo groups but significantly higher in the amitriptyline group. In contrast, a randomized, double-blind, placebo-controlled crossover study in 48 participants with migraine with and without aura found no difference in migraine attack frequency between extended-release melatonin 2 mg for 8 weeks and placebo [61]. However, placebo response was high. Adverse reactions were mild (fatigue, dizziness, nervousness, nightmares) and not significantly different than placebo. One open-label study ($n = 49$; 41 completed study) showed that 6 months of 4 mg melatonin resulted in less frequent migraines ($p < 0.001$) and chronic tension-type headaches ($p = 0.033$) and lower HIT-6 scores for both groups ($p < 0.001$ and $p = 0.002$, respectively) [60].

Melatonin benefited a small series of patients with indomethacin-responsive headaches, both hemicrania continua ($n = 11$) [63] and idiopathic stabbing headache ($n = 3$) [64]. The similar chemical structures of melatonin and indomethacin may explain the benefits seen [64]. Other studies have cited gastric protection with melatonin, suggesting it might be beneficial combined with nonsteroidal anti-inflammatory agents [65]. Although only a few studies have evaluated melatonin for cluster headache, with conflicting results, melatonin is considered a second-line therapy in cluster headache [66]. The evidence that melatonin levels may be low during a cluster attack strengthens the hypothesis that melatonin may act on cluster headaches [67]. One study of 20 participants (18 with episodic cluster and 2 with chronic cluster headaches) reported improvement after 14 days of 10 mg of melatonin taken once per day in the evening during a cluster period, compared to placebo [68]. Headache frequency was reduced in the melatonin group (ANOVA, $p < 0.03$) although no response was seen in the patients with chronic cluster. However, another study of nine participants (six with chronic cluster, three with episodic headaches) did not report a benefit from 2 mg melatonin given during a cluster period [69].

In an open-label trial of melatonin, 14 of 21 children with migraine with and without aura and chronic tension-type headache reported a >50% reduction of headache attack frequency compared to baseline [70]. One child complained of excessive daytime sleepiness. Clinical recommendations in the Journal of the European Paediatric Neurology Society state "there is still no definitive consensus about the therapeutic use of melatonin for headaches in children" [71].

Vitamin D

Vitamin D deficiency is prevalent in the USA despite its presence in food sources and exposure to sunlight. Vitamin D functions as a hormone, with receptors in nearly all cells of the body with many functions, including cell growth, bone health, immunity, and reducing inflammation [72]. A large cross-sectional population-based study ($n = 5938$) found an interaction with vitamin D levels and statin's benefit on migraine, such that statin use was associated with lower odds of having severe headaches/migraines only in those with high serum vitamin D levels [73]. Based on this observation, a RCT in migraineurs was conducted of simvastatin 20 mg twice daily plus vitamin D3 1000 IU twice daily vs. placebo. Patients continued their current migraine preventative. Those in the treatment group experienced approximately 3 less migraine days per month compared to placebo ($p < 0.001$) [74]. Unfortunately, given the intervention involved both vitamin D3 and simvastatin, it is unclear which treatment had the greatest effect or if both are required. A pediatric study ($n = 53$) demonstrated a decreased frequency of migraine days with supplementation of vitamin D plus amitriptyline, but the study was limited by the lack of control group [75]. A small case study ($n = 3$) reported the presence of severe vitamin D deficiency mimicking chronic tension-type headaches in children, with resultant improvement/near resolution after vitamin D supplementation [76].

Ginkgolide B (Ginkgo biloba)

Ginkgo biloba has been used in herbal medicine for thousands of years to treat dementia, anxiety, asthma, and schizophrenia, although with conflicting evidence. It is made from leaves from the maidenhair tree originating from China [77]. *Ginkgo* may have an effect through its impact on glutamate [78] and antiplatelet-activating factor [79].

Ginkgo biloba had some benefit as potential acute abortive for migraine aura in a small ($n = 25$) open preliminary trial [78]. Another open-label trial of *Ginkgo biloba* terpenes phytosome 60 mg plus coenzyme Q10 11 mg plus vitamin B2 8.7 mg was given twice daily for 4 months in 50 women with migraine with aura or migraine aura without headache [79]. Improvement in aura frequency and duration was seen. Abdominal complaint and vertigo were reported ($n = 3$), but overall was well tolerated. Two pediatric studies ($n = 119$ and $n = 24$) using combination products containing ginkgolide B, coenzyme Q10, riboflavin, and magnesium in migraine without aura found decreased migraine attack frequency [80, 81]. Another study compared Preparation A (ginkgolide B 80 mg, coenzyme Q10 20 mg, riboflavin 1.6 mg, and magnesium 300 mg) with Preparation B (L-tryptophan 250 mg, 5-hydroxytryptophan [*Griffonia simplicifolia*], vitamin PP, and vitamin B6 1 mg) in 374 school-aged children diagnosed with migraine without aura [82]. Both groups showed improvement in headache duration, pain intensity, disability, and behavioral reactions. Both groups had fewer headaches, especially the Preparation A group. However, the use of combination treatments makes it challenging to detect which component may be most helpful for migraine.

Combination Treatments

In a recent RCT, participants ($n = 130$) were given 400 mg riboflavin, 600 mg magnesium, and 150 mg coenzyme Q10, along with a multivitamin (containing 750 mg vitamin A, 200 mg vitamin C, 134 mg vitamin E, 5 mg thiamin, 20 mg niacin, 5 mg vitamin B6, 6 mg vitamin B12, 400 mg folic acid, 5 mg vitamin D, 10 mg pantothenic acid, 165 mg biotin, 0.8 mg iron, 5 mg zinc, 2 mg manganese, 0.5 mg copper, 30 mg chromium, 60 mg molybdenum, 50 mg selenium, 5 mg bioflavonoids) for 3 months [83]. Reduction in migraine days per month was not significant. However, reductions in migraine pain ($p = 0.03$) and HIT-6 scores ($p = 0.01$) were seen. In 1 RCT of 49 participants, no differences were seen between the treatment group (who received riboflavin 400 mg, magnesium 300 mg, and feverfew 100 mg) and the placebo group (who received placebo containing 25 mg riboflavin) regarding headache reduction, migraine days, migraine index, or triptan dose [46].

Homeopathy

Homeopathic remedies are based on the idea that giving minute amounts of a harmful substance will trigger the body's natural healing response against the harmful agent. Thousands of different homeopathic remedies/substances are used worldwide. Homeopathic treatments are created by "alternating steps of diluting and agitating a starting substance; the resulting "potencies" quickly reach dilutions beyond Avogadro's number where the probability that one molecule of the starting substance is still present approaches zero [84]." Although homeopathic experts claim that many remedies are helpful for migraine, there is currently a paucity of evidence-based research supporting its use. A systematic literature review found no evidence to support or refute the use of homeopathy for migraine, tension-type, or cervicogenic headache, [85] and the studies had numerous methodologic problems. A more recent meta-analysis included four RCTs of homeopathy and headache [86]; these showed a positive trend but no statistically significant benefit beyond placebo. Despite the lack of evidence, a survey of 124 Italian children with chronic headaches demonstrated that 47% use homeopathy [6]. Caution should be used with these products, as they have not been evaluated by the FDA for evidence, safety, or effectiveness [86].

Summary: Supplements and Chronic Daily Headache

The FDA has limited oversight on supplements, and given potential allegations of poor quality and safety of supplements, consumers need to look for the "stamp of approval" of third-party testing on bottles to confirm accuracy and quality of the product. Almost one-third of adults with severe headaches/migraines report using nutraceuticals. Many may seek herb/supplements for their supposed natural and safe profiles, although side effects also occur with supplements [87]. Few studies have evaluated the benefit of nutraceuticals specifically for chronic daily headache. Several supplements have Level B evidence of efficacy according to the 2012 AHS and the AAN guidelines, including feverfew (studied dose, 50–300 mg bid; 2.08–18.75 tid of MIG-99), riboflavin (studied dose, 400 mg daily), and magnesium (studied dose, 600 mg trimagnesium dicitrate daily). Coenzyme Q10 (studied dose 100 mg tid) was considered to have Level C evidence. Melatonin, vitamin D, and *Ginkgo biloba* have limited evidence of potential efficacy for headache. Homeopathy has limited evidence for use in headache. Despite its Level A evidence, controversy exists over the concern for hepatotoxicity with *Petasites* (butterbur); it is therefore not currently recommended [4, 12, 13]. Additional research is needed to further clarify benefits of supplements for chronic daily headache.

Conclusions to Parts I, II, and III: CAM and Chronic Daily Headache

Chronic daily headaches are often refractory to conventional treatment options, and CAM treatments may provide much-needed relief. However, research of CAM treatments specifically for chronic daily headaches is limited, so we have reviewed the research evidence for CAM for headache. Most of the studies have significant methodologic concerns, and larger, more rigorous studies are needed for all CAM modalities. Studies are limited by small sample sizes, heterogeneous interventions, limited headache outcomes, lack of active controls, and short-term follow-up. Despite these limitations, evidence for mind/body options such as meditation, yoga, tai chi, and deep breathing is promising, with the most research to date for mindfulness meditation. The strongest evidence for acupuncture is for chronic migraine, and cost analyses suggest it may have an overall cost benefit. There is some evidence for spinal manipulative therapy for chronic cervicogenic headache or chronic tension-type headache, but the potential for major adverse events, such as cervical dissection, limits more widespread recommendation for its use. No data support the use of massage for any chronic headache conditions. Other complementary therapies (aromatherapy, homeopathy, daith piercing, and oxygen administration) have minimal evidence to support their use for chronic daily headache. The supplements with the strongest level of evidence for benefit for headache (Level B) include feverfew, riboflavin, and magnesium, with CoQ10 having Level C evidence. Additional evidence is emerging for the potential benefits of supplemental vitamin D, melatonin, and *Ginkgo biloba*.

The research for CAM in general, and for headache, has been limited by methodologic concerns that reduce study quality, leading to challenges in interpreting and assessing interventions. Treatment modalities are often poorly defined and heterogeneous in delivery format, leading to difficulty in understanding what intervention was administered and how to replicate, recommend, or assess options for patients. Many studies had wait-list comparisons without an active control group, making it challenging to interpret the effect of the intervention above the placebo effect. Few studies have long-term follow-up. Most were conducted with the CAM therapy as an "add-on" therapy to usual care, making it difficult to compare it against usual care treatment options. Side effects are not always reported.

Unfortunately, many of the limitations with this research are inherent with this type of research (Table 20.1). Evaluating non-pharmacologic treatment options with research standards created for pharmacologic treatments is difficult. For example, although the "placebo" pill is the standard accepted control for drugs, there is no ideal placebo group for most CAM therapies. Blinding participants to active non-pharmacologic treatment options is challenging,

Table 20.1 Difficulties with non-pharmacological research

Limited ability to blind participants
Difficulty finding a credible control
Small sample sizes
Selection bias
Behavioral treatments often not comparable with medical treatments
Inability to reproduce intervention

Reproduced with permission from John Wiley & Sons, Inc. from the journal *Headache* [88]

if not impossible. Participants interested in this type of research may be different from most patients, leading to selection bias. Interventions may not be easily reproduced, and non-drug treatments are often not comparable with medical treatments [88].

Since the research into most CAM therapies has really just begun, few studies specifically evaluate CAM for chronic daily headache syndromes, so extrapolation of the information from headache studies is required. Many studies done in headache evaluating CAM therapies were not conducted with well-defined headache research parameters. For example, many studies did not clarify if the intervention was assessing episodic or chronic headaches. Most did not use ICHD diagnostic criteria.

Despite these limitations and challenges, the research suggests that many CAM therapies may be beneficial, with minimal side effects. Patients with headaches, especially chronic daily headaches, are especially desperate. Although CAM treatments may be helpful, the placebo rates are quite high in many studies. Further, broad recommendations of potentially non-therapeutic interventions may damage the trust instilled in the doctor-patient relationship. Further research is critical to having a better understanding of the value of these types of therapies for chronic daily headache.

For pregnant or nursing women, CAM therapies may be quite helpful at a time when pharmacologic options are much more dangerous [50]. Pediatric patients are often open and willing to consider CAM therapies to avoid medications. Sometimes more traditional treatment options, even non-pharmacologic options such as biofeedback, are difficult for patients due to cost and availability. This point is illustrated with data from the 2007 NHIS analyses that demonstrated that <1% of patients with severe headaches/migraines used the well-researched intervention of biofeedback, while 9% used yoga, 17% meditated, and 24% did deep breathing exercises [88].

While most CAM therapies have minimal side effects compared to pharmacologic options, the potential side effects from CAM are not negligible. The time, energy, and cost associated with many of these interventions are an important consideration in the recommendation and adherence to CAM therapies, especially since many of these treatment options are out of pocket. While several of the cost analysis studies for acupuncture demonstrated increased costs of the procedure, when the entire condition is considered and quality-adjusted life years taken into account, the value becomes apparent. Even so, the amount of money spent on CAM is tremendous, with an estimated $33.9 billion in out-of-pocket costs spent by US adults [89].

Despite the significant amount of research discussed in this chapter, there are still many unanswered questions about most CAM therapies for chronic daily headache [90]. Uncertainty persists as to optimal dosages (frequency, duration, length of treatment), which types of patients and headaches are most responsive to these interventions, and mechanisms of action [90].

Despite all these limitations and persistent questions, CAM therapies may be a viable treatment option for adults with chronic daily headache. Given the significant risks associated with many pharmacologic treatments, especially opioids and the potential for medication-overuse headache, CAM treatments may be especially helpful. The study assessing mindfulness therapy vs. pharmacologic treatments after medication-overuse headache withdrawal is especially encouraging, suggesting that non-pharmacologic treatments may be comparable to pharmacologic treatments for medication-overuse headache.

One of the most important aspects of many CAM therapies is the opportunity for patients to be active in their own treatment plans and to learn techniques that improve their own sense of self-efficacy. Many CAM therapies may not be most effective as individual treatments but, as an approach to care, with patients encouraged to use many CAM therapies discussed in this chapter together, using an "integrative" approach. One study even retrospectively assessed for this possibility through chart reviews comparing a multimodal approach that included osteopathic manipulative treatments, mindfulness, and qigong to standard pharmacologic treatments in 83 adolescents with chronic tension-type headache [91].

Although both were effective, multimodal treatment was statistically more beneficial than the pharmacologic option in headache outcomes.

CAM in the "real world" takes into account patient preference and considers CAM as an integral part of every treatment plan, as first line rather than last resort [92]. Understanding CAM therapies is critical for providers to advocate for their patients' health care, as Dr. Rob Cowan points out, because "we don't need to embrace every alternative medical system to serve our patients, but there exists a wide variety of modalities which, whether we incorporate them into our practices or not, need to be on our radar, and which with we need more than a passing familiarity. Moreover, we need to provide some guidance to our patients in these areas if we are truly able to be their advocate in healthcare" [92, 93]. The goal of these chapters is to equip providers with the knowledge to appropriately counsel patients on these treatment options and to make patients and providers aware of the possibilities that CAM therapies may offer to those who need additional treatment options.

Chronic daily headache is a challenging condition to treat, with high associated disability and psychological comorbidities. One patient describes her experience with integrative medicine in an eloquent letter published in *Headache* and concludes by stating "Since I have begun to incorporate Integrative Medicine, I have started telling myself to stop waiting until I am 100% healthy to live my life. If all I have is 40%, then I make sure it is the best 40%" [94]. Hopefully, a better understanding of CAM therapies and an integrative medicine approach will give all chronic daily headache patients and providers hope to achieve that goal [90].

Acknowledgments Dr. Wells is supported by the National Center for Complementary and Integrative Health of the National Institutes of Health under Award Number K23AT008406. The content is solely the responsibility of the authors and does not necessarily represent the official views of the National Institutes of Health. We gratefully acknowledge the editorial assistance of Karen Klein, MA, in the Wake Forest Clinical and Translational Science Institute, funded by the National Center for Advancing Translational Sciences (NCATS), National Institutes of Health, through Grant Award Number

UL1TR001420. We also thank Mark McKone, Librarian at Carpenter Library, Wake Forest School of Medicine, for his help with the use of Zotero. We are appreciative of the help from Nakiea Choate from the Department of Neurology at Wake Forest Baptist for her administrative support.

References

1. Kalra EK. Nutraceutical–definition and introduction. AAPS PharmSci. 2003;5(3):E25.
2. Office of dietary supplements–Dietary supplement health and education act of 1994 [Internet]. [cited 2017 Apr 26]. Available from: https://ods.od.nih.gov/About/DSHEA_Wording.aspx
3. Wallace TC. Twenty years of the dietary supplement health and education act–how should dietary supplements be regulated? J Nutr. 2015;145(8):1683–6.
4. Rajapakse T, Pringsheim T. Nutraceuticals in migraine: a summary of existing guidelines for use. Headache. 2016;56(4):808–16.
5. US Food and Drug Administration. Label claims for conventional foods and dietary supplements [Internet]. [cited 2017 Jun 13]. Available from: https://www.fda.gov/food/ingredientspackaginglabeling/labelingnutrition/ucm111447.htm.
6. Dalla Libera D, Colombo B, Pavan G, Comi G. Complementary and alternative medicine (CAM) use in an Italian cohort of pediatric headache patients: the tip of the iceberg. Neurol Sci. 2014;35(Suppl 1):145–8.
7. US Food and Drug Administration. FDA investigates elevated lead levels linked to ton shen health/life rising dietary supplements [Internet]. [cited 2017 Jun 13]. Available from: https://www.fda.gov/food/recallsoutbreaksemergencies/outbreaks/ucm518288.htm.
8. The New York Times. New York Attorney General Targets Supplements at Major Retailers [Internet]. [cited 2017 Jun 13]. Available from: https://well.blogs.nytimes.com/2015/02/03/new-york-attorney-general-targets-supplements-at-major-retailers/.
9. Wells RE, Bertisch SM, Buettner C, Phillips RS, McCarthy EP. Complementary and alternative medicine use among adults with migraines/severe headaches. Headache. 2011;51(7):1087–97.
10. Toldo I, Rattin M, Perissinotto E, De Carlo D, Bolzonella B, Nosadini M, et al. Survey on treatments for primary headaches in 13 specialized juvenile headache centers: the first multicenter Italian study. Eur J Paediatr Neurol. 2016;21(3):507–21.
11. Rossi P, Di Lorenzo G, Malpezzi MG, Faroni J, Cesarino F, Di Lorenzo C, et al. Prevalence, pattern and predictors of use of complementary and alternative medicine (CAM) in migraine patients attending a headache clinic in Italy. Cephalalgia. 2005;25(7):493–506.
12. Tepper SJ. Nutraceutical and other modalities for the treatment of headache. Continuum Minneap Minn. 2015;21(4 Headache):1018–31.
13. Mauskop A. Evidence-based guideline update: NSAIDs and other complementary treatments for episodic migraine prevention in adults: report of the quality standards Subcommittee of the American Academy of neurology and the American headache society. Neurology. 2013;80(9):868.
14. Pareek A, Suthar M, Rathore GS, Bansal V. Feverfew (Tanacetum parthenium L.): a systematic review. Pharmacogn Rev. 2011;5(9):103–10.
15. Wider B, Pittler MH, Ernst E. Feverfew for preventing migraine. In: Cochrane database of systematic reviews. Hoboken, N.J: John Wiley & Sons, Ltd; 2015.
16. Pittler MH, Ernst E. Feverfew for preventing migraine. Cochrane Database Syst Rev. 2004;1:CD002286.
17. Diener HC, Pfaffenrath V, Schnitker J, Friede M. Hennecke-von Zepelin H-H. Efficacy and safety of 6.25 mg t.I.D. Feverfew CO2-extract (MIG-99) in migraine prevention–a randomized, double-blind, multicentre, placebo-controlled study. Cephalalgia. 2005;25(11):1031–41.
18. Johnson ES, Kadam NP, Hylands DM, Hylands PJ. Efficacy of feverfew as prophylactic treatment of migraine. Br Med J Clin Res Ed. 1985;291(6495):569–73.
19. Murphy JJ, Heptinstall S, Mitchell JR. Randomised double-blind placebo-controlled trial of feverfew in migraine prevention. Lancet. 1988;2(8604):189–92.
20. Palevitch D, Earon G, Carasso R. Feverfew (Tanacetum parthenium) as a prophylactic treatment for migraine: a double-blind placebo-controlled study. Phytother Res. 1997;11(7):508–11.
21. De Weerdt CJ, Bootsma HP, Hendriks H. Herbal medicines in migraine prevention randomized double-blind placebo-controlled crossover trial of a feverfew preparation. Phytomedicine. 1996;3(3):225–30.
22. Pfaffenrath V, Diener HC, Fischer M, Friede M, Hennecke-von Zepelin HH. Investigators. The efficacy and safety of Tanacetum parthenium (feverfew) in migraine prophylaxis--a double-blind, multicentre, randomized placebo-controlled dose-response study. Cephalalgia. 2002;22(7):523–32.
23. Cady RK, Goldstein J, Nett R, Mitchell R, Beach ME, Browning R. A double-blind placebo-controlled pilot study of sublingual feverfew and ginger (LipiGesicTM M) in the treatment of migraine. Headache. 2011;51(7):1078–86.
24. Loder E, Burch R, Rizzoli P. The 2012 AHS/AAN guidelines for prevention of episodic migraine: a summary and comparison with other recent clinical practice guidelines. Headache. 2012;52(6):930–45.
25. Pringsheim T, Davenport WJ, Mackie G, Worthington I, Aubé M, Christie SN, et al. Canadian headache society guideline for migraine prophylaxis. Can J Neurol Sci. 2012;39(2 Suppl 2):S1–59.
26. Evers S, Afra J, Frese A, Goadsby PJ, Linde M, May A, et al. EFNS guideline on the drug treatment of migraine--revised report of an EFNS task force. Eur J Neurol. 2009;16(9):968–81.
27. Colombo B, Saraceno L, Comi G. Riboflavin and migraine: the bridge over troubled mitochondria. Neurol Sci. 2014;35(1):141–4.

28. Mauskop A. Nonmedication, alternative, and complementary treatments for migraine. Continuum Minneap Minn. 2012;18(4):796–806.

29. Smith CB. Riboflavin in migraine. Can Med Assoc J. 1946;54(6):589.

30. Schoenen J, Jacquy J, Lenaerts M. Effectiveness of high-dose riboflavin in migraine prophylaxis. A randomized controlled trial. Neurology. 1998;50(2):466–70.

31. Sándor PS, Afra J, Ambrosini A, Schoenen J. Prophylactic treatment of migraine with betablockers and riboflavin: differential effects on the intensity dependence of auditory evoked cortical potentials. Headache. 2000;40(1):30–5.

32. Boehnke C, Reuter U, Flach U, Schuh-Hofer S, Einhäupl KM, Arnold G. High-dose riboflavin treatment is efficacious in migraine prophylaxis: an open study in a tertiary care Centre. Eur J Neurol. 2004;11(7):475–7.

33. MacLennan SC, Wade FM, Forrest KML, Ratanayake PD, Fagan E, Antony J. High-dose riboflavin for migraine prophylaxis in children: a double-blind, randomized, placebo-controlled trial. J Child Neurol. 2008;23(11):1300–4.

34. Bruijn J, Duivenvoorden H, Passchier J, Locher H, Dijkstra N, Arts W-F. Medium-dose riboflavin as a prophylactic agent in children with migraine: a preliminary placebo-controlled, randomised, double-blind, cross-over trial. Cephalalgia. 2010;30(12):1426–34.

35. Condò M, Posar A, Arbizzani A, Parmeggiani A. Riboflavin prophylaxis in pediatric and adolescent migraine. J Headache Pain. 2009;10(5):361.

36. Melnikova AM-E, Schäppi MG, Korff C. Riboflavin in cyclic vomiting syndrome: efficacy in three children. Eur J Pediatr. 2016;175(1):131–5.

37. Rosanoff A, Weaver CM, Rude RK. Suboptimal magnesium status in the United States: are the health consequences underestimated? Nutr Rev. 2012;70(3):153–64.

38. Mauskop A, Varughese J. Why all migraine patients should be treated with magnesium. J Neural Transm. 2012;119(5):575–9.

39. Taylor FR. Nutraceuticals and headache: the biological basis. Headache. 2011;51(3):484–501.

40. Trauninger A, Pfund Z, Koszegi T, Czopf J. Oral magnesium load test in patients with migraine. Headache. 2002;42(2):114–9.

41. Samaie A, Asghari N, Ghorbani R, Arda J. Blood magnesium levels in migraineurs within and between the headache attacks: a case control study. Pan Afr Med J. 2012;11:46.

42. Assarzadegan F, Asgarzadeh S, Hatamabadi HR, Shahrami A, Tabatabaey A, Asgarzadeh M. Serum concentration of magnesium as an independent risk factor in migraine attacks: a matched case-control study and review of the literature. Int Clin Psychopharmacol. 2016;31(5):287–92.

43. Mauskop A, Altura BT, Altura BM. Serum ionized magnesium levels and serum ionized calcium/ionized

44. Peikert A, Wilimzig C, Köhne-Volland R. Prophylaxis of migraine with oral magnesium: results from a prospective, multi-center, placebo-controlled and double-blind randomized study. Cephalalgia. 1996;16(4):257–63.

45. Chiu H-Y, Yeh T-H, Huang Y-C, Chen P-Y. Effects of intravenous and oral magnesium on reducing migraine: a meta-analysis of randomized controlled trials. Pain Physician. 2016;19(1):E97–112.

46. Maizels M, Blumenfeld A, Burchette R. A combination of riboflavin, magnesium, and feverfew for migraine prophylaxis: a randomized trial. Headache. 2004;44(9):885–90.

47. Pfaffenrath V, Wessely P, Meyer C, Isler HR, Evers S, Grotemeyer KH, et al. Magnesium in the prophylaxis of migraine–a double-blind placebo-controlled study. Cephalalgia. 1996;16(6):436–40.

48. Wang F, Van Den Eeden SK, Ackerson LM, Salk SE, Reince RH, Elin RJ. Oral magnesium oxide prophylaxis of frequent migrainous headache in children: a randomized, double-blind, placebo-controlled trial. Headache. 2003;43(6):601–10.

49. Grazzi L, Andrasik F, Usai S, Bussone G. Magnesium as a preventive treatment for paediatric episodic tension-type headache: results at 1-year follow-up. Neurol Sci. 2007;28(3):148–50.

50. Wells RE, Turner DP, Lee M, Bishop L, Strauss L. Managing migraine during pregnancy and lactation. Curr Neurol Neurosci Rep. 2016;16(4):40.

51. Markley HG. CoEnzyme Q10 and riboflavin: the mitochondrial connection. Headache. 2012;52(Suppl 2):81–7.

52. Hershey AD, Powers SW, Vockell A-LB, Lecates SL, Ellinor PL, Segers A, et al. Coenzyme Q10 deficiency and response to supplementation in pediatric and adolescent migraine. Headache. 2007;47(1):73–80.

53. Parikh S, Saneto R, Falk MJ, Anselm I, Cohen BH, Haas R. A modern approach to the treatment of mitochondrial disease. Curr Treat Options Neurol. 2009;11(6):414–30.

54. Orr SL. Diet and nutraceutical interventions for headache management: a review of the evidence. Cephalalgia. 2016;36(12):1112–33.

55. Littarru GP, Tiano L. Clinical aspects of coenzyme Q10: an update. Nutr Burbank Los Angel Cty Calif. 2010;26(3):250–4.

56. Sándor PS, Di Clemente L, Coppola G, Saenger U, Fumal A, Magis D, et al. Efficacy of coenzyme Q10 in migraine prophylaxis: a randomized controlled trial. Neurology. 2005;64(4):713–5.

57. Slater SK, Nelson TD, Kabbouche MA, LeCates SL, Horn P, Segers A, et al. A randomized, double-blinded, placebo-controlled, crossover, add-on study of CoEnzyme Q10 in the prevention of pediatric and adolescent migraine. Cephalalgia. 2011;31(8):897–905.

58. Rozen TD, Oshinsky ML, Gebeline CA, Bradley KC, Young WB, Shechter AL, et al. Open label trial of

coenzyme Q10 as a migraine preventive. Cephalalgia. 2002;22(2):137–41.

59. Shoeibi A, Olfati N, Soltani Sabi M, Salehi M, Mali S, Akbari OM. Effectiveness of coenzyme Q10 in prophylactic treatment of migraine headache: an open-label, add-on, controlled trial. Acta Neurol Belg. 2016;117(1):103–9.

60. Bougea A, Spantideas N, Lyras V, Avramidis T, Thomaidis T. Melatonin 4 mg as prophylactic therapy for primary headaches: a pilot study. Funct Neurol. 2016;31(1):33–7.

61. Alstadhaug KB, Odeh F, Salvesen R, Bekkelund SI. Prophylaxis of migraine with melatonin: a randomized controlled trial. Neurology. 2010;75(17):1527–32.

62. Gonçalves AL, Martini Ferreira A, Ribeiro RT, Zukerman E, Cipolla-Neto J, Peres MFP. Randomised clinical trial comparing melatonin 3 mg, amitriptyline 25 mg and placebo for migraine prevention. J Neurol Neurosurg Psychiatry. 2016;87(10):1127–32.

63. Rozen TD. How effective is melatonin as a preventive treatment for hemicrania continua? A clinic-based study. Headache. 2015;55(3):430–6.

64. Rozen TD. Melatonin as treatment for idiopathic stabbing headache. Neurology. 2003;61(6):865–6.

65. Bandyopadhyay D, Ghosh G, Bandyopadhyay A, Reiter RJ. Melatonin protects against piroxicam-induced gastric ulceration. J Pineal Res. 2004;36(3):195–203.

66. Leroux E, Ducros A. Cluster headache. Orphanet J Rare Dis. 2008;3:20.

67. Leone M, Lucini V, D'Amico D, Moschiano F, Maltempo C, Fraschini F, et al. Twenty-four-hour melatonin and cortisol plasma levels in relation to timing of cluster headache. Cephalalgia. 1995;15(3):224–9.

68. Leone M, D'Amico D, Moschiano F, Fraschini F, Bussone G. Melatonin versus placebo in the prophylaxis of cluster headache: a double-blind pilot study with parallel groups. Cephalalgia. 1996;16(7):494–6.

69. Pringsheim T, Magnoux E, Dobson CF, Hamel E, Aubé M. Melatonin as adjunctive therapy in the prophylaxis of cluster headache: a pilot study. Headache. 2002;42(8):787–92.

70. Miano S, Parisi P, Pelliccia A, Luchetti A, Paolino MC, Villa MP. Melatonin to prevent migraine or tension-type headache in children. Neurol Sci. 2008;29(4):285–7.

71. Bruni O, Alonso-Alconada D, Besag F, Biran V, Braam W, Cortese S, et al. Current role of melatonin in pediatric neurology: clinical recommendations. Eur J Paediatr Neurol. 2015;19(2):122–33.

72. Pfotenhauer KM, Shubrook JH. Vitamin D deficiency, its role in health and disease, and current supplementation recommendations. J Am Osteopath Assoc. 2017;117(5):301–5.

73. Buettner C, Burstein R. Association of statin use and risk for severe headache or migraine by serum vitamin D status: a cross-sectional population-based study. Cephalalgia. 2015;35(9):757–66.

74. Buettner C, Nir R-R, Bertisch SM, Bernstein C, Schain A, Mittleman MA, et al. Simvastatin and vitamin D for migraine prevention: a randomized, controlled trial. Ann Neurol. 2015;78(6):970–81.

75. Cayir A, Turan MI, Tan H. Effect of vitamin D therapy in addition to amitriptyline on migraine attacks in pediatric patients. Braz J Med Biol Res. 2014;47(4):349–54.

76. Prakash S, Makwana P, Rathore C. Vitamin D deficiency mimicking chronic tension-type headache in children. BMJ Case Rep. 2016;2016:bcr2015213833.

77. Kreijkamp-Kaspers S, McGuire T, Bedford S, Loadsman P, Pirotta M, Moses G, et al. Your questions about complementary medicines answered: gingko biloba. Aust Fam Physician. 2015;44(8):565–6.

78. Allais G, D'Andrea G, Maggio M, Benedetto C. The efficacy of ginkgolide B in the acute treatment of migraine aura: an open preliminary trial. Neurol Sci. 2013;34(Suppl 1):S161–3.

79. D'Andrea G, Bussone G, Allais G, Aguggia M, D'Onofrio F, Maggio M, et al. Efficacy of Ginkgolide B in the prophylaxis of migraine with aura. Neurol Sci. 2009;30(Suppl 1):S121–4.

80. Esposito M, Carotenuto M. Ginkgolide B complex efficacy for brief prophylaxis of migraine in school-aged children: an open-label study. Neurol Sci. 2011;32(1):79–81.

81. Usai S, Grazzi L, Andrasik F, Bussone G. An innovative approach for migraine prevention in young age: a preliminary study. Neurol Sci. 2010;31(Suppl 1):S181–3.

82. Esposito M, Ruberto M, Pascotto A, Carotenuto M. Nutraceutical preparations in childhood migraine prophylaxis: effects on headache outcomes including disability and behaviour. Neurol Sci. 2012;33(6):1365–8.

83. Gaul C, Diener H-C, Danesch U. Migravent® study group. Improvement of migraine symptoms with a proprietary supplement containing riboflavin, magnesium and Q10: a randomized, placebo-controlled, double-blind, multicenter trial. J Headache Pain. 2015;16:516.

84. Witt CM, Lüdtke R, Willich SN. Homeopathic treatment of patients with migraine: a prospective observational study with a 2-year follow-up period. J Altern Complement Med. 2010;16(4):347–55.

85. Owen JM, Green BN. Homeopathic treatment of headaches: a systematic review of the literature. J Chiropr Med. 2004;3(2):45–52.

86. Homeopathy [Internet]. NCCIH. 2012 [cited 2017 Mar 27]. Available from: https://nccih.nih.gov/health/homeopathy.

87. Wells RE, Baute V, Wahbeh H. Complementary and integrative medicine for neurologic conditions. Med Clin North Am. 2017;101(5):881–9.

88. Wells RE, Loder E. Mind/body and behavioral treatments: the evidence and approach. Headache. 2012;52(Suppl 2):70–5.

89. Nahin RL, Barnes PM, Stussman BJ, Bloom B. Costs of complementary and alternative medicine (CAM) and frequency of visits to CAM practitioners: United States, 2007. Natl Health Stat Rep. 2009;18:1–14.

90. Wells RE, Smitherman TA, Seng EK, Houle TT, Loder EW. Behavioral and mind/body interventions in headache: unanswered questions and future research directions. Headache. 2014;54(6):1107–13.

91. Przekop P, Przekop A, Haviland MG. Multimodal compared to pharmacologic treatments for chronic tension-type headache in adolescents. J Bodyw Mov Ther. 2016;20(4):715–21.

92. Cowan RP. CAM in the real world: you may practice evidence-based medicine, but your patients don't. Headache. 2014;54(6):1097–102.

93. Tepper SJ. Editorial: complementary and alternative medicine (CAM), Ayurvedic medicine, and research into behavioral and mind/body interventions in headache. Headache. 2014;54(6):1114.

94. Oinonen SM. Integrative medicine: a necessary component in completing treatment for my chronic migraines. Headache. 2017;57(5):809–11.

Animal Models in Chronic Daily Headache (CDH) and Pathophysiology of CDH

21

Xianghong Arakaki, Noah B. Gross, Alfred N. Fonteh, and Michael G. Harrington

Abbreviations

5,7-DHT	5,7-Dihydroxytryptamine creatinine sulfate
BAEP	Brainstem auditory-evoked potential
BBB	Blood-brain barrier
BoNT-A	Botulinum neurotoxin type A
CBF	Cerebral blood flow
CDH	Chronic daily headache
CGRP	Calcitonin gene-related peptide
CM	Chronic migraine
CSD	Cortical spreading depression
CTTH	Chronic tension-type headache
EPs	Evoked potentials
FHM	Familial hemiplegic migraine
fMRI	Functional magnetic resonance imaging
IM	Inflammatory mediator
IP	Intraperitoneal
IS	Inflammatory soup
MOH	Medication overuse headache
NDPH	New daily persistent headache
NO	Nitric oxide
NTG	Nitroglycerin
nVNS	Noninvasive vagus nerve stimulation
ONS	Occipital nerve stimulation
PAG	Periaqueductal gray
RVM	Rostral ventromedial medulla
SD	Sprague-Dawley
TCC	Trigeminocervical complex
tDCS	Transcranial direct current stimulation
TENS	Transcutaneous electrical nerve stimulation
TMS	Transcranial magnetic stimulation
TNC	Trigeminal nucleus caudalis
VPM	Ventral posteromedial nucleus (of the thalamus)

X. Arakaki (✉) · N. B. Gross · A. N. Fonteh
M. G. Harrington
Neurosciences, Huntington Medical Research Institutes (HMRI), Pasadena, CA, USA
e-mail: xianghong@hmri.org

Introduction of Animal CM Model

Chronic migraine (CM) is a primary headache disorder, characterized by a transformation from a sporadic or "episodic" state to a more frequent or "chronic" state. This subgroup of episodic migraine patients, about 3% per year, evolve from having less headache days than non-headache days to having more headache days than non-headache days in any given month of the year [1]. Therapeutic approaches for CM patients are limited, and less than 50% of the individuals with CM are satisfied with their acute treatment [2]. To explore interventions for CM sufferers, research that explores neurobiological mechanisms of migraine transformation is critical but not practical in clinical studies. Animal models are ideally suited for this type of investigation and have played crucial roles in our understanding of CM pathophysiology, elucidating many of the mechanisms underlying migraine transition to aid in treatment [3]. However, few treatments currently exist for CM, which only bolsters the idea that more valid and reliable animal models for CM are needed. To have positive translational significance, these models should mimic the features of human CM by having similar mechanisms as well as sharing similar responses to interventions [4]. Therefore, three important prerequisites for animal models of CM should be to (1) reflect the recurrent activation of the trigeminal nociceptive system shown in all CM patients, (2) model the prominent phenotypic traits such as allodynia/hyperalgesia and photophobia [5], and (3) demonstrate positive responses to migraine treatments.

CM is a heterogeneous condition, and medications are effective for some but not all patients. Multiple models can be used to reveal the diverse mechanisms underlying this complex condition across diverse CM patient populations. Currently, there exist a few animal models for CM, although in their relative infancy, these models are beginning to shed light on this devastating neurological condition and treatment options. These paradigms include but are not limited to the following four different categories [5]: (1) repeated trigeminal nociceptive stimulation by applying inflammatory soup (IS) or inflammatory mediator (IM) epidurally via a small craniotomy applied to the animal's dorsal skull region [6–11]; (2) repeated trigeminal nociceptive stimulation by a nitric oxide (NO) donor, the most commonly used is nitroglycerin (NTG) [12–14]; (3) chronic modulation of the endogenous pain-modulating system, such as by serotonin (5-HT) depletion/chronic hyperleptinemia [15, 16]; and (4) chronic state of allodynia/hyperalgesia by genetic manipulations [17–30]. The first two paradigms to model CM are to repeatedly stimulate the nociceptive receptors of trigeminovascular neurons and produce a chronic pain state [6–14]. Chronic modification of pain modulatory pathways includes modification of ascending or descending pain modulatory pathways by altering neurotransmitters such as serotonin level [15, 16]. Genetic manipulation includes familial hemiplegic migraine (FHM)-associated dysfunction of channels and pumps [17–19], genes associated

with reduced threshold for cortical spreading depression (CSD) [20–22], genes associated with migraine trigeminal nociception and pain [23–29], as well as individual rats with migraine traits and yet unidentified genetic factors [30].

To highlight the importance of animal models in CM research, we will discuss the following aspects: anatomical networks and details of CM models induced by repeated nociceptive stimulations, clinical manifestations of CM models, electrophysiological mechanisms and non-pharmacological approaches, biochemical mechanisms and pharmacological approaches, genetic manipulations, and limitations of animal models. Examples of CM animal models are listed in Table 21.1.

Anatomy (Neural Substrate and Their Connections) and CM Models from Trigeminal Nociceptive Activation

Neurogenic Theory of Migraine

Over the past 150 years, many theories have been proposed to explain the pathophysiology of migraine. Based on extensive studies of migraine in animal models, it is widely accepted that migraine is a neurogenic disorder, originating in the brain, and involves activation and sensitization of the trigeminovascular pathways, brainstem nuclei, and diencephalic nuclei [31]. The head pain associated with a migraine attack, including the frontal, temporal, parietal, occipital, and upper cervical region, is thought to result from activation of the trigeminovascular system [31, 32]. Animal studies have also been instrumental in characterizing the anatomy and brain circuits that underlie migraine pathophysiology, as will be described in detail in the next section [31, 32].

Neural Circuitry Implicated in CM

CM is a disabling and complex neurological disorder, where multiple sensory pathways, limbic

Table 21.1 Representative animal models for CM

Animal species	Approach for CM	Migraine outcome	References
Male Sprague-Dawley (SD) rats	Epidural cannula infusion: 10 miroL inflammatory mediator (IM), 15 infusions over 3 weeks (2.5 h before testing). Single-unit recording in ventral posteromedial nucleus (VPM) of the thalamus	VPM neurons in CM rats fire faster than sham during mechanical stimulation, which was reduced after occipital nerve stimulation (ONS)	[6]
Male SD rats	Epidural cannula infusion: 10 miroL inflammatory mediator (IM), 14–17 daily infusions	Mechanical allodynia occurred in CM, which was reduced after acute ONS Thermal allodynia was not affected by ONS	[7]
Male SD rats	IS (inflammatory soup) of low intensity and high intensity or artificial cerebrospinal fluid (aCSF) through cannula at 2- or 3-day intervals for 4 times; cranial/extracephalic allodynia (by von Frey withdrawal thresholds); neuronal excitability (single-unit recording and c-Fos) and diffuse noxious inhibitory control (single-unit recording)	Single high IS or repetitive low IS produces reversible cephalic allodynia; repetitive high IS causes reversible cephalic and extracephalic allodynia; repeated high IS causes trigeminal neuronal hyperexcitability and impairs descending pain inhibition and results in development of central sensitization and cutaneous allodynia, which might facilitate subsequent migraine attacks and contribute to progression to CM	[9]
Male SD rats	IS (contained 1 mM histamine, serotonin, and bradykinin and 0.1 mM prostaglandin E2 in phosphate-buffered saline pH 7.4)	Repeated dura nociceptive stimulation caused maladaptive neuroplasticity in the brain that is similarly observed in CM patients: long-lasting allodynia; hypersensitivity to Nit roglycerin (NTG) (long-lasting decreased mechanical threshold and long-lasting higher TNC glutamatergic transmission by microdialysis) that is similarly seen in CM patients	[10]
Male and female C57BL6/J mice	Repeated systematic administration of NTG	Repeated NTG-induced acute hyperalgesia with each NTG application and progressive chronic basal hypersensitivity; known acute medication sumatriptan reduced the acute but not chronic hyperalgesia; known preventive medication topiramate inhibited the acute and chronic hyperalgesia	[12]
Male and female mice	Repeated systematic administration of NTG	Repeated NTG-induced acute hyperalgesia with each NTG application and progressive chronic basal hypersensitivity; known preventive medication propranolol inhibited the acute and chronic hyperalgesia; daily administration of acute medication sumatriptan resulted in acute and chronic hyperalgesia similar to that after repeated NTG application, consistent with medication-overuse headache (MOH)	[13]
Male SD rats	Repeated systematic administration of isosorbide dinitrate (ISDN), a NO donor at low (L-ISDN) or high (H-ISDN) dose	Repeated L-ISDN causes reversible cephalic cutaneous allodynia. H-ISDN causes both cephalic and extracephalic cutaneous allodynia, measured by von Frey filaments	[14]
Wistar rats, both genders	Repeated lateral ventricle injection of 5,7-dihydroxytryptamine creatinine sulfate (5,7-DHT)	Serotonin neurons and fibers degenerate; cerebral blood flow (CBF) velocity increased; cortical depolarization wave width extended	[15]
SD rats and Zucker fatty (ZF) rats, Zucker lean (ZL) rats	ICV leptin intraperitoneal (IP) leptin daily × 7 days; KCl-induced cortical spreading depression (CSD) recordings; measure CBF/direct current potential changes/CSD number/CSD duration	Number of CSD increased significantly in rats with 7 daily IP leptin injections or in ZF rats. Therefore, the cortex tends to be more susceptible to CSD in chronic hyperleptinemia	[16]
Mice	Knock-in mutation in the CACNA1A gene for alpha 1 subunit of neuronal Cav2.1 Ca^{2+} channels	Reduced threshold and increased propagation velocity of CSD	[17]
Mice	Knock-in mutation in the alpha 2 isoform of the ATP1A2 gene	Reduced threshold and increased propagation velocity of CSD	[18]
Mice	Knockout mutation in the ATP1A2 gene	Light sensitivity, over-activation of amygdala and piriform after conditioned fear stimuli	[19]

systems, autonomic networks, and cortical functions are involved. The nociceptive innervation of the intracranial vasculature and meninges is mainly through the ophthalmic (V1) division of the trigeminal nerve but also, to a lesser extent, through the maxillary (V2) and mandibular divisions (V3). There is also neuronal innervation of the dura mater from the cervical dorsal root ganglia [31]. The axon terminals of nociceptive nerve fibers that innervate the dura mater contain the vasoactive neuropeptides calcitonin gene-related peptide (CGRP), substance P, and neurokinin A, which are released upon stimulation and cause vasodilation of dural and pial vessels [31, 33–35]. The central neural circuitry of the trigeminovascular system includes a central afferent projection from the trigeminal ganglion that enters the caudal medulla of the brainstem, via the trigeminal tract, which terminates in the trigeminocervical complex (TCC), including the dorsal horns of the upper cervical spinal cord C1–C2, and the caudal division of the spinal trigeminal nucleus (TNC). The TCC makes reciprocal ascending and descending projections with several brainstem nuclei (periaqueductal gray (PAG), rostral ventromedial medulla (RVM)) and higher brain centers, including reciprocal connections with the hypothalamus and ascending projections to the thalamus (ventroposteriomedial and posterior), which in turn project widely throughout the cerebral cortex, where somatosensory and insular cortices form reciprocal projections with the TNC [31, 36] (Fig. 21.1).

The severe and throbbing pain in migraine is thought to result from activation of the nociceptive inputs from intra- and extracranial structures that converge in, and are relayed to higher brain centers through the TCC. All nociceptive information from craniovascular structures is relayed through the TCC and via ascending connections to other areas of the brainstem, diencephalon, and cerebral cortex, for modulation and interpretation of pain and other sensory-associated information. Pain processing is complex and involves a network of central neural activation primarily composed of the brainstem nuclei, midbrain, thalamus, hypothalamus, and cortical regions including the cingulate and insular cortices, somatosensory cortices, and prefrontal cortex.

Activation of these structures is thought to contribute to the perception of pain during migraine (sensory pathways) and also to endocrine (autonomic networks), cognitive (cortical functions), and affective (limbic systems) symptoms that last throughout the migraine "attack."

There is still much debate surrounding the role of brainstem and diencephalic activation during migraine. How does regional activation in the brain indicate where migraine may be triggered? Does migraine result from activation of the trigeminovascular system, which drives other symptoms in migraine? These questions have received some traction in human imaging studies where the hypothalamus shows temporally—and regionally—specific activation in episodic and chronic migraineurs, suggesting that the anterior hypothalamus underlies migraine initiation and the posterior hypothalamus is thought to underlie the transition from episodic to CM [37]. These questions have been under the intense scrutiny of migraine researchers in both human and animal studies seeking to discover more efficacious treatment options for episodic and chronic migraineurs. Animal studies, however, have the potential to more rapidly advance our understanding of migraine pathophysiology and drive preclinical drug screenings that will stand a better chance of successful clinical human phase trials.

Based on recently acquired empirical knowledge of migraine pathophysiology, the most common animal models for CM include either repeated systemic administration of pharmacological triggers of migraine, such as the NO donor NTG [12–14], or repeated epidural administration of inflammatory substances [6–11]. CM models induced by isosorbide dinitrate (ISDN) will also be mentioned in a later section. Although other NO donors such as sodium nitroprusside or diethylenetriamine/nitric oxide are being used in migraine research, they were either used in vivo [38] or in an acute mice model [39], which therefore is not a focus here.

NTG, or glyceryl trinitrate (GTN), is a potent vasodilator that evokes a delayed migraine in people who suffer with migraines [40–43], but not in non-migraineurs, and has been utilized in multiple human experimental paradigms [41]. NTG is an

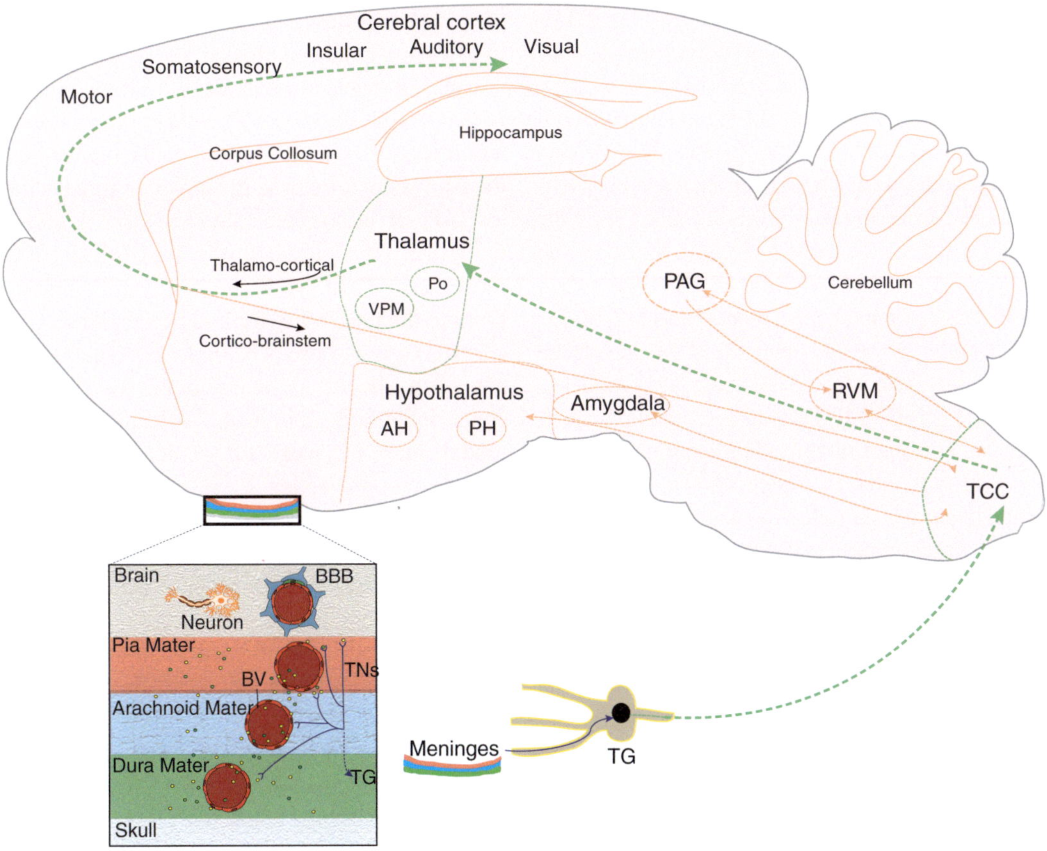

Fig. 21.1 Schematic diagram of the trigeminovascular system depicting principal rodent cephalic pain pathways. (Inset) The incipient events of a migraine headache include activation of nociceptors that innervate the meningeal blood vessels. Activation of meningeal nociceptors leads to the release of vasoactive proinflammatory peptides such as calcitonin gene-related peptide (CGRP) and substance P (SP) from their terminal nerve endings (colored circles near terminals), which produce neurogenic inflammation, characterized by vasodilation of meningeal blood vessels (BV), with possible deleterious effects on the blood-brain barrier (BBB), which is depicted by astrocytic end feet (blue) and pericytes (green) that directly appose brain capillaries. Pain information flows from the meningeal nociceptors via the trigeminal nerves (TNs) and proceeds to the trigeminal gan- glion (TG). Pain information is subsequently transmitted to the trigeminocervical complex (TCC) and then to several pain-processing nuclei, some of which have reciprocal modulatory connections with TCC (indicated by arrows). The major brain centers are depicted as mentioned in the main text. These include the rostral ventromedial medulla (RVM), the periaqueductal gray (PAG), the amygdala, the hypothalamus comprised of the anterior (AH) and posterior (PH) nuclei, the thalamus including the ventroposteriomedial (VPM) and posterior (Po) nuclei, and the cerebral cortex, comprised here of motor, somatosensory, insular, auditory, and visual cortices. Green dotted arrows indicate the main trigeminal pathway from TG to cortex; light brown-colored arrows show some modulatory pathways for trigeminovascular circuits

organic nitrate with a short plasma half-life (1–4 min) but longer half-life in lipophilic tissues such as the brain [44]. It is rapidly metabolized into NO in mammalian cells via both enzymatic and nonenzymatic processes. The breakdown metabolite, NO, is a free-radical species that acts as a smooth muscle relaxant and as a neuronal sec- ond messenger with diverse effects on signaling cascades in the central and peripheral nervous tissue [45]. NO donors are known migraine triggers in migraineurs, and inhibition of the enzyme, NO synthase, has antimigraine effects [46]. NTG-triggered hyperalgesia in rodents has been reliably used as a model for sensory hypersensitivity associated with migraine [47, 48]. The NTG-triggered migraine model has been used in mice [49] and rats [50], and has been shown to produce migraine-associated photophobia and altered meningeal blood flow [51], and prototypic allodynia and hyperalgesia that have been shown to be alleviated or reversed in rats or mice [14, 30, 52] by the antimigraine medications that target the serotonin system (i.e., triptans) and the CGRP system (i.e., CGRP receptor antagonist, olcegepant) [12, 50].

In order to better recreate CM, headache researchers have adapted the acute NTG model to examine chronic NTG effects on rodent pain sensitivity. The intermittent administration of NTG over several days has been shown to produce acute hyperalgesia following each NTG injection and a basal hypersensitivity that progressively worsens over time [12, 13]. Repeated NTG injections evoke mechanical hyperalgesia that was blocked by sumatriptan and long-lasting basal hyperalgesia that was blocked by the migraine prophylactic, topiramate. This chronic basal hypersensitivity was mediated by NO and cGMP signaling pathways because this NTG effect was enhanced by the phosphodiesterase-5 inhibitor sildenafil [12]. The observed long-lasting basal hyperalgesia reported following repeated NTG injections is consistent with clinical observations of people with CM that experience more allodynia, or pain to previously innocuous stimuli, during and between migraine attacks. Additionally, women are more susceptible to developing CM, and recent animal studies suggest that female rodents are more sensitive to repeated NTG than males: chronic basal hypersensitivity develops faster in female mice [12, 53]. These results are noteworthy because NTG-triggered sexual dimorphism in migraine-associated brain regions is related to estrogen levels, which further substantiates the chronic NTG model as a valid tool for studying sex differences in migraine [12, 54]. More detailed pharmacological value of this model will be discussed later in the biochemical mechanism section of this chapter.

There are also conflicting reported effects of systemic administration of NO donors on cutaneous sensitivity, including a decrease [52, 55, 56] or no change [57]. Those differences might stem from different doses of NTG used or difficulties in assessing cutaneous sensitivity in mice.

An important caveat in the NTG animal model is that a high dose of NTG (10 mg/kg) is often administered, which is substantially higher than the equivalent dose used in human migraine studies [41]. It is possible that this high dose has untoward physiological effects distinct from those associated with migraine in humans. Despite the possibility for additional physiological effects, high-dose NTG-induced hyperalgesia has been shown to be inhibited by systemic sumatriptan and topiramate, indicating that this model may be used for screening potential migraine prophylactics.

Another widely used animal model for studying CM is the aforementioned repeated dural application of IS. A large body of evidence from both animal studies and clinical observation suggests that a sterile meningeal inflammation is a key mechanism that underlies the sustained activation and sensitization of meningeal afferents during migraine attacks [34, 35]. In experimental animals, activation of meningeal nociceptors leads to the release of vasoactive proinflammatory substances such as CGRP from nerve endings, which produces vasodilation of meningeal blood vessels, plasma extravasation, and local activation of dural mast cells and subsequent release of cytokines and inflammatory mediators [34]. Several early studies in rodents have shown that a single dural application of IS (i.e., histamine, serotonin, bradykinin, prostaglandin E2) induces activation and mechanical sensitization of meningeal nociceptors and central trigeminovascular neurons [58, 59]. After brief local application of IS to the dura, second-order trigeminovascular neurons in the TCC showed long-lasting increased responses to innocuous mechanical or thermal facial skin stimulation, and third-order trigeminovascular neurons in the posterior thalamus showed long-lasting sensitized responses to both cephalic and extracephalic skin stimulations [8, 31]. Recently, this single application IS model has been modified to assess CM, in which various research groups have developed a rat model of trigeminal allodynia that closely mimics clinical observations in CM patients, characterized by chronic trigeminal allodynia, photophobia, increased sensitivity to migraine triggers, and similar pain-relieving responses to migraine treatments [10, 60, 61]. Using this rat model to deliver repeated dural stimulation represents the recurrent episodic nature of migraine attacks. After receiving five or more infusions, similar to repeated NTG injections, the rats exhibit trigeminal hypersensitivity at the baseline measure (prior to subsequent IS application), which represents a transition from an episodic to a chronic state of trigeminal sensitivity. After eight to ten IS infusions, the rats transition to a state of chronic trigeminal sensitization, where microdialysis in the TNC showed significantly increased levels of the excitatory neurotransmitter, glutamate, and sensitized behavioral responses that outlast the final infusion by as long as 3 months [10, 61].

Particularly interesting is the opportunity to utilize these CM animal models to investigate a controversial topic in the migraine field, the role of blood-brain barrier (BBB) permeability during both the episodic stage (following the second infusion, when dural stimulation only features an acute effect on trigeminal sensitivity, but does not induce long-lasting sensitivity) and the chronic stage (1 week after the tenth infusion, when the animals have developed long-lasting trigeminal sensitivity). It has recently been demonstrated using the sodium fluorescein permeability assay in many brain regions of the rats that during the chronic stage, astrocyte and microglial activation, BBB permeability, and trigeminal sensitivity were increased but only in the TNC. Furthermore, the tetracycline-derived antibiotic with anti-inflammatory properties, minocycline, prevented these chronic stage changes [61].

Preclinical Behavioral Manifestations of CM Models (Aura/CSD, Allodynia/Hyperalgesia, and Sensitivity to NTG)

There are a few preclinical behavioral features that are used for evaluating animal CM model, which include aura (CSD), allodynia and hyperalgesia, and sensitivity to NTG.

CSD and Aura

Migraine symptoms include aura and severe headache. CSD is a slowly propagating depolarization wave traveling at the speed around 3 mm/min across the cortex followed by neuronal activity suppression, which has been considered to underlie migraine aura [62] and can potentially activate the trigeminovascular pathway through trigeminal nociceptors [63, 64].

One animal model shows CM manifestation using repeated induction of CSD. For example, the frequency of CSD increased significantly in rats with seven daily intraperitoneal (IP) leptin injections or in ZF rats. Therefore, the cortex tends to be more susceptible to CSD in chronic hyperleptinemia [16]. This chronic hyperleptinemia may inhibit the serotonergic system [65, 66] and orexin-A secretion [67, 68], resulting in CSD enhancement and therefore increasing cortical susceptibility to migraine attacks by increasing long-term potentiation [69] and inflammatory cytokines [70] and facilitating migraine chronification [16]. Assessment of cortical depolarization wave width has also been assessed in a rat CM model [15].

Allodynia and Hyperalgesia

The preclinical CM and chronic pain features resulting from intrinsic neuronal hyperexcitability include allodynia and hyperalgesia [11]. Allodynia is pain perception to normal tactile stimuli; hyperalgesia is greater and longer pain perception or hypersensitivity to noxious stimuli [71].

CM is a product of progression from episodic to chronic state. The risk factors associated with the progression have become an increasing focus. The risk factors can reveal CM mechanisms and provide knowledge to slow down or reverse migraine progression for migraine management [1]. One of the important factors being investigated is allodynia [1]. The prevalence of cutaneous allodynia is significantly higher in CM than in episodic migraine and higher in a migraine group than in other headaches including other chronic daily headaches and episodic tension-type headache [72, 73]. The severity of cutaneous allodynia is also increased in CM relative to episodic migraine [72, 74–76]. Cutaneous allodynia is an indicator for CM [77, 78], which was found in more than 70% CM patients [72, 75]. Thus, allodynia can be a risk factor for transformation from episodic to CM [1]. Measurements of cutaneous sensitivity can therefore help model migraine transformation [13].

Similar to CM patterns in human studies, repeated dura nociceptive stimulation caused maladaptive neuroplasticity in the form of long-lasting allodynia in the rat brain [10]. Single high IS or repetitive low IS produces reversible cephalic allodynia; repetitive high IS causes reversible cephalic and extracephalic allodynia; and repeated high IS causes trigeminal neuronal hyperexcitability and impairs descending pain inhibition, resulting in the development of central sensitization and cutaneous allodynia and potentially facilitating subsequent migraine attacks and progression to CM [9, 10]. Repeat administration of the NO donor L-ISDN causes reversible cephalic cutaneous allodynia; H-ISDN causes both cephalic and extracephalic cutaneous allodynia, measured by von Frey filaments [14]. Those findings are consistent with migraineurs that do not have allodynia during early migraine stage but develop cephalic and later extracephalic allodynia as migraine attack frequency increases [1].

Animal studies on cutaneous hypersensitivity suggest that (a) the development of initial allodynia resulted from sensitization of trigeminovascular neurons that innervate the meninges [32]; (b) the cephalic allodynia is related to sensitization of second-order trigeminovascular neurons in the TNC that receive sensory input from both meninges and the scalp and facial skin [79]; and (c) the extracephalic allodynia results from sensitization of third-order trigeminovascular neurons in the posterior thalamic nuclei that accepts sensory input from the cephalic and extracephalic skin [8, 32]. Besides the trigeminal pain matrix, the activation of descending pain facilitation processes from the rostral ventromedial medulla (RVM) [80] and inhibition of descending pain inhibitory controls [9] are also involved.

Hypersensitivity to NTG

Besides being used as a CM trigger, NTG administration has also been suggested for migraine diagnosis [81, 82]. For instance, repeated migraine attacks sensitize the human brain to exogenous NO [83].

Similar hypersensitivity to NTG was shown in animals. For example, an animal CM model induced by repeated IS application and low dose of NTG induce long-lasting decreased mechanical threshold and long-lasting higher TNC glutamatergic transmission by microdialysis [10]. Greater NTG-induced hyperalgesia and reduced CSD threshold have been observed in a transgenic mouse model of familial migraine, with mutation in the gene encoding casein kinase I delta [20].

Treatment Assessment Based on the Symptoms

Migraine phenotypic traits such as allodynia/hyperalgesia have been used to evaluate treatment effects. For example, mechanical allodynia but not thermal allodynia in CM was reduced after acute occipital nerve stimulation (ONS), suggesting a greater involvement of A-α−/β-fiber than C fibers [7]. Further details of pharmacological and non-pharmacological treatment are discussed below.

Electrophysiological Mechanisms and Non-pharmacological Treatment

Repeated nociceptive activation can cause long-lasting neuroplasticity, eliciting allodynia or hyperalgesia [71] that underlies the mechanisms of migraine progression from episodic to CM. The anatomical network described above, especially the trigeminovascular pathway, provides a structural basis for studying electrophysiological mechanisms and developing and evaluating CM treatment.

Neuronal Hyperexcitability

In addition to allodynia [30, 52, 79], another important approach to study neuronal hypersensitivity is to record neuronal excitability directly by electrophysiological techniques, such as measuring action potential and bursting activities using single-unit recording. For instance, in the rat CM model induced by repeated epidural IM infusion, VPM neurons had higher firing frequency and bursting activity than those in sham rats from facial mechanical stimulation [6].

Neuronal hypersensitivity underlies the allodynia symptoms. For example, rat trigeminovascular neurons from posterior thalamus receive convergent afferents from both cranial meninges and the skin. These thalamic neurons were sensitized for cephalic and extracephalic innocuous and noxious stimulus after activation from dural exposure to IS [8]. This is consistent with higher posterior thalamic activation during migraine shown by fMRI [8]. Thalamic sensitization was associated with activation of pain-facilitating RVM "on" cells and suppression of RVM "off" cells [80].

Botulinum neurotoxin type A (BoNT-A) is the only approved prophylactic CM medication [84, 85]. Electrophysiology techniques have been used to explore the mechanism of BoNT-A effects in dural application of IS [11]: when applied after dural application of IS, BoNT-A reversed mechanical sensitization of meningeal C- but not Aδ-nociceptions; when applied before dural IS, BoNT-A prevented meningeal nociceptive sensitization from IS [11]. Further, extracranial suture injection of BoNT-A to rats inhibited trigeminal nerve nociceptive C-fiber responses to meningeal chemical stimulation through the capsaicin receptor TRPVI agonist (capsaicin) or a TRPAI agonist (mustard oil) after 7 days: no effect was seen on C-fiber responses or mechanical/chemical responses on both C- and Aδ-fibers [86]. Those studies provide mechanistic support for BoNT-A's prophylactic effect on CM, although no CM model was involved [85, 87]. This is also a great example of animal models used to compliment clinical applications.

Evoked Potentials (EPs)

Although "lack of habituation" of EPs has been considered as a biological hallmark of episodic migraine during the interictal stage, and different characteristics of EPs have been reported extensively in humans [88], studies about EPs in migraine animal model are still very limited. Brainstem auditory-evoked potential (BAEP) measurements in a NTG-induced acute migraine model have similar findings in humans: prolonged BAEP later peak (waves 4, 5, and 6) latencies after NTG injection are consistent with abnormal monoaminergic transmission in upper brainstem [89, 90]. This EP approach in animal models has great potential clinical value for CM research, because the measurements are non-invasive and are translational/reverse translational to clinical CM studies.

CSD

As mentioned previously, the frequency of CSD events was used to monitor migraine progression, which can be enhanced by chronic hyperleptinemia [16].

Treatment Using Electrophysiological Approach

The pharmacological CM treatment is challenging and often refractory because of a limited effect and with many intolerable adverse effects [91]. Medical treatments are less likely to work when administered after the development of allodynia and central sensitization [92]. However, neurostimulation used after the development of allodynia and central sensitization [92] has gained increasing attention as an alternative technique and has now been widely explored for the treatment of CM [93, 94]. Neurostimulation has been applied to the central nervous system for pain modulation, either invasively (e.g., deep brain stimulation) [93], minimally invasively (e.g., subcutaneous occipital nerve stimulation) [93–97], or noninvasively by transcranial direct current stimulation (tDCS), transcranial magnetic stimulation

(TMS), or transcutaneous nerve stimulation (TENS) [98]. For example, ONS treatment significantly reduced the higher firing and bursting activities of VPM neurons from the CM model induced by multiple epidural IMs, but not from the sham rats [6], supporting the gate control by ONS, where analgesic effects from nerve stimulation work during pain states via gate mechanisms [6, 99]. Another example, noninvasive vagus nerve stimulation (nVNS), was evaluated in patients with CM using stimulation parameters based on clinical studies [100] and preclinical models of migraine [101, 102] and provided persistent prophylactic effect which was well tolerated and safe [103]. In spite of the advantages of neurostimulation treatment, and because of limited knowledge of detailed mechanisms, pharmacological treatments are still most commonly used in the clinic.

Biochemical Mechanisms and Pharmacological Treatment

Animal Studies Reveal Molecular Mechanisms

The major hypothesized migraine mechanisms involve primary CNS [104] changes associated with neurotransmitters, neuropeptides, receptors and ion channels, and pumps and result in susceptible individuals who are more sensitive to changes in physiological and environmental factors [105]. Initiation of migraine attacks involves CSD and activation of trigeminal nerves. At the molecular level, neurotransmitters and neuropeptides acting on their specific receptors are released upon nerve activation. Receptor-mediated signaling events that may alter intracellular calcium or initiate the formation of mediators of inflammation accompany nerve activation in migraine. Several episodic and CM (M/CM) animal models that relate to neurotransmitters or neuropeptide signaling pathways have resulted in preclinical discoveries of migraine therapies (Table 21.2).

Since migraine pathophysiology involves the interaction of several molecules (Table 21.2), readouts from animal studies can be used translationally to determine how these molecules affect humans. A multifocal study by Ghosh et al. suggests interaction of hormonal, inflammatory, and GWAS variants but not neurotransmitters in migraine [121]. However, both animal and human studies have identified migraine-associated variants regulating neurotransmitter pathways, pain-sensing pathways, synaptic function [122], and transmembrane remodeling enzymes [123]. In FHM2 knock-in mouse model, there is evidence of a link between female sex hormone cycle, glutamate signaling, and psychiatric behaviors [124].

Discovery of Mechanism-Based CM Therapy

Examining the molecular mechanisms that may underlie migraine pathophysiology has resulted in several pharmacological treatment strategies. Animal models are extensively used to examine pain syndromes (nociceptive, inflammatory pain, neuropathic pain), and similarities with migraine drug development have recently been reviewed [125]. For example, migraine medications such as triptans [126, 127] were contributed by studies in animal models of migraine. This has also recently been exemplified with the promising new migraine treatment that targets CGRP using monoclonal antibodies where studies progressed from preclinical animal studies to currently ongoing clinical phase 3 human trials [128–130]. With several underlying mechanisms, animal studies suggest that poly-prophylactic or poly-therapies may be indicated to manage CM, and these may also impact recognized migraine comorbidities where similar pathways are altered. A mouse model for CM developed by chronic intermittent administration of NTG has been used to test preventive therapies in male and female animals. This model has been shown and established to screen and test preventive CM treatment [12, 13]. Known acute medication sumatriptan reduced the acute but not chronic hyperalgesia [12], consistent with sumatriptan unable to prevent migraine progression [131]; known preventive medication topiramate inhibited the acute and chronic hyperalgesia [12]. The acute hyperalgesia and sustained basal hypersensitivity induced in the same CM model were blocked by known preventive medication

Table 21.2 Animal models, potential mechanism, and therapeutic significance in M/CM

Molecules	Model and mechanism	Migraine clinical significance
Neurotransmitters Serotonin, glutamate, GABA, dopamine	Rat microdialysis with dural inflammation and quantification of extracellular concentrations of neurotransmitters [106]. Serotonin levels change in animal migraine models [107]	Increase in glutamate but no change in the excitatory amino acid (aspartic acid) or the inhibitory neurotransmitters, gamma-aminobutyric acid, or glutamine, suggests that glutamate is important in allodynia and hyperalgesia [106]. 5-HT receptor antagonists have clinical utility in migraine [107]
Neuropeptides CGRP, natriuretic peptide bradykinin	CSD induced by the application of KCl to the cortex increased CGRP Chronic paracetamol treatment enhanced CGRP [108] expression Natriuretic peptide P2X3 receptor inhibition	Increased trigeminovascular nociception is associated with CGRP expression [108]
Neuromodulators Cations (Na^+, Ca^{2+})	Increases in rat brain sodium after NTG (IP) is associated with enhanced excitability [56] Localization of Na^+/K^+-ATPase isoforms in rat brain [109] NTG mouse model for mechanical hyperalgesia hypersensitivity [110] Enhanced motor nerve Ca^{2+} influx through mutated Ca^{2+} presynaptic Ca^{2+}v2.1 channels	Specific Na^+/K^+-ATPase isoforms are targets for brain sodium regulation Sensitive to sumatriptan, hypersensitivity that is prevented by topiramate [110]
Mediators of inflammation Prostaglandins, PAF, endocannabinoids	Production of prostaglandins in animal models Systemic NTG produces hyperalgesia in the rats 4 h after its administration [111]. An inhibitor or fatty acid amide hydrolase had antinociceptive effects and blocked NTG-induced hyperalgesia [112]	NSAIDs that prevent prostaglandin production by inhibiting cyclooxygenase are widely used in animal models Pretreatment with endocannabinoid reduced nociception, hyperalgesia, and neuronal activation [111]
Hormones, estrogen	Sex and estrogen influence neuronal activation in NTG-treated rats [54] Changes in female hormones modulates CSD in mice [113]	Gender differences call for customized therapies
Medication (triptan) overuse headache (MOH)	Lower CSD threshold, reduced Fos expression, deranges 5HT modulating pathways [114]	Triptan overuse effects are reversed by topiramate [115]
Receptor-mediated signaling pathways	CM rat model of repeated infusion of inflammatory soup increased protein kinase C gamma. PKC gamma activation increased CGRP and Fos [116] Involvement of phosphorylated extracellular signal-regulated kinase (p-ERK), CGRP, and cyclooxygenase-2 (COX-2) in pain and nociceptive pathways [117, 118], brain-derived neurotrophic factor (BDNF), tropomyosin receptor kinases (TrkB), and c-AMP-responsive element-binding protein (CREB) [118]. Activation of PI3-K/PTEN pathway [119]	PKC gamma inhibition reduced phosphorylation of GluT1 and allodynia [116] PTEN and many signaling pathways affected in M/CM are promising therapeutic targets [120]

propranolol (β-blocker), while valproate had no effect [13]. Amiloride inhibited NTG-induced hyperalgesia; memantine was ineffective, while administration of sumatriptan did not alter NTG-induced hyperalgesia but resulted in acute and chronic hyperalgesia [13]. These studies establish the repeated NTG-induced CM model as a tool for verifying potential mechanisms and testing migraine-preventive therapies. Therefore, animal models can have both translational and reverse translational values for CM studies.

Medication overuse headache (MOH) typically occurs in genetically susceptible individuals suffering from migraine or tension-type headache. Excessive use of headache medications, i.e., triptans or opioids (more than 10 days/month/>3 months), leads to a gradual exacerbation of episodic migraine frequency, transforming the individual into a chronic headache sufferer. This condition has recently been examined in animal models with repeated administration of migraine-relieving drugs (e.g., sumatriptan) which resulted in enduring central sensitization, measured by increased cutaneous allodynia, and increased susceptibility to CSD, similar to that after repeated NTG application, consistent with MOH [13, 115, 132]. The pathophysiology and mechanisms of MOH are also explored: Fos expression in TNC of sumatriptan-treated rats was reduced by topiramate, suggesting that the underlying mechanism of triptan-induced MOH involved increased activation of TNC [115]; the humanized CGRP antibody (TEVA 48125) has been shown to reduce NO- and stress-mediated reinstatement of allodynia in a sumatriptan MOH model [133]. In addition to the TNC, chronic medication overuse affects several brain regions related to headache pathology. In addition to the upregulation of CGRP, substance P, and NO synthase and increase in the receptive field, the main mechanism underlying headache chronification seems to be the derangement of 5-HT-dependent signaling pathways [114].

To summarize, animal models provide knowledge bases for exploring migraine biochemical mechanisms and developing antimigraine pharmacological treatment options. For example, current rescue medication for CM such as serotonin agonist (triptans) or CGRP receptor antagonist (gepants) is developed from animal models; mechanisms of prophylactic medication topiramate are explored in animal models, leading to its improved prophylactic applications in clinical applications [134]. Those are positive translational examples for CM preclinical studies, in addition to reverse translational applications of biochemical and pharmacological treatment.

Genetic Models

Four genes implicated in familial hemiplegic migraine (FHM-1 to FHM-4, reviewed in [135–137]) represent models to investigate the role of specific genes in FHM. The next seven murine mutants include models that demonstrate a lower threshold for central sensitization and/or sensory nociception that are surrogate analogues for migraine. Finally, an inherited cranial nociceptive trait in SD rats is included; while no gene locus or linkage has been identified, this approach has potential to investigate a more natural migraine-type predisposition that is distinct from transgenic mice models.

FHM-1 is present in about 50% of FHM patients: two mice models have been developed from the knock-in of human mutations R192Q [17] or S218L [138] that are encoded in the α1 subunit of the voltage-gated Cav2.1 Ca^{2+} channel CACNA1A. The homozygous R192Q mice have a milder phenotype in both humans and mice, and the mice were shown to have a reduced threshold and increased velocity of CSD, widely considered to be the neurophysiological correlate of the migraine aura. R192Q mice had gain-of-function effects in the CACNA1A channel's current density and enhancement of neurotransmission at the neuromuscular junction, and the CSD effects enhanced circadian phase resetting and potentiated trigeminal nociception [17, 139–147]. These studies reveal inflammatory, receptor, channel, signaling, and calcitonin G-related peptide (CGRP) roles in FHM-1 [17, 139–147]. The S218L mice have a more severe phenotype, similar to humans. S218L mice have a gene dosage effect where the homozygous state is often lethal [138, 148].

FHM-2, present in about 25%V of FHM patients, is based on mutations in the α_2 isoform of the ATP1A2 gene for the Na+/K+-ATPase. This isoform is expressed in the brain predominantly in astrocytes [18] but also in the epithelial cells of the choroid plexus [109]. Only heterozygous knock-in or knockout mice are viable, as homozygous animals die around birth, probably from respiratory failure [149].

Heterozygous knock-in of either of the human $\alpha_2^{+/R887}$ or $\alpha_2^{+/G301R}$ mutations leads to a reduced induction threshold and increased propagation velocity of CSD [18] resembling the effect of the human FHM-2 mutations. The varying phenotype from both of these knock-in mutations has the commonality of altered CSD with a greater effect in females, which are notable features of migraine. Features of these mice are reminiscent of some other migraine behaviors: $\alpha_2^{+/R887}$ mice had minimal clinical alteration with elevated fear response and increased anxiety on SHIRPA protocol assessment; $\alpha_2^{+/G301R}$ mice had depression-like behavior, such as increased immobility compared to WT mice [124] and displayed stress-induced anhedonia and increased acoustic startle responses, implying abnormal levels of fear and anxiety. Females but not males were hypoactive in the open field test with excessive grooming and compulsive behaviors: female $\alpha_2^{+/G301R}$ mice buried significantly more marbles compared to both WT and male $\alpha_2^{+/G301R}$ mice [124].

Heterozygous knockout of the ATP1A2 generated $\alpha_2^{+/-}$ mice models, which displayed increased fear and anxiety as the main abnormal behavioral phenotype [19, 149, 150]. Compared to WT littermates, $\alpha_2^{+/-}$ mice spent less time in the illuminated room during the light/dark test, and the latency to enter the illuminated room was also significantly higher [19], suggesting increased fear and anxiety behaviors. We suggest this result also represents behavior analogous to the light sensitivity of migraine. In the open field test, $\alpha_2^{+/-}$ mice were found to be less active compared to WT mice [149], a commonly used indicator of enhanced fear behavior [149]. c-Fos expression was elevated in the amygdala and piriform cortex in adult $\alpha_2^{+/-}$ mice after conditioned fear stimuli, indicating neuronal hyperactivity in the amyg-

dala and piriform cortex [19]. A dysfunction in the removal of neurotransmitters from synapses could be the underlying cause of neuronal hyperactivity and of the observed neurodegeneration in the amygdala and piriform cortex. Uptake of glutamate and GABA into crude synaptosome preparations from $\alpha_2^{-/-}$ fetuses was impaired compared to WT preparations, and consequently, both glutamate and GABA levels were increased in brains from $\alpha_2^{-/-}$ fetuses relative to WT littermates [19]. We suggest this is an interesting analogue of the altered amygdala reports in migraine [19, 54, 151, 152].

Further evidence of a role for the Na+/K+-ATPase α_2 isoform in the animal migraine analogue comes from our recent studies where we found that $\alpha_2^{+/-}$ mice have reduced mechanical aversive threshold to von Frey hairs and increased c-Fos immunoreactivity in the TNC [153].

FHM-3 (the voltage-gated sodium channel SCN1A, $Na_v1.1$) mutations are much less commonly found in FHM, when these SCN1A mice have been studied for their prominent epilepsy syndromes thus far. A principal mechanism for the effect of SCN1A mutations on lowering the epilepsy threshold is from loss of function in inhibitory neurons, which may illuminate migraine phenotype studies [154–156].

FHM-4 (proline-rich transmembrane protein 2, PRRT2) mutations are found in the majority of patients with benign familial infantile epilepsy, infantile convulsions and choreoathetosis, and paroxysmal kinesigenic dyskinesia but more recently with FHM [157]. PRRT2 knockout mice have been recently reported [158] and display paroxysmal neurological features with increased sensitivity that include jumping in response to sounds that are not displayed in the WT.

Additional genetic models that resulted in reduced CSD threshold or increased CSD include casein kinase Iδ (CKIδ) [20], neurogenic locus notch homolog protein 3 (Notch 3) [21], or the ligand-gated cation channel receptor P2X7 [22]. CGRP receptors are overexpressed and sensitized in a mice model with genetic manipulation of the gene nestin/human receptor activity-modifying protein-1 (hRAMP1) [23]. Migraine-susceptible genes associated with trigeminal nociception include acid-sensing ion channel 1 (ASIC1) [24] and transient receptor potential M8 (TRPM8) [25–28].

Neurofibromatosis type 1 (NF1) is linked to inactivating mutations or homozygous deletion of the NF1 gene, with numerous effects including migraine and pain. Moutal and colleagues demonstrate a peptide, t-CNRP1, that mimics the antinociceptive signaling of neurofibromin, the NF1 translated protein, and reduces in vivo responses to noxious stimuli [29].

Genetic effect in rats is recognized but not yet localized. Oshinsky and colleagues [30] reported individual Sprague-Dawley rats that were intermittently and spontaneously more susceptible to mechanical trigeminal (periorbital) aversive nociception. This allodynia was reversed by rescue or prophylactic antimigraine medications and, on the other hand, triggered with NTG or CGRP. They reported that this trait was maintained in breeding. While not yet identified, a rat model of migraine would have great value in further identifying the genetic factors involved in migraine.

Limitations of CM Animal Models

While animal models have revealed CM pathophysiology, identified novel therapeutic targets, and estimated treatment effects, there are several limitations:

1. Pain is a subjective and complicated experience with sensory, emotional, and cognitive components that are difficult to replicate in animal models.
2. Trigeminovascular nociceptive activation used in the CM models, such as IM/IS or NTG, is not endogenous and cannot fully mimic the events that trigger human migraine attacks.
3. Interpretations of the behavioral readouts or CM phenotypic traits are challenging [159].
4. Genetic models represent one particular gene that occurs in FHM and cannot represent common CM cases that are not genetically linked.
5. Animal brains are different from human brains and have less complicated social and emo-

tional circuits that can be important in some subpopulations with CM.
6. CM comorbidities are complex and difficult to replicate in animal models.
7. Several potential medications (such as substance P antagonists) have failed in clinical trials in spite of strong animal model support [160, 161].
8. Some treatment approaches, such as mindfulness-based training that is effective in CM patients [162], cannot be studied in animal models.

Summary and Conclusion

CM has a complex underlying pathophysiology that is not easily unraveled by a single animal model. Several important animal models involving NTG sensitization, application of inflammatory agents, or genetic manipulations are revealing complex molecular abnormalities that contribute to the CM mechanisms. Various models reveal molecules/signaling pathways and putative mechanisms with potential therapeutic significance (Tables 21.1 and 21.2). Animal models have not always led to successful translation in humans. Animal models cannot replace the study and treatment of migraine. However, their undisputed utility means that animal models are unraveling disease mechanisms and contributing to the development of therapeutic tools with translational implications and will eventually guide the dire need for personalized therapies [123, 163].

References

1. Bigal ME, Lipton RB. What predicts the change from episodic to chronic migraine? Curr Opin Neurol. 2009;22(3):269–76.
2. Bigal ME, Serrano D, Reed M, Lipton RB. Chronic migraine in the population: burden, diagnosis, and satisfaction with treatment. Neurology. 2008; 71(8):559–66.
3. McGonigle P, Ruggeri B. Animal models of human disease: challenges in enabling translation. Biochem Pharmacol. 2014;87(1):162–71.
4. McGonigle P. Animal models of CNS disorders. Biochem Pharmacol. 2014;87(1):140–9.

5. Storer RJ, Supronsinchai W, Srikiatkhachorn A. Animal models of chronic migraine. Curr Pain Headache Rep. 2015;19(1):467.

6. Walling I, Smith H, Gee LE, Kaszuba B, Chockalingam A, Barborica A, et al. Occipital nerve stimulation attenuates neuronal firing response to mechanical stimuli in the ventral posteromedial thalamus of a rodent model of chronic migraine. Neurosurgery. 2017.

7. De La Cruz P, Gee L, Walling I, Morris B, Chen N, Kumar V, et al. Treatment of allodynia by occipital nerve stimulation in chronic migraine rodent. Neurosurgery. 2015;77(3):479–85. discussion 85.

8. Burstein R, Jakubowski M, Garcia-Nicas E, Kainz V, Bajwa Z, Hargreaves R, et al. Thalamic sensitization transforms localized pain into widespread allodynia. Ann Neurol. 2010;68(1):81–91.

9. Boyer N, Dallel R, Artola A, Monconduit L. General trigeminospinal central sensitization and impaired descending pain inhibitory controls contribute to migraine progression. Pain. 2014;155(7):1196–205.

10. Oshinsky ML, Gomoncharoensiri S. Episodic dural stimulation in awake rats: a model for recurrent headache. Headache. 2007;47(7):1026–36.

11. Burstein R, Zhang X, Levy D, Aoki KR, Brin MF. Selective inhibition of meningeal nociceptors by botulinum neurotoxin type A: therapeutic implications for migraine and other pains. Cephalalgia. 2014;34(11):853–69.

12. Pradhan AA, Smith ML, McGuire B, Tarash I, Evans CJ, Charles A. Characterization of a novel model of chronic migraine. Pain. 2014;155(2):269–74.

13. Tipton AF, Tarash I, McGuire B, Charles A, Pradhan AA. The effects of acute and preventive migraine therapies in a mouse model of chronic migraine. Cephalalgia. 2016;36(11):1048–56.

14. Dallel R, Descheemaeker A, Luccarini P. Recurrent administration of the nitric oxide donor, isosorbide dinitrate, induces a persistent cephalic cutaneous hypersensitivity: a model for migraine progression. Cephalalgia. 2017;333102417714032.

15. Cui Y, Li QH, Yamada H, Watanabe Y, Kataoka Y. Chronic degeneration of dorsal raphe serotonergic neurons modulates cortical spreading depression: a possible pathophysiology of migraine. J Neurosci Res. 2013;91(6):737–44.

16. Kitamura E, Kanazawa N, Hamada J. Hyperleptinemia increases the susceptibility of the cortex to generate cortical spreading depression. Cephalalgia. 2015;35(4):327–34.

17. van den Maagdenberg AM, Pietrobon D, Pizzorusso T, Kaja S, Broos LA, Cesetti T, et al. A Cacna1a knockin migraine mouse model with increased susceptibility to cortical spreading depression. Neuron. 2004;41(5):701–10.

18. Leo L, Gherardini L, Barone V, De Fusco M, Pietrobon D, Pizzorusso T, et al. Increased susceptibility to cortical spreading depression in the mouse model of familial hemiplegic migraine type 2. PLoS Genet. 2011;7(6):e1002129.

19. Ikeda K, Onaka T, Yamakado M, Nakai J, Ishikawa TO, Taketo MM, et al. Degeneration of the amygdala/piriform cortex and enhanced fear/anxiety behaviors in sodium pump alpha2 subunit (Atp1a2)-deficient mice. J Neurosci. 2003;23(11):4667–76.

20. Brennan KC, Bates EA, Shapiro RE, Zyuzin J, Hallows WC, Huang Y, et al. Casein kinase i delta mutations in familial migraine and advanced sleep phase. Sci Transl Med. 2013;5(183):183ra56. 1–11.

21. Eikermann-Haerter K, Yuzawa I, Dilekoz E, Joutel A, Moskowitz MA, Ayata C. Cerebral autosomal dominant arteriopathy with subcortical infarcts and leukoencephalopathy syndrome mutations increase susceptibility to spreading depression. Ann Neurol. 2011;69(2):413–8.

22. Chen SP, Qin T, Seidel JL, Zheng Y, Eikermann M, Ferrari MD, et al. Inhibition of the P2X7-PANX1 complex suppresses spreading depolarization and neuroinflammation. Brain. 2017;140(6):1643–56.

23. Marquez de Prado B, Hammond DL, Russo AF. Genetic enhancement of calcitonin gene-related Peptide-induced central sensitization to mechanical stimuli in mice. J Pain. 2009;10(9):992–1000.

24. Fu H, Fang P, Zhou HY, Zhou J, Yu XW, Ni M, et al. Acid-sensing ion channels in trigeminal ganglion neurons innervating the orofacial region contribute to orofacial inflammatory pain. Clin Exp Pharmacol Physiol. 2016;43(2):193–202.

25. Anttila V, Stefansson H, Kallela M, Todt U, Terwindt GM, Calafato MS, et al. Genome-wide association study of migraine implicates a common susceptibility variant on 8q22.1. Nat Genet. 2010;42(10):869–73.

26. Chasman DI, Schurks M, Anttila V, de Vries B, Schminke U, Launer LJ, et al. Genome-wide association study reveals three susceptibility loci for common migraine in the general population. Nat Genet. 2011;43(7):695–8.

27. Freilinger T, Anttila V, de Vries B, Malik R, Kallela M, Terwindt GM, et al. Genome-wide association analysis identifies susceptibility loci for migraine without aura. Nat Genet. 2012;44(7):777–82.

28. Kayama Y, Shibata M, Takizawa T, Ibata K, Shimizu T, Ebine T, et al. Functional interactions between transient receptor potential M8 and transient receptor potential V1 in the trigeminal system: relevance to migraine pathophysiology. Cephalalgia. 2017;333102417712719.

29. Moutal A, Wang Y, Yang X, Ji Y, Luo S, Dorame A, et al. Dissecting the role of the CRMP2-neurofibromin complex on pain behaviors. In: Pain; 2017.

30. Oshinsky ML, Sanghvi MM, Maxwell CR, Gonzalez D, Spangenberg RJ, Cooper M, et al. Spontaneous trigeminal allodynia in rats: a model of primary headache. Headache. 2012;52(9):1336–49.

31. Pietrobon D, Moskowitz MA. Pathophysiology of migraine. Annu Rev Physiol. 2013;75:365–91.

32. Bernstein C, Burstein R. Sensitization of the trigeminovascular pathway: perspective and implications to migraine pathophysiology. J Clin Neurol. 2012;8(2):89–99.

33. Levy D. Migraine pain and nociceptor activation—where do we stand? Headache. 2010;50(5):909–16.

34. Levy D. Migraine pain, meningeal inflammation, and mast cells. Curr Pain Headache Rep. 2009;13(3):237–40.

35. Waeber C, Moskowitz MA. Migraine as an inflammatory disorder. Neurology. 2005;64(10 Suppl 2):S9–15.

36. Noseda R, Burstein R. Migraine pathophysiology: anatomy of the trigeminovascular pathway and associated neurological symptoms, cortical spreading depression, sensitization, and modulation of pain. Pain. 2013.

37. Schulte LH, Allers A, May A. Hypothalamus as a mediator of chronic migraine: evidence from high-resolution fMRI. Neurology. 2017;88(21):2011–6.

38. Capuano A, De Corato A, Lisi L, Tringali G, Navarra P, Dello Russo C. Proinflammatory-activated trigeminal satellite cells promote neuronal sensitization: relevance for migraine pathology. Mol Pain. 2009;5:43.

39. Galeotti N, Ghelardini C. St. John's wort reversal of meningeal nociception: a natural therapeutic perspective for migraine pain. Phytomedicine. 2013;20(10):930–8.

40. Ashina M, Simonsen H, Bendtsen L, Jensen R, Olesen J. Glyceryl trinitrate may trigger endogenous nitric oxide production in patients with chronic tension-type headache. Cephalalgia. 2004;24(11):967–72.

41. Olesen J. The role of nitric oxide (NO) in migraine, tension-type headache and cluster headache. Pharmacol Ther. 2008;120(2):157–71.

42. Iversen HK, Olesen J, Tfelt-Hansen P. Intravenous nitroglycerin as an experimental model of vascular headache. Basic characteristics. Pain. 1989;38(1):17–24.

43. Afridi SK, Kaube H, Goadsby PJ. Glyceryl trinitrate triggers premonitory symptoms in migraineurs. Pain. 2004;110(3):675–80.

44. Torfgard K, Ahlner J, Axelsson KL, Norlander B, Bertler A. Tissue levels of glyceryl trinitrate and cGMP after in vivo administration in rat, and the effect of tolerance development. Can J Physiol Pharmacol. 1991;69(9):1257–61.

45. Moncada S, Palmer RM, Higgs EA. Nitric oxide: physiology, pathophysiology, and pharmacology. Pharmacol Rev. 1991;43(2):109–42.

46. Lassen LH, Ashina M, Christiansen I, Ulrich V, Olesen J. Nitric oxide synthase inhibition in migraine. Lancet. 1997;349(9049):401–2.

47. Tassorelli C, Joseph SA. Systemic nitroglycerin induces Fos immunoreactivity in brainstem and forebrain structures of the rat. Brain Res. 1995;682(1–2):167–81.

48. Bergerot A, Holland PR, Akerman S, Bartsch T, Ahn AH, MaassenVanDenBrink A, et al. Animal models of migraine: looking at the component parts of a complex disorder. Eur J Neurosci. 2006;24(6):1517–34.

49. Bates EA, Nikai T, Brennan KC, Fu YH, Charles AC, Basbaum AI, et al. Sumatriptan alleviates nitroglycerin-induced mechanical and thermal allodynia in mice. Cephalalgia. 2010;30(2):170–8.

50. Capuano A, Greco MC, Navarra P, Tringali G. Correlation between algogenic effects of calcitonin-gene-related peptide (CGRP) and activation of trigeminal vascular system, in an in vivo experimental model of nitroglycerin-induced sensitization. Eur J Pharmacol. 2014;740:97–102.

51. Markovics A, Kormos V, Gaszner B, Lashgarara A, Szoke E, Sandor K, et al. Pituitary adenylate cyclase-activating polypeptide plays a key role in nitroglycerol-induced trigeminovascular activation in mice. Neurobiol Dis. 2012;45(1):633–44.

52. Farkas S, Bolcskei K, Markovics A, Varga A, Kis-Varga A, Kormos V, et al. Utility of different outcome measures for the nitroglycerin model of migraine in mice. J Pharmacol Toxicol Methods. 2016;77:33–44.

53. Victor TW, Hu X, Campbell JC, Buse DC, Lipton RB. Migraine prevalence by age and sex in the United States: a life-span study. Cephalalgia. 2010;30(9):1065–72.

54. Greco R, Tassorelli C, Mangione AS, Smeraldi A, Allena M, Sandrini G, et al. Effect of sex and estrogens on neuronal activation in an animal model of migraine. Headache. 2013;53(2):288–96.

55. Greco R, Tassorelli C, Armentero MT, Sandrini G, Nappi G, Blandini F. Role of central dopaminergic circuitry in pain processing and nitroglycerin-induced hyperalgesia. Brain Res. 2008;1238:215–23.

56. Harrington MG, Chekmenev EY, Schepkin V, Fonteh AN, Arakaki X. Sodium MRI in a rat migraine model and a NEURON simulation study support a role for sodium in migraine. Cephalalgia. 2011;31(12):1254–65.

57. Bree D, Levy D. Development of CGRP-dependent pain and headache related behaviours in a rat model of concussion: implications for mechanisms of post-traumatic headache. Cephalalgia. 2016.

58. Burstein R, Yamamura H, Malick A, Strassman AM. Chemical stimulation of the intracranial dura induces enhanced responses to facial stimulation in brain stem trigeminal neurons. J Neurophysiol. 1998;79(2):964–82.

59. Levy D, Strassman AM. Mechanical response properties of A and C primary afferent neurons innervating the rat intracranial dura. J Neurophysiol. 2002;88(6):3021–31.

60. Boyer N, Signoret-Genest J, Artola A, Dallel R, Monconduit L. Propranolol treatment prevents chronic central sensitization induced by repeated dural stimulation. Pain. 2017.

61. Fried NT, Maxwell CR, Elliott MB, Oshinsky ML. Region-specific disruption of the blood-brain barrier following repeated inflammatory dural stimulation in a rat model of chronic trigeminal allodynia. Cephalalgia. 2017;333102417703764.

62. Charles AC, Baca SM. Cortical spreading depression and migraine. Nat Rev Neurol. 2013;9(11):637–44.

63. Zhang X, Levy D, Noseda R, Kainz V, Jakubowski M, Burstein R. Activation of meningeal nociceptors by cortical spreading depression: implications for migraine with aura. J Neurosci. 2010;30(26):8807–14.

64. Zhang X, Levy D, Kainz V, Noseda R, Jakubowski M, Burstein R. Activation of central trigeminovascular neurons by cortical spreading depression. Ann Neurol. 2011;69(5):855–65.

65. Supornsilpchai W, Sanguanrangsirikul S, Maneesri S, Srikiatkhachorn A. Serotonin depletion, cortical spreading depression, and trigeminal nociception. Headache. 2006;46(1):34–9.

66. Oury F, Karsenty G. Towards a serotonin-dependent leptin roadmap in the brain. Trends Endocrinol Metab. 2011;22(9):382–7.

67. Kitamura E, Hamada J, Kanazawa N, Yonekura J, Masuda R, Sakai F, et al. The effect of orexin-A on the pathological mechanism in the rat focal cerebral ischemia. Neurosci Res. 2010;68(2):154–7.

68. Jequier E. Leptin signaling, adiposity, and energy balance. Ann N Y Acad Sci. 2002;967:379–88.

69. Berger M, Speckmann EJ, Pape HC, Gorji A. Spreading depression enhances human neocortical excitability in vitro. Cephalalgia. 2008;28(5):558–62.

70. Vezzani A, Friedman A. Brain inflammation as a biomarker in epilepsy. Biomark Med. 2011;5(5):607–14.

71. Woolf CJ, Salter MW. Neuronal plasticity: increasing the gain in pain. Science. 2000;288(5472):1765–9.

72. Bigal ME, Ashina S, Burstein R, Reed ML, Buse D, Serrano D, et al. Prevalence and characteristics of allodynia in headache sufferers: a population study. Neurology. 2008;70(17):1525–33.

73. Lipton RB, Bigal ME, Ashina S, Burstein R, Silberstein S, Reed ML, et al. Cutaneous allodynia in the migraine population. Ann Neurol. 2008;63(2):148–58.

74. Ashkenazi A, Silberstein S, Jakubowski M, Burstein R. Improved identification of allodynic migraine patients using a questionnaire. Cephalalgia. 2007;27(4):325–9.

75. Burstein R, Yarnitsky D, Goor-Aryeh I, Ransil BJ, Bajwa ZH. An association between migraine and cutaneous allodynia. Ann Neurol. 2000;47(5):614–24.

76. Lovati C, D'Amico D, Bertora P, Rosa S, Suardelli M, Mailland E, et al. Acute and interictal allodynia in patients with different headache forms: an Italian pilot study. Headache. 2008;48(2):272–7.

77. Louter MA, Bosker JE, van Oosterhout WP, van Zwet EW, Zitman FG, Ferrari MD, et al. Cutaneous allodynia as a predictor of migraine chronification. Brain. 2013;136(Pt 11):3489–96.

78. Mathew PG, Cutrer FM, Garza I. A touchy subject: an assessment of cutaneous allodynia in a chronic migraine population. J Pain Res. 2016;9:101–4.

79. Burstein R, Jakubowski M. Analgesic triptan action in an animal model of intracranial pain: a race against the development of central sensitization. Ann Neurol. 2004;55(1):27–36.

80. Edelmayer RM, Vanderah TW, Majuta L, Zhang ET, Fioravanti B, De Felice M, et al. Medullary pain facilitating neurons mediate allodynia in headache-related pain. Ann Neurol. 2009;65(2):184–93.

81. Sances G, Tassorelli C, Pucci E, Ghiotto N, Sandrini G, Nappi G. Reliability of the nitroglycerin provocative test in the diagnosis of neurovascular headaches. Cephalalgia. 2004;24(2):110–9.

82. Dalsgaard-Nielsen T. Migraine diagnostics with special reference to pharmacological tests. Int Arch Allergy Appl Immunol. 1955;7(4–6):312–22.

83. Olesen J, Iversen HK, Thomsen LL. Nitric oxide supersensitivity: a possible molecular mechanism of migraine pain. Neuroreport. 1993;4(8):1027–30.

84. Aurora SK, Dodick DW, Turkel CC, DeGryse RE, Silberstein SD, Lipton RB, et al. OnabotulinumtoxinA for treatment of chronic migraine: results from the double-blind, randomized, placebo-controlled phase of the PREEMPT 1 trial. Cephalalgia. 2010;30(7):793–803.

85. Diener HC, Dodick DW, Aurora SK, Turkel CC, DeGryse RE, Lipton RB, et al. OnabotulinumtoxinA for treatment of chronic migraine: results from the double-blind, randomized, placebo-controlled phase of the PREEMPT 2 trial. Cephalalgia. 2010;30(7):804–14.

86. Zhang X, Strassman AM, Novack V, Brin MF, Burstein R. Extracranial injections of botulinum neurotoxin type A inhibit intracranial meningeal nociceptors' responses to stimulation of TRPV1 and TRPA1 channels: are we getting closer to solving this puzzle? Cephalalgia. 2016;36(9):875–86.

87. Naumann M, Carruthers A, Carruthers J, Aurora SK, Zafonte R, Abu-Shakra S, et al. Meta-analysis of neutralizing antibody conversion with onabotulinumtoxinA (BOTOX(R)) across multiple indications. Mov Disord. 2010;25(13):2211–8.

88. Kalita J, Bhoi SK, Misra UK. Is lack of habituation of evoked potential a biological marker of migraine? Clin J Pain. 2014;30(8):724–9.

89. Arakaki X, Galbraith G, Pikov V, Fonteh AN, Harrington MG. Altered brainstem auditory evoked potentials in a rat central sensitization model are similar to those in migraine. Brain Res. 2014;1563:110–21.

90. Sand T, Zhitniy N, White LR, Stovner LJ. Brainstem auditory-evoked potential habituation and intensity-dependence related to serotonin metabolism in migraine: a longitudinal study. Clin Neurophysiol. 2008;119(5):1190–200.

91. Blumenfeld AM, Bloudek LM, Becker WJ, Buse DC, Varon SF, Maglinte GA, et al. Patterns of use and reasons for discontinuation of prophylactic medications for episodic migraine and chronic migraine: results from the second international burden of migraine study (IBMS-II). Headache. 2013;53(4):644–55.

92. Burstein R, Collins B, Jakubowski M. Defeating migraine pain with triptans: a race against the development of cutaneous allodynia. Ann Neurol. 2004;55(1):19–26.

93. Perini F, De Boni A. Peripheral neuromodulation in chronic migraine. Neurol Sci. 2012;33(Suppl 1):S29–31.

94. Notaro P, Buratti E, Meroni A, Montagna MC, Rubino FG, Voltolini A. The effects of peripheral occipital nerve stimulation for the treatment of patients suffering from chronic migraine: a single center experience. Pain Physician. 2014;17(3):E369–74.

95. Nnoaham KE, Kumbang J. Transcutaneous electrical nerve stimulation (TENS) for chronic pain. Cochrane Database Syst Rev. 2008(3):CD003222.

96. McQuay HJ, Moore RA, Eccleston C, Morley S, Williams AC. Systematic review of outpatient services for chronic pain control. Health Technol Assess. 1997;1(6):i–iv. 1–135.

97. Vincent MB, Ekman R, Edvinsson L, Sand T, Sjaastad O. Reduction of calcitonin gene-related peptide in jugular blood following electrical stimulation of rat greater occipital nerve. Cephalalgia. 1992;12(5):275–9.

98. Didier HA, Di Fiore P, Marchetti C, Tullo V, Frediani F, Arlotti M, et al. Electromyography data in chronic migraine patients by using neurostimulation with the Cefaly(R) device. Neurol Sci. 2015;36(Suppl 1):115–9.

99. Wall PD. The gate control theory of pain mechanisms. A re-examination and re-statement. Brain. 1978;101(1):1–18.

100. Goadsby PJ, Grosberg BM, Mauskop A, Cady R, Simmons KA. Effect of noninvasive vagus nerve stimulation on acute migraine: an open-label pilot study. Cephalalgia. 2014;34(12):986–93.

101. Chen SP, Ay I, de Morais AL, Qin T, Zheng Y, Sadeghian H, et al. Vagus nerve stimulation inhibits cortical spreading depression. Pain. 2016;157(4):797–805.

102. Oshinsky ML, Murphy AL, Hekierski H Jr, Cooper M, Simon BJ. Noninvasive vagus nerve stimulation as treatment for trigeminal allodynia. Pain. 2014;155(5):1037–42.

103. Silberstein SD, Calhoun AH, Lipton RB, Grosberg BM, Cady RK, Dorlas S, et al. Chronic migraine headache prevention with noninvasive vagus nerve stimulation: the EVENT study. Neurology. 2016;87(5):529–38.

104. Goadsby PJ, Holland PR, Martins-Oliveira M, Hoffmann J, Schankin C, Akerman S. Pathophysiology of migraine: a disorder of sensory processing. Physiol Rev. 2017;97(2):553–622.

105. Goadsby PJ. Pathophysiology of migraine. Neurol Clin. 2009;27(2):335–60.

106. Oshinsky ML, Luo J. Neurochemistry of trigeminal activation in an animal model of migraine. Headache. 2006;46(Suppl 1):S39–44.

107. Johnson KW, Phebus LA, Cohen ML. Serotonin in migraine: theories, animal models and emerging therapies. Prog Drug Res. 1998;51:219–44.

108. Yisarakun W, Chantong C, Supornsilpchai W, Thongtan T, Srikiatkhachorn A, Reuangwechvorachai P, et al. Up-regulation of calcitonin gene-related peptide in trigeminal ganglion following chronic exposure to paracetamol in a CSD migraine animal model. Neuropeptides. 2015;51:9–16.

109. Arakaki X, McCleary P, Techy M, Chiang J, Kuo L, Fonteh AN, et al. Na,K-ATPase alpha isoforms at the blood-cerebrospinal fluid-trigeminal nerve and blood-retina interfaces in the rat. Fluids Barriers CNS. 2013;10(1):14.

110. Moye LS, Pradhan AAA. Animal model of chronic migraine-associated pain. Curr Protoc Neurosci. 2017;80:9.60.1–9.

111. Greco R, Mangione AS, Sandrini G, Maccarrone M, Nappi G, Tassorelli C. Effects of anandamide in migraine: data from an animal model. J Headache Pain. 2011;12(2):177–83.

112. Greco R, Bandiera T, Mangione AS, Demartini C, Siani F, Nappi G, et al. Effects of peripheral FAAH blockade on NTG-induced hyperalgesia—evaluation of URB937 in an animal model of migraine. Cephalalgia. 2015;35(12):1065–76.

113. Bolay H, Berman NE, Akcali D. Sex-related differences in animal models of migraine headache. Headache. 2011;51(6):891–904.

114. Bongsebandhu-phubhakdi S, Srikiatkhachorn A. Pathophysiology of medication-overuse headache: implications from animal studies. Curr Pain Headache Rep. 2012;16(1):110–5.

115. Green AL, Gu P, De Felice M, Dodick D, Ossipov MH, Porreca F. Increased susceptibility to cortical spreading depression in an animal model of medication-overuse headache. Cephalalgia. 2014;34(8):594–604.

116. Wu B, Wang S, Qin G, Xie J, Tan G, Zhou J, et al. Protein kinase C gamma contributes to central sensitization in a rat model of chronic migraine. J Mol Neurosci. 2017.

117. Dong X, Hu Y, Jing L, Chen J. Role of phosphorylated extracellular signal-regulated kinase, calcitonin gene-related peptide and cyclooxygenase-2 in experimental rat models of migraine. Mol Med Rep. 2015;12(2):1803–9.

118. Guo JQ, Deng HH, Bo X, Yang XS. Involvement of BDNF/TrkB and ERK/CREB axes in nitroglycerin-induced rat migraine and effects of estrogen on these signals in the migraine. Biol Open. 2017;6(1):8–16.

119. Liu YY, Jiao ZY, Li W, Tian Q. PI3K/AKT signaling pathway activation in a rat model of migraine. Mol Med Rep. 2017.

120. Qin G, Xie J, Chen L, Wu B, Gui B, Zhou J. PTEN inhibition preserves trigeminal nucleus caudalis neuron activation through tyrosine phosphorylation of the NR2B subunit at Tyr1472 of the NMDA receptor in a rat model of recurrent migraine. Neurol Res. 2016;38(4):320–6.

121. Ghosh J, Pradhan S, Mittal B. Multilocus analysis of hormonal, neurotransmitter, inflammatory pathways and genome-wide associated variants in migraine susceptibility. Eur J Neurol. 2014;21(7):1011–20.

122. Di Guilmi MN, Wang T, Inchauspe CG, Forsythe ID, Ferrari MD, van den Maagdenberg AM, et al. Synaptic gain-of-function effects of mutant Cav2.1 channels in a mouse model of familial hemiplegic migraine are due to increased basal [Ca2+]i. J Neurosci. 2014;34(21):7047–58.

123. Ferrari MD, Klever RR, Terwindt GM, Ayata C, van den Maagdenberg AM. Migraine pathophysiology:

lessons from mouse models and human genetics. Lancet Neurol. 2015;14(1):65–80.

124. Bottger P, Glerup S, Gesslein B, Illarionova NB, Isaksen TJ, Heuck A, et al. Glutamate-system defects behind psychiatric manifestations in a familial hemiplegic migraine type 2 disease-mutation mouse model. Sci Rep. 2016;6:22047.

125. Munro G, Jansen-Olesen I, Olesen J. Animal models of pain and migraine in drug discovery. Drug Discov Today. 2017;22(7):1103–11.

126. Connor HE, Feniuk W, Beattie DT, North PC, Oxford AW, Saynor DA, et al. Naratriptan: biological profile in animal models relevant to migraine. Cephalalgia. 1997;17(3):145–52.

127. Humphrey PP, Feniuk W, Marriott AS, Tanner RJ, Jackson MR, Tucker ML. Preclinical studies on the anti-migraine drug, sumatriptan. Eur Neurol. 1991;31(5):282–90.

128. Tepper SJ, Stillman MJ. Clinical and preclinical rationale for CGRP-receptor antagonists in the treatment of migraine. Headache. 2008;48(8):1259–68.

129. Tso AR, Goadsby PJ. Anti-CGRP monoclonal antibodies: the next era of migraine prevention? Curr Treat Options Neurol. 2017;19(8):27.

130. Karsan N, Goadsby PJ. Calcitonin gene-related peptide and migraine. Curr Opin Neurol. 2015;28(3):250–4.

131. Bigal ME, Lipton RB. Excessive acute migraine medication use and migraine progression. Neurology. 2008;71(22):1821–8.

132. De Felice M, Ossipov MH, Wang R, Lai J, Chichorro J, Meng I, et al. Triptan-induced latent sensitization: a possible basis for medication overuse headache. Ann Neurol. 2010;67(3):325–37.

133. Kopruszinski CM, Xie JY, Eyde NM, Remeniuk B, Walter S, Stratton J, et al. Prevention of stress- or nitric oxide donor-induced medication overuse headache by a calcitonin gene-related peptide antibody in rodents. Cephalalgia. 2017;37(6):560–70.

134. Silberstein SD. Topiramate in migraine prevention: a 2016 perspective. Headache. 2017;57(1):165–78.

135. Chen SP, Tolner EA, Eikermann-Haerter K. Animal models of monogenic migraine. Cephalalgia. 2016;36(7):704–21.

136. Friedrich T, Tavraz NN, Junghans C. ATP1A2 mutations in migraine: seeing through the facets of an ion pump onto the neurobiology of disease. Front Physiol. 2016;7:239.

137. Isaksen TJ, Lykke-Hartmann K. Insights into the pathology of the alpha2-Na(+)/K(+)-ATPase in neurological disorders; lessons from animal models. Front Physiol. 2016;7:161.

138. van den Maagdenberg AM, Pizzorusso T, Kaja S, Terpolilli N, Shapovalova M, Hoebeek FE, et al. High cortical spreading depression susceptibility and migraine-associated symptoms in Ca(v)2.1 S218L mice. Ann Neurol. 2010;67(1):85–98.

139. van Oosterhout F, Michel S, Deboer T, Houben T, van de Ven RC, Albus H, et al. Enhanced circadian phase resetting in R192Q Cav2.1 calcium channel migraine mice. Ann Neurol. 2008;64(3):315–24.

140. Eising E, Shyti R, t Hoen PAC, Vijfhuizen LS, SMH H, LAM B, et al. Cortical spreading depression causes unique dysregulation of inflammatory pathways in a transgenic mouse model of migraine. Mol Neurobiol. 2017;54(4):2986–96.

141. Franceschini A, Nair A, Bele T, van den Maagdenberg AM, Nistri A, Fabbretti E. Functional crosstalk in culture between macrophages and trigeminal sensory neurons of a mouse genetic model of migraine. BMC Neurosci. 2012;13:143.

142. Franceschini A, Vilotti S, Ferrari MD, van den Maagdenberg AM, Nistri A, Fabbretti E. TNFalpha levels and macrophages expression reflect an inflammatory potential of trigeminal ganglia in a mouse model of familial hemiplegic migraine. PLoS One. 2013;8(1):e52394.

143. Gnanasekaran A, Bele T, Hullugundi S, Simonetti M, Ferrari MD, van den Maagdenberg AM, et al. Mutated CaV2.1 channels dysregulate CASK/P2X3 signaling in mouse trigeminal sensory neurons of R192Q Cacna1a knock-in mice. Mol Pain. 2013;9:62.

144. Gnanasekaran A, Sundukova M, van den Maagdenberg AM, Fabbretti E, Nistri A. Lipid rafts control P2X3 receptor distribution and function in trigeminal sensory neurons of a transgenic migraine mouse model. Mol Pain. 2011;7:77.

145. Nair A, Simonetti M, Birsa N, Ferrari MD, van den Maagdenberg AM, Giniatullin R, et al. Familial hemiplegic migraine Ca(v)2.1 channel mutation R192Q enhances ATP-gated P2X3 receptor activity of mouse sensory ganglion neurons mediating trigeminal pain. Mol Pain. 2010;6:48.

146. Vilotti S, Vana N, Van den Maagdenberg AM, Nistri A. Expression and function of calcitonin gene-related peptide (CGRP) receptors in trigeminal ganglia of R192Q Cacna1a knock-in mice. Neurosci Lett. 2016;620:104–10.

147. Hullugundi SK, Ferrari MD, van den Maagdenberg AM, Nistri A. The mechanism of functional up-regulation of P2X3 receptors of trigeminal sensory neurons in a genetic mouse model of familial hemiplegic migraine type 1 (FHM-1). PLoS One. 2013;8(4):e60677.

148. Eikermann-Haerter K, Dilekoz E, Kudo C, Savitz SI, Waeber C, Baum MJ, et al. Genetic and hormonal factors modulate spreading depression and transient hemiparesis in mouse models of familial hemiplegic migraine type 1. J Clin Invest. 2009;119(1):99–109.

149. Moseley AE, Williams MT, Schaefer TL, Bohanan CS, Neumann JC, Behbehani MM, et al. Deficiency in Na,K-ATPase alpha isoform genes alters spatial learning, motor activity, and anxiety in mice. J Neurosci. 2007;27(3):616–26.

150. Lingrel JB, Williams MT, Vorhees CV, Moseley AE. Na,K-ATPase and the role of alpha isoforms in behavior. J Bioenerg Biomembr. 2007;39(5–6):385–9.

151. Burstein R, Jakubowski M. Neural substrate of depression during migraine. Neurol Sci. 2009;30(Suppl 1):S27–31.

152. Desouza DD, Woldeamanue YW, Peretz AM, Sanjanwala BM, Cowan RP, editors. Interactions between affective measures and amygdala volume in chronic migraine: associations in the absence of group volumetric differences. 18th International Headache Congress; 2017 September 7–10. Vancouver: Cephalalgia; 2017.

153. Michael G. Harrington XA, Alfred N. Fonteh, Natalie Chen, Eduard, Chekmenev VS, Jiarong Chiang. Na,K-ATPase is a regulator of rodent central sensitization: implications for migraine. American Society for Biochemistry and Molecular Biology, 14th International Conference on Na,K-ATPase August 3, 2014 - September 5, 2014; De Werelt Conference Centre, Lunteren, NL2014.

154. Kalume F, Yu FH, Westenbroek RE, Scheuer T, Catterall WA. Reduced sodium current in Purkinje neurons from Nav1.1 mutant mice: implications for ataxia in severe myoclonic epilepsy in infancy. J Neurosci. 2007;27(41):11065–74.

155. Ogiwara I, Miyamoto H, Morita N, Atapour N, Mazaki E, Inoue I, et al. Nav1.1 localizes to axons of parvalbumin-positive inhibitory interneurons: a circuit basis for epileptic seizures in mice carrying an Scn1a gene mutation. J Neurosci. 2007;27(22):5903–14.

156. Yu FH, Mantegazza M, Westenbroek RE, Robbins CA, Kalume F, Burton KA, et al. Reduced sodium current in GABAergic interneurons in a mouse model of severe myoclonic epilepsy in infancy. Nat Neurosci. 2006;9(9):1142–9.

157. Riant F, Roze E, Barbance C, Meneret A, Guyant-Marechal L, Lucas C, et al. PRRT2 mutations cause hemiplegic migraine. Neurology. 2012;79(21):2122–4.

158. Michetti C, Castroflorio E, Marchionni I, Forte N, Sterlini B, Binda F, et al. The PRRT2 knockout mouse recapitulates the neurological diseases associated with PRRT2 mutations. Neurobiol Dis. 2017;99:66–83.

159. Berge OG. Predictive validity of behavioural animal models for chronic pain. Br J Pharmacol. 2011;164(4):1195–206.

160. May A, Goadsby PJ. Pharmacological opportunities and pitfalls in the therapy of migraine. Curr Opin Neurol. 2001;14(3):341–5.

161. Goldstein DJ, Wang O, Saper JR, Stoltz R, Silberstein SD, Mathew NT. Ineffectiveness of neurokinin-1 antagonist in acute migraine: a crossover study. Cephalalgia. 1997;17(7):785–90.

162. Grazzi L, Sansone E, Raggi A, D'Amico D, De Giorgio A, Leonardi M, et al. Mindfulness and pharmacological prophylaxis after withdrawal from medication overuse in patients with chronic migraine: an effectiveness trial with a one-year follow-up. J Headache Pain. 2017;18(1):15.

163. Kojic Z, Stojanovic D. Pathophysiology of migraine—from molecular to personalized medicine. Med Pregl. 2013;66(1–2):53–7.

Economic Impact of Chronic Headaches

22

Anna Pace

Chronic daily headache has been reported to affect 3–4% of the adult and elderly population of the world [1]. Chronic daily headache comprises a heterogeneous group of various headache types, where patients report 15 days or more out of every month with headache for at least 3 months. The majority of patients with chronic daily headache meet the criteria for chronic migraine, and/or medication overuse headache, but other headache disorders included in this group are chronic tension-type headache, chronic trigeminal autonomic cephalgias, and new daily persistent headache [1].

Chronic daily headache causes a significant degree of disability in many patients and is an important public health concern, as chronic daily headaches often affect young and middle-aged patients at the time of their prime productivity [2]. Primary headaches are prevalent, and even the smallest economic loss for a patient suffering from chronic headaches, whether due to increased healthcare utilization or due to lost productivity at work or school, can have a significant impact on both the patient and the economy. Much of the literature evaluating the economic burden of chronic daily headache focuses on chronic migraine and/or medication overuse headache related to chronic migraine, as migrainous

headaches are a common reason for patients to seek medical help.

There have been two major studies looking at the cost and economic burden of chronic migraine in the USA, Europe, and throughout the world. The first study was the American Migraine Prevalence and Prevention Study, or AMPP, initiated in 2004 and surveyed over 120,000 households for patients who self-reported chronic severe headache [3]. Using ICHD-2 criteria, patients were categorized as having either episodic migraine (EM) or chronic migraine (CM) based on reported frequency. After this first screen, patients were then surveyed regarding other variables, including primary care visits, emergency room visits, neurologist or headache specialist outpatient visits, pain management visits, medication use, and overnight hospitalizations. Participants were also surveyed about "productivity loss," where patients had to report the number of days in the prior 3 months where they missed work or school, and how many days their productivity at work or school, was reduced by more than half, or 50%, on the days they had headache. Cost assumptions were made based on healthcare and medication use and productivity loss based on a PharMetrics Patient-Centric database and allowed amounts per diagnosis code [3].

Results showed that those who suffered from chronic migraine had more primary care visits, neurologist or headache specialist visits, pain management visits, and ER visits, compared to those with episodic migraine. The mean number

A. Pace
Department of Neurology, Icahn School of Medicine at Mount Sinai, New York, NY, USA
e-mail: anna.pace@mssm.edu

of hours lost from work or school due to chronic migraine was 85.7 h per person per year, and the mean number of hours with reduced productivity due to headache was 256 h per person per year [4]. Patients with chronic migraine incurred a mean yearly cost of $7750 per person per year, including both direct and indirect costs, compared to $1757 in costs incurred by those patients whose migraines are episodic [3]. The researchers' analysis showed that the majority of the total costs incurred by the patients were due to lost productive time at work or school (69.6%, or estimated $5,392.03 per year, out of $7750) [3].

The second study examining the economic impact of chronic migraine was the International Burden of Migraine Study, which utilized a web-based questionnaire to recruit patients with episodic migraine and chronic migraine in North America, Germany, France, Italy, Spain, the UK, Australia, Taiwan, and Brazil [5–7]. The two-part screen included surveying participants recruited through a portal of registered panelists who were willing to fill out health surveys and, then based on their responses to the main survey about headache and frequency, were categorized as having either episodic migraine or chronic migraine; a similar distinction was made in the AMPP study mentioned previously. The second part of the administered survey involved a 70-item questionnaire to elucidate healthcare usage, costs, socioeconomic information, and disability or quality of life related to migraine. Costs were estimated based on each country's national formulary systems with the exception of Italy, which utilized a private site for healthcare professionals to estimate healthcare and medication costs [6].

The IBMS researchers showed that those patients with chronic migraine utilized healthcare resources significantly more than those patients who had episodic migraine throughout all of the countries participating in the study. This includes more primary care visits and neurologist outpatient visits, as well as emergency department visits, though inpatient hospitalizations were only found to be higher for patients with CM in the UK and not in the other participating countries [5–7]. More diagnostic testing was performed for patients with CM compared to those with EM in the UK, France, Spain, the USA, and Canada. Acute medication use was statistically significantly higher in patients with CM only in Italy (56.4% in patients with CM vs. 35.5% in patients with EM), and prophylactic medication use was higher in patients with CM in Spain, the USA, and Canada. Direct costs related to chronic migraine estimated by the IBMS are reported to be approximately three times that of the direct costs related to episodic migraine, with the biggest difference in costs seen in the UK, where patients with CM incurred a 3.6-fold higher cost than patients with EM [5–7].

The IBMS researchers found that patients with CM had an estimated overall productivity loss of 67.67 days over a 3-month period, whereas patients with EM had an estimated productivity loss of 13.57 days per 3-month period. There is a high rate of disability seen in patients with CM throughout the various participating countries, with CM sufferers noted to be less likely to be employed full time than those with EM, especially in the USA [5–7]. The US data for the IBMS study showed that total annual cost for people with chronic migraine is $8243 compared to people with episodic migraine, who incur an annual cost of $2649 [4]. Contrasting to findings in AMPP, direct medical costs were considered to be the majority contributor to total headache-related costs for both those with CM (60%) and for those with EM (64.3%) [5–7]. This data, collected over many participating countries, suggests that the economic burden of chronic migraine is a significant worldwide problem.

Very few studies have looked specifically at the economic burden of chronic tension-type headaches, though one report from a study in Turkey compared the economic impact of primary chronic migraine as opposed to chronic tension-type headache at university-based hospitals [8]. In the study, published in the *Journal of Headache and Pain* in 2006, 937 patients were recruited, and patients were categorized by primary headache disorder based on ICHD criteria. Participants were then surveyed regarding the frequency of headache, frequency of medication use, and outpatient or hospital visits for headache [8]. Costs were estimated based on physician costs for outpatient visits and medication costs in relation to monthly average analgesic consumption and preventive medication use. Indirect costs were calculated based on mean loss of days at work or efficiency loss, and the minimum wage of $14.08 USD was used in the calculations for lost work days [8]. The ratio of total cost per headache patient was compared to the GNP for Turkey per capita to calculate the ratio of costs to average income. Researchers found that patients with migraine (with or without aura) had the highest mean direct costs, at $250 and $225.60, respectively, per year [8]. Patients with chronic tension-type headache had a mean total direct cost of $104.80 per year, with medication use being the primary driver of costs incurred by these patients [8]. Patients with chronic daily headache, either tension type or migraine, or patients with both, had the most work days lost due to headache, with more days of reduced efficiency per year, compared to episodic headache syndromes [8]. While the total direct cost for patients with chronic tension-type headache is lower than that for chronic migraine in this Turkish population, these results still emphasize the significant economic burden of chronic daily headache.

Chronic headache is a major public health problem, not just in the USA but around the world. Research has continued to show that chronic headaches, especially chronic migraine, take a large economic toll on worldwide healthcare systems and especially on patients who suffer from them, whether through direct medication use costs, or costs of specialist visits, or indirectly by affecting productivity and efficiency at work or school.

References

1. Lanteri-Minet M, Duru G, Mudge M, Cottrell S. Quality of life impairment, disability and economic burden associated with chronic daily headache, focusing on chronic migraine with or without medication overuse: a systematic review. Cephalalgia. 2011;31(7):837–50.
2. Lanteri-Minet M. Economic burden and costs of chronic migraine. Curr Pain Headache Rep. 2014;18:385.
3. Munaka J, Hazard E, Serrano D, Klingman D, Rupnow MFT, Tierce J, Reed M, Lipton R. Economic burden of transformed migraine: results from the american migraine prevalence and prevention (AMPP) study. Headache. 2009;49:498–508.
4. Messali A, Sanderson JC, Blumenfeld AM, Goadsby P, Buse D, Varon SF, Stokes M, Lipton R. Direct and indirect costs of chronic and episodic migraine in the United States: a web-based survey. Headache. 2016;56:306–22.
5. Bloudek LM, Stokes M, Buse DC, Wilcox TK, Lipton RB, Goadsby PJ, Varon SF, Blumenfeld AM, Katsar Z. Cost of healthcare for patients with migraine in five European countries: results from the International Burden of Migraine Study (IBMS). J Headache Pain. 2012;13:361–78.
6. Stokes M, Becker WJ, Lipton RB, Sullivan SD, Wilcox TK, Wells L, Manack A, Proskorovsky I, Gladstone J, Buse DC, Varon SF, Goadsby PJ, Blumenfeld AM. Cost of health care among patients with chronic and episodic migraine in Canada and the USA: results from the International Burden of Migraine Study (IBMS). Headache. 2011;51:1058–77.
7. Blumenfeld AM, Varon SF, Wilcox TK, Buse DC, Kawata AK, Manack A, Goadsby PJ, Lipton RB. Disability, HRQoL and resource use among chronic and episodic migraineurs: results from the International Burden of Migraine Study (IBMS). Cephalalgia. 2011;31(3):301–15.
8. Karli N, Zarifoglu M, Ertas M, Saip S, Öztürk V, Biçakçi S, Boz C, Selçuki D, Oguzhanoglu A, Neyal M, Siva A, Irkeçk C, Kaleagasi H, Kansu T, Sarica Y, Tasdemir N, Uzuner N. Economic impact of primary headaches in Turkey: a university hospital based study: part II. J Headache Pain. 2006;7:75–82.

From Episodic to Chronic: A Discussion on Headache Transformation

23

Anna Pace and Bridget Mueller

"Chronic daily headache" (CDH) encompasses various headache syndromes, including chronic migraine, chronic tension-type headache, hemicrania continua, and new daily persistent headache. While there are some patients who initially present with a primary chronic daily headache, most patients begin with episodic headache and then progress, or transform, into chronic headache over time. Chronic daily headache has been reported to affect 3–4% of the population worldwide, and patients with CDH represent a significant number of referrals to tertiary care centers for headache. Chronic daily headache can lead to a significant degree of disability in many patients, especially when affecting young patients in the prime of their workforce capabilities.

According to proposed criteria by Silberstein et al. in 1994, used frequently by headache specialists, chronic headache can be subdivided into four entities—transformed migraine (TM), chronic tension-type headache (CTTH), hemicrania continua (HC), and new daily persistent headache (NDPH) [1]. Transformed migraine is found in patients who previously had a history of episodic migraine but have experienced more frequent attacks over time and whose nausea, vomiting, photophobia, and phonophobia have become less prominent features

of their headaches. These patients have this progression over at least 3 months, to result in daily or almost daily head pain for greater than 1 months' time [1]. The group then subdivides into those with or without medication overuse: medication overuse is defined as involving simple analgesic use >5 days a week, combination analgesic use >3 days a week, or using narcotics at least 2 days a week for >1 month [1]. For chronic tension-type headache, which often evolves from episodic tension-type headache, Silberstein et al. proposes criteria to include an average headache frequency of more than 15 days a month with the duration of each attack lasting longer than 4 h a day, for 6 months' time [1]. Patients should have a history of episodic tension-type headache in the past, with an evolution of their headaches increasing in frequency over a 3-month period; headache should involve a bilateral pressing/tightening type pain and associated with no more than one of nausea, photophobia, or phonophobia, and no vomiting. CTTH is also subdivided into patients with or without medication overuse, as previously described with TM. Hemicrania continua is defined as a strictly unilateral headache present for at least 1 month, with continuous pain that may have "jabs and jolts" superimposed, and may be associated with or without medication overuse. It has no precipitating mechanisms and is often unremitting [1]. New daily persistent headache is described as a headache that is acute on onset and is constant and unremitting, for >15 days a month for at least 1 month, and patients with NDPH do not have a previous

A. Pace (✉) · B. Mueller
Department of Neurology, Icahn School of Medicine at Mount Sinai, New York, NY, USA
e-mail: anna.pace@mssm.edu;
bridget.mueller@mountsinai.org

© Springer International Publishing AG, part of Springer Nature 2019
M. W. Green et al. (eds.), *Chronic Headache*, https://doi.org/10.1007/978-3-319-91491-6_23

313

history of migraine or tension-type headache that has increased in frequency or decreased in severity over the past 3 months [1]. The focus of the following discussion will be primarily transformed migraine and chronic tension-type headache.

Pathophysiology of Chronic Headache

Serotonin Receptors

The pathophysiology of headache transformation is not completely well understood, but there have been proposed mechanisms of this headache process. One study published in *Headache* in 1994 proposed that an upregulation of 5HT-2 serotonin receptors may be implicated in transformed migraine [2]. This study, which looked at six patients with transformed migraine and seven controls, measured the 5HT-2 serotonin receptors on platelet membranes and found a significant increase in the maximal number of receptors on the platelets in migraineurs compared to the control patients [2]. The researchers deduced that, since there is a significant similarity in receptor characterization between platelet membranes and aminergic neurons, it could be postulated that aminergic neurons would also have higher levels of serotonin receptors. This was suggested to play a role in transformed migraine, as patients with episodic migraine have a decrease in 5HT-2 receptors on platelets during periods of headache freedom. Therefore, the increase in receptors may contribute to the lack of pain freedom in patients with transformed migraine. The researchers also postulated that the increase in serotonergic receptors may be due to "serotonergic hypofunction," whereby there is a hyposecretion of serotonergic vesicles presynaptically which leads to decreased serotonin levels over time and results in the upregulation of postsynaptic serotonergic receptors [2].

CSF Glutamate

Researchers Gallai and colleagues in 2003 found that there were elevated levels of CSF glutamate

and CSF nitrites, as well as subsequent increases in CSF cyclic guanosine monophosphate compounds (cGMP), in patients with chronic daily headache compared to healthy controls [3]. These findings help support the theory that the release of glutamate and nitrous oxide may play a role in chronic daily headache development. Substance P and calcitonin gene-related peptide (CGRP) were also found to be elevated in measured CSF samples of patients with CDH, though the study researchers did not find a relationship between these levels and that of the elevated levels of glutamate and nitrites [3]. The study investigators propose in patients with chronic daily headache that there is activation of NMDA and other non-NMDA receptors, which results in the release of glutamate and production of NO species that contribute to central sensitization, with the subsequent release of cGMP correlating with sustained nociception [3].

Calcitonin Gene-Related Peptide (CGRP)

Calcitonin gene-related peptide (CGRP) has also been implicated in headache chronification. In a study conducted by researchers in Spain and published in *Neurology* in 2013, women with episodic migraine and women with chronic migraine underwent testing to determine CGRP levels in the blood interictally between migraine attacks [4]. These patients were compared to healthy controls and patients with episodic cluster headaches. Results showed that the women with chronic migraine had significantly higher levels of plasma CGRP compared to women with episodic migraine, women with episodic cluster, and women who were in the healthy control group [4]. These levels were not affected by rescue medication use, comorbid psychiatric conditions, vascular risk factors, or age [4]. Researchers hypothesize that the presence of persistently elevated CGRP levels may be a marker for headache chronification.

Genetics

There are suggestions in the literature that there may be underlying genetic predispositions to headache chronification, though there have been no concrete studies evaluating specific gene patterns implicated in chronic daily headache. One study by Cevoli and colleagues in 2008 evaluated family history for chronic headache and family history of drug overuse as possible contributors to headache transformation in patients [5]. One hundred five patients with chronic headache, either with tension-type (CTTH), chronic migraine (CM), or with medication overuse headache (MOH), were interviewed directly by investigators about family history of headache, psychiatric disorders, and substance abuse or dependence. Patients were asked to provide details about their first-degree and second-degree relatives regarding timing and onset of headache and headache frequency, substance use, and history of psychiatric disorders, the latter two being classified by DSM-IV criteria [5]. Researchers found that 38.1% of patients with chronic headache reported a family history of chronic headache, compared to only 13.7% of patients with episodic headache reporting a family history of chronic headache. Patients with chronic headache also reported an increased family history of medication overuse and substance abuse than those patients with episodic headache, but there was no significant difference noted in family history of psychiatric disorders when compared between the two groups. History was not distinguished between first-degree and second-degree relatives for the participants in the study. Investigators postulate, due to the high family history of chronic headache in patients with chronic headache, that there may be an underlying genetic etiology or predisposition that may contribute to chronification of headaches [5].

Another study in 2010 by Arruda, Bigal, and others surveyed 1994 children with headache to determine if maternal headache history and frequency could predict the frequency of headaches in the pediatric participants [6]. Participants, ages 5–12, were chosen based on their headache frequency as reported by their mothers, and divided into low frequency (1–4 headache days per month), intermediate frequency (5–9 headache days per month), high frequency (10–14 headache days per month), and CDH (15+ headache days per month) [6]. The mothers of the participants were also surveyed with the same questionnaire and divided into the same frequency categories. Analyses found that if the mother was classified as having low-frequency headache, the prevalence of low-frequency headaches in the children was 27.3% and the prevalence of intermediate-/high-frequency headache was 4.8%, with the prevalence of CDH at 0.6% [6]. If the mother had high-frequency headaches, the prevalence of high-frequency headaches in the children was 16.1%, and the prevalence of CDH in the children was 1.3% [6]. If the mother had CDH, the prevalence of intermediate-/high-frequency headaches in the children was 15.8%, and the children were found to have a 12-fold increased risk of CDH, compared to children of mothers with low-frequency headaches [6]. While this study is not able to provide definitive evidence that CDH is genetic, the results imply some inheritable basis for headache chronification in families [6].

Quality of Life in CDH

When looking at quality of life for patients with episodic migraine versus chronic migraine, Meletiche et al. studied a group of 90 migraineurs by administering questionnaires including the Short Form 36 (SF36) and the Migraine Disability Assessment (MIDAS) [7]. These questionnaires look to quantify various domains of quality of life in these migraine patients, including assessing social functioning, general health, mental health, vitality, physical functioning, and bodily pain. When patients were grouped by ICH-D criteria as episodic migraine or transformed migraine (the latter following proposed criteria by Silberstein et al. [1]), the researchers found that patients with transformed migraines had significantly lower scores on seven out of the eight tested domains on the SF36 assessment and significantly higher scores on the MIDAS compared to patients with episodic migraine [7].

There is a significant economic burden of transformed migraine when compared to episodic migraine. According to the American

Migraine Prevalence and Prevention Study (AMPP), those migraineurs with transformed migraines utilize more primary care and neurologist outpatient visits, visiting emergency rooms more frequently, and incurred a 4.4-fold higher cost annually compared to patients with episodic migraine, and this cost includes both direct and indirect costs [8]. Patients with TM had more missed days at work or school due to their daily pain and were less productive when able to attend work or school compared to patients with episodic migraine [8].

This important data suggests that chronic headache, and specifically transformed migraine, is a major public health problem [8]. With the report of decreasing quality of life and an increased economic burden in patients with transformed migraine, it is evident that neurologists should look to identify risk factors for headache chronification and attempt to prevent this progression by helping to modify those risk factors. The transformation from episodic headache into a chronic headache disorder likely involves both an underlying genetic vulnerability and specific environmental risk factors. Medication overuse, obesity, sleep disturbances, stress, depression, and menstrual-related migraines have been shown to be potent triggers for headache progression.

pies showed improvement in headache frequency, duration, and intensity [10]. The effectiveness of detoxification was again demonstrated in a controlled open-label trial that randomized chronic headache patients to either complete detoxification or restriction to medication 2 days per week [11]. Patients who stopped all acute pharmacotherapy interventions experienced twice as many headache-free days per month compared to patients who decreased medication usage to the recommended frequency of two to three times per week. In addition, 70% of detoxified patients reverted to episodic headaches, while only 42% of restricted patients reverted [11].

Not all drugs are created equal. Barbiturates and opioids increase the risk of transformation to chronic migraine by at least twofold, at any frequency of use [12]. Barbiturates exhibit a dose-response effect, with the heaviest users experiencing progression from episodic headaches to chronic headaches most frequently. These effects persisted after adjusting for headache severity. Triptans did not increase transition to chronic headache. Interestingly, NSAID use was associated with a decreased risk of headache progression in patients with low frequency of headaches and an increased risk of headache progression in patients with high-frequency attacks [12, 13].

Risk Factors for Transformation

Medication Overuse

Patients with chronic daily headache disorders are often self-medicating at frequencies that qualify as overuse. Population studies estimate ~30% of patients with transformed migraine is overusing pain-relieving medication [9, 10]. At headache tertiary centers, 80–85% of patients are overusing medication at time of presentation [10].

"Detox studies" have shown that medication overuse is often a reversible cause of headache transformation. In a large retrospective study, patients with chronic migraine and medication overuse who stopped all acute pharmacothera-

Obesity

Obesity dramatically increases the risk of episodic migraines progressing to chronic daily headaches. In a longitudinal population study that followed episodic migraineurs over 1 year, obese migraineurs (BMI > 30) had a five-fold increased risk in headache transformation, while overweight individuals (BMI 25–29) had a three-fold increased risk of headache transformation [14]. The episodic migraineur and episodic chronic tension-type headache patient are not affected by obesity equally. While even modest weight gain significantly increases the risk of developing a transformed migraine, only morbid obesity increases the risk for progression to chronic tension-type headache [15, 16].

The pathophysiology underlying the association between obesity and headache transformation is likely multifactorial. It is well established that both migraine and obesity share a proinflammatory state. In addition, the hypothalamus and its associated peptides and neurotransmitters including 5-HT, adiponectin, and leptin play critical roles in headaches and energy balance. Interestingly, in addition to migraineurs having increased serum levels of leptin and adiponectin compared with healthy controls, chronic migraineurs have increased leptin and adiponectin compared to episodic migraine patients [17].

Studies performed in obese migraineurs who underwent bariatric surgery suggest weight reduction is an effective way to decrease headache frequency in chronic migraine patients. Three months following surgery, five of the six chronic migraineurs reported at least a 50% reduction in headache frequency [18]. Additional studies are needed to replicate these results and determine if modest weight loss achieved through behavioral measures also influences headache frequency in chronic migraineurs.

Sleep

Poor sleep is a widespread complaint in patients with chronic headache. Approximately two-thirds of patients with chronic migraine suffer from insomnia on a daily or near-daily basis [19]. As measured by the Pittsburgh Sleep Quality Index, higher migraine frequency correlates with poorer sleep quality. Further, patients with chronic migraine report non-restorative sleep and a higher number of night awakenings compared to patients with episodic migraine [20].

The relationship between sleep and chronic headache presents the classic "chicken or the egg" question: do headaches interfere with sleep or does poor sleep produce headaches? In a randomized placebo-controlled study, chronic migraineurs who followed behavioral sleep modifications aimed at improving sleep quality and increasing sleep duration were more likely to revert to episodic migraine, suggesting a causal relationship between poor sleep and the development of chronic migraine [21]. Interestingly, the degree of improvement in headache symptoms was proportionate to the number of sleep behaviors changed, further supporting a causal link between poor sleep and the development of a chronic headache disorder.

The importance of screening headache patients for obstructive sleep apnea (OSA) has been highlighted by several studies [22, 23]. A retrospective study examining the prevalence of OSA in patients with various headache disorders found 83% of chronic migraine patients without aura suffered from OSA while 50% of episodic migraineurs suffered from OSA [22]. Overall, chronic migraineurs without aura were 20 times more likely to have OSA than patients with other headache types including tension-type and episodic migraines. The effectiveness of continuous positive airway pressure (CPAP) to improve headaches was examined. Almost half of the chronic migraineurs without aura reported a 50% reduction in headache severity and frequency with CPAP, indicating CPAP may be an important tool for treating chronic headache disorders [22].

Acute Stress

It is a common complaint heard in the clinic: "Stress gives me headaches." In fact, more than 90% of headache patients report that stress affects their headaches [24]. Determining the role of acute stress in progression of headaches is complex as experiencing pain can produce stress. Numerous studies have attempted to parse this relationship by establishing temporality of events. A retrospective study found 44.8% of patients with transformed headache report a stressful event correlated with transformation from episodic to a chronic disorder [25]. Health problems accounted for 35.6% of stressful events, marriage disputes accounted for 13.6% of events, bereavement accounted for 13.6% of events, and work accounted for 11.4% of events. A smaller percentage of patients said stress related to education, legal concerns, and immigration preceded worsening of their headaches. Events in this study were characterized by severity using the Paykel score [26]. Approximately one-third of transformed migraine patients reported a major stressful event, characterized as bereavement, legal concerns, serious illness, change or loss of job, and retirement, preceding progression. Two-thirds of patients said minor stressors such as interpersonal conflict and suboptimal work conditions coincided with headache transformation.

There are several biological mechanisms likely underlying the relationship between stress and headache. Acute stress activates an opioid-mediated pain response, which temporarily decreases sensation of pain; this may be an evolutionarily preserved adaptive response permitting improved response to a perceived threat. However, recurring stimulation of this pain center can produce central sensitization leading to hyperalgesia [27]. In addition, animal studies have shown that chronic stress, but not acute stress, results in increased sensitivity to pain in peripheral nociceptors, which may play an important role in headache transformation [28].

While acute stress may play a role in headache transformation, therapies focused solely on stress reduction have had minimal success in alleviating pain burden and reverting chronic to episodic headache. Only 13% of those suffering from chronic headaches reported reduction in headache burden following behavioral therapy, while 52% of patients with episodic headaches reported improvement in headache [29]. A combination of pharmacologic and behavioral stress reduction appears to be more effective than either therapy alone. Patients with chronic tension-type headache who received behavioral intervention and antidepressant therapy were significantly more likely (64% of patients) to show a clinically significant decrease in headache activity than patients who received antidepressant medication (38% of patients) or cognitive behavioral therapy (35% of patients) alone [30].

In addition to the direct influence of stress on progression of headache disorders, stress likely exerts important indirect effects by influencing factors known to contribute to headache progression. Stress can lead to poor sleep as well as increase the risk for obesity and medication overuse [31, 32]. Clinicians should be encouraged to screen for stress in their headache patients and consider a multipronged management approach to help patients reduce stress.

Depression

There is extensive literature showing a bidirectional link between migraine and depression [33]. Psychiatric comorbidity has been shown to be a risk factor for headache progression, and, not surprisingly, living with chronic pain adversely affects mood. Patients with chronic daily headache have higher levels of anxiety and depressive disorders than episodic migraineurs. In episodic migraineurs, 1 year of depression (as determined by PHQ-9 scale) was a significant predictor of progression to a chronic headache disorder. This effect was present after controlling for sociodemographic variables, headache frequency, comorbidities, and medications. Further, authors demonstrated a dose-dependent effect of depression on transformation risk, with the most severely depressed patients having odds risk of 2.65 and mild depression with an odds risk of 1.77 [34].

As postulated by Lipton and Silberstein, there are several hypotheses to account for the linkage between depression and onset of chronic migraine, including shared risk factors, depression resulting from increasing number of headache episodes, and a direct influence of depression on headache progression through sensitization of central pain pathways [35].

Chronic stress is a well-established risk factor for both depression and chronic migraine. Chronic stress has been shown to induce neuroinflammation in the brain, which may lead to hyperalgesia through suppression of the nociceptive threshold [36].

There is also evidence that depression may result from increasing headache burden. Treating chronic migraine with onabotulinumtoxinA produced not only a reduction in headache burden but also alleviation of depression, demonstrating that decreasing headache frequency leads to improved psychological outcome even in the absence of interventions aimed at improving mood [37].

Finally, depression may influence headache progression through centrally mediated alterations in pain sensitization. Imaging studies show depressed patients have increased amygdala activity and neuroplastic changes, which may contribute to central pain activation and sensitization [38]. Similarly, rodents with chemically induced chronic migraine show evidence of depression and anxiety behaviors as well as decreased levels of dopamine and serotonin in the frontal cortex [39].

These hypotheses are not mutually exclusive, and it is probable that, for any specific individual suffering from episodic headaches and depression, one or all three of these factors can influence headache progression.

Menstrual-Related Migraines

It has been known for decades that the premenstrual decline in estrogen can precipitate a migraine [40]. In one study, 70% of female migraineurs report headache episodes associated with their menses. The attacks occurring during menstruation are reported to be longer, more painful, and resistant to therapy [41]. Patients with MRM often present to a headache center in the setting of a chronic headache disorder. In a retrospective study, Calhoun and colleagues tried to determine whether alleviation of menstrual-related migraines (MRM) reverted a chronic headache disorder to an episodic disorder [21]. Ninety-two percent of patients with MRM met the criteria for chronic migraine disorder, and 72% met the criteria for medication overuse. Treatment of MRM achieved with oral contraceptive therapy to prevent the premenstrual decline in estrogen led to resolution of MRM in 81% of compliant subjects. Further, alleviation of MRM led to reversion of chronic migraine to episodic migraine in 59% of patients, while only 18% of patients with persistent MRM showed reversion to an episodic phenotype. Interestingly, the resolution of MRM often correlated with decreased headache frequency outside the menstrual week. This improvement likely stemmed from the significant decrease in medication overuse. Women with persistent MRM used 41.6 acute agents per month, while women with resolved MRM only averaged 15.7 acute agents per month. This data suggests that hormonal therapy should be considered in women not only to reduce MRM but also medication overuse headaches.

Conclusion

While the exact pathophysiology of headache transformation is not entirely well understood, there have been many studies providing evidence that there are several modifiable risk factors that can contribute to headache chronification. Understanding how risk factors shift an episodic disorder to unremitting, daily or near-daily headache may lead to novel treatment and prevention strategies, and help provide headache patients with an improved quality of life.

References

1. Silberstein SD, Lipton RB, Solomon S, Mathew NT. Classification of daily and near-daily headaches: proposed revisions to the IHS criteria. Headache. 1994;34(1):1–7.
2. Srikiatkhachorn A, Govitrapong P, Limthavon C. Up-regulation of 5HT-2 serotonin receptor: a possible mechanism of transformed migraine. Headache. 1994;34:8–11.
3. Gallai V, Alberti A, Coppola F, Floridi A, Sarchielli P. Glutamate and nitric oxide pathway in chronic daily headache: evidence from cerebrospinal fluid. Cephalalgia. 2003;23:166–74.
4. Cernuda-Morollón E, Ramon C, Vega J, Martínez-Camblor P, Pascual J. Interictal increase of CGRP levels in peripheral blood as a biomarker for chronic migraine. Neurology. 2013;81:1191–6.
5. Cevoli S, Sancisi E, Grimaldi D, Pierangeli G, Zanigni S, Nicodemo M, Cortelli P, Montagna P. Family history for chronic headache and drug overuse as a risk factor for headache chronification. Headache. 2009;49:412–8.
6. Arruda MA, Guidetti V, Galli F, Albuquerque RCAP, Bigal ME. Frequency of headaches in children is influenced by headache status in the mother. Headache. 2010;50:973–80.
7. Meletiche D, Lofland J, Young W. Quality-of-life differences between patients with episodic and transformed migraine. Headache. 2001;41:573–8.
8. Munakata J, Hazard E, Serrano D, Klingman D, Rupnow M, Tierce J, Reed M, Lipton R. Economic burden of transformed migraine: results from the American Migraine Prevalence and Prevention (AMPP) study. Headache. 2009;49:498–508.
9. Scher AI, Stewart WF, Liberman J, Lipton RB. Prevalence of frequent headache in a population sample. Headache. 1998;38(7):497–506.

10. Bigal ME, Rapoport AM, Sheftell FD, Tepper SJ, Lipton RB. Transformed migraine and medication overuse in a tertiary headache centre—clinical characteristics and treatment outcomes. Cephalalgia. 2004;24(6):483–90.

11. Carlsen LN, Munksgaard SB, Jensen RH, Bendtsen L. Complete detoxification is the most effective treatment of medication overuse headache: a randomized controlled open-label trial. Cephalalgia. 2017;333102417737779.

12. Bigal ME, Serrano D, Buse D, Scher A, Stewart WF, Lipton RB. Acute migraine medications and evolution from episodic to chronic migraine: a longitudinal population-based study. Headache. 2008;48(8):1157–68.

13. Thorland K, Sun-Edelstein C, Druyts E, Kanters S, Ebrahim S, Bhambri R. Risk of medication overuse headache across classes of treatments for acute migraine. J Headache Pain. 2016;17:107.

14. Scher AI, Stewart WF, Ricci JA, Lipton RB. Factors associated with the onset and remission of chronic daily headache in a population-based study. Pain. 2003;106:81–9.

15. Bigal ME, Liberman JN, Lipton RB. Obesity and migraine: a population study. Neurology. 2006;66:545–50.

16. Bigal ME, Lipton RB. Obesity is a risk factor for transformed migraine but not chronic tension-type headache. Neurology. 2006;67:252–7.

17. Domínguez C, Vieites-Prado A, Pérez-Mato M, Sobrino T, Rodríguez-Osorio X, López A, Campos F, Martínez F, Castillo J, Leira R. Role of adipocytokines in the pathophysiology of migraine. A cross-sectional study. Cephalalgia. 2017;333102417731351.

18. Novack V, Fuchs L, Lantsberg L, Kama S, Lahoud U, Horev A, Loewenthal N, Ifergane G. Changes in headache frequency in premenopausal obese women with migraine after bariatric surgery: a case series. Cephalalgia. 2011;31(13):1336–42.

19. Sancisi E, Cevoli S, Vignatelli L, Nicodemo M, et al. Increased prevalence of sleep disorders in chronic headache: a case-control study. Headache. 2010;50(9):1464–72.

20. Kelman L, Rains JC. Headache and sleep: examination of sleep patterns and complaints in a large clinical sample of migraineurs. Headache. 2005;45:904–10.

21. Calhoun AH, Ford S. Behavioral sleep modification may revert transformed migraine to episodic migraine. Headache. 2007;47(8):1178–83.

22. Johnson KG, Zimeba AM, Garb JL. Improvement in headaches with continuous positive airway pressure for obstructive sleep apnea: a retrospective analysis. Headache. 2013;53(2):333–43.

23. Rains JC, Poceta JS. Headache and sleep disorders: review and clinical implications for headache management. Headache. 2006;46(9):1344–63.

24. Penzien DB, Rains JC, Holroyd KA. Psychological assessment of the recurrent headache sufferer. In: Tollinson CD, Kunkel RS, editors. Headache: diagnosis and treatment. Baltimore, MD: Williams and Williams; 1993. p. 39–49.

25. D'Amico D, Libro G, Prudenzano MP, Peccarisi C, et al. Stress and chronic headache. J Headache Pain. 2000;1:S49–52.

26. Paykel ES, Prusoff BA. Scaling of life events. Arch Gen Psychiatry. 1971;25(4):340–7.

27. Silberstein S, Olesen J. Chronic migraines. In: Olesen J, Goadsby PJ, Ramadan NM, Tfelt-Hansen P, Welch KMA, editors. The headaches. Philadelphia, PA: Lippincott Williams & Wilkins; 2006. p. 613–7.

28. Costa A, Smeraldi C, Tassorellia R, Grecoa G. Effects of acute and chronic restraint stress on nitroglycerin-induced hyperalgesia in rats. Neurosci Lett. 2005;383:22–9.

29. Blanchard EB, Appelbaum KA, Radnitz CL, et al. The refractory headache patient—I: chronic, daily, high intensity headache. Behav Res Ther. 1989;27:403–10.

30. Holroyd KA, Malinoski PE, O'Donnell FJ, et al. Antidepressant medication and cognitive behavioral therapy for CTTH: predictors of treatment response and dose-response relationships. Headache. 2002;42:456–7.

31. Nash JM, Thebarge RW. Understanding psychological stress, its biological processes, and impact on primary headache. Headache. 2006;46:1377–86.

32. Lake AE. Screening and behavioral management: medication overuse headache—the complex case. Headache. 2008;48:26–31.

33. Radat F, Swendsen J. Psychiatric comorbidity in migraine: a review. Cephalgia. 2005;25(3):165–78.

34. Ashina S, Serrano D, Lipton RB Maizels M, Manack AN, Turkel CC, Reed ML, Buse DC. Depression and risk of transformation of episodic to chronic migraine. Headache Pain. 2012;13:615–24.

35. Lipton RB, Silberstein SD. Why study the comorbidity of migraine? Neurology. 1994;44:S4–5.

36. Rivat C, Becker C, Blugeot A, et al. Chronic stress induces transient spinal neuroinflammation, triggering sensory hypersensitivity and long-lasting anxiety-induced hyperalgesia. Pain. 2010;150:358–68.

37. Boudreau GP, Grosberg BM, McAllister PJ, Sheftell FD, Lipton RB, Buse DC. Open-label, multicenter study of the efficacy and outcome of onabotulinum-toxin-A treatment in patients with chronic migraine and comorbid depressive disorders. J Headache Pain. 2010;11:S50.

38. Neugebauer V, Li W, Bird GC, Han JS. The amygdala and persistent pain. Neuroscientist. 2004;10:221–34.

39. Zhang M, Liu Y, Zhao M, Wenjing T, Xiaolin W, Zhao D, Shengyuan Y. Depression and anxiety behaviour in a rat model of chronic migraine. Headache Pain. 2017;18(1):27.

40. Somerville BW. The influence of progesterone and estradiol upon migraine. Headache. 1972;12(3):93–102.

41. MacGregor EA, Frith A, Ellis J, Aspinall L, Hackshaw A. Incidence of migraine relative to menstrual cycle phases of rising and falling estrogen. Neurology. 2006;67(12):2154–8.

Chronic Daily Headache and Comorbid Disorders

Sara Siavoshi, Carrie Dougherty, and Jessica Ailani

Introduction

Chronic daily headache (CDH), comprised of the headache disorders chronic migraine (CM), chronic tension-type headache (CTTH), new daily persistent headache (NDPH), and hemicrania continua (HC), has a prevalence between 4 and 6% worldwide [1]. In a disease state that will be encountered by most healthcare providers during their career, it is important not only to understand and identify CDH but also recognize its comorbid conditions. Diagnosis and treatment of comorbid disorder in CDH can impact headache-related disability, health-related quality of life, and treatment outcomes [2]. Understanding comorbid conditions can also lead to insight about shared genetic and environmental causes of each individual disease, as well as genetic and pathophysiological mechanisms for co-occurrence.

This chapter will review comorbid disorders seen in CDH with a particular emphasis on CM. It will discuss mood disorders (depression, anxiety, childhood maltreatment, and post-traumatic stress disorder), musculoskeletal (MSK) disorders (temporal mandibular dysfunction cervicalgia, and connective tissue disorder), other neurological disorders (head injury, epilepsy, and ischemic stroke), and medical disorders (sleep disorders, obesity, asthma and allergic rhinitis, and cardiovascular disease).

Most comorbid disorders in CDH are best studied in CM, though they are likely seen in CTTH as well. NDPH may share mood and MSK comorbidities, but currently there is little evidence to suggest comorbid conditions in both NDPH and HC. This may be related to the lower prevalence of these disorders in comparison with CM.

S. Siavoshi
Department of Neurosciences, University of California San Diego, San Diego, CA, USA

C. Dougherty
Department of Neurology, Medstar Georgetown Headache Center, MedStar Georgetown University Hospital, Washington, DC, USA

J. Ailani (✉)
Department of Neurology, Medstar Georgetown Headache Center, Medstar Georgetown University Hospital, Washington, DC, USA
e-mail: jessica.x.ailani@gunet.georgetown.edu

Mood Disorders

Clinic-based studies show an association between CDH and at least one psychiatric disorder in a majority of cases [3, 4]. In this section, we will review depression, anxiety, childhood maltreatment, and post-traumatic stress disorder in persons with CDH.

Depression

Depression is known to be comorbid with migraine. Population studies show that depression is diagnosed in 40–47% of people with migraine [2]. Depression is comorbid in non-migrainous headache as well. Persons with non-migrainous headache are 4% more likely to be diagnosed with depression [5]. More frequent migraine headache is associated with higher rates of depression [6, 7]. Persons with CM are more likely than those with episodic migraine (EM) to meet criteria for depression (41.2–47% vs. 25%) and are two times more likely to have received a diagnosis of depression [6, 7]. Compared with persons with non-migrainous headache, depression risk was 3.83-fold higher in persons with CM [8].

Depression may be a risk factor for chronification of migraine [9]. This is when persons with EM transition to CM. Increased depression severity correlated with an increased risk of chronification, with moderate and severe depression carrying the highest risk [9].

Depression can also add further burden to chronic headache by impacting employment status, reducing earnings, and restricting career achievement [10].

Depression does not seem to impact remission of CM to EM; improved mood unrelated to headache burden did not lead to reduced headache frequency [11]. The opposite may be true of impact of headache frequency on mood. A small study evaluating onabotulinumtoxinA for CM found reducing headache frequency also reduced depression [12].

Anxiety

Anxiety disorders include general anxiety disorder (GAD), panic attacks, obsessive-compulsive disorder, and specific phobias. Anxiety disorders are more prevalent in CM than EM and are also a risk factor for disease chronification [6, 7, 9]. A study done by Guidetti et al. found that over time anxiety disorders were predictive of either unchanged or worsening headache in 70% of migraineurs [13]. General anxiety disorder is the most prevalent reported psychiatric disorder in CDH and is five times higher in migraineurs than non-migraineurs [3, 14].

Depression and anxiety affect serotonin and dopamine signaling, both of which are involved in the pathophysiology of various headache disorders, which may explain their shared co-occurrence in CDH [2].

Childhood Maltreatment

Childhood maltreatment can refer to sexual, physical, or emotional abuse in childhood and other maltreatment, such as neglect [15]. It is a public health concern that is often silent [16]. There are close to one million cases of childhood maltreatment substantiated per year in the USA, but true burden is likely much greater [16]. Rates of childhood maltreatment in CDH are reported to be between 27 and 40% [16].

There are unique challenges to evaluating childhood maltreatment in population and clinic-based studies compared to evaluating other mood disorders. Most studies of childhood maltreatment and CDH are retrograde identification of maltreatment, which can carry potential bias related to recollection to painful experiences [15]. Prospective studies are difficult, as maltreatment is rarely reported at the time of occurrence [15]. This may lead to under- or overrepresentation of disease comorbidity.

Community studies of childhood maltreatment are rare. Juang et al. studied childhood adversities in CDH in young adolescents in public schools and found frequencies of physical abuse and parental divorce were significantly higher in persons with CDH than controls [17].

There are several clinic-based studies evaluating childhood maltreatment in CM. Tietjen et al., in a cross-sectional multi-headache clinic (11 sites) study, reported that childhood maltreatment was significantly associated with CM and transformation of migraine. Emotional abuse in childhood was associated with earlier-onset headache as well as continuous daily headache, severe headache-related disability, and migraine-associated allodynia [18].

The relationship between childhood maltreatment and CDH is likely due to alterations in brain physiology caused by early stress that trigger a change in the pain matrix. In childhood maltreatment, early-life stressors can cause long-term changes to the hypothalamic-pituitary-adrenal (HPA) axis function and regulation. This dysfunction has been associated with CM [16]. Early-life stress can also cause changes in a range of neurotransmitters involved in migraine (dopamine, serotonin, GABA-A), as well as increase release of pro-inflammatory cytokines [16].

Post-traumatic Stress Disorder

Post-traumatic stress disorder (PTSD) occurs as a result of being exposed to extreme traumatic experiences that cause feelings of helplessness and fear [19]. Persons with PTSD will emotionally re-experience the event, avoid stimuli, have a negative mood or poor cognition, and have symptoms of overstimulation [15]. Prevalence of PTSD is between 1 and 8% in the population [15]. Studies evaluating the correlation between PTSD and CDH find the lifetime prevalence of PTSD in persons with CDH to be 19.2% compared to 4.5% in persons without headache [20]. Clinic-based studies have found a greater frequency of comorbid PTSD and depression in CDH compared to EM [19].

PTSD is related to serotonergic function and may also cause dysregulation of the HPA axis [15]. This may explain the coexistence of PTSD in patients with migraine.

Musculoskeletal Disorders

Muscle tension was long thought to be involved in the pathophysiology of tension headaches [21]. While this has been disproven, many patients with CDH experience comorbid MSK disorder. This may be related to the trigeminal cervical complex and its descending pathway through C1–C3 triggering pain in the upper neck and related areas [21]. In this section, we will review CDH and comorbid temporal mandibular dysfunction (TMD), cervicalgia, and connective tissue disorders.

Temporal Mandibular Dysfunction

CM patients are more likely to have tenderness at the temporomandibular joint and on masticatory muscles relative to EM and controls without headaches [22]. Bevilaqua-Grossi et al. demonstrated that cutaneous allodynia occurs more frequently in EM patients with TMD than those without, and thus TMD was proposed as a risk factor for transformation to CM [23]. A cross-sectional survey study found that individuals with TMD are significantly more likely to have CDH, with more symptoms of TMD imparting greater risk [24]. A subsequent controlled study in clinic confirmed that TMD is strongly associated with both migraine and CDH, but not episodic tension-type headache (ETTH), and that increasing TMD severity is associated with increasing headache frequency [25]. Sleep bruxism is also associated with CM, but not EM or ETTH [26].

Cervicalgia

Neck pain accompanies chronic migraine (CM) so frequently that it is difficult to conceptualize the two as separate conditions. A prospective study of 113 migraineurs, nearly half of whom were chronic, found that neck pain occurs more frequently in migraine than nausea, a defining associated symptom [27]. The prevalence of neck pain increases with migraine chronicity [27]. Neck-related disability and pain thresholds demonstrate similar trends. Florencio et al. reported that individuals with CM were at a significantly increased risk for cervical disability relative to episodic migraineurs [28]. Patients with transformed migraine (TM) have significantly lower pain thresholds in the neck both between and during migraine than their EM counterparts [28].

Neck pain in migraine is likely a manifestation of allodynia due to activation of upper cervical afferents in the trigeminal nucleus caudalis (TNC) [29]. Allodynia is a known risk factor for the development of chronic migraine [30]. These studies support the notion that neck pain is implicit in the pathophysiology of chronic migraine and not a separate co-occurring condition.

Connective Tissue Disorders and Pain Disorders

Pain disorders, including musculoskeletal pain, fibromyalgia, and joint hypermobility syndrome (JHS; type III Ehlers-Danlos syndrome), are comorbid with migraine [31–34].

The Nord-Trøndelag Health Study found the prevalence of both migraine and non-migrainous headache was increased in persons with musculoskeletal symptoms lasting for ≥3 months, compared to persons without musculoskeletal symptoms. The prevalence of chronic headache (headache on >14 days per month) was 4.6 times higher in persons with musculoskeletal symptoms than in those without such symptoms [33].

Marcus and colleagues reported that out of 100 fibromyalgia patients evaluated, 76 reported headache. Of the 76 patients with headache, 48 (63%) received a diagnosis of migraine, either in isolation or combined with tension-type headache [34].

Castori and colleagues assessed the prevalence of headaches in 21 patients with JHS from a group of 40 individuals with suspected hereditary connective tissue disorder. Of the 21 patients with JHS, 18 (86%) reported recurrent headaches [35]. Bendik and colleagues assessed the prevalence, frequency, and disability of migraine in female patients with migraine compared to a control population. Of the 28 patients with JHS, 21 (75%) had migraine compared with 43% of controls [31]. Migraine was more prevalent, frequent, and disabling in female JHS patients as compared with controls [31].

Central sensitization may mediate migraine, musculoskeletal pain, and fibromyalgia [36, 37]. Central sensitization arises when central pain pathways develop lower thresholds for activation. This may result from dysregulated pain-producing mechanisms. It is not known, however, whether central sensitization is secondary to ongoing painful input or whether it is a primary disease mechanism [38]. JHS, like migraine, may be mediated through mechanisms involving autonomic dysfunction or dysregulated cytokine signaling.

Neurological Disorders

Headache is the most common neurological disorder and affects both the central and peripheral nervous system. It is therefore not surprising that other neurological disorders can be found more often in patients with CDH. In this section, we will review CDH and comorbid association with head injury, epilepsy, and stroke.

Head Injury

Several studies have suggested that head injury and whiplash are risk factors for the development of CDH [39–44]. In some instances, CDH occurs in direct relationship to head trauma and is then characterized as post-traumatic headache (PTH). The Frequent Headache Epidemiology Study, a population interview survey, found that head and neck injury account for 15% of CDH [45]. The same study also noted that in CDH there is a higher frequency of lifetime incidence of history of head trauma, in which the onset of headache was not temporally related to the injury [45]. The lifetime risk of CDH increased with the number of head/neck injuries [45].

The literature on PTH has shown that headaches following head injury exhibit increased prevalence of CDH than headaches that are not associated with head trauma [46, 47]. In a cross-sectional study of soldiers returning from combat deployment, 27% of subjects with PTH experienced CDH, as compared to 14% of subjects with non-traumatic headaches [47]. A subsequent study by the authors similarly showed that 20% of patients with headache following deployment-related concussion met criteria for CDH [47]. This is noted in the civilian population as well with 46% of patients with mild TBI reporting a headache frequency of 15 days per month or more [47].

The theoretical mechanisms by which head injury can precipitate or potentiate headache frequency include post-injury inflammation, increased neuronal and glial excitability, and enhanced release of calcitonin gene-related peptide from trigeminal afferents [47].

Epilepsy

There are several studies that have shown migraine to be comorbid with epilepsy [48–53]. Both epilepsy and migraine are thought to arise, in part, due to neuronal hyperexcitability—the proposed point of convergence for these comorbid disorders. Based on this insight, many of the treatments for both disorders target neuronal hyperexcitability [54]; however not all antiepileptic drugs provide effective prophylaxis for migraine.

Ischemic Stroke

Persons with migraine have been shown to be at increased risk for ischemic stroke [55–66], and there is a relationship between stroke and migraine with aura [56, 57, 59, 61, 63–65], particularly in women [56, 57, 63, 64]. Several studies have also shown an increased incidence of white matter abnormalities in migraineurs with aura [67, 68]. It has been suggested that prothrombotic states, some of which predispose to stroke, are risk factors for transformation from EM to CM [69].

Six hypotheses have been proposed to explain the mechanisms by which migraine may lead to ischemic stroke:

1. Migraine directly causes ischemic stroke.
2. Migraine-specific physiology disrupts vascular lesions, which can lead to an ischemic stroke (e.g., vomiting during a migraine leads to carotid or vertebral artery dissection which then acts as a source for ischemic stroke).
3. Migraine is associated with a higher prevalence of an unfavorable cardiovascular risk profile.
4. Migraine and ischemic stroke are linked through shared genetic mechanisms.
5. Anti-migraine medications, such as triptans and ergots, are vasoconstrictors which increase the risk of ischemic events. This theory is contradicted by a 2004 study that showed that triptan usage was not associated with an increased risk of stroke, MI, or cardiovascular death [70]. The CAMERA-2 study also found no association between white matter abnormality progression and triptan therapy [71].
6. Migraine is associated with an increased prevalence of patent foramen ovale (PFO) [72]. Evidence for this is inconsistent.

Despite evidence in support of these various hypotheses, the precise mechanism leading to comorbidity of ischemic stroke and migraine remains unknown.

While there is a risk of ischemic stroke in patients with migraine with aura, a clear increased risk of ischemic stroke has not been seen in patients with CDH. For patients with CDH, ischemic stroke risk counseling should be provided to patients who have concurrent migraine with aura, especially women.

Medical Disorders

Patients with frequent headache will often experience disruptions of routine functions, such as sleep. Some patients with particular medical conditions may be at a higher risk for frequent headaches, such as patients who have thyroid disorders, who are obese, or who have asthma or allergies. This section will review CDH and comorbid sleep disorders, obesity, asthma and allergies, and cardiovascular disease.

Thyroid Disorders

In the Fernald Medical Monitoring Program (FMMP), patients with a self-report of "frequent" headache disorder had a 21% increased risk of developing new-onset hypothyroidism, while those with self-report of "frequent" possible migraine showed an increased risk of 41%. Age was found to be a predictor of hypothyroidism, as HRs progressively increased from the youngest to the oldest participants [73]. In a clinic-based study, the correlation between age and hypothyroidism was found to be stronger in CM than in EM [74].

In a prospective study of 102 adults with hypothyroidism, 30% of those that endorsed headaches with onset after the first symptoms of hypothyroidism also reported resolution of headache symptoms after initiation of thyroid hormone therapy [75].

One theory of shared pathophysiology is that upregulation of the immune system in headache disorders provokes an attack on the thyroid gland. This is supported by a study that shows interictal periods of elevated CRP and altered proportions of T lymphocytes in migraineurs [76].

Sleep Disorders

Findings from the National Comorbidity Survey-Replication Study demonstrated a significant association between frequent severe headache and sleep disorders. Compared with persons without headache, those with frequent severe headache reported more difficulty initiating and staying asleep, early morning awakening, and daytime fatigue. Migraine, specifically, was associated with an increased risk of sleep disorders [77]. The correlation between sleep disorders and migraine may be affected by migraine frequency. A study of 332 patients, assessed using the Pittsburgh Sleep Quality Index (PSQI), found that patients with more migraine days per month had higher PSQI scores, indicative of poorer sleep [78].

The relationship between migraine and obstructive sleep apnea was evaluated in a cross-sectional population-based study, and results were not statistically significant. There was, however, a statistically significant relationship between migraine and excessive daytime sleepiness [79].

The Nord-Trøndelag Health Study of 297 participants showed a strong association between severe sleep disturbances and chronic headaches, with CM being more strongly associated than EM. Sleep maybe a precipitant as well as a palliative agent for migraine [80]. Shared neurophysiologic mechanisms in sleep disorders and migraine include involvement of the hypothalamus and the neurotransmitters, serotonin and melanin [80]. Migraines are thought to be triggered in the hypothalamus, as it is highly active

during attacks [81]. The hypothalamic suprachiasmatic nuclei that control circadian rhythms are integral to sleep patterns [80]. Finally, the hypothalamus has extensive connections with the limbic system, the pineal gland, and brainstem nuclei involved in the sleep-waking cycles and pain modulation [82].

Obesity

Like many comorbidities of migraine, obesity is more prevalent in persons with CM than in those with EM [68]. Like many other comorbidities, obesity has been demonstrated to be a risk factor for progression from EM to CM [83]. The link between obesity and migraine has been investigated in a number of population-based studies [6, 83, 84]. Bigal and colleagues found that higher-BMI patients experienced a greater frequency of migraine attacks. In the normal-weight group, 4.4% had 10–15 headache days per month, increasing to 5.8% of the overweight, 13.6% of the obese, and 20.7% of the morbidly obese group. Body mass index was also a predictor of headache severity. A significantly higher proportion of overweight, obese, and morbidly obese persons reported severe headaches compared with persons in the normal-weight group. Finally, obese and morbidly obese patients experienced more headache-related disabilities, including more missed workdays, and their headache pain was more frequently exacerbated by physical activity [85].

An analysis of data from the American Migraine Prevalence and Prevention (AMPP) study of 120,000 US households found that high-frequency headaches (10–14 days per month) occurred in 7.4% of overweight persons, 8.2% of obese persons, and 10.4% of morbidly obese persons, compared with 6.5% of persons in the normal-weight group. Headache-related disability was associated with BMI as well. Compared with migraineurs in the normal-weight group, overweight, obese, and morbidly obese subjects were significantly more disabled [86].

Significant BMI reduction has been demonstrated to benefit headache frequency. Bond and colleagues demonstrated a reduced frequency of headache in persons with CM in a small study of severely obese individuals who underwent bariatric surgery. Twenty-four patients with migraine were assessed before and 6 months after bariatric surgery. The mean number of headache days was reduced from 11.1 preoperatively to 6.7 postoperatively, after a mean percent excess weight loss of 49.4%. Reduction in pain severity was also observed, and the number of patients reporting moderate to severe disability decreased from 50.0% before surgery to 12.5% after surgery [87].

Migraine and obesity may in fact be biochemically linked [85]. Obesity is a pro-inflammatory state. Several inflammatory mediators, such as interleukins and calcitonin gene-related peptide (CGRP), which are important in migraine, are also increased in obese persons [88]. Adiponectin, a protein hormone secreted by fat cells, may modulate pain during migraine. Adiponectin levels are increased in obesity; and at low and abnormal levels, adiponectin is nociceptive. Similarly, orexins modulate both pain and metabolism, and dysfunctional orexin pathways may be a risk factor for both migraine and obesity [88].

Obesity is a modifiable risk factor for headache chronification. Prevention and treatment should be considered as part of CDH treatment.

Allergic Rhinitis and Asthma

The relationship between migraine and non-migrainous headache and hay fever, a form of allergic rhinitis [89], was assessed in the Head-HUNT study, a cross-sectional population-based study. Persons with both migraine and non-migrainous headache were more likely to have hay fever than those without headaches. This effect was greater in individuals with more than 14 days of headache per month [90]. Buse and colleagues demonstrated that the rates of allergies and hay fever are higher in persons with CM than in those with EM (59.9% vs. 50.7%) [68].

The AMPP study found that 66.8% of 5849 migraineurs had rhinitis (most commonly mixed rhinitis). Those with rhinitis were more likely to have higher headache frequency and a higher level of disability [91].

In a small clinic-based study of 76 persons diagnosed with allergic rhinitis, immunotherapy (allergy shots) decreased the frequency and disability of migraine headaches by 52% and 45%, respectively, in those migraineurs who were younger than 40 years of age [92].

Several large population-based studies have found an increased risk of asthma in migraineurs [93–96]. Findings from the 2005 AMPP study indicate that persons with CM are more likely to have asthma than those with EM. Self-report of a physician diagnosis of asthma occurred in 24.4% of respondents with CM compared with 17.2% of respondents with EM [68]. Martin and colleagues reported that the risk for CM increased by 2.1-fold in episodic migraineurs with asthma as compared to those without asthma [97].

Mast cells play an important role in both migraine and asthma or allergic rhinitis. The dura mater is highly innervated by pain fibers and densely populated by mast cells [98]. Animal studies suggest that mast cell degranulation in the dura could activate trigeminal nociceptors, contributing to migraine pathogenesis. Animal studies further show that plasma protein extravasation, including extravasation of neurotransmitters involved in pain mechanisms, is increased in pre-sensitized animals upon exposure to an allergen [99]. It is also possible that allergic disorders may indirectly contribute to the onset of migraine. Allergic disorders may modulate comorbidities and possible precipitants of CDH such as sleep, depression, or anxiety. It has also been proposed that the comorbidity with migraine may be due to immune system dysfunction in migraineurs. The clinical manifestations of allergic rhinitis include itching, runny nose, and mucous secretion. This response is mediated in part by the release of histamines in response to an inciting allergen [100]. Since histamines have been implicated in the pathogenesis of migraine headaches, and the nasal passage is in close proximity to the central nervous system, it has been hypothesized that allergic rhinitis may trigger migraine headaches [92].

Comorbid asthma in migraine may affect treatment choices. Beta-blockers can trigger bronchospasm in patients with asthma [101]. Nonsteroidal anti-inflammatory drugs (NSAIDs) may worsen asthma, especially in persons with nasal polyps and exercise-induced asthma [102].

Irritable Bowel Syndrome and Other Gastrointestinal Disorders

Various population-based studies have found migraineurs to be two to three times more likely to develop IBS. Migraine and IBS have been observed to be comorbid conditions [103–107]. Lau et al. found this effect to be more pronounced as headache frequency increased [103].

Celiac disease, an autoimmune disorder of the small intestine, has been reported to be comorbid with migraine [108–110]. A small study also found weak evidence that a gluten-free diet might reduce migraine frequency [108].

Aberrant autonomic dysfunction may pose a link between migraine and GI disorders. This mechanism is supported by studies that show delayed gastric emptying during interictal migraine periods [111, 112]. Another theory for shared migraine and GI pathogenesis is that of the "gut-brain axis," a term that represents the bidirectional relationship between the gut microbiome and brain function and links alterations in GI flora to neurological disorder like migraine [113].

Oral administration of migraine medications may have limited effectiveness in the context of delayed gastric emptying, nausea, and vomiting associated with migraine and should prompt consideration of alternative delivery routes [114].

Cardiovascular Diseases

Population-based studies demonstrate that migraine is significantly associated with cardiovascular risk factors, including an unfavorable cholesterol profile, elevated blood pressure, and diabetes [68, 115–117]. Both men and women with migraine with aura have increased risk of angina. Women with migraine with aura have been found to have an increased risk of cardiovascular events including angina and myocardial infarction (MI) [118, 119]. The results of the AMPP and IBMS studies showed that cardiovascular diseases and risk factors are significantly more likely to be associated with CM than with EM [7, 68]. Furthermore, heart disease, angina, and stroke were more prevalent in those with CM than in those with EM. Compared to those with EM, respondents with CM had a higher frequency of high blood pressure (33.7% vs. 27.9%) and high cholesterol (34.2% vs. 25.6%) [68].

The mechanisms that link migraine to ischemic vascular disease and its risk factors are unknown. Migraine with aura has been associated with several risk factors for heart disease including unfavorable cholesterol profiles, elevated blood pressure, history of early myocardial infarction, and both CHD and early-onset CHD [116].

Potential theories explaining cardiovascular disease risk in migraineurs include both intrinsic and extrinsic mechanisms. Intrinsic mechanisms may include changes in vascular reactivity, endothelial disturbance, and platelet dysfunction. Altered platelet aggregation in migraineurs combined with changes in blood flow may predispose to ischemic disease [117]. An insufficiency or dysfunction of endothelial precursor cells (EPCs), which are programmed to renew the endothelium, is a possible mechanism of vascular pathology in migraine [117]. However in contrast, Oterino and colleagues showed that a higher number of activated EPCs were found in migraineurs as compared to controls. This was explained by the mobilization of EPCs after vascular injury in migraine [120]. Additionally, elevated prothrombotic or vasoactive peptides have been observed in migraine including prothrombin factor 1.2, factor V Leiden, serotonin, and von Willebrand factor [118].

Sedentary lifestyle and medication effect are extrinsic mechanisms of cardiovascular disease risk in this population. However, in the Women's Health Study, the increased risk of vascular events remained even after correcting for external cardiovascular risk factors [121]. Specifically in regard to risk associated with migraine medications, a systematic review of observational studies found pooled odds ratios for serious ischemic events associated with migraine medications to be significantly increased for ergotamines, but not for triptans [122]. Similarly, a large cohort of over 63,000 migraine patients found no association between triptan prescription and stroke or MI risk [70].

Conclusion

CDH is often accompanied by multiple comorbidities that can complicate treatment and result in significantly higher healthcare-related expenses [123]. Comorbidities in CM also increase the likelihood of disability, the rate of which exceeds 40% in patients with four or more chronic conditions [123]. The high rates of disability highlight the complexity of treating these patients and the shortcomings of available therapeutics. Improvement in outcomes will depend on further research to better define the pathophysiological mechanisms that may link CDH to comorbid conditions and guide evidence-based, disease-specific interventions.

References

1. Castillo J, Munoz P, Guitera V, Pascual J. Epidemiology of chronic daily headache in the general population. Headache. 1999;39:190–6.
2. Buse DC, Silberstein SD, Manack AN, Papapetropoulos S, Lipton RB. Psychiatric comorbidities of episodic and chronic migraine. J Neurol. 2013;260:1960–9.
3. Verri AP, Proletti CA, Galli C, Grenella F, Sandrini G, Nappi G. Psychiatric co-morbidity in chronic daily headache. Cephalalgia. 1998;18:45–9.
4. Singh AK, Shukla R, Trivedi JK, Singh D. Association of psychiatric co-morbidity and efficacy of treatment in chronic daily headache in Indian population. J Neurosci Rural Pract. 2013;4:132–9.
5. Zwart JA, Drb G, Hagen K, Odegard KJ, Dahl AA, Bovim G, Stovner LJ. Depression and anxiety disorders associated with headache frequency. The Nord-Trøndelag Health Study. Eur J Neurol. 2003;10:147–52.
6. Buse DC, Manack A, Serrano D, Turkel C, Lipton RB. Sociodemographic and comorbidity profiles of chronic migraine and episodic migraine sufferers. J Neurol Neurosurg Psychiatry. 2010;81:428–32.

7. Blumendfeld A, Varon S, Wilcox TK, Buse D, Kawata AK, Manack A, Goadsby PJ, Lipton RB. Disability, HR QoL and resource use among chronic and episodic migraineurs: results from the International Burden of Migraine Study (IBMS). Cephalalgia. 2011;31:301–15.
8. Chen YC, Tang CH, Ng K, Wang SJ. Comorbidity profiles of chronic migraine sufferers in a national database in Taiwan. J Headache Pain. 2012;13:311–9.
9. Ashina S, Serrano D, Lipton RB, Maizels M, Manack AN, Turkel CC, Reed ML, Buse DC. Depression and risk of transformation of episodic to chronic migraine: results of the American Migraine Prevalence and Prevention study. J Headache Pain. 2012;13:615–24.
10. Zebenholzer K, Lechner A, Broessner G, Lampl C, Luthringshausen G, Al W, Obmann S, Berek K, Wober C. Impact of depression and anxiety on burden and management of episodic and chronic headaches—a cross sectional multicenter study in eight Austrian headache centers. J Headache Pain. 2016;17:15.
11. Manack A, Buse DC, Serrano D, et al. Rates, predictors, and consequences of remission from chronic migraine to episodic migraine. Neurology. 2011;76:711–8.
12. Boudreau GP, Grossberg BM, McAllister PJ, Sheftell FD, Lipton RB, Buse DC. Open-label, multicenter study of the efficacy and outcome of onabotulinum—a treatment in patients with chronic migraine and comorbid depressive disorders. J Headache Pain. 2017;18:23.
13. Guidetti V, Galli F, Fabrizi P, Giannantoni AS, Napoli L, Bruni O, Trillo S. Headache and psychiatric comorbidity: clinical aspects and outcome in an 8-year follow up study. Cephalalgia. 1998;18:455–62.
14. Merikangas KR, Angst J, Isler H. Migraine and psychopathology. Results of the Zurich cohort study of young adults. Arch Gen Psychiatry. 1990;47(9):849–53.
15. Juang KD, Yang C. Psychiatric comorbidity of chronic daily headache: focus on traumatic experiences in childhood, post-traumatic stress disorder and suicidality. Curr Pain Headache Rep. 2014;18:405.
16. Tietjen GE, Peterlin BL. Childhood abuse and migraine: epidemiology, sex differences, and potential mechanisms. Headache. 2011;51:869–79.
17. Juang KD, Wang SJ, Fuh JL, Lu SR, Chen YS. Association between adolescent chronic daily headache and childhood adversity: a community-based study. Cephalalgia. 2004;24:54–9.
18. Tietjen GE, Brandes JL, Peterlin BL, Eloff A, Dafer R, Stein MR, Drexler E, Martin VT, Hutchinson S, Aurora SK, Recober A, Herial NA, Utley C, White L, Khuder SA. Childhood maltreatment and migraine (Part II). Emotional abuse as a risk factor for headache chronification. Headache. 2010;50(50):32–41.
19. Peterlin BL, Tietjen GE, Meng S, Lidicker J, Bigal M. Post-traumatic stress disorder in episodic and chronic migraine. Headache. 2008;48:517–22.

20. Peterlin BL, Rosso AL, Sheftell FD, Libon DJ, Mossey JM, Merikangas KR. Post-traumatic stress disorder, drug abuse and migraine: new findings from the National Comorbidity Survey Replication. Cephalalgia. 2011;31:235–44.

21. Fumal A, Schoenen J. Tension-type headache: current research and clinical management. Lancet Neurol. 2008;7(1):70–83.

22. Stuginski-Barbosa J, Macedo HR, Bigal ME, Speciali JG. Signs of temporomandibular disorders in migraine patients: a prospective, controlled study. Clin J Pain. 2010;26(5):418–21.

23. Bevilaqua-Grossi D, Lipton RB, Napchan U, Grosberg B, Ashina S, Bigal ME. Temporomandibular disorders and cutaneous allodynia are associated in individuals with migraine. Cephalalgia. 2010;30(4):425–32.

24. Gonçalves DA, Speciali JG, Jales LCF, et al. Temporomandibular symptoms, migraine and chronic daily headaches in the population. Neurology. 2009;73(8):645–6.

25. Gonçalves DA, Camparis CM, Speciali JG, Franco AL, Castanharo SM, Bigal ME. Temporomandibular disorders are differentially associated with headache diagnosis: a controlled study. Clin J Pain. 2011;27(7):611–5.

26. Fernandes G, Franco AL, Gonçalves DA, Speciali JG, Bigal ME, Camparis CM. Temporomandibular disorders, sleep bruxism, and primary headaches are mutually associated. J Orofac Pain. 2013;27(1):14–20.

27. Calhoun AH, Ford S, Millen C, Finkel AG, Truong Y, Nie Y. The prevalence of neck pain in migraine. Headache. 2010;50(8):1273–7.

28. Florencio LL, Chaves TC, Carvalho GF, Goncalves MC, Casmiro EC, Dach F, Bigal ME, Bevilaqua-Gross D. Neck pain disability is related to the frequency of migraine attacks: a cross-sectional study. Headache. 2014;54(7):1203–10.

29. Piovesan EJ, Kowacs PA, Tatsui CE, Lange MC, Ribas LC, Werneck LC. Referred pain after painful stimulation of the greater occipital nerve in humans: evidence of convergence of cervical afferences on trigeminal nuclei. Cephalalgia. 2001;21(2):107–9.

30. Bigal ME, Ashina S, Burstein R, et al. AMPP Group. Prevalence and characteristics of allodynia in headache sufferers: a population study. Neurology. 2008;70:1525–33.

31. Bendik EM, Tinkle BT, Al-shuik E, et al. Joint hypermobility syndrome: a common clinical disorder associated with migraine in women. Cephalalgia. 2011;31:603–13.

32. Evans RW, de TM. Migraine and fibromyalgia. Headache. 2011;51:295–9.

33. Hagen K, Einarsen C, Zwart JA, Svebak S, Bovim G. The co-occurrence of headache and musculoskeletal symptoms amongst 51 050 adults in Norway. Eur J Neurol. 2002;9:527–33.

34. Marcus DA, Bernstein C, Rudy TE. Fibromyalgia and headache: an epidemiological study supporting migraine as part of the fibromyalgia syndrome. Clin Rheumatol. 2005;24:595–601.

35. Castori M, Sperduti I, Celletti C, Camerota F, Grammatico P. Symptom and joint mobility progression in the joint hypermobility syndrome (Ehlers-Danlos syndrome, hypermobility type). Clin Exp Rheumatol. 2011.

36. Aurora SK, Kulthia A, Barrodale PM. Mechanism of chronic migraine. Curr Pain Headache Rep. 2011;15:57–63.

37. Staud R, Rodriguez ME. Mechanisms of disease: pain in fibromyalgia syndrome. Nat Clin Pract Rheumatol. 2006;2:90–8.

38. Kindler LL, Bennett RM, Jones KD. Central sensitivity syndromes: mounting pathophysiologic evidence to link fibromyalgia with other common chronic pain disorders. Pain Manag Nurs. 2011;12:15–24.

39. Weiss HD, Stern BJ, Goldberg J. Post-traumatic migraine: chronic migraine precipitated by minor head or neck trauma. Headache. 1991;31:451–6.

40. Jensen OK, Nielsen FF. The influence of sex and pretraumatic headache on the incidence and severity of headache after head injury. Cephalalgia. 1990;10:285–93.

41. Yamaguchi M. Incidence of headache and severity of head injury. Headache. 1992;32:427–31.

42. Scher AI, Lipton RB, Stewart W. Risk factors for chronic daily headache. Curr Pain Headache Rep. 2002;6(6):486–91.

43. Moscato D, Peracchi MI, Mazzotta G, Savi L, Battistella PA. Post-traumatic headache from moderate head injury. J Headache Pain. 2005;6:284–6.

44. Bekkelund SI, Salvesen R. Prevalence of head trauma in patients with difficult headache: the North Norway Headache Study. Headache. 2003;43:59–62.

45. Couch JR, Lipton RB, Stewart WF, et al. Head or neck injury increases the risk of chronic daily headache: a population-based study. Neurology. 2007;69(11):1169–77.

46. Theeler BJ, Flynn FG, Erickson JC. Headaches after concussion in US soldiers returning from Iraq or Afghanistan. Headache. 2010;50:1262–72.

47. Theeler BJ, Lucas S, Riechers R, Ruff RL. Post-traumatic headaches in civilian and military personnel: a comparative clinical review. Headache. 2013;53:881–900.

48. Ottman R, Lipton RB. Comorbidity of migraine and epilepsy. Neurology. 1994;44:2105–10.

49. Gameleira FT, Ataíde L Jr, Raposo MC. Relations between epileptic seizures and headaches. Seizure. 2013;22:622–6.

50. Ottman R, Lipton RB. Is the comorbidity of epilepsy and migraine due to a shared genetic susceptibility? Neurology. 1996;47:918–24.

51. Ottman R, Lipton RB, Ettinger AB, et al. Comorbidities of epilepsy: results from the Epilepsy Comorbidities and Health (EPIC) survey. Epilepsia. 2011;52:308–15.

52. Winawer MR, Connors R, Investigators EPGP. Evidence for a shared genetic susceptibility to migraine and epilepsy. Epilepsia. 2013;54:288–95.

53. Velioğlu SK, Boz C, Ozmenoğlu M. The impact of migraine on epilepsy: a prospective prognosis study. Cephalalgia. 2005;25:528–35.

54. Goadsby PJ, Lipton RB, Ferrari MD. Migraine—current understanding and treatment. N Engl J Med. 2002;346:257–70.

55. Katsarava Z, Weimar C. Migraine and stroke. J Neurol Sci. 2010;299:42–4.

56. Donaghy M, Chang CL, Poulter N. Duration, frequency, recency, and type of migraine and the risk of ischaemic stroke in women of childbearing age. J Neurol Neurosurg Psychiatry. 2002;73:747–50.

57. Rist PM, Buring JE, Kase CS, Schurks M, Kurth T. Migraine and functional outcome from ischemic cerebral events in women. Circulation. 2010;122:2551–7.

58. Carolei A, Marini C, De Matteis G. History of migraine and risk of cerebral ischaemia in young adults. The Italian National Research Council Study Group on Stroke in the Young. Lancet. 1996;347(9014):1503–6.

59. Stang PE, Carson AP, Rose KM, et al. Headache, cerebrovascular symptoms, and stroke: the Atherosclerosis Risk in Communities study. Neurology. 2005;64:1573–7.

60. Buring JE, Hebert P, Romero J, Kittross A, Cook N, Manson J, Peto R, Hennekens C. Migraine and subsequent risk of stroke in the Physicians' Health Study. Arch Neurol. 1995;52(2):129–34.

61. Chang CL, Donaghy M, Poulter N. Migraine and stroke in young women: case-control study. The World Health Organisation Collaborative Study of Cardiovascular Disease and Steroid Hormone Contraception. BMJ. 1999;318(7175):13–8.

62. Li H, Yu Y. Association between ischemic stroke and migraine in elderly Chinese: a case-control study. BMC Geriatr. 2013;13:126.

63. Spector JT, Kahn SR, Jones MR, Jayakumar M, Dalal D, Nazarian S. Migraine headache and ischemic stroke risk: an updated meta-analysis. Am J Med. 2010;123:612–24.

64. Schürks M, Rist PM, Bigal ME, Buring JE, Lipton RB, Kurth T. Migraine and cardiovascular disease: systematic review and meta-analysis. BMJ. 2009;339:b3914.

65. Etminan M, Takkouche B, Isorna FC, Samii A. Risk of ischaemic stroke in people with migraine: systematic review and meta-analysis of observational studies. BMJ. 2005;330(7482):63. [Review. Erratum in: BMJ. 2005 Mar 12;330(7491):596. BMJ. 2005 Feb 12;330(7487):345].

66. Monteith T, Gardener H, Rundek T, Dong C, Yoshita M, Elkind MS, DeCarli C, Sacco RL, Wright CB. Migraine, white matter hyperintensities, and subclinical brain infarction in a diverse community: the northern Manhattan study. Stroke. 2014;45(6):1830–2.

67. Bashir A, Lipton RB, Ashina S, Ashina M. Migraine and structural changes in the brain: a systematic review and meta-analysis. Neurology. 2013;81(14):1260–8.

68. Kruit MC, van Buchem MA, Hofman PA, et al. Migraine as a risk factor for subclinical brain lesions. JAMA. 2004;291:427–34.

69. Bigal ME, Lipton RB. Modifiable risk factors for migraine progression. Headache. 2006;46:1334–43.

70. Hall GC, Brown MM, Mo J, MacRae KD. Triptans in migraine: the risks of stroke, cardiovascular disease, and death in practice. Neurology. 2004;62:563–8.

71. Palm-Meinders IH, Koppen H, Terwindt GM, et al. Structural brain changes in migraine. JAMA. 2012;308:1889–97.

72. Kurth T, Diener HC. Current views of the risk of stroke for migraine with and migraine without aura. Curr Pain Headache Rep. 2006;10:214–20.

73. Martin AT, Pinney SM, Xie C, Herrick RL, Bai Y, Buckholz J, Martin VT. Headache disorders may be a risk factor for the development of new onset hypothyroidism. Headache. 2017;57:21–30.

74. Bigal ME, Sheftell FD, Rapoport AM, Tepper SJ, Lipton RB. Chronic daily headache: identification of factors associated with induction and transformation. Headache. 2002;42:575–81.

75. Moreau T, Manceau E, Giroud-Baleydier F, Dumas R, Giroud M. Headache in hypothyroidism. Prevalence and outcome under thyroid hormone therapy. Cephalalgia. 1998;18:687–9.

76. Sarchielli P, Alberti A, Baldi A, et al. Proinflammatory cytokines, adhesion molecules, and lymphocyte integrin expression in the internal jugular blood of migraine patients without aura assessed ictally. Headache. 2006;46:200–7.

77. Lateef T, Swanson S, Cui L, Nelson K, Nakamura E, Merikangas K. Headaches and sleep problems among adults in the United States: findings from the National Comorbidity Survey-Replication study. Cephalalgia. 2011;31:648–53.

78. Sadeghniiat K, Rajabzadeh A, Ghajarzadeh M, Ghafarpour M. Sleep quality and depression among patients with migraine. Acta Med Iran. 2013;51(11):784–8.

79. Kristiansen HA, Kværner KJ, Akre H, Øverland B, Russell MB. Migraine and sleep apnea in the general population. J Headache Pain. 2011;12:55–61.

80. Kelman L, Rains JC. Headache and sleep: examination of sleep patterns and complaints in a large clinical sample of migraineurs. Headache. 2005;45:904–10.

81. Nobre ME, Leal AJ, Filho PM. Investigation into sleep disturbance of patients suffering from cluster headache. Cephalalgia. 2005;25:488–92.

82. Rains JC, Poceta JS, Penzien DB. Sleep and headaches. Curr Neurol Neurosci Rep. 2008;8:167–75.

83. Bigal ME, Lipton RB. Obesity is a risk factor for transformed migraine but not chronic tension-type headache. Neurology. 2006;67:252–7.

84. Peterlin BL, Rosso AL, Rapoport AM, Scher AI. Obesity and migraine: the effect of age, gen-

der and adipose tissue distribution. Headache. 2010;50:52–62.

85. Bigal ME, Liberman JN, Lipton RB. Obesity and migraine: a population study. Neurology. 2006;66:545–50.

86. Bigal ME, Tsang A, Loder E, Serrano D, Reed ML, Lipton RB. Body mass index and episodic headaches: a population-based study. Arch Intern Med. 2007;167:1964–70.

87. Bond DS, Vithiananthan S, Nash JM, Thomas JG, Wing RR. Improvement of migraine headaches in severely obese patients after bariatric surgery. Neurology. 2011;76:1135–8.

88. Bigal ME, Lipton RB, Holland PR, Goadsby PJ. Obesity, migraine, and chronic migraine: possible mechanisms of interaction. Neurology. 2007;68:1851–61.

89. Gibson MM, Day JH. Allergic rhinitis. Can Fam Physician. 1982;28:1805–11.

90. Aamodt AH, Stovner LJ, Langhammer A, Hagen K, Zwart JA. Is headache related to asthma, hay fever, and chronic bronchitis? The Head-HUNT study. Headache. 2007;47:204–12.

91. Martin VT, Fanning KM, Serrano D, Buse DC, Reed ML, Bernstein JA, Lipton RB. Chronic rhinitis and its association with headache frequency and disability in persons with migraine: results of the American Migraine Prevalence and Prevention (AMPP) study. Cephalalgia. 2014;34(5):336–48.

92. Ku M, Silverman B, Prifti N, Ying W, Persaud Y, Schneider A. Prevalence of migraine headaches in patients with allergic rhinitis. Ann Allergy Asthma Immunol. 2006;97:226–30.

93. Davey G, Sedgwick P, Maier W, Visick G, Strachan DP, Anderson HR. Association between migraine and asthma: matched case-control study. Br J Gen Pract. 2002;52:723–7.

94. Karlstad O, Nafstad P, Tverdal A, Skurtveit S, Furu K. Comorbidities in an asthma population 8-29 years old: a study from the Norwegian Prescription Database. Pharmacoepidemiol Drug Saf. 2012;21:1045–52.

95. Fernández-de-Las-Peñas C, Hernández-Barrera V, Carrasco-Garrido P, et al. Population-based study of migraine in Spanish adults: relation to socio-demographic factors, lifestyle and co-morbidity with other conditions. J Headache Pain. 2010;11(2):97–104.

96. Le H, Tfelt-Hansen P, Russell MB, Skytthe A, Kyvik KO, Olesen J. Co-morbidity of migraine with somatic disease in a large population-based study. Cephalalgia. 2011;31:43–64.

97. Martin V, Fanning K, Buse D, Serrano D, Reed M, Lipton R. Asthma is a risk factor for the new onset chronic migraine: results from the American Migraine Prevalence and Prevention (AMPP) study. Headache. 2016;56(1):118–31.

98. Artico M, Cavallotti C. Catecholaminergic and acetylcholine esterase containing nerves of cranial and spinal dura mater in humans and rodents. Microsc Res Tech. 2001;53:212–20.

99. Markowitz S, Saito K, Moskowitz MA. Neurogenically mediated plasma extravasation in dura mater: effect of ergot alkaloids. A possible mechanism of action in vascular headache. Cephalalgia. 1988;8:83–91.

100. Small P, Kim H. Allergic rhinitis. Allergy Asthma Clin Immunol. 2011;7(Suppl 1):S3.

101. Ramadan NM, Silberstein SD, Freitag FG, Gilbert TT, Frishberg BM, Consortium UH. Evidence-based guidelines for migraine headache in the primary care setting: pharmacological management for prevention of migraine. 2000. http://www.aan.com/professionals/practice/pdfs/gl0090.pdf.

102. Sturtevant J. NSAID-induced bronchospasm—a common and serious problem. A report from MEDSAFE, the New Zealand Medicines and Medical Devices Safety Authority. N Z Dent J. 1999;95:84.

103. Cl L, Lin CC, Chen WH, Wang HC, Kao CH. Association between migraine and irritable bowel syndrome: a population-based retrospective cohort study. Eur J Neurol. 2014;21(9):1198–204.

104. Faresjö Å, Grodzinsky E, Hallert C, Timpka T. Patients with irritable bowel syndrome are more burdened by co-morbidity and worry about serious diseases than healthy controls—eight years follow-up of IBS patients in primary care. BMC Public Health. 2013;13:832.

105. Cole JA, Rothman KJ, Cabral HJ, Zhang Y, Farraye FA. Migraine, fibromyalgia, and depression among people with IBS: a prevalence study. BMC Gastroenterol. 2006;6:26.

106. Chang FY, Lu CL. Irritable bowel syndrome and migraine: bystanders or partners? J Neurogastroenterol Motil. 2013;19(3):301–11.

107. Park JW, Cho YS, Lee SY, Kim ES, Cho H, Shin HE, Suh GI, Choi MG. Concomitant functional gastrointestinal symptoms influence psychological status in Korean migraine patients. Gut Liver. 2013;7(6):668–74.

108. Gabrielli M, Cremonini F, Fiore G, Addolorato G, Padalino C, Candelli M, De Leo ME, Santarelli L, Giacovazzo M, Gasbarrini A, Pola P, Gasbarrini A. Association between migraine and Celiac disease: results from a preliminary case-control and therapeutic study. Am J Gastroenterol. 2003;98(3):625–9. [Erratum in: Am J Gastroenterol. 2003;98(7):1674].

109. Zelnik N, Pacht A, Obeid R, Lerner A. Range of neurologic disorders in patients with celiac disease. Pediatrics. 2004;113(6):1672–6.

110. Dimitrova AK, Ungaro RC, Lebwohl B, Lewis SK, Tennyson CA, Green MW, Babyatsky MW, Green PH. Prevalence of migraine in patients with celiac disease and inflammatory bowel disease. Headache. 2013;53(2):344–55.

111. Aurora SK, Kori SH, Barrodale P, SA MD, Haseley D. Gastric stasis in migraine: more than just a par-

oxysmal abnormality during a migraine attack. Headache. 2006;46(1):57–63.

112. Christensen CJ, Johnson WD, Abell TL. Patients with cyclic vomiting pattern and diabetic gastropathy have more migraines, abnormal electrogastrograms, and gastric emptying. Scand J Gastroenterol. 2008;43(9):1076–81.

113. van Hemert S, Breedveld AC, Rovers JM, Vermeiden JP, Witteman BJ, Smits MG, de Roos NM. Migraine associated with gastrointestinal disorders: review of the literature and clinical implications. Front Neurol. 2014;5:241.

114. Parkman HP. Migraine and gastroparesis from a gastroenterologist's perspective. Headache. 2013;53(Suppl 1):4–10.

115. Scher AI, Terwindt GM, Picavet HS, Verschuren WM, Ferrari MD, Launer LJ. Cardiovascular risk factors and migraine: the GEM population-based study. Neurology. 2005;64:614–20.

116. Bigal ME, Kurth T, Santanello N, et al. Migraine and cardiovascular disease: a population-based study. Neurology. 2010;74:628–35.

117. Mitchell P, Wang JJ, Currie J, Cumming RG, Smith W. Prevalence and vascular associations with migraine in older Australians. Aust N Z J Med. 1998;28(5):627–32.

118. Kurth T, Gaziano JM, Cook NR, Logroscino G, Diener HC, Buring JE. Migraine and risk of cardiovascular disease in women. JAMA. 2006;296(3):283–91. [Erratum in: JAMA. 2006 Aug 9;296(6):654. JAMA. 2006;296(3):1 p following 291].

119. Rose KM, Carson AP, Sanford CP, Stang PE, Brown CA, Folsom AR, Szklo M. Migraine and other headaches: associations with Rose angina and coronary heart disease. Neurology. 2004;63(12):2233–9.

120. Oterino A, Toriello M, Palacio E, Quintanilla VG, Ruiz-Lavilla N, Montes S, Vega MS, Martinez-Nieto R, Castillo J, Pascual J. Analysis of endothelial precursor cells in chronic migraine: a case-control study. Cephalalgia. 2013;33(4):236–44.

121. T K, Schürks M, Logroscino G, Gaziano JM, Buring JE. Migraine, vascular risk, and cardiovascular events in women: prospective cohort study. BMJ. 2008;337:a636.

122. Roberto G, Raschi E, Piccinni C, et al. Adverse cardiovascular events associated with triptans and ergotamines for treatment of migraine: systematic review of observational studies. Cephalalgia. 2015;35(2):118–31.

123. Thorpe KE. Prevalence, health care spending and comorbidities associated with chronic migraine patients. The Headache & Migraine Policy Forum. 2017. Accessed 14 Feb 2017. https://www.headachemigraineforum.org/resources?category=Policy+Papers.

Neurostimulation in the Management of Chronic Migraine

25

Derrick Alan Shumate and Frederick G. Freitag

Introduction

There are effective and tolerable acute and preventive management strategies for migraine and chronic migraine. Many patients benefit from non-pharmacologic strategies such as biofeedback and cognitive behavioral therapy. In tertiary headache centers, the use of both pharmacological and non-pharmacological interventions is commonplace. Therapies such as onabotulinumtoxinA injections [1, 2] and topiramate [3, 4] have been shown to be effective for the management of chronic migraine along with other therapies including tricyclic antidepressants and beta-blockers; however, patient preference, lack of response, and intolerance often preclude the use of established pharmacotherapies. Among the potential non-pharmacologic treatments for chronic migraine, there is developing substantial interest in the role of neurostimulation.

The term "neurostimulation" encompasses a variety of treatments, utilizing both invasive and noninvasive methods. They are used in the management of a diverse group of both painful and non-painful neurological and psychiatric conditions. Deep brain stimulation techniques have been employed in the management of various movement disorders including Parkinson's disease [5], essential tremor [6, 7], medically refractory dystonia [8], and Tourette syndrome [9, 10]. Posterior hypothalamic deep brain stimulation has been examined as a potential treatment for refractory cluster headaches, chronic paroxysmal hemicranias, and intractable short-lasting unilateral neuralgiform headache with conjunctival injection and tearing [11–15]. More recently, the ventral tegmentum has been considered a potential site for stimulation in cluster headache [16]. Implantable vagus nerve stimulation has been shown to be effective in the management of epilepsy [17–20], depression [21–23], and headache and other pain disorders [24–26].

We will discuss noninvasive vagal nerve stimulation in the management of migraine later in this chapter. Neuromodulation is being employed as potential therapies in several headache disorders. We examine in this chapter specific stimulation modalities for the treatment of migraine including occipital nerve stimulation (ONS), single-pulse transcranial magnetic stimulation (sTMS), repetitive-pulse transcranial magnetic stimulation, transcranial direct current stimulation (tDCS), transcutaneous supraorbital nerve stimulation, transcutaneous vagal nerve stimulation (VNS), and sphenopalatine ganglion stimulation.

D. A. Shumate · F. G. Freitag (✉)
Neurology, Medical College of Wisconsin,
Milwaukee, WI, USA
e-mail: ffreitag@mcw.edu

Implantable Occipital Nerve Stimulation

The basis for the utilization of percutaneous occipital nerve stimulation in the management of migraine has its roots in the work of Weiner and Reed who proposed ONS might be an effective means by which to manage intractable occipital neuralgia [27]; however, after review of the cases from the study and resultant diagnostic scrutiny, functional neuroimaging was recommended and performed. Eight of the 13 patients underwent positron emission tomography (PET) with findings consistent with those changes seen in migraine [28]. There were significant changes in regional cerebral blood flow (rCBF) in the dorsal rostral pons, anterior cingulate cortex (ACC), cuneus, and left pulvinar, correlating to pain and stimulation-induced paresthesia scores. The activation pattern in the dorsal rostral pons is the same as that seen in chronic migraine.

Early case series [29] showed a reduction in headache days from 75.6 to 38.1 for a 90-day period and an improvement of 88.7% in the Migraine Disability Assessment (MIDAS) scores with implanted peripheral nerve stimulation at C1 through C3. Open-label studies by Dodick et al. [30] and Schwedt et al. [31] suggested implanted occipital nerve stimulation may be an effective tool for the management of chronic migraine showing significant improvement across multiple efficacy measures including headache frequency, pain intensity, MIDAS scores, and Headache Impact Test-6 (HIT-6) and Beck Depression Inventory-II (BDI-II) scores.

One hundred and thirty-two patients who suffered from chronic migraine were enrolled in the Precision Implantable Stimulator for Migraine, or PRISM, study [32] in which a 12-week blinding phase was then followed by an open treatment phase. Implantation was pursued if the preceding 5–10-day stimulation trial with external leads was successful at alleviating pain. The reduction in headache days per month was not statistically significant at 12-week follow-up; however, there appeared to be a trend toward more benefit in those patients without medication overuse versus those who had been overusing

medications with reductions of −5.9 vs. −2.6 and − 5.9 vs. −4.8, respectively.

In the ONSTIM feasibility study [33], patients with chronic migraine who experienced at least a 50% reduction in headache within 24 h of a greater occipital nerve block were randomized to receive one of three treatments: adjustable implanted occipital nerve stimulation, preset stimulation, or medical management. Multiple efficacy measures were evaluated at 3 months, including reduction in headache days per month and decrease in overall pain intensity compared to baseline values. The percent reduction in headache days per month was 27.0 ± 44.8% for the adjustable stimulation group, 8.8 ± 28.6% for the preset stimulation group, and 4.4 ± 19.1% for the medical management group. The reduction in headache intensity was 1.5 ± 1.6 for the adjustable stimulation group, 0.5 ± 1.3 for the preset stimulation groups, and 0.6 ± 1.0 for the medical management group. However, analysis showed no statistically significant improvement in the adjustable stimulation group over baseline when compared to the preset stimulation and medical management groups. Lead migration was the most common adverse event and occurred in 12 of 51, or 24%, of patients. Incision site complications were another adverse event reported in 4% of patients.

In the St. Jude study [34], Silberstein et al. randomized 57 patients in a 2:1 manner to either active occipital nerve stimulation or sham protocol. Patients underwent implantation if they experienced at least a 50% reduction in pain or paresthesia in the area of pain during a trial phase. The primary endpoint was defined as the difference in the percentage of responders who achieved a ≥ 50% reduction in daily visual analog pain scale scores. The active ONS group demonstrated a 17.1% reduction versus 13.5% with sham protocol, which was not statistically significant; however, differences between the two groups in 40%, 30%, and 20% reduction were significant. There was a significant difference in reduction of number of headache days, reduction in MIDAS scores, and patient reports of pain relief. Persistent implant site pain was the most commonly reported device-related adverse event.

Dodick et al. [35] conducted a multicenter, double-blinded, sham-controlled study of the effectiveness of ONS that included analyses of 125 patients with intractable chronic migraine as well as an intent-to-treat (ITT) population of 157 patients after a 2-week blind period followed by a 50-week open period. The number of headache days was significantly reduced by 7.7 (±8.7) days in the intractable chronic migraine group and reduced by 6.7 (±8.4) days in the intent-to-treat group. Reduction in headache intensity, MIDAS scores, and Pain and Distress (PAD) scores and direct patient reports of improvement in quality of life and pain relief were also significantly improved. Adverse events were common and reported by 70.7% of patients. Two hundred and nine adverse events were reported in total. Among them were 38 cases of persistent pain or numbness, 5 wound site complications, 11 infections, 8 battery failures, 29 lead migrations, and 7 lead breakages or lead fractures.

The reduction in pain intensity and attack frequency seen in some patients may be attributable to activation of central pain modulation centers similar to that seen on FDG-PET results of patients with cluster headache that have undergone peripheral occipital nerve stimulation [36]. All patients compared with controls in the trials demonstrated several areas of hypermetabolism including the ipsilateral hypothalamus, midbrain, and ipsilateral lower pons. After ONS all areas normalized except for the hypothalamus. The perigenual anterior cingulate cortex (PACC) was hyperactive in ONS responders compared to non-responders. ONS may also provide pain relief via modulation of the trigeminocervical complex as trigeminal nociceptive fibers are in proximity to, and intertwined with, those from the C2 level [37, 38]. Implanted occipital nerve stimulation will likely maintain a limited role in the management of refractory chronic migraine as implantation and device-related adverse effects are common [33, 35] and insurance coverage is uncommon.

Of note, two smaller unblinded studies by Reed et al. and Hann [39, 40] have suggested that combined implanted supraorbital nerve and occipital nerve stimulation may benefit those suffering from chronic migraine; however, adverse events were common with 42.8% reporting lead migraine and 14.2% infection in the latter study.

Transcutaneous Supraorbital Nerve Stimulation

Transcutaneous supraorbital nerve stimulation may be effective for the prevention of migraine. In a study of 67 migraine patients, Schoenen et al. [41] observed a greater reduction in migraine days per month, from 6.9 to 4.8, in the group treated with 20 min of stimulation daily for 1 month with Cefaly®, a novel transcutaneous supraorbital nerve stimulation device, versus sham in which migraine days were reduced from 6.5 to 6.2 days. Post hoc statistical analysis of data from the aforementioned study [41] suggested that those patients who suffered from more migraine attacks at baseline may have experienced a greater reduction in migraine days [42]. The patient satisfaction rate, among a population of both episodic migraine and chronic migraine sufferers, was 54% [43]. This may suggest a greater role for such technology in chronic than episodic migraine, but to date, there are no studies to support such a supposition.

It is hypothesized that transcutaneous supraorbital nerve stimulation, as with occipital nerve stimulation, likely owes its beneficial effects in migraine to modulation of central pain centers. It appears to be well tolerated and effective in migraine prophylaxis with a possible tendency toward greater benefit in those suffering from more frequent headache attacks. Additional translational and controlled clinical studies, specifically in the chronic migraine population, could be revealing.

Transcranial Stimulation Methods

The effects of TMS can be divided into two types depending on the mode of stimulation: a single- or paired-pulse TMS. sTMS causes neurons in the neocortex under the site of stimulation to depolarize and discharge an action potential. If used in the primary motor cortex, it produces muscle activity, referred to as a motor evoked potential (MEP), which can be recorded on electromyography. If used on the occipital cortex, "phosphenes" (flashes of light) might be perceived by the subject. In most other areas of the cortex, the participant does not consciously experience any effect, but his or her behavior may be slightly altered (e.g., slower reaction time on a cognitive task), or changes in brain activity may be detected using sensing equipment.

Repetitive TMS (rTMS) produces longer-lasting effects, which persist past the initial period of stimulation. rTMS can increase or decrease the excitability of the corticospinal tract depending on the intensity of stimulation, coil orientation, and frequency. The mechanism of these effects is not clear, though it is widely believed to reflect changes in synaptic efficacy akin to long-term potentiation (LTP) and long-term depression (LTD).

The transcranial stimulation techniques, including single-pulse transcranial magnetic stimulation, repetitive-pulse transcranial magnetic stimulation, and transcranial direct current stimulation, likely influence migraine through normalization of cortical hyper-reactivity which is thought to be present in migraine sufferers as evidenced by defective habituation [44–46] across multiple sensory modalities [47], including nociceptive inputs [48], observed in multiple evoked potentials studies of patients with migraine. Repetitive-pulse transcranial magnetic stimulation may also reduce migraine attack frequency through the upregulation of inhibitory input, thereby restoring habituation [44]. In the following section, we will discuss recent clinical data pertaining to, and possible utility of, the various methods.

Repetitive-Pulse Transcranial Magnetic Stimulation

Brighina et al. [49] examined the potential effectiveness of daily high-frequency repetitive transcranial magnetic stimulation for the prevention of both episodic migraine and chronic migraine. Stimulation was delivered over the left dorsolateral prefrontal cortex. Six chronic migraine patients were randomized to receive active TMS, and another six were randomized to sham protocol. Migraine attack frequency was reduced by 53% in the active treatment group and by 7% with sham. In a randomized, double-blind, sham-controlled study of 100 patients, 60 of whom suffered from chronic migraine. Misra et al. [50] observed a 78.7% reduction in headache frequency in those patients who received three treatments of high frequency over the left frontal cortex on alternating days versus a 33.3% reduction with sham protocol. Headache severity was also reduced with active versus sham treatment by 76.6% versus 27.1%, respectively. All patients reported some discomfort related to TMS, but no serious adverse events were reported. Conversely, in a small study, Conforto et al. [51] randomized seven chronic migraine patients to receive 23 sessions of rTMS over the left dorsolateral prefrontal cortex and found active TMS to be less effective than sham.

Single-Pulse Transcranial Magnetic Stimulation

Clark et al. [52] conducted an open-label study, which examined the tolerability and efficacy of single-pulse transcranial magnetic stimulation for the acute management of migraine in 41 patients suffering from migraine without aura, migraine with aura, and probable migraine. One to three trials of two pulses were applied over the area of perceived pain in those patients with migraine without aura and over the visual cortex in patients who suffered from migraine with aura. Reduction in pain intensity was used as the primary outcome measure and was reduced by 75% for up to 20 min poststimulation. Thirty-two percent of subjects reported no headache recurrence for up to 24 h after one treatment. Additional treatments appeared to convey benefit as 24-h headache freedom was observed in 29% of those who received two treatments and 40% of those who received three treatments. This particular TMS paradigm appeared to be well tolerated without any serious adverse events. Dizziness, drowsiness, and feeling tired were reported.

Lipton et al. [53] conducted a randomized, double-blind, sham-controlled study of the effects of single-pulse transcranial magnetic stimulation in which 164 patients who suffered from migraine with aura used a portable device to administer either a single magnetic field pulse or sham treatment over the area of the visual cortex without 1 h of aura onset. Patients treated up to three attacks of migraine with aura over a 3-month span. Pain freedom at 2 h was the primary outcome measure and was observed in 39% of those who received active TMS versus 22% in the sham group. Sustained headache freedom at 24 and 48 h were secondary outcome measures and were both superior with active treatment versus sham protocol at 29% versus 16% and 27% versus 13%, respectively.

In their open-label study, Bhola et al. [54] examined the effectiveness of single-pulse magnetic transcranial stimulation delivered via the portable Spring® TMS device for the acute treatment of migraine. One hundred and ninety patients, including 59 with either migraine without aura or migraine with aura and 131 with chronic migraine who had found previous acute pharmacotherapies ineffective, intolerable, or medically contraindicated, participated in the study. Patients were instructed to treat individual migraine attacks with 2 consecutive pulses followed by additional "as needed" pulses at 15-min intervals to a maximum of either 16 single pulses or 8 double pulses. There was no limit on the number of attacks treated or the days of utilization. The specific stimulation parameters mirrored those in the study by Lipton et al. [53]. Fifty-nine percent of patients reported a reduction in migraine days after 12 weeks. Sixty-two percent reported reduced or alleviated pain with stimulation.

potential treatment for migraine. Antal et al. [55] conducted a randomized, sham-controlled trial of 26 patients with migraine with aura (14) and migraine without aura (12). Attack frequency and attack duration were not significantly reduced in either the real stimulation or sham protocol group. Similarly, Rocha et al. [56] did not observe a reduction in migraine frequency, intensity, or duration in their randomized, sham-controlled trial in which patients received 12 20-min cathodal stimulation sessions over the visual cortex.

Conversely, Dasilva et al. [57] examined the potential effectiveness of anodal stimulation over the contralateral motor cortex and cathodal stimulation over the contralateral orbitofrontal area of 13 chronic migraine patients with some promising results. Ten 20-min sessions of 2 mA stimulation were administered over a 4-week span in the active group, whereas those patients in the sham protocol also received 2 mA stimulation but only for 30 s. Improvements in both headache duration and pain intensity were observed in the active tDCS group.

In a randomized, sham-controlled study, Auvichayapat et al. [58] observed a statistically significant reduction in migraine frequency, intensity, and the number of acute medications utilized in 37 patients with episodic migraine who administered either active anodal tDCS treatment or sham therapy over the motor cortex for 20 min daily for 20 days consecutively. Treatment was well tolerated without any reported serious adverse events.

Repetitive transcranial magnetic stimulation may prevent migraine attacks; however, the availability and portability of the delivery system may be prohibitive. Single-pulse transcranial magnetic stimulation, such as with the Spring® TMS device, may have a role in both acute and preventive treatment of migraine and is portable.

Transcranial Direct Current Stimulation

Transcranial direct current stimulation is thought to potentially provide relief from migraine by normalization of cortical hypersensitivity. Cathodal transcranial direct current stimulation which is inhibitory has also been studied as a

Transcutaneous Vagus Nerve Stimulation

As mentioned earlier in this chapter, vagus nerve stimulation has been utilized in the management of epilepsy and depression for several years. The complete mechanism by which vagal nerve stimulation may acutely abort or prevent migraine attacks has not been elucidated. VNS may in part owe its therapeutic effect to its synapses within the trigeminal nucleus caudalis and the ability to inhibit glutamate release from within this structure [59], thereby potentially limiting propagation of pain messaging.

One small case series demonstrated the potential benefit of implantable vagus nerve stimulation in six patients with either refractory chronic cluster or migraine [60]. Nesbitt et al. [61] utilized a portable noninvasive VNS device for both the acute management and prevention of headache attacks in eight patients with episodic cluster headache and 11 patients with chronic cluster headache. Forty-seven percent of attacks were aborted within an average of 11 ± 1 min initiating treatment. The average attack frequency was reduced from 4.5 per 24 h to 2.6 per 24 h. Gaul et al. [62] conducted a prospective, randomized, controlled study (PREVA study) of adjunctive transcutaneous vagus nerve stimulation versus standard-of-care treatment alone in 114 chronic cluster headache sufferers and found that the number of attacks per week was significantly reduced in the adjunctive vagus nerve stimulation group versus standard-of-care treatment alone at −5.9 vs. −2.1 attacks/week, respectively. Patients also experienced improvement in quality of life measures and a reduction in the use of abortive pharmacotherapies.

In an open-label study by Goadsby et al. [63], 30 patients with either migraine without aura or migraine with aura utilized transcutaneous vagus nerve stimulation for the acute management of migraine. Stimulation was delivered in two 90-s bursts to the right vagus nerve. Thirty-eight percent of patients with attacks of mild severity and 22% of patients with moderate-to-severe pain experienced pain freedom at 2 h. Barbanti et al. [64] conducted another open-label study of transcutaneous vagus nerve stimulation for the acute management of high-frequency migraine and chronic migraine. 56.3% of patients in the active VNS group experienced pain relief at 1 h, 64.6% had pain relief at 2 h, and 35.4% and 39.6% were pain-free at 1 and 2 h, respectively. Two-hour pain relief and

pain freedom were lower in the chronic migraine group versus high-frequency migraine.

Silberstein et al. [65] conducted a randomized, sham-controlled study of noninvasive vagus nerve stimulation in 59 patients suffering from chronic migraine with a mean headache frequency of 21.5 days per month. Patients administered three stimulation sessions daily in which they received two 90-s bursts of stimulation to the right vagus nerve. At 2 months, the average reduction in headache days per month was −1.4 in the active VNS group versus −0.2 days with sham protocol. Fifteen patients randomized to active treatment completed an 8-month open-label period with a significant reduction in headache days of −7.9 per month from baseline. Similarly, efficacy improved over time in studies of VNS in depression and epilepsy [66, 67]. Adverse effects were similar between groups.

Sphenopalatine Nerve Stimulation

Sympathetic hypoactivity and parasympathetic activation are cardinal features of some primary headache disorders including cluster headache and the trigeminal autonomic cephalalgias, but increased parasympathetic activity may also be observed during the ictus of a migraine attack. This is likely due to the presence of parasympathetic efferents, originating in the superior salivatory nucleus, projecting from the sphenopalatine ganglion (SPG) to the meningeal blood vasculature, lacrimal gland, and nasal mucosa. Activation along this pathway may result in the propagation of neurogenic inflammation and ultimately headache through the release of vasoactive peptides [68, 69].

Various SPG blockade methods have been shown to be potentially effective at aborting cluster headache attacks including application of 4% lidocaine intranasal droplets [70], 4% lidocaine intranasal spray [71], intranasal application of cocaine or lidocaine using a cotton-tipped applicator [72, 73], and supra-zygomatic SPG blockade with alcohol [74]. Case series as well as prospective and retrospective studies have also suggested that patients with refractory cluster headache may benefit from radiofrequency abla- tion of the sphenopalatine ganglion [75–80]. Migraine has also been a potential target of SPG blockade using intranasal lidocaine [81–83] with relatively rapid onset of relief.

In a randomized, double-blind, placebo- controlled trial, Cady et al. [84] demonstrated the potential effectiveness of SPG blockade in the management of acute headache attacks in patients suffering from chronic migraine utilizing 0.3 ml of 0.5% bupivacaine delivered via the Tx360® device. The active treatment group demonstrated statistically significant reduction pain scores at 15 min, 30 min, and 24 h versus placebo (saline).

In a small open-label study of 11 patients with either episodic or chronic migraine, Tepper et al. [85] sought to determine if electrical stimulation of the SPG could abate an intractable migraine attack. Ten patients underwent stimulation. Two patients achieved pain freedom, three reported pain reduction, and five denied any change in headache severity.

Conclusion

Chronic migraine is prevalent, frequently dis- abling, and often challenging to manage despite the utilization of a multifaceted approach consisting of both pharmacologic treatments and non-pharmacological interven- tions. The emergence of new neurostimulation methods provides multiple potential treatment opportunities for both the acute and prophy- lactic management of chronic migraine and is employed in those scenarios in which pharma- cotherapies have been poorly tolerated or inef- fective or patient preference dictates the use of non-pharmacologic treatment.

Implantable occipital nerve stimulation may be effective; however, it will likely main- tain a limited role in the management of refractory chronic migraine as implantation and device-related adverse effects are com- mon and insurance coverage is uncommon. Transcutaneous supraorbital nerve stimulation appears to be well tolerated and effective in migraine prophylaxis with a possible tendency toward greater benefit in those suffering from more frequent headache attacks; however,

additional translational and controlled clinical studies, specifically in the chronic migraine population, are needed to confirm.

Transcranial magnetic stimulation methods may prevent migraine through normalization of cortical hyper-reactivity, which is thought to be present in migraine sufferer, and by upregulation of inhibitory input. Repetitive transcranial magnetic stimulation is possibly efficacious for the prevention of migraine attacks; however, the availability and portabil- ity of the delivery system may prohibit wide- spread utilization at this time. Single-pulse transcranial magnetic stimulation may have a role in both acute and preventive treatment of migraine and is portable.

Sphenopalatine ganglion blockade meth- ods have been shown to possibly be effective for the management of both cluster headache and migraine; however, SPG neurostimulation trials in chronic migraine are limited and include one small open-label study. Additional studies are needed.

References

1. Dodick DW, Turkel CC, DeGryse RE, Aurora SK, Silberstein SD, Lipton RB, et al. OnabotulinumtoxinA for treatment of chronic migraine: pooled results from the double-blind, randomized, placebo-controlled phases of the PREEMPT clinical program. Headache. 2010;50(6):921–36.
2. Diener HC, Dodick DW, Aurora SK, Turkel CC, DeGryse RE, Lipton RB, et al. OnabotulinumtoxinA for treatment of chronic migraine: results from the double-blind, randomized, placebo-controlled phase of the PREEMPT 2 trial. Cephalalgia. 2010;30(7):804–14.
3. Silberstein SD, Lipton RB, Dodick DW, Freitag FG, Ramadan N, Mathew N, et al. Efficacy and safety of topiramate for the treatment of chronic migraine: a randomized, double-blind, placebo-controlled trial. Headache. 2007;47(2):170–80.
4. Diener HC, Bussone G, Van Oene JC, Lahaye M, Schwalen S, Goadsby PJ, et al. Topiramate reduces headache days in chronic migraine: a randomized, double-blind, placebo-controlled study. Cephalalgia. 2007;27(7):814–23.
5. Okum MS. Deep-brain stimulation for Parkinson's disease. New Engl J Med. 2012;367(16):1529–38.
6. Peng-Chen Z, et al. Unilateral thalamic deep brain stimulation in essential tremor demonstrates long-term

ipsilateral effects. Parkinsonism Relat Disord. 2013; 19:1113–7.

7. Pahwa R, et al. Long-term evaluation of deep brain stimulation of the thalamus. J Neurosurg. 2006;104(4):506–12.

8. Vadailhet M, Jutras MF, Grabli D, Roze E. Deep brain stimulation for dystonia. J Neurol Neurosurg Psychiatry. 2013;84(9):1029–42.

9. Vandewalle V, van der Linden C, Groenewegen J, Caemaert J. Stereotactic treatment of Gilles de la Tourette syndrome by high frequency stimulation of thalamus. Lancet. 1999;353(9154):724.

10. Schrock LE, et al. Tourette syndrome deep brain stimulation: a review and updated recommendations. Mov Discord. 2014;30(4):448–71.

11. Leone M, Franzini A, Bussone G. Stereotactic stimulation of posterior hypothalamic gray matter for intractable cluster headache. NEJM. 2001;345(19):1428–9.

12. Fontaine D, Lazorthes Y, Mertens P, Blond S, Géraud G, Fabre N, et al. Safety and efficacy of deep brain stimulation in refractory cluster headache: a randomized placebo-controlled double-blind trial followed by a 1-year open extension. J Headache Pain. 2010;11:23–31.

13. Walcott BP, Bamber NI, Anderson DE. Successful treatment of chronic paroxysmal hemicrania with posterior hypothalamic stimulation: technical case report. Neurosurgery. 2009;65:E997.

14. Bartsch T, Falk D, Knudsen K. Deep brain stimulation of the posterior hypothalamic area in intractable short-lasting unilateral neuralgiform headache with conjunctival injection and tearing (SUNCT). Cephalalgia. 2011;31:1405–8.

15. Lyons MK, Dodick DW, Evidente VG. Responsiveness of short-lasting unilateral neuralgiform headache with conjunctival injection and tearing to hypothalamic deep brain stimulation. J Neurosurg. 2009;110:279–81.

16. Akram H, Miller S, Lagrata S, Hyam J, Jahanshahi M, Hariz M, et al. Ventral tegmental area deep brain stimulation for refractory chronic cluster headache. Neurology. 2016;86(18):1676–82.

17. Ben-Menachem E, Mañon-Espaillat R, Ristanovic R, Wilder BJ, Stefan H, Mirza W, Tarver WB, Wernicke JF. Vagus nerve stimulation for treatment of partial seizures: a controlled study of effect on seizures. First International Vagus Nerve Stimulation Study Group. Epilepsia. 1994;35(3):616–26.

18. George R, Salinsky M, Kuzniecky R, Rosenfeld W, Bergen D, Tarver WB, Wernicke JF. Vagus nerve stimulation for treatment of partial seizures: 3. Long-term follow-up on first 67 patients exiting a controlled study. First International Vagus Nerve Stimulation Study Group. Epilepsia. 1994;35(3):637–43.

19. Handforth A, DeGiorgio CM, Schachter SC, Uthman BM, Naritoku DK, Tecoma ES, Henry TR, Collins SD, Vaughn BV, Gilmartin RC, Labar DR, Morris GL 3rd, Salinsky MC, Osorio I, Ristanovic RK, Labiner DM, Jones JC, Murphy JV, Ney GC, Wheless JW. Vagus nerve stimulation therapy for partial-onset seizures: a randomized active-control trial. Neurology. 1998;51(1):48–55.

20. CM DG, Schachter SC, Handforth A, Salinsky M, Thompson J, Uthman B, Reed R, Collins S, Tecoma E, Morris GL, Vaughn B, Naritoku DK, Henry T, Labar D, Gilmartin R, Labiner D, Osorio I, Ristanovic R, Jones J, Murphy J, Ney G, Wheless J, Lewis P, Heck C. Prospective long-term study of vagus nerve stimulation for the treatment of refractory seizures. Epilepsia. 2000;41(9):1195–200.

21. Cimpianu CL, Strube W, Falkai P, Palm U, Hasan A. Vagus nerve stimulation in psychiatry: a systematic review of the available evidence. J Neural Transm (Vienna). 2017;124(1):145–58.

22. Eljamel S. Vagus nerve stimulation for major depressive episodes. Prog Neurol Surg. 2015;29:53–63.

23. Tronnier VM. Vagus nerve stimulation: surgical technique and complications. Prog Neurol Surg. 2015;29:29–38.

24. Chakravarthy K, Chaudhry H, Williams K, Christo PJ. Review of the uses of vagal nerve stimulation in chronic pain management. Curr Pain Headache Rep. 2015;19(12):54.

25. Ben-Menachem E, Revesz D, Simon BJ, Silberstein S. Surgically implanted and non-invasive vagus nerve stimulation: a review of efficacy, safety and tolerability. Eur J Neurol. 2015;22(9):1260–8.

26. Multon S, Schoenen J. Pain control by vagus nerve stimulation: from animal to man...and back. Acta Neurol Belg. 2005;105(2):62–7.

27. Weiner RL, Reed KL. Peripheral neurostimulation for control of intractable occipital neuralgia. Neuromodulation. 1999;2:217–22.

28. Matharu MS, Bartsch T, Ward N, Frackowiak RSJ, Weiner RL, Goadsby PJ. Central neuromodulation in chronic migraine patients with suboccipital stimulators: a PET study. Brain. 2004;127:220–30.

29. Popeney CA, Alo KM. Peripheral neurostimulation for the treatment of chronic, disabling transformed migraine. Headache. 2003;43:369–75.

30. Dodick DW, Trentman T, Zimmerman R, Eross EJ. Occipital nerve stimulation for intractable chronic primary headache disorders. Cephalalgia. 2003;23:701.

31. Schwedt TJ, Dodick DW, Hentz J, Trentman TL, Zimmerman RS. Occipital nerve stimulation for chronic headache—long-term safety and efficacy. Cephalalgia. 2007;27:153–7.

32. Lipton R, Goadsby P, Cady R, Aurora S, Grosberg B, Freitag F, et al. PRISM study: occipital nerve stimulation for treatment-refractory migraine. Cephalalgia. 2009;29(suppl 1):30.

33. Joel R, Saper JR, Dodick DW, Silberstein SD, McCarville S, Mark Sun M, Goadsby PJ. Occipital nerve stimulation for the treatment of intractable chronic migraine headache: ONSTIM feasibility study. Cephalalgia. 2011;31(3):271–85.

34. Silberstein SD, Dodick DW, Saper J, Huh B, Slavin KV, Sharan A, et al. Safety and efficacy of peripheral nerve stimulation of the occipital nerves for the man-

agement of chronic migraine: results from a randomized, multicenter, double-blinded, controlled study. Cephalalgia. 2012;32(6):1165–79.

35. Dodick DW, Silberstein SD, Reed KL, Deer TR, Slavin KV, Huh B, et al. Safety and efficacy of peripheral nerve stimulation of the occipital nerves for the management of chronic migraine: long-term results from a randomized, multicenter, double-blinded, controlled study. Cephalalgia. 2015;35(4):344–58.

36. Magis D, Bruno MA, Fumal A, Gerardy PY, Hustinx R, Laureys S, Schoenen J. Central modulation in cluster headache patients treated with occipital nerve stimulation: an FDG-PET study. BMC Neurol. 2011;11:25.

37. Goadsby PJ, Hargreaves R. Refractory migraine and chronic migraine: pathophysiological mechanisms. Headache. 2008;48:799–804.

38. Bartsch T, Goadsby PJ. Anatomy and physiology of pain referral in primary and cervicogenic headache disorders. Headache Curr. 2005;2:42–8.

39. Reed K, Black S, Banta C, Will K. Combined occipital and supraorbital neurostimulation for the treatment of chronic migraine headaches: initial experience. Cephalalgia. 2009;30(3):260–71.

40. Hann S, Sharan A. Dual occipital and supraorbital nerve stimulation for chronic migraine: a single-center experience, review of literature, and surgical considerations. Neurosurg Focus. 2013;35(3):E9.

41. Schoenen J, Vandermissen B, Jeangette S, et al. Migraine prevention with a supraorbital transcutaneous stimulator: a randomized controlled trial. Neurology. 2013;80:697–704.

42. Schoenen J. Addendum to migraine prevention with a supraorbital transcutaneous stimulator: a randomized controlled trial. Neurology. 2015;86:2–3.

43. Magis D, Sava S, d'Elia TS, Baschi R, Schoenen J. Safety and patients' satisfaction of transcutaneous supraorbital neurostimulation (tSNS) with the Cefaly® device in headache treatment: a survey of 2,313 headache sufferers in the general population. J Headache Pain. 2013;14(1):1.

44. Brighina F, Palermo A, Fierro B. Cortical inhibition and habituation to evoked potentials: relevance for pathophysiology of migraine. J Headache Pain. 2009;10(2):77–84.

45. Schoenen J, Wang W, Albert A, Delwaide PJ. Potentiation instead of habituation characterizes visual evoked potentials in migraine patients between attacks. Eur J Neurol. 1995;2:115–22.

46. Schoenen J. Neurophysiological features of the migrainous brain. Neurol Sci. 2006;27(suppl 2):S77–81.

47. Coppola G, Pierelli F, Schoenen J. Habituation and migraine. Neurobiol Learn Mem. 2009;92(2):249–59.

48. de Tommaso M. Laser-evoked potentials in primary headaches and cranial neuralgias. Expert Rev Neurother. 2008;8:1339–45.

49. Brighina F, Piazza A, Vitello G, et al. rTMS of the prefrontal cortex in the treatment of chronic migraine: a pilot study. J Neurol Sci. 2004;227:67–71.

50. Misra U, Kalita J, Bhoi S. High-rate repetitive transcranial magnetic stimulation in migraine prophylaxis: a randomized, placebo-controlled study. J Neurol. 2013;260:2793–801.

51. Conforto A, Amaro E, Gonçalves A. Randomized, proof-of-principle clinical trial of active transcranial magnetic stimulation in chronic migraine. Cephalalgia. 2014;34:464–72.

52. Clark B, Upton A, Kamath M, et al. Transcranial magnetic stimulation for migraine: clinical effects. J Headache Pain. 2006;341–6.

53. Lipton R, Dodick D, Silberstein S, et al. Single-pulse transcranial magnetic stimulation for acute treatment of migraine with aura: a randomized, double-blind, parallel-group, sham-controlled trial. Lancet Neurol. 2010;9:373–80.

54. Bhola R, Kinsella E, Giffin N, et al. Single-pulse transcranial magnetic stimulation (sTMS) for the acute management of migraine: evaluation of outcome data for the UK post market pilot program. J Headache Pain. 2015;16:535.

55. Antal A, Kriener N, Lang N, et al. Cathodal transcranial direct current stimulation of the visual cortex in the prophylactic treatment of migraine. Cephalalgia. 2011;31:820–9.

56. Rocha S, Melo L, Boudoux C, et al. Transcranial direct current stimulation in the prophylactic treatment of migraine based on interictal visual cortex excitability abnormalities: a pilot randomized controlled trial. J Neurol Sci. 2015;349:33–9.

57. Dasilva A, Mendonca M, Zaghi S, et al. tDCS-induced analgesia and electrical fields in pain-related neural networks in chronic migraine. Headache. 2012;52:1283–95.

58. Auvichayapat P, Janyacharoen T, Rotenberg A, et al. Migraine prophylaxis by anodal transcranial direct current stimulation, a randomized, placebo-controlled trial. J Med Assoc Thail. 2012;95:1003–12.

59. Oshinsky ML, Murphy AL, Hekierski H, Cooper M, Simon BJ. Noninvasive vagus nerve stimulation as treatment for trigeminal allodynia. Pain. 2014;155(5):1037–42.

60. Mauskop A. Vagus nerve stimulation relieves chronic refractory migraine and cluster headaches. Cephalalgia. 2005;25(2):82–6.

61. Nesbitt A, Marin J, Tompkins E, Rutteledge M, Goadsby P. Initial use of a novel noninvasive vagus nerve stimulator for cluster headache treatment. Neurology. 2015;84:5–1.

62. Gaul C, Diener HC, Silver N, et al. Non-invasive vagus nerve stimulation for PREVention and Acute treatment of chronic cluster headaches (PREVA): a randomized controlled study. Cephalalgia. 2016;26:534–46.

63. Goadsby P, Grosberg B, Mauskop A, et al. Effect of noninvasive vagus nerve stimulation on acute migraine: an open-label pilot study. Cephalalgia. 2014;34:986–93.

64. Barbanti P, Grazzi L, Egeo O, et al. Non-invasive vagus nerve stimulation for acute treatment of high-frequency and chronic migraine: an open-label study. J Headache Pain. 2015;16:542.

65. Silberstein SD, Calhoun AH, Lipton RB, Grosberg BM, Cady RK, Dorlas S, et al. Chronic migraine headache prevention with noninvasive vagus nerve stimulation: the EVENT study. Neurology. 2016;87(5):529–38.
66. Murphy JV. Left vagal nerve stimulation in children with medically refractory epilepsy: The Pediatric VNS Study Group. J Pediatr. 1999;134:563–6.
67. Aaronson ST, Carpenter LL, Conway CR, et al. Vagus nerve stimulation therapy randomized to different amounts of electrical charge for treatment-resistant depression: acute and chronic effects. Brain Stimul. 2013;6:631–40.
68. Goadsby PJ, Edvinsson L. Human in vivo evidence for trigeminovascular activation in cluster headache neuropeptide changes and effects of acute attacks therapies. Brain. 1994;117(3):427–34.
69. May A, Goadsby PJ. The trigeminovascular system in humans: pathophysiologic implications for primary headache syndromes of the neural influences on the cerebral circulation. J Cereb Blood Flow Metab. 1999;19(2):115–27.
70. Kittrelle JP, Grouse DS, Seybold ME. Cluster headache: local anesthetic abortive agents. Arch Neurol. 1985;42(5):496–8.
71. Robbins L. Intranasal lidocaine for cluster headache. Headache. 1995;35(2):83–4.
72. Barre F. Cocaine as an abortive agent in cluster headache. Headache. 1982;22(2):69–73.
73. Costa A, Pucci E, Antonaci F, Sances G, Granella F, Broich G, Nappi G. The effect of intranasal cocaine and lidocaine on nitroglycerin-induced attacks in cluster headache. Cephalalgia. 2000;20(2): 85–91.
74. Devoghel JC. Cluster headache and sphenopalatine block. Acta Anaesthesiol Belg. 1981;32:101–7.
75. Sanders M, Zuurmond WW. Efficacy of sphenopalatine ganglion blockade in 66 patients suffering from cluster headache: a 12- to 70-month follow-up evaluation. J Neurosurg. 1997;87(6):876–80.
76. Narouze S, Kapural L, Casanova J, Mekhail N. Sphenopalatine ganglion radiofrequency ablation for the management of chronic cluster headache. Headache. 2009;49(4):571–7.
77. Chua NH, Vissers KC, Wilder-Smith OH. Quantitative sensory testing may predict response to sphenopalatine ganglion pulsed radiofrequency treatment in cluster headaches: a case series. Pain Pract. 2011;11(5):439–45.
78. Van Bets B, Raets I, Gypen E, Mestrum R, Heylen R, Van Zundert J. Pulsed radiofrequency treatment of the pterygopalatine (sphenopalatine) ganglion in cluster headache: a 10 year retrospective analysis: 14AP7-5. Eur J Anaesthesiol. 2014;31:233.
79. Fang L, Jingjing L, Ying S, Lan M, Tao W, Nan J. Computerized tomography-guided sphenopalatine ganglion pulsed radiofrequency treatment in 16 patients with refractory cluster headaches: twelve- to 30-month follow-up evaluations. Cephalalgia. 2016;36(2):106–12.
80. Loomba V, Upadhyay A, Kaveeshvar H. Radiofrequency ablation of the sphenopalatine ganglion using cone beam computed tomography for intractable cluster headache. Pain Physician. 2016;19:E1093–6.
81. Kudrow L, Kudrow DB, Sandweiss JH. Rapid and sustained relief of migraine attacks with intranasal lidocaine: preliminary findings. Headache. 1995;35(2):79–82.
82. Maizels M, Scott B, Cohen W, Chen W. Intranasal lidocaine for treatment of migraine: a randomized, double-blind, controlled trial. JAMA. 1996;276(4):319–21.
83. Maizels M, Geiger AM. Intranasal lidocaine for migraine: a randomized trial and open-label follow-up. Headache. 1999;39(8):543–51.
84. Cady R, Saper J, Dexter K, Manley HR. A double-blind, placebo-controlled study of repetitive transnasal sphenopalatine ganglion blockade with Tx360® as acute treatment for chronic migraine. Headache. 2015;55(1):101–16.
85. Tepper SJ, Rezai A, Narouze S, Steiner C, Mohajer P, Ansarinia M. Acute treatment of intractable migraine with sphenopalatine ganglion electrical stimulation. Headache. 2009;49(7):983–9.

Postsurgical Headaches and Their Management

Michael Doerrler and José Biller

Anatomy

To understand the pathophysiology of postsurgical headaches, it is important to define the pain-sensitive structures of the skull and brain. Much of the anatomy of sensitive structures in the head was identified by Harold Wolff, Bronson Ray, and Wilder Penfield in the mid-twentieth century [1]. The brain parenchyma is shown to lack the capacity to sense pain. However, many structures surrounding the brain do have this ability. These structures include the basal dura; meninges; venous sinuses; cranial nerves V, IX, and X; upper cervical nerves; dural arteries; carotid arteries; vertebral arteries; basilar artery; circle of Willis; and proximal portions of the major intracranial vessels [1, 2]. Studies show the major contributors to intracranial nociception are trigeminal afferents. These nerve fibers primarily sense mechanical, thermal, and chemical stimulation.

Further contributing to the nociceptive system are the afferent nerve fibers which primarily enter the trigeminal ganglion and dorsal root ganglion of the upper cervical roots. The fibers involved include small unmyelinated C fibers, lightly myelinated A-delta fibers, and silent nociceptors, which respond only to extreme stimuli [2]. C fibers have been associated with slow-building aching, throbbing, or burning pain. A-delta fibers are thought to transmit sharper pain sensations [2].

Most of the sensation from the face and head is conveyed by the trigeminal sensory afferent nerves. These fibers terminate in the trigeminal brainstem nuclear complex (TBNC) [3]. The TBNC is divided in the principal sensory nucleus and the spinal trigeminal nucleus. These fibers enter the brainstem in the sensory root of the trigeminal nerve. The ascending fibers terminate in the principal nucleus, and the descending fibers make up the trigeminal spinal tract. The termination of these fibers is topographically organized, with the mandibular afferents terminating in the dorsomedial medullary dorsal horn (MDH) [3]. The ophthalmic fibers terminate in the ventrolateral MDH. Most nociceptive fibers from the face and head appear to terminate in the subnucleus caudalis rat models, but this still remains to be fully defined in a human model [3].

TBNC fibers largely (60–80%) project to the contralateral thalamus. They cross and ascend with the medial lemniscus. This conglomeration of medial lemniscus and trigeminothalamic fibers projects to the ventro-postero-medial nucleus of the thalamus (VPM) [3]. Only a small percentage of the neurons in the VPM respond to nociceptive stimulation. These neurons primarily exist in the outer regions of the VPM. These neurons appear to receive fibers from the caudal aspect of the TBNC. These caudal nociceptive TBNC projections also go to the posterior thalamus and the internal medullary lamina. The thalamus and the

M. Doerrler (✉) · J. Biller
Department of Neurology, Loyola University Chicago Stritch School of Medicine, Maywood, IL, USA

© Springer International Publishing AG, part of Springer Nature 2019
M. W. Green et al. (eds.), *Chronic Headache*, https://doi.org/10.1007/978-3-319-91491-6_26

TBNC appear to be the primary drivers in nociceptive stimulation as there are few cortical neurons capable of responding to nociceptive events [3]. The neurons that do respond in the cortex are primarily for spatial localization and facilitating cortical arousal.

The trigeminothalamic system of nociception does, however, have multiple opportunities for pain modulation. Projections from the somatosensory cortex and other cortical input appear to modulate the intensity and scope of noxious stimulation. It is also hypothesized that input from the thalamus behaves similarly. Fibers from the TBNC also project to the periaqueductal gray, a known site of enkephalin production and pain modulation [3] (Fig. 26.1).

Nociception in this system can also be a peripheral process, transmitted by small unmyelinated afferents in muscle groups dissected during the procedure. The suboccipital musculature

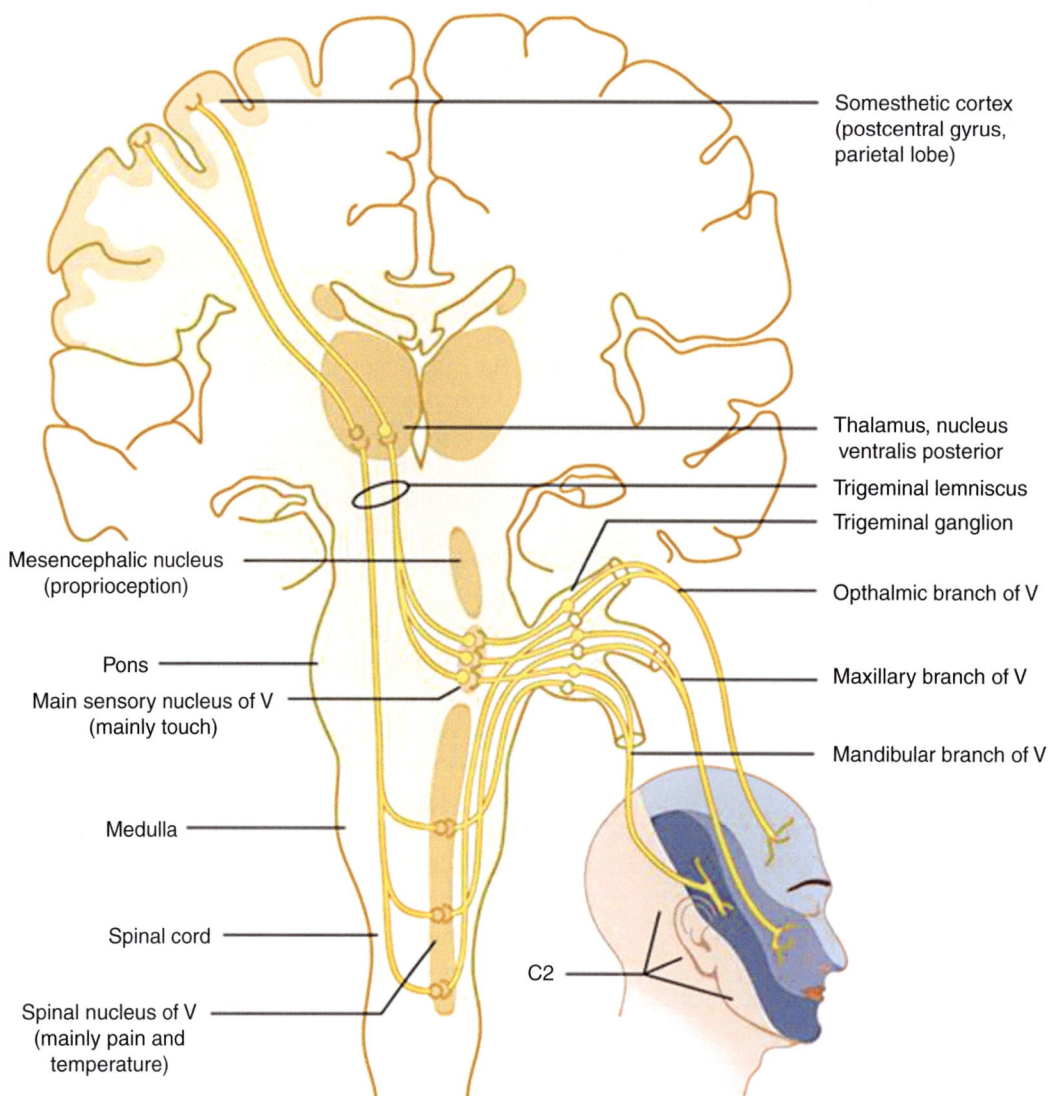

Fig. 26.1 The trigeminal brainstem nuclear complex, as illustrated in this image, is the pathway thought to be a major driver of postsurgical headaches. Nuclei send information to the VPM via the anterior trigeminothalamic pathway [3]. Reproduced with permission from Biller J, Gruener G, Brazis PW. DeMyer's The Neurologic Examination. 7th ed. New York, NY: McGraw-Hill; 2017

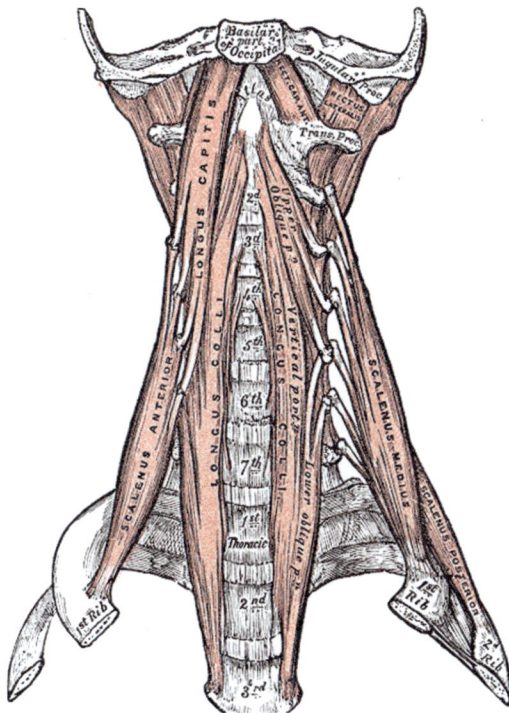

Fig. 26.2 Suboccipital musculature in relation to the occipital bone. These muscles are frequently reflected during suboccipital procedures. Surgical procedures in this area are much more likely to be associated with postoperative headaches [4]. Source: Plate 387, Gray's Anatomy of the Human Body (1918)

(particularly the capitis muscles and levator scapulae) is more frequently associated with short-term and long-term pain when compared to supratentorial procedures [4] (Fig. 26.2).

Craniotomy Technique

While the location and reason may vary, the purpose of a craniotomy remains the same: to expose a variable amount of intracranial structures to allow visualization and intervention. It is beyond the scope of this text to provide a "how-to" for this procedure, but a basic understanding of which structures are disturbed is important. As an example, a fronto-temporo-sphenoidal craniotomy will be detailed; the principle remains the same throughout the skull.

With the patient supine, an incision is made from the zygoma to above the hairline, down to the forehead. The skin and galea are elevated and skin clips are placed. The incision is then carried through the pericranium, temporalis fascia, and muscle line. The temporalis muscle is then stripped from the zygomatic process of the frontal bone to gain further access to the temporal fossa, the pterion, and the greater wing of the sphenoid [5]. With the skull exposed, four burr holes are made in the skull. A drill is then used to cut the interposing bone between the burr holes. Once the bone is fractured by the drill, it can be removed from the rest of the skull. The underlying dura is now exposed and can be incised. The dura is incised in a semicircular fashion, reflected, and retracted, exposing the Sylvain cistern underneath [5].

After the intracranial procedure is complete, the dura is replaced and reconnected with simple interrupted sutures. Gelfoam is then placed over the dural incision to act as a seal and prevent subgaleal accumulation and CSF hypotension [6]. The bone flap is then replaced and connected to the skull by means of microplates. The temporalis muscle, temporal fascia, and galea are all closed separately [6]. Finally the skin is closed and the surgical site cleaned and dressed.

For craniectomy, the bone flap is left off. Depending on the underlying pathology, procedure can vary where they might be expanded by the placement of a dural graft.

Postsurgical Headaches

Acute Headaches

Postsurgical causes for headache can be multifactorial. Headaches related to surgery can be initially subdivided into acute (occurring within <48 h of surgery) and chronic (new-onset headache in the postoperative period lasting greater than 2 months). In the acute setting, up to 60% of post-craniotomy/post-craniectomy cases suffer from surgery-related pain. The pain is more commonly described as superficial, rather than deep pain. This indicates that the acute pain experienced by patients is more likely to be somatic pain rather than visceral pain [7]. The likely etiology of the pain is injury to the scalp musculature and associated soft tissue structures. The suboccipital and sub-temporal routes are associated with the highest incidence of acute postoperative pain [7]. This is likely due to insult to the muscle groups in these regions [7, 8]. However, some studies show a higher level of pain using a frontal approach. There is some suggestion that location is not as important as the amount of tissue injury and the sub-temporal and suboccipital approaches have more tissue to injure [8]. Cerebrospinal fluid (CSF) leakage can also account for some pain that patients experience. These headaches are usually orthostatic in nature and resolve when lying flat.

Acute Postcraniotomy Headache [9]
Diagnostic criteria:

A. Headache of variable intensity, maximal in the area of the craniotomy, fulfilling criteria C and D
B. Craniotomy performed for a reason other than head trauma
C. Headache develops within 7 days after craniotomy
D. One or other of the following:
   1. Headache resolves within 3 months after craniotomy
   2. Headache persists but 3 months have not yet passed since craniotomy

Note: 1. When the craniotomy was for head trauma, code as 5.1.1 acute post-traumatic headache attributed to moderate or severe head injury.

Treatment

Historically, surgeons presumed craniotomy patients would not feel much pain due to the poor innervation of the dura and underlying brain tissue. As a result, analgesia was given on an "as-needed" basis and there are still many questions that remain [8]. Presently, the main forms of acute pain control consist of local analgesia in the form of a scalp nerve block and systemic analgesia, commonly an opioid medication. A survey of UK neurosurgical departments in 2005 shows that 48% of services are prescribed on an as-needed basis [10]. The other finding was that all centers used opioids with variable therapies, as there is no standardized protocol for post-craniotomy analgesia [10].

Opioid Medications

The opioid class is the mainstay of postoperative pain and has many side effects. Commonly, it can cause decreased level of consciousness and respiratory depression. Increased cerebral blood flow and by extension increased intracranial pressure also occur [10]. In addition, their use can blunt the clinical significance of the neurologic examination. Use of these medications has been associated with prolonged ICU stays and ICU complications.

Acetaminophen with Codeine

Codeine-based analgesia has been widely used for post-craniotomy pain control. It has a lower risk of respiratory depression and sedation. It also preserves pupillary light reflexes better than other opioid medications [8, 10]. The main drawback of the medication is sub-optimal pain control. However, this appears to be mediated by individual demethylation processes and is highly variable [10]. Other concerns about its use are common to all opioids, including constipation, dependence, and addiction.

Tramadol

Tramadol is an analgesic medication that acts on opiate and non-opiate pathways. It is a μ-opiate receptor agonist but also acts to increase CNS levels of serotonin and noradrenaline [8]. It is less effective than morphine and has fewer side effects. There is no ceiling effect and depression of respiratory function is rare [8]. When compared to other opioids for postoperative analgesia, it decreases length of stay and overall hospitalization costs [11]. The main drawbacks include nausea and vomiting after bolus and a small increase in seizure risk [8, 10].

Morphine PCA

A morphine PCA affords the patient some control over the levels of analgesia, while also allowing a baseline of pain control as well. This gives the patient some psychological relief while simultaneously decreasing the total morphine requirement for the patient. Jellish et al. found that in 2 years of using a dosage of 1.5 mg with an 8-min lockout (4 h max dose no greater than 40 g), there were no incidences of respiratory depression or re-intubation related to analgesic use [12].

Nonsteroidal Anti-inflammatory Drug (NSAID) Medications

In the acute postoperative period, NSAID use is controversial. They do decrease pain without the systemic side effects of opioid medications; however they do inhibit the cyclooxygenase pathway (COX-1 and COX-2). This inhibition of the COX-1 pathway can cause a clinically significant defect in the hemostatic system [10]. This increases the risk of intracranial hematoma and other potential sites for bleeding [8]. Preoperative diclofenac has been shown to decrease pain scores postoperatively [4]. In a study comparing ketoprofen to acetaminophen, it was found that those on ketoprofen have decreased oxycodone needs compared to the acetaminophen group [4]. It also has the potential to cause renal insufficiency. Due to these risks, neurosurgeons have shied away from their use for acute postoperative pain relief.

Local Anesthetics

The goal of local anesthesia is to block the nerves supplying the superficial tissues. This is achieved by preventing nociceptive nerves from depolarizing and sending signals to the spinal cord and brain. The most challenging aspect of local anesthesia is to localize the appropriate nerves for blockade and to apply the block without causing unintended motor and sensory compromise [8]. Blockade is not without its drawbacks. The most important drawback is the ephemeral nature of the block, typically lasting only a few hours. However, 0.75% ropivacaine can last up to 48 h [7]. Potential risks include systemic toxicity with repeated administrations, hematoma, infection, and, rarely, intra-arterial/subarachnoid injection [8]. These blocks can be done preoperatively to diminish the effects of intraoperative stimulation on the circulatory system and postoperatively. In one study preoperative blocks decreased pain scores up to 12 h postoperatively, and morphine use was decreased in the first 24 h [4].

Dexmedetomidine

Dexmedetomidine (trade name, Precedex) is a highly selective α-2 agonist which has been shown to have antinociceptive effects through binding of these receptors both centrally and peripherally. It decreases pain scores up to 24 h postoperatively compared to placebo [4]. It also decreases postoperative nausea and vomiting. Dexmedetomidine is associated with decreased morphine use compared to placebo. Hemodynamic stability, a significant postoperative concern, is improved compared to placebo [4]. Dexmedetomidine can cause bradycardia, and, in some cases, bradycardia secondary to dexmedetomidine has been confused for a Cushing's reflex (also known as vasopressor response to increased intracranial pressure characterized by increased blood pressure, irregular breathing, and bradycardia). There is a theoretical risk of delayed emergence from general anesthesia, but some studies found no significant difference between dexmedetomidine and placebo [4].

Chronic Headaches

Chronic headaches are known complications following craniotomy/craniectomy. These headaches are defined as occurring postoperatively, lasting greater than 2 months and not attributable to any other cause. The incidence of chronic post-craniotomy headaches has been estimated between 12% and 34% [7]. These headaches can present as chronic persistent head pain, tension headaches, orthostatic headaches, headaches with nuchal rigidity, local pain syndromes, or even headache syndromes similar to migraines or trigeminal autonomic cephalalgias. The exact incidence of these subtypes is not fully defined. Some studies show that in acoustic neuroma resection, postoperative headache incidence is 46.7% for tension-type headaches, occipital neuralgia 16.6%, trigeminal neuropathy 16.6%, neuropathy of the intermedian nerve 10%, and cervicogenic headache 10% [13].

The exact cause of chronic post-craniotomy headaches is unclear but believed to be multifactorial. Contributing causes include nerve entrapment, persistent dural traction, CSF leakage, scar tissue formation, aseptic meningitis, persistent musculoskeletal dysfunction, and even central sensitization [7, 8, 14]. It has been hypothesized that post-craniotomy headaches lie on the spectrum of post-traumatic headaches, with the surgery as trauma [15]. There is an increased headache incidence in sub-tentorial craniotomies/craniectomies, in particular suboccipital [8]. Aside from location, approach and technique seem to play a role. In regard to vestibular schwannoma resection, bone flap replacement has a much higher incidence of headache (94% replaced vs. 27% not replaced). Duraplastic closure has a much lower incidence of headaches than with direct dura closure (0% vs. 100%) [7]. Drilling of the internal auditory canal and the use of fibrin glue also may have an association with increased incidence of postsurgical headaches [7]. The multitude of potential contributing factors for chronic postsurgical headaches means that effective treatment can be a difficult road to travel. However, most patients have some response to a combination of pharmacologic and non-pharmacologic therapies.

Chronic Postcraniotomy Headache [9]
Diagnostic criteria:

A. Headache of variable intensity, maximal in the area of the craniotomy, fulfilling criteria C and D
B. Craniotomy performed for a reason other than head trauma
C. Headache develops within 7 days after craniotomy
D. Headache persists for >3 months after craniotomy

Note: 1. When the craniotomy was for head trauma, code as 5.2.1 chronic post-traumatic headache attributed to moderate or severe head injury.

Treatment

As the exact mechanism of postsurgical headaches is unclear, the treatment is often geared to the syndrome that the symptoms most resemble. Patients will often be given or self-treat with systemic anal-gesics including acetaminophen, NSAIDs, or opioids. While this may be effective in some patients, it can result in rebound headaches if the medications are taken frequently. Cervicogenic headaches may respond to trigger point injections [7]. Botulinum toxin type A (Botox) injections could be a potential avenue of therapy; however, some small studies have not shown benefit [7]. For other neuropathic pain, mainstay treatments such as tricyclic antidepressants, gabapentin, carbamazepine, and duloxetine are tried based on patient's medical comorbidities. Lamotrigine is reportedly effective in trigeminal nerve pain disorders and may be of clinical value in patients suffering from chronic post-craniotomy headaches [7]. However, it is not considered a first-line agent. Patients with migraine-like symptoms can be treated similarly to migraines, but in post-craniotomy/trauma patients, sodium valproate has been shown to be effective [8]. Opioids are used but are typically ineffective in chronic neuropathic pain as there is a downregulation of μ-receptors as the disease state progresses, making the opioids less effective. Tramadol, a weak opioid agonist, can be effective as it also acts on serotonin and norepinephrine uptake [7]. There have been instances were ketamine has been used for refractory post-craniotomy pain. It acts as an NMDA receptor antagonist. Its use is limited as the medication is foul tasting and has side effects of hallucinations and feelings of unreality [7].

Local allodynia can be treated with a variety of topical anesthetics or nerve blocks [8]. Most of these act as sodium channel blockers (e.g., lidocaine) to reduce the spontaneous firing of peripheral nerves.

While pharmacologic therapy alone can be effective, non-pharmacologic therapies can be added to increase the odds of a favorable outcome in appropriate patients [8]. These therapies include TENS, acupuncture, radiofrequency ablation, cryoablation, and physical therapy.

Hemicrania Continua

Hemicrania continua was originally described by Drs. Sjaastad and Spierings as a steady, non-paroxysmal, moderate to severe headaches that responded reliably to indomethacin [16]. The pain these patients suffer is always unilateral and does not alternate, unlike the typical migraine phenotype. These headaches have also been described sometimes as being associated with ipsilateral autonomic symptoms (lacrimation, rhinorrhea, etc.). A small case series done by Gantenbein et al. in 2015 described three patients with hemicrania-like syndromes. While resistant to most NSAIDs, they had full relief on indomethacin [15]. These patients had different surgical approaches for different underlying pathologies; it was felt that they shared common underlying pathophysiology through the cervico-trigeminothalamic pathway [15]. In these patients, MR imaging should be performed to exclude other structural causes of secondary hemicrania continua. These causes include carotid artery (ICA) dissection, pineal mass or cyst, pituitary mass, ipsilateral mass, unruptured ipsilateral intracranial aneurysm, and posterior fossa infarctions [17–20]. When evaluating these patients for postoperative hemicrania continua, the differential may also include side-locked chronic migraine or other trigeminal autonomic cephalalgias [21].

Scalp Neuralgias

Neuropathic pain can form at the site of craniotomy or craniectomy most likely due to localized trauma, gliosis, nerve entrapment, and localized sensitization [22]. Diagnosis of scalp neuralgias is primarily clinical. The pain will be isolated to a specific superficial nerve distribution. The most common scalp neuralgias are supraorbital and occipital. The supraorbital can become entrapped by the frontalis muscle, and the occipital nerve may become entrapped by the semispinalis capitis muscle [23]. Another possible cause of neuralgia in patients with occipital neuralgia and postsurgical anatomy would be a close proximity of the occipital nerve and the occipital artery [23].

The treatment for this can be localized, through nerve blocks, lidocaine patches, and in some cases nerve release procedures. The treatment can also be systemic through typical neuropathic pain agents including GABAergic agents, tricyclic antidepressants, and the like.

Hemicrania Continua [9]
Description: Persistent strictly unilateral headache responsive to indomethacin.
   Diagnostic criteria:

A. Headache for >3 months fulfilling criteria B–D
B. All of the following characteristics:
   1. Unilateral pain without side shift
   2. Daily and continuous, without pain-free periods
   3. Moderate intensity, but with exacerbations of severe pain
C. At least one of the following autonomic features occurs during exacerbations and ipsilateral to the side of pain:
   1. Conjunctival injection and/or lacrimation
   2. Nasal congestion and/or rhinorrhea
   3. Ptosis and/or miosis
D. Complete response to therapeutic doses of indomethacin
E. Not attributed to another disorder

CSF Hypotension Syndrome

This is a pattern of headaches that can occur in the post-craniotomy/craniectomy setting as a result of imperfect dural healing or gaps in the dura postoperatively. These headaches commonly are worsened upon standing, but there have been reports of worsening upon lying as well. Associated symptoms include photophobia, phonophobia, meningismus, nausea, vomiting, loss of hearing, blurred vision, double vision, and in rare extreme cases depressed level of consciousness [24]. Spontaneous CSF hypotension is either idiopathic or associated with systemic connective tissue diseases, such as Marfan syndrome and Ehlers-Danlos syndrome, or malformations of the dura [24]. Postsurgical CSF leak can be attributed to any number of reasons, including dural dehiscence, size of the dural defect, surgical approach, and dural friability limiting repair [25]. In vestibular schwannoma (also known as acoustic neuroma) resection, there appears to be increased need for surgical repair of the trans-labyrinthine approach compared to the retrosigmoid approach, but there was no difference in incidence of the rate of leaks [25]. It is uncommon for spontaneous CSF leaks to cause CSF rhinorrhea, but more common in a surgical scenario. This is particularly true for the translabyrinthine approach [25].

Diagnosis includes a thorough history and physical examination MRI, and lumbar puncture (LP) (Fig. 26.3). A brain MRI should be performed with and without contrast, and depending on the location of the surgery, spinal imaging may also be needed. MR brain findings can include diffuse uninterrupted smooth pachymeningeal enhancement, sagging of brain structures (especially midline), subdural fluid collections, pituitary enlargement, and decreased ventricle size [24]. Should spinal imaging be needed, MRI may show extra arachnoid/dural fluid collection or dural enhancement. If a spinal source of the hypotension is suspected, however, the gold standard is myelography.

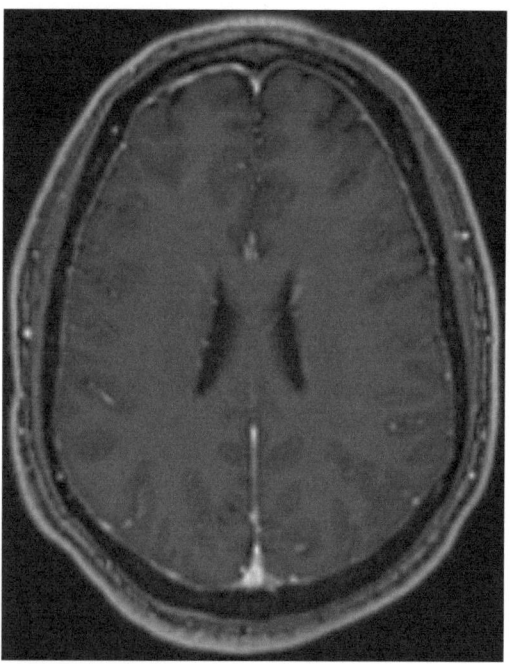

Fig. 26.3 MR brain post-contrast sequence in a patient with CSF hypotension. Note smooth continuous dural enhancement

Initial management is typically conservative including hydration, salt tabs, bed rest, and caffeine. However, should conservative management fail, intervention may be required. If a spinal source is suspected, blood patching or fibrin glue may be used [24]. However, in the postsurgical CSF hypotension, surgical repair may be required if conservative measures do not work. Surgical management can include re-approximating the dural edges, grafting with autogenic tissues (fat or muscles), or grafting with allogenic dural matrix.

Headache Attributed to Low Cerebrospinal Fluid Pressure [9]
Diagnostic criteria:

A. Any headache fulfilling criterion C
B. Low CSF pressure (<60 mm CSF) and/or evidence of CSF leakage on imaging
C. Headache has developed in temporal relation to the low CSF pressure or CSF leakage or led to its discovery
D. Not better accounted for by another ICHD-3 diagnosis

Medication Overuse Headaches

In treating patients with chronic headaches, one must resolve not to do further harm by causing more headaches. Almost any pharmacologic treatment for headaches increases the risk of developing medication overuse headache (MOH). However, some medications are more prone to causing this than others. MOH are defined as chronic headaches (>15 days per month) that develop as a consequence of taking analgesic medication too frequently [26]. Often, these patients will note an increase in headache frequency, sometimes to the point of being a daily persistent headache. They will worsen when not taking the abortive medication, but will never truly be headache free. For patients seeing primary care services, MOH is most commonly caused by over-the-counter (OTC) analgesics. Patients being seen in secondary and tertiary medical settings (commonly the postsurgical population) are most often afflicted by MOH caused by centrally acting agents. For all chronic headache patients in the United States, 23% are though to suffer from MOH. About 50% of patients with 15 or more headaches per month have MOH [26]. Not all patients with headaches on medication develop headache and the exact pathogenesis is unclear. Some feel that it is due to the difference in mechanism of medication, pathology of underlying headaches, or some as of yet undescribed pathway. In the general migraine population, different medications convey different risks of headache progression. Opioid medication use increased risk in patients using it more than 8 days out of a month. Barbiturates increased risk in patients exposed greater than 5 days out of a month [27]. NSAIDs were protective of headache progression in patients suffering from less than 10 days of headache out of the month but increased risk in patients suffering from more frequent headaches [27]. It is unclear what the frequency of postsurgical patients with chronic headaches suffer from MOH or if they suffer it in a similar manner as patients in the general population.

As MOH is a heterogeneous disorder, there is no international consensus on treatment. However, the mainstay is removal of the overused agent [26]. Commonly patients experience a withdrawal 2–10 days after discontinuation of medication. This typically manifests as a worsening of the headaches, nausea, vomiting, sleep difficulties, and anxiety. Duration of withdrawal appears to vary depending on the overused drug with triptans being about 4 days and analgesics being about 10 days [26]. A suggested strategy is to withdraw the offending agent, to provide pharmacologic and non-pharmacologic support for withdrawal symptoms, and to prevent relapse of MOH. In one study, simply giving the patient information about overuse headaches cut the occurrence by 42% [26]. There is currently no consensus whether to bridge a patient on prophylactic medication during detoxification.

Medication Overuse Headache [28]
Diagnostic criteria:

A. Headache occurring on ≥15 days per month in a patient with a pre-existing headache disorder
B. Regular overuse for >3 months of one or more drugs that can be taken for acute and/or symptomatic treatment of headache
C. Not better accounted for by another ICHD-3 diagnosis

Other Postsurgical Syndromes Associated with Headaches

Frontotemporal Brain Sagging Syndrome

Patients can present with behavior typical of behavioral variant of frontotemporal dementia (bvFTD) but can lack the obvious imaging changes, as well as have other findings on imaging as well to suggest a different clinical entity. This syndrome has been called frontotemporal brain sagging syndrome (FBSS). It typically presents with an insidious decline in cognition and behavior, daytime somnolence, and headaches [29]. They have cognitive decline in a similar manner as bvFTD, but do not have the typical patterns of atrophy and have sagging of midline structures associated with CSF hypotension.

Typical behavioral symptoms included are disinhibition and apathy with concomitant onset of daytime sleepiness. Some patients can have an orthostatic component to their headache. In one case series, only one of eight patients had verified CSF hypotension [29]. On MRI they were found to have a range of findings including sagging of the brainstem and cerebellum and trans-tentorial herniation of medial temporal lobe and corpus callosum (Fig. 26.4). Pachymeningeal enhancement, subdural fluid collections, and atrophy were uncommon. These patients were found to have decreased frontal and temporal metabolism

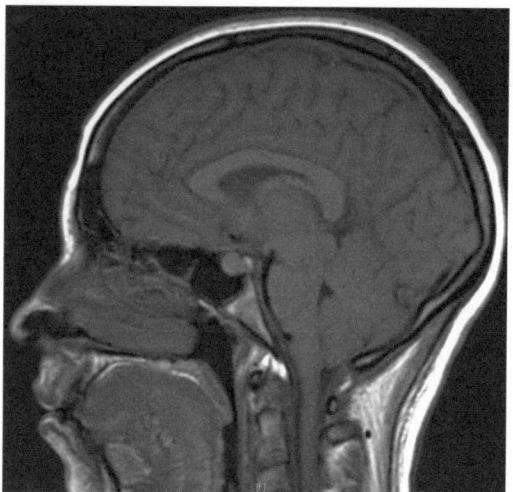

Fig. 26.4 A sagittal T1 MR brain showing an example of midline structure sagging in a patient with CSF hypotension

on PET scan. Notably this hypometabolism resolved after leak repair [29].

A variety of therapies were tried in these patients including corticosteroids, direct dural repair, and blood patching. Some patients transiently improved, but ultimately all declined despite therapy [29]. It is felt that this disease process could represent a chronic CSF leak that could either be spontaneous or iatrogenic. It is thought that this is a treatable disease process and bears further research.

Syndrome of the Trephine

The syndrome of the trephine (SoT) also known as *motor trephine syndrome*, *sunken brain and scalp flap syndrome*, or *sinking skin flap syndrome* is a rare syndrome involving a persistent cranial vault defect after large craniectomy (Fig. 26.5). It was first described in 1977 by Yamaura et al. [30]. These patients principally present with severe headaches, mental status changes, focal deficits, or seizures. Uncommonly these patients can present with dysautonomia. These symptoms include paroxysmal changes in heart rate, respiratory rate, temperature, blood pressure, and diaphoresis [31]. Autonomic symptoms portent a worse outcome compared to its absence. The onset of this syndrome is typically late (months to over a year)

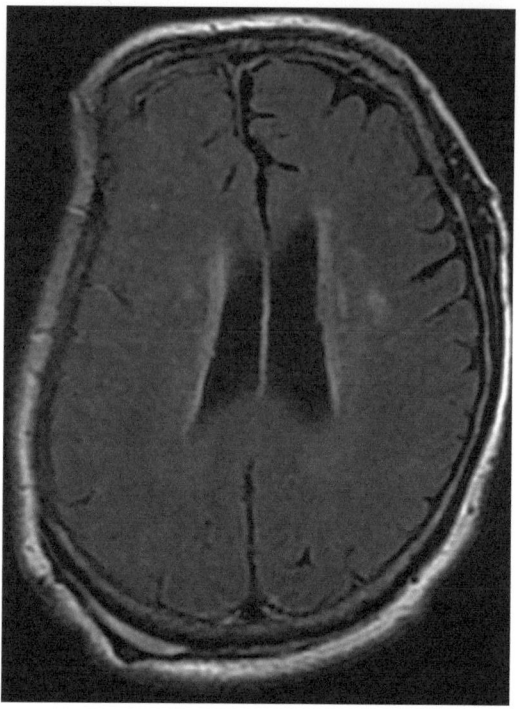

Fig. 26.5 MRI brain FLAIR sequence showing paradoxical herniation of a patient with a chronic right hemicraniectomy who had worsening of left-sided weakness during periods of prolonged standing

after the hemicraniectomy without subsequent replacement of the bone flap.

The pathophysiology of the syndrome is felt to be caused by persistent atmospheric pressure. A contributing component could be over-shunting by a VP shunt [31]. It may even have an orthostatic component. Untreated, SoT can progress to a paradoxical herniation causing further neurologic dysfunction, coma, and death [31]. The treatment is replacement of the bone flap or reduction of shunt flow volume.

Carotid Endarterectomy-Related Headaches

There is a headache entity seen in patients that undergo carotid endarterectomies. It is classified as a unilateral and ipsilateral headache that begins within 1 week of a carotid endarterectomy. It typically will resolve within 1 month. It also cannot be attributed to any other pathology besides the surgery [32]. It can have an extremely variable presentation that has had descriptions outside of the International Headache Society (IHS) guidelines. Commonly it can present with a migrainous pulsation without other associated migrainous features, as a "cluster-like" headache with ipsilateral lacrimation and erythema, or just a mild self-limited headache. It has even been described as a bilateral phenomenon [32, 33]. There does not appear to be any relationship with the occurrence of the headache and the preoperative history, degree of stenosis, or even past history of headache. These headaches are typically self-limiting and, once resolved, did not reoccur [32]. As such, these patients do not need long-term pharmacologic therapy for these headaches. This headache should not be confused for another post-endarterectomy syndrome, cerebral hyperperfusion syndrome (CHS). CHS can occur in patients with chronic high-grade stenosis with decreased ipsilateral blood flow and presents with a severe headache, seizures, and decreased level of consciousness. It can also be associated with intraparenchymal hemorrhage [34].

Post-endarterectomy Headache [28]
Diagnostic criteria:

A. Any new headache fulfilling criterion C
B. Carotid endarterectomy has been performed
C. Evidence of causation demonstrated by at least two of the following:
  1. Headache develops within 1 week of carotid endarterectomy
  2. Headache resolves within 1 month after carotid endarterectomy
  3. Headache is unilateral, on the side of the carotid endarterectomy, and has one of the following three characteristics:
    a) Diffuse mild pain
    b) Cluster headache-like pain occurring once or twice a day in attacks lasting 2–3 h
    c) Pulsating severe pain
D. Not better accounted for by another ICHD-3 diagnosis, and arterial dissection has been excluded by appropriate investigations.

References

1. Cutrer FM. Pain sensitive cranial structures: chemical anatomy. In: Silberstein SD, Lipton RB, Dalessio DJ, editors. Wolff's headache and other head pain. 7th ed. New York, NY: Oxford UP; 2001. p. 50–5.
2. Dunne PB. Anatomy and physiology of headache. In: Tollison CD, Kunkel RS, editors. Headache: diagnosis and treatment. Baltimore: Williams & Wilkins; 1993. p. 13–7. Print.
3. Renehan WE, Jacquin MF. Anatomy of central nervous system pathways related to head pain. In: Olesen J, Tfelt-Hansen P, KMA W, editors. The headaches. New York, NY: Raven; 1993. p. 77–86.
4. Dunn LK, Naik BI, Nemergut EC, Durieux ME. Postcraniotomy pain management: beyond opioids. Curr Neurol Neurosci Rep. 2016;16(10):93.
5. Yasargil MG, Smith RD. Management of aneurysms of anterior circulation by intracranial procedures. In: Youmans JR, editor. Youmans neurological surgery. Vol 3. 2nd ed. Philadelphia, PA: W.B. Saunders; 1982. p. 1663–96.
6. Salcman M, Kempe LG, Heros RC, Laws ER, Sonntag VKH. Pterional or frontotemporal craniotomy, opening and closure. In: Kempe's operative neurosurgery. Vol 1. New York: Springer; 2004. p. 1–17.
7. deGray LC, Matta BF. Acute and chronic pain following craniotomy: a review. Anaesthesia. 2005;60(7):693–704.
8. Haldar R, Kaushal A, Gupta D, Srivastava S, Singh PK. Pain following craniotomy: reassessment of the available options. Biomed Res Int. 2015;2015:509164. https://doi.org/10.1155/2015/509164. Epub 2015 Oct 1
9. Olesen J, et al. The international classification of headache disorders. 2nd ed (ICHD-II). Revue Neurologique. 2005;161.6-7:689–91. Web.
10. Santos CMT, et al. Options to manage postcraniotomy acute pain: no protocol available. Rev Chil Neurocirugía. 2013;39:22–7. Web.
11. Rahimi SY, Alleyne CH, Vernier E, Witcher MR, Vender JR. Postoperative pain management with tramadol after craniotomy: evaluation and cost analysis. J Neurosurg. 2010;112(2):268–72.
12. Jellish WS, Murdoch J, Leonetti JP. Perioperative management of complex skull base surgery: the anesthesiologist's point of view. Neurosurg Focus. 2002;12(5):1–7.
13. Schankin CJ, Straube A. Secondary headaches: secondary or still primary? J Headache Pain. 2012;13(4):263–70.
14. Ferreira KDS, Dach F, Speciali JG. Scar neuromas as triggers for headache after craniotomy: clinical evidence. Arq Neuropsiquiatr. 2012;70(3):206–9.
15. Gantenbein AR, Sarikaya H, Riederer F, Goadsby PJ. Postoperative hemicrania continua-like headache—a case series. J Headache Pain. 2015;16:526.
16. Sjaastad O, Spierings EL. "Hemicrania continua": another headache absolutely responsive to indomethacin. Cephalalgia. 1984;4(1):65–70.
17. EJ E, Swanson JW, Dodick DW. Hemicrania continua: an indomethacin-responsive case with an underlying malignant etiology. Headache. 2002;42(6):527–9.

18. Rogalewski A, Evers S. Symptomatic hemicrania continua after internal carotid artery dissection. Headache. 2005;45(2):167–9.
19. Levy MJ. The clinical characteristics of headache in patients with pituitary tumours. Brain. 2005;128(8):1921–30.
20. Valença MM, Andrade-Valença LP, da Silva WF, Dodick DW. Hemicrania continua secondary to an ipsilateral brainstem lesion. Headache. 2007;47(3):438–41.
21. Kaup AO, Mathew NT, Levyman C, Kailasam J, Meadors LA, Villarreal SS. 'Side locked' migraine and trigeminal autonomic cephalgias: evidence for clinical overlap. Cephalalgia. 2003;23(1):43–9.
22. Chien GC, Mathur S, Harvey RL, Harden RN. Topical diclofenac treatment for post-incisional neuropathic pain. Pain Med. 2013;14(6):950–1.
23. Shimizu S. Scalp neuralgia and headache elicited by cranial superficial anatomical causes: supraorbital neuralgia, occipital neuralgia, and post-craniotomy headache. Rinsho Shinkeigaku. 2014;54(5):387–94.
24. Mokri B. Spontaneous low pressure, low CSF volume headaches: spontaneous CSF leaks. Headache. 2013;53(7):1034–53.
25. Brennan JW, Rowed DW, Nedzelski JM, Chen JM. Cerebrospinal fluid leak after acoustic neuroma surgery: influence of tumor size and surgical approach on incidence and response to treatment. J Neurosurg. 2001;94(2):217–23.
26. Kristoffersen ES, Lundqvist C. Medication-overuse headache: epidemiology, diagnosis and treatment. Ther Adv Drug Saf. 2014;5(2):87–99.
27. Bigal ME, Lipton RB. Excessive acute migraine medication use and migraine progression. Neurology. 2008;71(22):1821–8.
28. ICHD-3 beta—the international classification of headache disorders. 3rd ed (Beta Version). International Headache Society, n.d. Web. 15 Mar 2017. https://www.ichd-3.org/.
29. Wicklund MR, Mokri B, Drubach DA, Boeve BF, Parisi JE, Josephs KA. Frontotemporal brain sagging syndrome: an SIH-like presentation mimicking FTD. Neurology. 2011;76(16):1377–82.
30. Yamaura A, Sato M, Meguro K, Nakamura T, Uemura K. Cranioplasty following decompressive craniectomy—analysis of 300 cases (author's transl). No Shinkei Geka. 1977;5(4):345–53.
31. Romero FR, Zanini MA, Ducati LG, Gabarra RC. Sinking skin flap syndrome with delayed dysautonomic syndrome—an atypical presentation. Int J Surg Case Rep. 2013;4(11):1007–9.
32. Tehindrazanarivelo AD, Lutz G, PetitJean C, Bousser MG. Headache following carotid endarterectomy: a prospective study. Cephalalgia. 1992;12(6):380–2.
33. De Marinis M, Zaccaria A, Faraglia V, Fiorani P, Maira G, Agnoli A. Post-endarterectomy headache and the role of the oculosympathetic system. J Neurol Neurosurg Psychiatry. 1991;54(4):314–7.
34. Moulakakis KG, Mylonas SN, Sfyroeras GS, Andrikopoulos V. Hyperperfusion syndrome after carotid revascularization. J Vasc Surg. 2009;49(4):1060–8.

Chronic Daily Headache Classification

27

Maggie W. Waung and Morris Levin

Introduction

Chronic daily headache affects approximately 3–5% of the population [1–3], extracting significant morbidity and healthcare costs. Despite the highly negative impact of chronic daily headache on global health, relatively little is understood about the underlying mechanisms of headache chronification and maintenance. The limited mechanistic understanding of long-standing headache poses significant challenges to the classification and diagnosis of chronic headache. This chapter discusses goals and pitfalls of headache classification, provides a brief history of chronic daily headache classification, and summarizes the current knowledge of the major chronic daily headache categories. Chronic headaches of long duration will be presented, with attention given to chronic daily headache in children and the elderly.

M. W. Waung (✉)
Department of Neurology, University of California San Francisco, San Francisco, CA, USA
e-mail: Maggie.Waung@ucsf.edu

M. Levin
Department of Neurology, UCSF Headache Center, University of California San Francisco, San Francisco, CA, USA

Goals of Classification

Many aspects of chronic daily headache classification have drawn heated debate, and we will attempt to draw attention to the most salient debates for the reader. A number of these contentions arise from different viewpoints on the goals of classification. For some, the major agenda of headache classification is to allow rigorous epidemiological characterization in order to facilitate quality research, enable the study of pathophysiology, and guide targeted treatment discovery. However, another goal for headache classification is more practical, to allow clinicians a guide for diagnosis and treatment of their headache population. While these goals are not always in opposition, there can be conflict when classifications are overly stringent for research purposes versus overly broad or simplistic for ease of diagnosis.

It has been proposed that a valid classification should reflect underlying biological mechanisms, demonstrate consistent clinical characteristics, and predict treatment response [4]. Functional classifications also tend to be relatively straightforward and easy to apply [5]. In examining the history of headache classification, it becomes clear that the back-and-forth between researchers and clinicians in the iterative shaping of disease classification is critical for promoting the ongoing discovery and understanding of headache mechanisms. Hopefully, discussion of the insights and

© Springer International Publishing AG, part of Springer Nature 2019
M. W. Green et al. (eds.), *Chronic Headache*, https://doi.org/10.1007/978-3-319-91491-6_27

criticisms of chronic daily headache classification will illuminate the progress we have made in our understanding of the basic mechanisms of chronic headaches but also shine a spotlight on areas that need further research and understanding.

History of CDH Classification

Classification of chronic daily headache has a history of confusing taxonomy and nomenclature. In the early 1980s, Mathew et al. [6] drew a connection between patients with daily headaches and a history of episodic or menstrual-related migraine and coined the term "transformed migraine." At the time, it was generally believed that daily headaches were more related to "muscle contraction headache" or tension headache. In the early 1990s, the idea of *transformed migraine* [7] became associated with chronic daily headache as patients with episodic migraine developed more severe and more frequent headaches. These transformed headaches were either related or unrelated to excessive drug use.

By the mid-1990s, Manzoni et al. divided chronic daily headache into chronic tension-type, chronic migraine, and migraine with interparoxysmal headaches, as headaches on at least 6 days a week for at least 1 year [8], while the Silberstein and Lipton (S-L) criteria defined chronic daily headache as headache lasting at least 4 h per day for at least 15 days per month for at least 1 month, with a history of transformation [9]. Silberstein et al. further subcategorized chronic daily headache into transformed migraine, new daily persistent headache, chronic tension-type headache, and hemicrania continua [10].

Although discussion of chronic daily headache classification was ongoing, it was not included in the first edition of the International Classification of Headache Disorders (ICHD-I) criteria published in 1988 [11]. Not until 2004 with the publication of ICHD-II [12] did chronic migraine replace transformed migraine as headaches lasting for greater than 3 months. In addition to chronic migraine, definitions emerged for chronic tension-type headache, new daily persistent headache, hemicrania continua, and medication-overuse headache.

The ICHD-II criteria for chronic migraine were deemed to be overly restrictive, as Bigal et al. demonstrated by classifying 638 CDH patients over 20 years, with only 9 patients fulfilling the ICHD-II criteria for transformed migraine compared to 158 using the S-L criteria [13]. The authors of this comparative study went on to argue that the rarity of chronic migraine under the ICHD-II criteria would hamper clinical trials in this group. The ICHD-II criteria for chronic headaches were further criticized due to their focus on classification of attack phenomenology for a snapshot in time and for not taking into account the progressive clinical course of patients, whose symptoms may develop insidiously over several years [14]. Many chronic migraine patients often have several headache types, and many headaches did not fit the criteria for migraine, begging the question, "Why call it 'chronic migraine' when the majority of headaches are usually tension-type?" [15]. In 2006, a proposal was put forth to ignore the classification of specific attacks in the diagnosis of chronic migraine with the justification that "most attacks of migraine without aura initially develop and go through a phase that phenomenologically fulfills criteria for tension-type headache before the headache gets worse, and early intake of triptan may abort the attack before typical characteristics of migraine develop."

The 2006 ICHD-IIR diagnostic criteria defined chronic migraine as:

1. Headache on ≥ or equal to 15 days per month for ≥3 months.
2. Occurring in patient with at least five attacks fulfilling criteria for migraine without aura.
3. On ≥8 days per month for ≥3 months, headache has fulfilled criteria for pain and associated symptoms of migraine without aura, or patient has been successfully treated with an ergot or triptan and no medication overuse and not attributed to another causative disorder.

In 2010, a multiaxial classification for CDH was proposed largely based on the structure of classification for psychiatric diseases [16]. This classification addresses some of the criticisms arising from chronic daily headache and medication-overuse headache classification and attempts to break down complexities of CDH into different axes for a more comprehensive assessment of headaches. The proposed classification envisioned six different components of CDH classification:

Axis I: main headache category
Axis II: subtypes
Axis III: associated conditions
Axis IV: contributory factors and triggers (including medication overuse)
Axis V: functional impairment
Axis VI: pain severity

In the same year, the US Food and Drug Administration (FDA) approved a definition of chronic migraine for prescribing onabotulinum-toxinA as "≥15 days per month with headache lasting 4 h a day or longer," further complicating chronic migraine classification for the clinician. ICHD-III (beta edition) was published in 2013 [17] and will be used in this chapter for further discussion of the chronic daily headache subtypes.

CDH Differential Diagnoses

Chronic daily headache affects up to 4.7% of the adult population [2] and can be classified into two major categories, primary or secondary headaches (Table 27.1).

In this chapter, we will discuss the major primary and secondary chronic headaches of long

Table 27.1 Primary and secondary causes of chronic daily headache

Primary causes	Secondary causes
Chronic migraine with and without aura	Medications and toxins
Chronic tension-type headache	Persistent toxin exposure
Chronic cluster headache	Medication-overuse headache
Hemicrania continua	Posttraumatic head or neck injury
New daily persistent headache	Post-craniotomy headache
	Cervicogenic headache
	Chronic subdural hematoma
	Headache due to past ischemic stroke
	Headache due to past nontraumatic intracranial hemorrhage (subarachnoid, intracerebral, or acute subdural hemorrhage)
	Headache due to vascular malformations (unruptured saccular aneurysm, arteriovenous malformation, dural arteriovenous fistula, cavernous angioma, encephalotrigeminal or leptomeningeal angiomatosis)
	Headache due to past cervical or vertebral artery dissection
	Cerebral venous thrombosis
	Cerebral arteritis (primary central nervous system or systemic)
	Headache due to past reversible cerebral vasoconstriction syndrome
	Idiopathic intracranial hypertension (pseudotumor cerebri)
	Spontaneous cerebrospinal fluid leak
	Intracranial hypotension following lumbar puncture, trauma, or durotomy
	Solid brain parenchymal tumor (primary, metastatic, lymphoma)
	Skull-based tumor (primary, metastatic)
	Meningeal neoplastic disease
	Neurosarcoidosis
	Chronic viral or other meningoencephalitis (HIV, malaria, EBV)
	Headache due to systemic infection in the absence of meningitis or meningoencephalitis
	Intracranial abscesses (bacterial, fungal, cysticercosis)
	Hypophysitis
	Chronic sinusitis

Adapted with permission from Levin [18]
HIV human immunodeficiency virus, *EBV* Epstein-Barr virus

duration. We will not address the short-lasting headaches that may also develop into chronic forms such as chronic paroxysmal hemicrania, chronic short-lasting unilateral neuralgiform headache attacks with cranial autonomic symptoms (SUNA), and chronic short-lasting unilateral neuralgiform headache attacks with conjunctival injection and tearing (SUNCT).

Chronic Migraine with and Without Aura

Chronic migraine is the most common chronic daily headache, classified as pain and associated symptoms of migraine without aura for 15 or more days per month over 3 months or longer, without medication overuse. As mentioned above, it was first included in the ICHD-II in 2004 under complications of migraine.

ICHD-III Beta: Diagnostic Criteria

A. Headache (tension-type-like and/or migraine-like) on ≥15 days per month for >3 months [2] and fulfilling criteria B and C

B. Occurring in a patient who has had at least five attacks fulfilling criteria B–D for 1.1 migraine without aura and/or criteria B and C for 1.2 migraine with aura

C. On ≥8 days per month for >3 months, fulfilling any of the following [3]:
   1. Criteria C and D for 1.1 migraine without aura
   2. Criteria B and C for 1.2 migraine with aura
   3. Believed by the patient to be migraine at onset and relieved by a triptan or ergot derivative

D. Not better accounted for by another ICHD-III diagnosis

Other Features

A diagnosis of chronic migraine excludes tension-type headache and requires a headache diary for at least 1 month to establish frequency of symptoms. The phenotype of individual headaches can vary within the same patient [19], and migraine features such as throbbing pain, nausea, photophobia, and phonophobia are less prominent in patients with chronic migraine compared to episodic migraine [20, 21].

Epidemiology

Chronic migraine affects 1–3% of the global population [22, 23], which is more common than other neurological disorders including epilepsy or Parkinson's disease. The ratio of female to males with chronic migraine mirrors the gender distribution in episodic migraine (approximately 2.5 to 3:1 female to male) [23]. The age distribution of chronic migraine skews slightly older compared to episodic migraine with peak prevalence in the fifth decade [23]. In the United States, chronic migraine disproportionately affects individuals with low household incomes while having no increased prevalence for any particular race and ethnicity after adjusting for socioeconomic factors [23].

Risk Factors

The American Migraine Prevalence and Prevention (AMPP) study found several risk factors for chronification of headache, including lower socioeconomic status, obesity, snoring, comorbid pain, head or neck injury, stressful life events, high caffeine intake, overuse of certain medications [24], and persistent frequent nausea [25]. In the Chronic Migraine Epidemiology and Outcomes (CaMEO) study, episodic migraine patients with comorbid pain were also more likely to develop chronic migraine [26]. The presence of anxiety, depression, and allodynia [27] also correlates with an increased risk of migraine chronification.

In patients with episodic migraine, approximately 2–3% of patients convert to chronic migraine per year [28]. Interestingly, ineffective treatment of episodic migraine was associated with a higher risk of chronic migraine, suggesting that adequate treatment of episodic migraine may prevent headache chronification, although refractory episodic migraines may be a marker of impending chronic migraine [29]. Other than reducing medication overuse, so far there is no definitive data demonstrating that modification of risk factors can influence the natural history of chronic migraine.

Comorbidities

AMPP Data—Psychiatric and pain disorders associated significantly more often with CM than EM include (Table 27.2):

Pathophysiology

The underpinnings of chronic migraine are thought to involve both central and peripheral mechanisms, with central nervous system alterations supported by advanced imaging studies and CSF studies, while peripheral changes may be implicated by serum biomarker studies. Central changes in cortical and subcortical structure, metabolism, functional connectivity, and nociceptive pain processing have been documented in chronic migraine patients compared to healthy controls and episodic migraine patients [32–37].

Structural MRI studies looking at cortical surface area, cortical thickness, and regional volumes demonstrate changes in multiple brain regions, including several known to be involved in pain processing such as the anterior cingulate, the medial orbital frontal cortex, the insula, and the temporal pole. Principle component analysis of structural imaging data enabled the development of a set of anatomical classifiers to differentiate between chronic and episodic migraine patients [38]. Furthermore, the anatomical differentiation between chronic and episodic migraine using this model is most accurate when using a threshold 15 headache days per month [38], further supporting the current definition of chronic migraine.

A few studies have utilized MRI to characterize alterations in iron homeostasis in the brainstem of patients with chronic migraine. Increased iron deposition in the periaqueductal gray positively correlates with the duration of migraine [34] and increased deposition of iron in the basal ganglia can differentiate between chronic vs. episodic migraineurs [39]. Resting-state functional connectivity of areas involved in pain such as the periaqueductal gray and anterior insula correlates with the frequency of attacks [40] and duration of chronic migraine [33].

Table 27.2 Comorbid conditions with increased prevalence on chronic migraine compared to episodic migraine patients

Comorbidities	Associated with		Odds ratio	95% confidence interval	p value
	CM (%)	EM (%)			
Arthritis	33.6	22.2	1.71	1.43–2.05	0.001
Chronic pain disorders other than migraine	31.5	15.1	2.49	2.08–2.97	0.001
Anxiety	30.2	18.8	1.80	1.51–2.15	0.001
Depression	30.2	17.2	2.00	1.67–2.4	0.001
Bipolar disorder	4.6	2.8	1.56	1.06–2.31	0.024
Obesity	5.0	21.0	1.24	1.03–1.50	0.020
Circulation problems	17.3	11.4	1.51	1.21–1.87	0.001
Heart disease	9.6	6.3	1.43	1.08–1.90	0.012
High blood pressure	33.7	27.8	1.23	1.03–1.47	0.021
Stroke	4.0	2.2	1.65	1.09–2.52	0.019
Allergies or Hay fever	59.9	50.7	1.47	1.25–1.73	0.001
Asthma	24.4	17.2	1.53	1.27–1.84	0.001
Bronchitis	19.2	12.9	1.54	1.25–1.89	0.001
Chronic bronchitis	9.2	4.5	1.99	1.49–2.65	0.001
Emphysema or COPD	4.9	2.6	1.73	1.18–2.54	0.005
Sinusitis	45.2	37.0	1.39	1.18–1.63	0.001
PTSD[a]	42.9	9.5			0.023

Data compiled from [30] and [31][a]

Neurophysiological studies illustrate alterations in the brainstem and cortical areas of patients with chronic migraine. Laser-evoked potentials (LEPs) that elicit nociceptive brain responses via activation of Aδ and C thermal nociceptors may be increased at baseline in chronic migraine patients [36] and lead to increased activation of the rostral anterior cingulate cortex compared to episodic migraine patients, which correlates with migraine frequency [37]. Visual evoked potentials measured via magnetoencephalography demonstrated increased occipital cortex excitability in interictal chronic migraine patients, which are similar to visual processing changes seen in patients with episodic migraine during an attack [41]. Furthermore, hyperexcitability of the occipital cortex in chronic migraine patients was demonstrated using magnetic suppression of perceptual accuracy with transcranial magnetic stimulation (TMS) [35].

Several small studies have examined a variety of molecules related to inflammation and pain processing, revealing altered molecular signaling pathways in chronic migraine compared to healthy controls. Patients with chronic migraine have interictal elevation of serum CGRP compared to EM patients [42]. Other biomarkers reported to be elevated in serum or CSF of chronic migraine patients include tumor necrosis factor-α [43], corticotrophin-releasing factor [44], orexin-A [44], taurine, glycine, and glutamine [45]. Lower levels of glial cell line-derived neurotrophic factor and somatostatin were found in chronic migraine patients compared to age-matched controls [46]. The melatonin metabolite 6-sulfatoxymelatonin is elevated in urine of patients with chronic migraine compared with patients with episodic migraine and healthy controls [47], perhaps indicating aberrant hypothalamic signaling. Recently, adipokine dysfunction has been implicated in both episodic and chronic migraine, as levels of adiponectin, resistin, and leptin were found to be elevated in chronic migraineurs compared to healthy controls [48].

While the inheritability of episodic migraine is well accepted, genetic factors that may or may not predispose to chronic migraine are not well established. It is possible that while episodic migraine has a strong genetic influence, the development of chronic migraine may be more dependent on environmental or epigenetic factors. A European candidate genome-wide association study looking for genetic factors associated with migraine chronification did not find any significant associations [49], though clearly more genetic studies are needed.

Chronic Tension-Type Headache

Classification

The classification of tension-type headache is controversial, mainly because the current classification lumps a heterogeneous group of patients together whose headaches do not necessarily reflect common neurobiological underpinnings. The clinical features of tension-type headaches are characterized by the absence of migraine-like features, and not based upon positive attributes or unique defining characteristics. However, a few neurophysiological, imaging, and genetic studies point toward potential distinguishing features of chronic tension-type headache.

ICHD-III Beta: Diagnostic Criteria

A. Headache occurring on ≥15 days per month on average for >3 months (≥180 days per year), fulfilling criteria B–D

B. Lasting hours to days or unremitting

C. At least two of the following four characteristics:
   1. Bilateral location
   2. Pressing or tightening (non-pulsating) quality
   3. Mild or moderate intensity
   4. Not aggravated by routine physical activity such as walking or climbing stairs

D. Both of the following:
   1. No more than one of photophobia, phonophobia, or mild nausea
   2. Neither moderate or severe nausea nor vomiting

E. Not better accounted for by another ICHD-III diagnosis

Other Features

Aside from eliminating secondary causes, it is important to distinguish chronic tension-type headache from chronic migraine, although this can be challenging. Patients with chronic tension-type headache have been noted to exhibit increased pericranial tenderness compared to migraine [50, 51] and increased pain sensitivity, which positively correlates with CTTH duration [52]. Pain intensities in extracranial muscles, such as the trapezius, also demonstrate changes in the pain response curve and increased sensitivity in patients with chronic tension-type headache compared to healthy controls [53]. One study has also found that patients with CTTH are more likely to drink alcohol on a daily or near-daily basis [54], which may be a helpful distinguishing factor from chronic migraine. Patients with chronic daily headache can technically fulfill the criteria for both chronic tension-type headache (>15 headaches per month fulfilling criteria for tension-type headache) and chronic migraine (>15 headache days with >8 headaches fulfilling criteria for chronic migraine), and these patients are given the diagnosis of chronic migraine headache only [17].

Epidemiology

Chronic tension-type headache occurs in 2–3% of population-based studies [55–57]. There is a slightly higher incidence of CTTH in women compared to men (5:4 [3], 5:2 [50]), and the average age of onset of TTH is higher than in migraine, ranging from 25 to 30 years in cross-sectional epidemiologic studies [58]. The prevalence of chronic tension-type headache peaks between ages 30 and 39 and decreases slightly with age [59].

Risk Factors

Triggers reported most frequently for TTH are fatigue and stress, either mental or physical. Only migraineurs had episodes of tension-type head-ache precipitated by alcohol, over-matured cheese, chocolate, and physical activity [60]. Risk factors for developing TTH include poor self-rated health, inability to relax after work, and sleeping fewer hours per night [61].

Comorbidities

Chronic tension-type headaches have been linked to depression [62] and vitamin D deficiency [63].

Pathophysiology

High-quality studies addressing the pathophysiological mechanisms underlying chronic tension headache are lacking or produce conflicting results among different research groups.

Clinical features of prominent cranial muscle tenderness led to the hypothesis that muscle-related factors may contribute to tension-type headache. Electromyography (EMG) of pericranial muscles demonstrates higher activity on average in CTTH patients compared to healthy controls; however neither elevated EMG activity [64] or hardness of muscle [65] correlates with pain severity. Furthermore, onabotulinumtoxinA injections into pericranial muscles, while decreasing electromyographic activity in pericranial muscles, do not relieve headaches [66]. There is no elevation of inflammatory mediators (prostaglandin E2, ATP, glutamate, or bradykinin) in tender points of patients with TTH compared to healthy controls, suggesting that tender points are not areas of ongoing inflammation [67]. Neurogenic inflammation also does not appear to play a key role in CTTH, as plasma concentrations of CGRP [68], substance P, neuropeptide Y, and vasoactive intestinal peptide are not different in patients with CTTH compared to healthy controls [69, 70].

Central sensitization plays a role in the transformation of ETT to CTTH. Patients with CTTH have generalized decreases in mechanical pain thresholds [71] and higher pain ratings with suprathreshold electrical stimulation [72] throughout their body compared to ETT patients or healthy controls, suggestive of a defect of central pain modulation. Differences in brainstem reflexes, such as decreases in the R2 amplitude of the nociceptive-specific blink reflex [73] and abnormal trigemino-cervical reflexes [74] are observed in patients with CTTH compared to ETTH. EMG studies also support a role for altered descending modulation of pain. Altered pain-induced inhibition of voluntary muscle activity in the temporalis muscle in CTTH patients [75] indirectly implicates inhibitory interneuron deficits. Glyceryl trinitrate produces an immediate headache without pericranial sensitivity followed by a typical tension-type headache hours later [76], similar to migraine. Nitric oxide synthase inhibitors decrease muscle hardness in patients with CTTH, perhaps through inhibition of central sensitization.

Structural studies using voxel-based morphometry demonstrate decreases in brain regions involved in pain processing such as the dorsal rostral and ventral pons, the anterior cingulate cortex, and the insula, in CTTH as compared to healthy controls or MOH patients [77]. These changes correlated positively with increasing headache duration.

Genetic studies examining the inheritance of chronic tension-type headaches indicate that first-degree relatives have a two- to fourfold risk of developing CTTH compared to the general population, suggesting a genetic component that likely follows a multifactorial inheritance pattern [78, 79].

Prognosis

Poor outcome was associated with baseline chronic TTH, coexisting migraine, not being married, and sleeping problems [61]. Overall, there is a general sense that the course of chronic tension-type headache is not as severe or protracted as chronic migraine. In-depth epidemiological studies for chronic tension-type headache have been scarce in part due to lack of consensus on its definition.

Clearly, the mechanisms underlying chronic tension-type headache are not well understood, and this may reflect insufficiency in the nosology of this entity. This gap is reflected in the lack of specific treatments and outcome data for patients with chronic tension-type headache.

Chronic Cluster Headache

Cluster headache is characterized by severe, unilateral retro-orbital/temporal pain lasting for 15 min to 3 h, usually associated with cranial autonomic parasympathetic features. Chronic cluster headache is defined as cluster headache attacks without periods of remission.

Classification

ICHD-III beta: cluster headache attacks occurring for more than 1 year without remission or with remission periods lasting less than 1 month

> **Diagnostic Criteria**
> A. Attacks fulfilling criteria for 3.1 cluster headache and criterion B below
> B. Occurring without a remission period or with remissions lasting <1 month, for at least 1 year

Other Features

Bouts of pain in chronic cluster headache occur anywhere from every other day up to eight times a day with a periodicity. Cluster headaches frequently peak in the early morning, midafternoon, or late evening and can occur nocturnally out of sleep [80, 81]. While patients with migraine headaches prefer lying down in a dark room during their headaches, patients with cluster headache tend to be restless and agitated and describe pacing around. Pain in cluster headache is often described as excruciating, with a boring, non-throbbing quality [82]. Furthermore, patients with chronic cluster headache may have a persistent baseline headache between cluster attacks, which can be confused for chronic migraine or hemicrania continua.

Individuals with CCH are more likely to report radiation of the pain to the upper teeth, jaw, cheek, ear, and shoulder. Rhinorrhea and osmophobia are more commonly reported features in CCH compared to episodic cluster headache. Shifting of the affected side within the same bout of headaches is infrequent but occurs with higher frequency in patients with chronic compared to episodic cluster headache [81].

Chronic cluster headache can be chronic at outset (primary) or arise from episodic cluster headache (secondary). Primary CCH represents about 2/3 patients, while secondary CCH reflects 1/3 of patients with CCH. Notable triggers of chronic cluster headache bouts include stress, alcohol, and weather changes [80]. Light exposure, crossing multiple time zones, and head trauma are also reported triggers of cluster headaches.

Epidemiology

The prevalence of cluster headache is 124/100,000 in population-based studies [83]. In a clinic-based study, 4% of patients with episodic cluster headache (ECH) converted to chronic cluster headache (CCH) over a period of 16 years [84]. In another study, 13% of ECH converted to CCH over 10 years [85]. The mean age of onset of chronic cluster tends to be higher than with episodic cluster headache (37 vs. 28). There is a striking male predominance of chronic cluster headache, with the male to female ratio for chronic cluster headache ranging from 4:1 [86] to as high as 15:1 [83].

Risk Factors

Later onset of cluster headache, the presence of sporadic attacks, a high frequency of cluster periods, and short-lived duration of remission periods are risk factors predicting the transition from episodic to chronic cluster headache [87]. External and lifestyle factors such as head trauma, cigarette smoking, and alcohol intake have also been proposed to have a negative effect on the clinical course of cluster headache, but have not been proven [87].

Comorbidities

Unlike chronic migraine, which is associated with higher rates of depression and anxiety compared to episodic migraine, little is known about the medical and psychiatric comorbidities of cluster headache, much less chronic cluster headache. Some studies have demonstrated an increased rate of mood disorders and depression in patients with chronic cluster headache [80, 88]. A recent pilot study suggests a lower rate of anxiety and depression in chronic cluster headache patients compared to historical healthy controls [89]. More detailed and comprehensive multicenter studies are needed to better characterize the medical and psychiatric comorbidities related to chronic cluster headache.

Pathophysiology

The trigeminovascular system is thought to play a key role in cluster headache pathophysiology. In particular, autonomic features of cluster headache are thought to arise via activation of the trigeminal parasympathetic reflex through the superior salivatory nucleus (SSN), which sends efferent projections via the sphenopalatine ganglion (SPG) to meningeal nociceptors. Activation of meningeal nociceptors leads to subsequent activation of the trigeminal nucleus caudalis, which facilitates trigeminal pain and further perpetuates activation of the SSN. In support of this theory, low-frequency stimulation of the SPG can provoke cluster-like attacks in patients with cluster headache, while high-frequency stimulation successfully treats these provoked attacks [90].

Functional brain PET imaging of patients with episodic cluster headache has highlighted a region in the posterior hypothalamus that is active during attacks but quiescent interictally [91], and MR brain imaging studies have confirmed structural changes in the same area in chronic cluster patients [92]. In animal studies, the hypothalamus is capable of modulating sensory pain activity both in the trigeminal nucleus caudalis [93, 94] and through direct connections to the SSN [95]. The circadian periodicity of cluster headaches implicates changes in hypothalamic signaling to the brainstem as potential markers or causative factors in the development of cluster headache bouts. Furthermore, there is evidence of decreased CSF hypocretin-1 in episodic and chronic cluster headache patients compared to healthy controls [96]. Finally, a large case series of patients with chronic cluster headache treated with deep brain stimulation in the hypothalamus demonstrated a greater than 50% clinical improvement in a majority of patients.

Thus far, there are limited studies differentiating the pathophysiology of chronic compared to episodic cluster headache. In addition to the clinical differences between chronic and episodic headache noted above, there are indications of alterations in biochemical pathways, such as tyrosine metabolism [97], in chronic cluster that have distinct profiles compared to patients with episodic cluster headache. In contrast to migraine, lack of habituation of the trigeminal nociceptive system has not been consistently demonstrated in chronic cluster headache [98], but there may be evidence of lateralized central facilitation of trigeminal nociception, as measured via electrically evoked V1 pain-related evoked potentials. In patients with episodic cluster headache, this facilitation occurs at the level of the brainstem, while in chronic cluster headache patients, there are additional changes in the evoked potentials corresponding to supraspinal facilitation at the thalamic or cortical level [99].

Prognosis

Limited longitudinal data exists for chronic cluster headache; however 33% of chronic cluster patients remit to episodic cluster [85].

Hemicrania Continua

First described in the 1980s [100, 101], hemicrania continua is characterized as a persistent, strictly unilateral headache with ipsilateral cranial autonomic features that is absolutely sensitive to indomethacin. It is distinguished from chronic

paroxysmal hemicranias by the presence of continuous, background headache without fluctuating periodicity. Although controversial [102, 103], HC is generally accepted as a trigeminal autonomic cephalalgia (TAC) and was included as such in the ICHD-III beta criteria. Opponents against the classification of hemicrania continua as a TAC argue that cranial autonomic symptoms should not be viewed as prominent features of this headache subtype [102].

Classification

Diagnostic Criteria
A. Unilateral headache fulfilling criteria B–D
B. Present for >3 months, with exacerbations of moderate or greater intensity
C. Either or both of the following:
1. At least one of the following symptoms or signs, ipsilateral to the headache:
(a) Conjunctival injection and/or lacrimation
(b) Nasal congestion and/or rhinorrhea
(c) Eyelid edema
(d) Forehead and facial sweating
(e) Forehead and facial flushing
(f) Sensation of fullness in the ear
(g) Miosis and/or ptosis
2. A sense of restlessness or agitation or aggravation of the pain by movement
D. Responds absolutely to therapeutic doses of indomethacin[1]
E. Not better accounted for by another ICHD-III diagnosis
1. In an adult, oral indomethacin should be used initially in a dose of at least 150 mg daily and increased if necessary up to 225 mg daily. The dose by injection is 100–200 mg. Smaller maintenance doses are often employed.

Other Features

Chronic background pain in hemicrania continua is punctuated by exacerbations of variable frequency (as opposed to CPH and CH where duration of attacks is more stereotyped). Pain intensity can fluctuate, though in general the pain is described as more moderate, and patients with HC are able to continue working, though work quality may be impacted. Eye itching or foreign body sensation in the eye and facial and cheek swelling are commonly reported. Most patients follow an unremitting subtype (60–80%), though some patients begin with a remitting headache punctured by breaks of headache freedom lasting anywhere from 1 day to several weeks.

Pain is commonly located predominantly in the V1 distribution, including temporal, frontal, orbital, or retro-orbital regions [104, 105] with spreading of pain to other regions during exacerbations [104]. Side-switching of pain [106] can occur and rare reports of bilateral pain [107] sensitive to indomethacin have been reported. Background pain is typically of mild to moderate intensity with dull and pressure-like characteristics, but throbbing and stabbing background pain is also reported. Exacerbations are often described as throbbing and/or stabbing. Lacrimation is the most commonly reported cranial autonomic symptom, and nasal congestion, conjunctival injection, and ptosis are most commonly reported cranial autonomic symptoms. Agitation during attacks as well as worsening of headache with movement can be features.

There can be overlap with migrainous features, as many patients report photophobia, with a lesser extent reporting phonophobia. The Indotest is used diagnostically in hemicrania continua, as HC patients respond absolutely to adequate levels of indomethacin, and the reappearance of pain upon indomethacin withdrawal is a positive confirmatory test. An additional placebo control has been proposed to be added to the Indotest to ensure the specificity of indomethacin as an effective treatment.

Epidemiology

Given the rarity of the disease, the prevalence of hemicrania continua has been difficult to assess and only a few hundred cases have been published in the literature. However, one headache center diagnosed 34 new cases of HC over a 3-year period, suggesting the disorder is more common than once thought [108]. One relatively large prospective case series looking at chronic daily headache found the prevalence of HC to be 0.8% [109]. There is a slight skew toward female predominance for HC, with a male to female ration ranging from 1:1.8 to 1:2.8, and the pooled mean age at onset is 40 years old, but the range of reported HC cases includes patients from age 5 to 77 [110].

Hemicrania continua is often misdiagnosed with a mean time to diagnosis ranging from 5 to 12 years. Factors contributing to misdiagnosis include a paucity of autonomic symptoms, overuse of analgesics, and atypical aggravating factors [111]. Another potential contributing factor is missing the presence of background pain in the history, as patients can tend to focus on exacerbations. Instead, hemicrania continua is often confused with migraine, cluster headache, dental pain, and sinus headache [111].

Evaluation for secondary causes of headache with head imaging, as with all TACs, should be performed. There are numerous secondary causes of HC including head injury [112], postpartum [113], post craniotomy [114], venous malformation [115], ipsilateral brainstem infarction [116], leprosy [117], pituitary adenoma [118], osteoid osteoma [119], nonmetastatic lung cancer [120, 121], internal carotid artery dissection [122], and pineal cyst [123]. Furthermore, secondary HC may be responsive to indomethacin, so a positive indomethacin response should not be used as a rationale to forgo imaging studies.

Pathophysiology

Responsiveness to indomethacin suggests a specific underlying mechanism, but delineation of this mechanism has been elusive. PET studies have demonstrated significant activation in the contralateral posterior hypothalamus (similar to cluster headache) in patients during headaches compared to without headache on indomethacin, as well as ipsilateral dorsal rostral pons (similar to migraine) and ipsilateral ventrolateral midbrain and bilateral pontomedullary junction [124].

Prognosis

Most patients relapse with withdrawal of indomethacin; however 42% of patients could reduce their effective dose by more than 50% [125].

New Daily Persistent Headache

New daily persistent headache (NDPH) was first described in a case series by Vanast in 1986 [126]. Previously used terms for NDPH include chronic headache with acute onset and de novo chronic headache. New daily headache is characterized by a persistent headache, daily from its onset, which is clearly remembered. Patients can often recall the exact date, time, and what they were doing at the time. The pain lacks characteristic features and may be migraine-like and tension-type-like or have elements of both.

NDPH was first included in the ICHD-II classification; however this initial definition excluded migrainous features, including moderate or severe nausea or vomiting, and patients could have no more than one of photophobia, phonophobia, or mild nausea. In ICHD-III, the definition of NDPH was revised to allow inclusion of migrainous features. Patients with headaches that fulfill both criteria for NDPH and CM (or CTTH) are given the default diagnosis of NDPH. In contrast, patients that fulfill criteria for both NDPH and hemicrania continua are given the diagnosis of HC.

Classification

Diagnostic Criteria
A. Persistent headache fulfilling criteria B and C
B. Distinct and clearly remembered onset, with pain becoming continuous and unremitting within 24 h
C. Present for >3 months
D. Not better accounted for by another ICHD-III diagnosis

Other Features

Headache in NDPH is generally described as mild to severe intensity, with variable pain location, and often associated with migrainous features of vomiting, nausea, photophobia, and phonophobia.

While NDPH has a clear history of onset that distinguishes it from CM and CTTH, it is not clear whether NDPH is a distinct entity or whether it is a syndrome that encompasses a number of disorders [127]. It is important to exclude secondary causes, particularly spontaneous intracranial hypotension, as well as venous sinus thrombosis, intracranial hypertension, carotid or vertebral artery dissection, meningitis, sphenoid sinusitis, posttraumatic headache, and cervical facet syndrome. As such, patients should receive thorough head and neck imaging, including MRI with and without contrast, MRV, and MRA.

Epidemiology

The 1-year population prevalence of NDPH is anywhere from 0.03% [128] to 0.1% [2], and there is a slight female predominance [129]. Median age of onset of NDPH is in the 20s for women and in the 50s for men [129, 130].

Risk Factors

NDPH often follows a preceding viral illness, and EBV infection can be associated with NDPH. Suggested predisposing factors include cervical joint hypermobility or a stressful life event [131].

Comorbidities

NDPH patients have a higher prevalence of anxiety [132], depression, somatization, and pain catastrophization compared to healthy patients or patients with chronic low back pain [133]. Medication overuse is documented in over 1/3 of NDPH patients [130, 134].

Pathophysiology

The underlying mechanisms of NDPH are not well understood, which may reflect the notion that NDPH is an umbrella term for many distinct entities. Because NDPH is often linked to a preceding viral infection, it is postulated that CNS immune activation may play a role in the pathophysiology of NDPH. To support this idea, Rozen and Swiden found elevated levels of the pro-inflammatory cytokine TNFα in the CSF from 19 out of 20 patients with NDPH [43].

Prognosis

In general, the prognosis for NDPH is poor. Although the majority of patients with NDPH described by Vanast achieved complete headache remission over 2 years, other case studies have demonstrated that NDPH can persist for years and become refractory to treatment. A subset of patients with NDPH, more often those who have had symptoms for less than 6 months, can have a self-limited course, and a relapsing remitting form has also been described in a minority of patients [134]. Up to 76% of NDPH patients can experience persistent headache for more than 2 years, with only about 14% of patients achieving headache remission [134]. NDPH with a migrainous phenotype may portend a worse outcome compared to NDPH patients without migrainous features [130].

Medication-Overuse Headache

Medication-overuse headache is listed by the World Health Organization as the 20th leading cause of morbidity worldwide [135]. The category of medication-overuse headache is intrinsically controversial and poses several challenges to classification. Whether medication overuse is the root cause or manifesting symptom of worsening headaches is not known and highly debated. Thus far, discontinuation of acute medication has not been shown conclusively to produce improvement of headaches in a controlled study. Similarly, Scher and colleagues proposed that proving the existence of MOH would require the randomization of patients with episodic headaches to either limited or frequent use of acute medications in order to document the development of worsening headache with medication overuse [136]. Neither of these studies is feasible in the United States. Observational studies suggest that withdrawal of medications can lead to reduction of headaches in a subset of patients, although it is not clear whether this reduction in headaches reflects reversion to the mean or an intervention effect (either placebo or medication withdrawal itself).

The first formal definition of medication-overuse headache (MOH) appeared in the ICHD-II criteria and included typical headache features associated with the specific medications used. The idea of medication-specific clinical subtypes was challenged, as differential headache features did not bear out with rigorous clinical data collection. The number of days of medication overuse and the overall length of time of medication overuse are also not based on formal evidence, although certain medications do seem to have a higher propensity toward medication overuse, such as the barbiturates, opioids, and combination analgesics.

In 2005, a revision for the definition of MOH was developed based on constructive criticism given at the International Headache Research Seminar in Copenhagen in March 2004. This revision included "(i) elimination of the headache characteristics for each MOH subtype; and (ii) a new subform that takes into account patients over-using medications of different classes but not any single class (combination of acute medications)" [137]. In the 2006 ICHD-II revised criteria, the requirement for medication withdrawal was dispensed for the diagnosis of medication-overuse headache. These revised criteria (ICHD-IIR) were published in 2011. Critics of the revised criteria felt that although the criteria may be more applicable to clinical application, they may hamper rigorous research on the basic mechanisms of MOH, and the definition of MOH in large-scale epidemiological studies may make results more difficult to interpret.

Another limitation of the ICHD-II definition of MOH required two clinic visits and at least 2 months of medication withdrawal before the diagnosis could be given. For example, if medication overuse was present, then a diagnosis of probable chronic migraine and MOH were given. If headache improved after medication withdrawal, then MOH was confirmed. In the most recent proposed criteria for headache disorders, the ICHD-III beta, patients meeting criteria for chronic migraine and medication-overuse headache should be given both diagnoses. After drug withdrawal, the patient can be re-diagnosed accordingly, either as episodic migraine with medication-overuse headache or chronic migraine.

While medication-overuse headache is often thought of as a secondary headache, there is debate as to whether MOH is a complication of migraine and thus should be characterized under primary headache disorders, specifically as a complication of migraine. Medication overuse in itself is not sufficient to cause or exacerbate headache, and there is clinical evidence that MOH occurs predominantly in the background of migraine [138].

Classification

Headache occurring on 15 or more days per month developing as a consequence of regular overuse of acute or symptomatic headache medication (on 10 or more or 15 or more days per month, depending on the medication) for more than 3 months. It usually, but not invariably,

Diagnostic Criteria

A. Headache occurring on ≥ 15 days per month in a patient with a preexisting headache disorder
B. Regular overuse for >3 months of one or more drugs that can be taken for acute and/or symptomatic treatment of headache [1]
C. Not better accounted for by another ICHD-III diagnosis

resolves after the overuse is stopped.

General comment: In the criteria set out below for the various subtypes, the specified numbers of days of medication use considered to constitute overuse are based on expert opinion rather than on formal evidence.

Epidemiology

The prevalence of medication-overuse headache in the general population is close to 2% [139–141] with a male to female ratio of 1:3 [141, 142] and peak prevalence in the fifth decade [141].

Risk Factors and Comorbidities

There is an increased prevalence of active smokers and obesity in patients with medication-overuse headache [142]. MOH is also associated with increased frequency cardiovascular comorbidities such as hypertension, diabetes, and a history of myocardial infarction [142]. The prevalence of MOH is higher in individuals with lower education level and lower annual income [141].

Pathophysiology

Animal studies point toward medication overuse as a condition with discernible features and changes in neural circuitry. For example, upregulation of CGRP and neuronal nitric oxide synthase (nNOS) in trigeminal ganglia dural afferents occurs with both prolonged triptan and chronic opioid exposure [143, 144]. Intriguingly, subthreshold pain hypersensitivity can be unmasked even after cessation of medication exposure with either stress or administration of a NO donor [144]. Furthermore, imaging studies in humans demonstrate functional metabolic and connectivity differences between patients with chronic migraine and medication overuse [145, 146]. Clinical data indicates that MOH may require an underlying migraine (or other primary headache) phenotype [138, 147], arguing against a purely independent neurobiology.

A number of genetic polymorphisms related to dopaminergic signaling and addiction pathways have been associated with medication-overuse headache; however none of these associations have been replicated or validated in an independent cohort of medication-overuse patients [148]. While these studies suggest a possible genetic predisposition toward development of medication-overuse headache, better designed studies are required.

Prognosis

The prognosis of medication-overuse headache is linked to successful detoxification from medications. There is an estimated 20–40% relapse rate after medication detoxification within the first year [149–151].

Persistent Secondary Headaches

Persistent secondary headaches are most commonly a result of traumatic injury to the head and neck. ICHD-III separates out posttraumatic headache into three major categories based on the mechanism of trauma: injury to the head, injury attributed to whiplash, and injury attributed to craniotomy. Secondary headaches may also arise due to cranial or cervical vascular disorders, intracranial pathology, infection, disrupted homeostasis, or disorders of the cranium, cervical spine, temporomandibular joint, and eyes. These secondary headaches tend to improve with amelioration or treatment of the underlying disorder and will not be discussed here.

Persistent Headache Attributed to Traumatic Injury to the Head

By definition, persistent headache attributed to traumatic injury to the head or chronic posttraumatic headache (PTH) begins within 7 days of trauma or after consciousness is regained after trauma; however this cutoff is controversial, as new headaches have been reported to arise even 3 months after TBI [152]. These criteria were modified from the ICHD-I diagnostic criteria, which allowed for a time interval of up to 14 days. Similarly, the time landmark of 3 months delineating between acute and chronic PTH may be arbitrary [153]. Patients who experience worsening of a primary headache directly after head trauma are also given both a diagnosis of chronic migraine (or tension-type headache) and persistent PTH according to ICHD-III, and this was amended from the ICHD-II criteria, which maintained patients in this category under preexisting

Diagnostic Criteria

A. Any headache fulfilling criteria C and D.

B. Traumatic injury to the head has occurred.

C. Headache is reported to have developed within 7 days after one of the following:
1. The injury to the head
2. Regaining of consciousness following the injury to the head
3. Discontinuation of medication(s) that impair ability to sense or report headache following the injury to the head

D. Headache persists for >3 months after the injury to the head.

E. Not better accounted for by another ICHD-III diagnosis.

migraine exacerbated by headache attributable to head injury.

Classification

Description: headache of greater than 3 months' duration caused by traumatic injury to the head

Other Features

Chronic PTH does not have any unique clinical features. The most commonly reported characteristics of persistent headache due to TBI are migraine or tension-type headache features [154, 155], though characteristics of other primary headaches have been reported. Headaches are not necessarily localized to the site of head injury. PTH is often accompanied by post-concussive symptoms such as dizziness, tinnitus, photophobia, phonophobia, blurred vision, decreased smell, fatigue, impaired attention, decreased concentration, slowed mental processing, impaired memory, and irritability. These post-concussive symptoms are not distinctive for post-concussive syndrome, and most are indistinguishable from migraine.

Epidemiology

Posttraumatic headache occurs in 30–90% of patients after TBI, and 18–22% of patients continue to experience PTH headache after 1 year [156, 157]. In population-based surveys, the prevalence of PTH is found to be 0.2% [140]. People with pre-injury history of headache are more likely to develop PTH [158]. In the civilian population, the most common modes of head injury are motor vehicle accidents, falls, occupational accidents, and sports injuries. Blast injury from combat zones is the most common source of TBI leading to persistent headache in military personnel [159]. Some studies demonstrate that posttraumatic headaches are paradoxically more likely to occur after mild TBI [160, 161]. However, other studies have found similar rates of chronic PTH arising from mild compared to moderate/severe TBI [152, 162].

Comorbidities and Risk Factors in PTH Chronification

There is a 30% prevalence of PTSD in patients with chronic posttraumatic headache [163], and this tends to be higher in combat-related injuries. In deployed military personnel, PTSD symptoms were correlated with PTH severity [164]. Depression, anxiety, and cognitive complaints are also associated with PTH [165].

Risk factors for developing chronic PTH include insomnia, multiple concussions, and lower socioeconomic status [164, 166]. Older age (>60 years) may be protective against PTH [154].

Pathophysiology

A large component of acute pain after head or neck trauma is often attributed to musculoskeletal injuries, but trauma to the head can also result in cortical contusions or diffuse axonal injury due to shearing forces [167]. Injury to white matter tracts can be observed with diffusion tensor imaging as changes in fractional anisotropy (FA) that can persist for up to 6 months after traumatic brain injury [168]. Decreased FA in the splenium and increased FA in the genu of the corpus callosum are associated with patients with TBI who develop PTH [169].

On a cellular level, the physical impact of concussion in animal models causes sudden stretching of neuronal membranes, leading to unregulated flux of ions across channels and excessive release of excitatory neurotransmitters. Increased excitatory activity in cells trying to restore resting membrane potential leads to increased energy demand with decreased oxidative capacity from stunned mitochondria. This metabolic cascade of events renders neurons vulnerable to cell death, particularly in response to repeated injury [170, 171], which may be a mechanistic explanation for why cumulative head injury over time predisposes individuals to the development of posttraumatic headache.

Impairment of cerebral vascular autoregulation can also occur after brain injury, and higher cerebral vasoreactivity, as measured by transcranial Doppler coupled to end-tidal CO_2, correlates with increased severity of posttraumatic headaches [172].

Factors playing a role in PTH chronification include central sensitization from axonal injury of pain-inhibiting structures of the brainstem and abnormal cortical processing [153]. Underscoring persistent alterations in central pain processing mechanisms, quantitative sensory testing in chronic PTH patients demonstrates mechanical hyperalgesia and allodynia over the cranium [173] and changes in conditioned pain modulation, also known as diffuse noxious inhibitory control, which is lower in patients with chronic PTH [174]. A recent MRI study demonstrates differences in brain structure in patients with persistent PTH compared to patients with chronic migraine [175], likely indicating unique pathophysiology of PTH.

Prognosis

While most patients with PTH improve with time, up to 23% of patients continue to have headache at 1 year after injury [152]. Patients who continue to have frequent headaches at 1 year may continue to have chronic PTH after 5 years [176], though this has not been directly studied. Outcomes tend to be worse for older patients, female gender, and those with comorbid depression and anxiety. More severe headaches develop with penetrating TBI and pre-injury headaches [158].

Chronic Daily Headache in Children and Adolescents

Chronic daily headaches may also affect children and adolescents, with frequent headaches affecting children as young as 2 years old [177]. Identification of primary headache in children can be difficult for parents and healthcare providers due to the common belief that migraine only affects adults. As a result, a definite diagnosis for recurrent headache is often delayed by

12–36 months and more likely to be delayed for younger children [178]. CDH may significantly impact the quality of life in this age group, leading to frequent absenteeism from school and can also affect sleep [177]. Diagnosis and management of headaches in this age group can be challenging for a number of reasons. There are no specific CDH criteria for children, and many of the treatments used in adults for CDH are either not effective or not well-tolerated in children.

Clinical Features

As with adults, chronic migraine and chronic tension-type headaches are the most frequent subtype of headache in children [179]. Clinical features of migraine headache in children may differ from adults, in that headaches may be of shorter duration, headache location is more likely to be bilateral, and photophobia and phonophobia are more likely to be inferred by behavior [17]. Headache location tends to be more frontal and temporal, with a subset describing facial migraine pain. On the other hand, exclusive occipital pain is rare in children and should prompt further diagnostic investigation.

In young children, recognized variations of migraine include cyclical vomiting syndrome, abdominal migraine, benign paroxysmal vertigo, vestibular migraine, benign paroxysmal torticollis, infantile colic, and alternating hemiplegia of childhood [17].

Epidemiology

Chronic daily headache affects 1.5–3.5% of children and adolescents [180–182]. There is a higher prevalence of chronic daily headache in girls compared to boys, even prior to adolescence (approximately 2:1) [181, 182].

Chronic Daily Headache in Elderly

Although primary headache disorders generally begin at a younger age, they may become chronic at older ages, and 5.4% of all de novo headaches occur in patients 65 years and older [183]. Secondary headache is more common in the elderly, and new headaches arising in this population should prompt a thorough work-up. From population-based studies, around 4% of the total elderly population experiences chronic daily headache [184, 185]. There may be some phenotypic differences in elderly patients with primary headache disorders. For example, patients with migraines between 60 and 70 years of age were less likely to have unilateral headaches, nausea, vomiting, photophobia, and phonophobia compared to younger migraine patients. Instead, elderly patients with migraine were more likely to describe paleness, dry mouth, and anorexia as symptoms of migraine [186]. Furthermore, case reports have documented late-life migrainous accompaniments in the elderly, such as visual aura, sensory symptoms, motor weakness, vertigo, and other brainstem symptoms [187]. These symptoms can pose a diagnostic challenge in differentiating between migraine versus stroke or transient ischemic attacks.

Hypnic headache is a primary headache disorder described exclusively in the elderly with a mean age of onset of 60 years old. Pain in hypnic headache is described as diffuse, non-throbbing, and moderate in severity.

Important secondary causes to rule out include temporal arteritis, nocturnal seizures with post-

ictal headache, and obstructive sleep apnea with headache. Because hypnic headache arises during sleep at night, it can often be differentiated from cluster headache by the low degree of cranial autonomic features. The clinical prevalence of hypnic headache is 0.07–0.4%. A majority of patients with hypnic headache experience headaches upon wakening more than four times per week [188], with the length of headaches averaging between 15 and 180 min.

Because it is so rare and often misdiagnosed, the prognosis of hypnic headache is not well studied. A systematic analysis of published case reports on hypnic headache demonstrated spontaneous remission in about 5% of reported cases and 43% remission in patients treated with prophylactic agents [189].

Overall, treatment of headache in the elderly should take into account the higher frequency of coexisting medical conditions and polypharmacy. Elderly patients have decreased medication tolerance due to reduced hepatic and renal clearance, so lower doses of acute and preventive medications should be used and slowly titrated to effect.

Refractory Headaches

In general, refractory headaches have failed multiple classes of acute and preventive treatments at adequate doses for an adequate time period due to lack of efficacy. Surprisingly, a consensus on the definition of refractory headache has not been reached nor defined in the ICHD classifications. Schulman et al. have proposed criteria for refractory migraine based on surveying members of the American Headache Society: proposed criteria for refractory migraine include (1) the fulfillment of criteria for migraine or chronic migraine and (2) significant interference with function and quality of life despite adequate trials of abortive and preventive medications. Adequate trials of preventives include adequate doses of at least 2 months at maximally tolerated doses alone or in combination, from at least two different drug classes. For abortive medications, intranasal and injectable formulations of triptans and/or dihydroer-

---

Hypnic Headache Criteria

A. Recurrent headache attacks fulfilling criteria B through E

B. Developing only during sleep and causing wakening

C. Occurring on ≥10 days per month for more than 3 months

D. Lasting ≥15 min and for up to 4 h after waking

E. No cranial autonomic symptoms or restlessness

F. Not better accounted for by another ICHD-III diagnosis

gotamine (DHE) should be trialed in addition to either NSAIDs or combination analgesics [190]. This definition may be included into the ICHD as a separate chapter, a refractory subset for each headache type, an "R" modifier for refractoriness, or as a new axis [191].

One reason that no formal definition exists may be that refractory headaches reflect difficult to treat headaches of existing categories. Nevertheless, a formal operational definition will help provide a framework to generate better characterization and epidemiological data for refractory headaches to establish risk factors, evaluate unmet medical needs, and guide treatment. Furthermore, there may be common mechanisms of treatment refractory headaches that could be investigated in translational or laboratory settings.

Summary

Chronic daily headaches, i.e., headaches occurring on more days than not, as a group represent a serious world health problem affecting more than 100 million people worldwide. While treatable secondary causes must be excluded, most CDH is caused by primary headache disorders, whose definitions often overlap. Clearly, a deeper understanding of the distinctions between these disorders is needed. Ongoing discussion of clinical phenotypes in relationship to risk factors, epidemiology, and treatment response is critical, as is the continued study of underlying pathophysiological mechanisms of headache. When progress is made in these respects, perhaps more successful treatment outcomes will be achieved.

References

1. Scher AI, Stewart WF, Liberman J, Lipton RB. Prevalence of frequent headache in a population sample. Headache. 1998;38(7):497–506.
2. Castillo J, Munoz P, Guitera V, Pascual J. Kaplan Award 1998. Epidemiology of chronic daily headache in the general population. Headache. 1999;39(3):190–6.
3. Stovner L, Hagen K, Jensen R, et al. The global burden of headache: a documentation of headache prevalence and disability worldwide. Cephalalgia. 2007;27(3):193–210.
4. Lipton RB, Stewart WF, Merikangas KR. Reliability in headache diagnosis. Cephalalgia. 1993;13(Suppl 12):29–33.
5. Ramadan NM, Olesen J. Classification of headache disorders. Semin Neurol. 2006;26(2):157–62.
6. Mathew NT, Stubits E, Nigam MP. Transformation of episodic migraine into daily headache: analysis of factors. Headache. 1982;22(2):66–8.
7. Mathew NT. Transformed migraine. Cephalalgia. 1993;13(Suppl 12):78–83.
8. Manzoni GC, Granella F, Sandrini G, Cavallini A, Zanferrari C, Nappi G. Classification of chronic daily headache by International Headache Society criteria: limits and new proposals. Cephalalgia. 1995;15(1):37–43.
9. Silberstein SD, Lipton RB, Sliwinski M. Classification of daily and near-daily headaches: field trial of revised IHS criteria. Neurology. 1996;47(4):871–5.
10. Siberstein SD, Lipton RB, Solomon S, Mathew NT. Classification of daily and near-daily headaches: proposed revisions to the IHS criteria. Headache. 1994;34(1):1–7.
11. Headache Classification Committee of the International Headache Society. Classification and diagnostic criteria for headache disorders, cranial neuralgias and facial pain. Cephalalgia. 1988;8(Suppl 7):1–96.
12. Headache Classification Subcommittee of the International Headache Society. The international classification of headache disorders: 2nd edition. Cephalalgia. 2004;24(Suppl 1):9–160.
13. Bigal ME, Tepper SJ, Sheftell FD, Rapoport AM, Lipton RB. Chronic daily headache: correlation between the 2004 and the 1988 International Headache Society diagnostic criteria. Headache. 2004;44(7):684–91.
14. Manzoni GC, Torelli P. Epidemiological classification and social impact of chronic headache. Intern Emerg Med. 2010;5(Suppl 1):S1–5.
15. Solomon S. New appendix criteria open for a broader concept of chronic migraine. Cephalalgia. 2007;27(5):469; author reply 469–70.
16. Seshia SS, Wober-Bingol C, Guidetti V. The classification of chronic headache: room for further improvement? Cephalalgia. 2010;30(10):1268–70.
17. Headache Classification Committee of the International Headache Society. The international classification of headache disorders, 3rd edition (beta version). Cephalalgia. 2013;33(9):629–808.
18. Levin M. Chronic daily headache and the revised international headache society classification. Curr Pain Headache Rep. 2004;8(1):59–65.

19. Viana M, Sances G, Ghiotto N, et al. Variability of the characteristics of a migraine attack within patients. Cephalalgia. 2016;36(9):825–30.

20. Kelman L. Pain characteristics of the acute migraine attack. Headache. 2006;46(6):942–53.

21. Yalin OO, Uluduz D, Ozge A, Sungur MA, Selekler M, Siva A. Phenotypic features of chronic migraine. J Headache Pain. 2016;17:26.

22. Natoli JL, Manack A, Dean B, et al. Global prevalence of chronic migraine: a systematic review. Cephalalgia. 2010;30(5):599–609.

23. Buse DC, Manack AN, Fanning KM, et al. Chronic migraine prevalence, disability, and sociodemographic factors: results from the American Migraine Prevalence and Prevention Study. Headache. 2012;52(10):1456–70.

24. Scher AI, Midgette LA, Lipton RB. Risk factors for headache chronification. Headache. 2008;48(1):16–25.

25. Reed ML, Fanning KM, Serrano D, Buse DC, Lipton RB. Persistent frequent nausea is associated with progression to chronic migraine: AMPP study results. Headache. 2015;55(1):76–87.

26. Scher AI, Buse DC, Fanning KM, et al. Comorbid pain and migraine chronicity: the Chronic Migraine Epidemiology and Outcomes Study. Neurology. 2017;89:461.

27. Louter MA, Bosker JE, van Oosterhout WP, et al. Cutaneous allodynia as a predictor of migraine chronification. Brain. 2013;136(Pt 11):3489–96.

28. Bigal ME, Serrano D, Buse D, Scher A, Stewart WF, Lipton RB. Acute migraine medications and evolution from episodic to chronic migraine: a longitudinal population-based study. Headache. 2008;48(8):1157–68.

29. Lipton RB, Fanning KM, Serrano D, Reed ML, Cady R, Buse DC. Ineffective acute treatment of episodic migraine is associated with new-onset chronic migraine. Neurology. 2015;84(7):688–95.

30. Buse DC, Manack A, Serrano D, Turkel C, Lipton RB. Sociodemographic and comorbidity profiles of chronic migraine and episodic migraine sufferers. J Neurol Neurosurg Psychiatry. 2010;81(4):428–32.

31. Peterlin BL, Tietjen G, Meng S, Lidicker J, Bigal M. Post-traumatic stress disorder in episodic and chronic migraine. Headache. 2008;48(4):517–22.

32. Valfre W, Rainero I, Bergui M, Pinessi L. Voxel-based morphometry reveals gray matter abnormalities in migraine. Headache. 2008;48(1):109–17.

33. Schwedt TJ, Schlaggar BL, Mar S, et al. Atypical resting-state functional connectivity of affective pain regions in chronic migraine. Headache. 2013;53(5):737–51.

34. Welch KM, Nagesh V, Aurora SK, Gelman N. Periaqueductal gray matter dysfunction in migraine: cause or the burden of illness? Headache. 2001;41(7):629–37.

35. Aurora SK, Barrodale PM, Tipton RL, Khodavirdi A. Brainstem dysfunction in chronic migraine as evidenced by neurophysiological and positron emission tomography studies. Headache. 2007;47(7):996–1003; discussion 1004–7.

36. de Tommaso M, Valeriani M, Guido M, et al. Abnormal brain processing of cutaneous pain in patients with chronic migraine. Pain. 2003;101(1–2):25–32.

37. de Tommaso M, Losito L, Difruscolo O, Libro G, Guido M, Livrea P. Changes in cortical processing of pain in chronic migraine. Headache. 2005;45(9):1208–18.

38. Schwedt TJ, Chong CD, Wu T, Gaw N, Fu Y, Li J. Accurate classification of chronic migraine via brain magnetic resonance imaging. Headache. 2015;55(6):762–77.

39. Tepper SJ, Lowe MJ, Beall E, et al. Iron deposition in pain-regulatory nuclei in episodic migraine and chronic daily headache by MRI. Headache. 2012;52(2):236–43.

40. Mainero C, Boshyan J, Hadjikhani N. Altered functional magnetic resonance imaging resting-state connectivity in periaqueductal gray networks in migraine. Ann Neurol. 2011;70(5):838–45.

41. Chen WT, Wang SJ, Fuh JL, Lin CP, Ko YC, Lin YY. Persistent ictal-like visual cortical excitability in chronic migraine. Pain. 2011;152(2):254–8.

42. Cernuda-Morollon E, Larrosa D, Ramon C, Vega J, Martinez-Camblor P, Pascual J. Interictal increase of CGRP levels in peripheral blood as a biomarker for chronic migraine. Neurology. 2013;81(14):1191–6.

43. Rozen T, Swidan SZ. Elevation of CSF tumor necrosis factor alpha levels in new daily persistent headache and treatment refractory chronic migraine. Headache. 2007;47(7):1050–5.

44. Sarchielli P, Rainero I, Coppola F, et al. Involvement of corticotrophin-releasing factor and orexin-A in chronic migraine and medication-overuse headache: findings from cerebrospinal fluid. Cephalalgia. 2008;28(7):714–22.

45. Rothrock JF, Mar KR, Yaksh TL, Golbeck A, Moore AC. Cerebrospinal fluid analyses in migraine patients and controls. Cephalalgia. 1995;15(6):489–93.

46. Sarchielli P, Alberti A, Candeliere A, Floridi A, Capocchi G, Calabresi P. Glial cell line-derived neurotrophic factor and somatostatin levels in cerebrospinal fluid of patients affected by chronic migraine and fibromyalgia. Cephalalgia. 2006;26(4):409–15.

47. Masruha MR, Lin J, de Souza Vieira DS, et al. Urinary 6-sulphatoxymelatonin levels are depressed in chronic migraine and several comorbidities. Headache. 2010;50(3):413–9.

48. Rubino E, Vacca A, Govone F, et al. Investigating the role of adipokines in chronic migraine. Cephalalgia. 2017;37(11):1067–73.

49. Louter MA, Fernandez-Morales J, de Vries B, et al. Candidate-gene association study searching for genetic factors involved in migraine chronification. Cephalalgia. 2015;35(6):500–7.

50. Jensen R. Pathophysiological mechanisms of tension-type headache: a review of epidemio-

logical and experimental studies. Cephalalgia. 1999;19(6):602–21.

51. Buchgreitz L, Lyngberg AC, Bendtsen L, Jensen R. Frequency of headache is related to sensitization: a population study. Pain. 2006;123(1–2):19–27.

52. Buchgreitz L, Lyngberg AC, Bendtsen L, Jensen R. Increased pain sensitivity is not a risk factor but a consequence of frequent headache: a population-based follow-up study. Pain. 2008;137(3):623–30.

53. Ashina S, Babenko L, Jensen R, Ashina M, Magerl W, Bendtsen L. Increased muscular and cutaneous pain sensitivity in cephalic region in patients with chronic tension-type headache. Eur J Neurol. 2005;12(7):543–9.

54. Schramm SH, Obermann M, Katsarava Z, Diener HC, Moebus S, Yoon MS. Epidemiological profiles of patients with chronic migraine and chronic tension-type headache. J Headache Pain. 2013;14:40.

55. Rasmussen BK, Jensen R, Schroll M, Olesen J. Epidemiology of headache in a general population--a prevalence study. J Clin Epidemiol. 1991;44(11):1147–57.

56. Russell MB. Tension-type headache in 40-year-olds: a Danish population-based sample of 4000. J Headache Pain. 2005;6(6):441–7.

57. Schwartz BS, Stewart WF, Simon D, Lipton RB. Epidemiology of tension-type headache. JAMA. 1998;279(5):381–3.

58. Rasmussen BK. Epidemiology of headache. Cephalalgia. 1995;15(1):45–68.

59. Russell MB, Levi N, Saltyte-Benth J, Fenger K. Tension-type headache in adolescents and adults: a population based study of 33,764 twins. Eur J Epidemiol. 2006;21(2):153–60.

60. Ulrich V, Russell MB, Jensen R, Olesen J. A comparison of tension-type headache in migraineurs and in non-migraineurs: a population-based study. Pain. 1996;67(2–3):501–6.

61. Lyngberg AC, Rasmussen BK, Jorgensen T, Jensen R. Prognosis of migraine and tension-type headache: a population-based follow-up study. Neurology. 2005;65(4):580–5.

62. Yucel B, Kora K, Ozyalcin S, Alcalar N, Ozdemir O, Yucel A. Depression, automatic thoughts, alexithymia, and assertiveness in patients with tension-type headache. Headache. 2002;42(3):194–9.

63. Prakash S, Rathore C, Makwana P, Dave A, Joshi H, Parekh H. Vitamin D deficiency in patients with chronic tension-type headache: a case-control study. Headache. 2017;57(7):1096–108.

64. Schoenen J, Gerard P, De Pasqua V, Juprelle M. EMG activity in pericranial muscles during postural variation and mental activity in healthy volunteers and patients with chronic tension type headache. Headache. 1991;31(5):321–4.

65. Ashina M, Bendtsen L, Jensen R, Sakai F, Olesen J. Muscle hardness in patients with chronic tension-type headache: relation to actual headache state. Pain. 1999;79(2–3):201–5.

66. Rollnik JD, Karst M, Fink M, Dengler R. Botulinum toxin type A and EMG: a key to the understanding of chronic tension-type headaches? Headache. 2001;41(10):985–9.

67. Ashina M, Stallknecht B, Bendtsen L, et al. Tender points are not sites of ongoing inflammation - in vivo evidence in patients with chronic tension-type headache. Cephalalgia. 2003;23(2):109–16.

68. Ashina M, Bendtsen L, Jensen R, Schifter S, Jansen-Olesen I, Olesen J. Plasma levels of calcitonin gene-related peptide in chronic tension-type headache. Neurology. 2000;55(9):1335–40.

69. Ashina M, Bendtsen L, Jensen R, Lassen LH, Sakai F, Olesen J. Possible mechanisms of action of nitric oxide synthase inhibitors in chronic tension-type headache. Brain. 1999;122(Pt 9):1629–35.

70. Ashina M, Lassen LH, Bendtsen L, Jensen R, Olesen J. Effect of inhibition of nitric oxide synthase on chronic tension-type headache: a randomised crossover trial. Lancet. 1999;353(9149):287–9.

71. Schoenen J, Bottin D, Hardy F, Gerard P. Cephalic and extracephalic pressure pain thresholds in chronic tension-type headache. Pain. 1991;47(2):145–9.

72. Ashina S, Bendtsen L, Ashina M, Magerl W, Jensen R. Generalized hyperalgesia in patients with chronic tension-type headache. Cephalalgia. 2006;26(8):940–8.

73. Sohn JH, Choi HC, Kim CH. Differences between episodic and chronic tension-type headaches in nociceptivespecific trigeminal pathways. Cephalalgia. 2013;33(5):330–339.

74. Nardone R, Tezzon F. The trigeminocervical reflex in tension-type headache. Eur J Neurol. 2003;10(3):307-312].

75. Schoenen J, Jamart B, Gerard P, Lenarduzzi P, Delwaide PJ. Exteroceptive suppression of temporalis muscle activity in chronic headache. Neurology. 1987;37(12):1834–6.

76. Ashina M, Bendtsen L, Jensen R, Olesen J. Nitric oxide-induced headache in patients with chronic tension-type headache. Brain. 2000;123(Pt 9):1830–7.

77. Schmidt-Wilcke T, Leinisch E, Straube A, et al. Gray matter decrease in patients with chronic tension type headache. Neurology. 2005;65(9):1483–6.

78. Russell MB, Ostergaard S, Bendtsen L, Olesen J. Familial occurrence of chronic tension-type headache. Cephalalgia. 1999;19(4):207–10.

79. Russell MB, Iselius L, Ostergaard S, Olesen J. Inheritance of chronic tension-type headache investigated by complex segregation analysis. Hum Genet. 1998;102(2):138–40.

80. Donnet A, Lanteri-Minet M, Guegan-Massardier E, et al. Chronic cluster headache: a French clinical descriptive study. J Neurol Neurosurg Psychiatry. 2007;78(12):1354–8.

81. Bahra A, May A, Goadsby PJ. Cluster headache: a prospective clinical study with diagnostic implications. Neurology. 2002;58(3):354–61.

82. Kudrow L. Cluster headache: diagnosis and management. Headache. 1979;19(3):142–50.

83. Fischera M, Marziniak M, Gralow I, Evers S. The incidence and prevalence of cluster headache: a meta-analysis of population-based studies. Cephalalgia. 2008;28(6):614–8.
84. Pearce JM. Natural history of cluster headache. Headache. 1993;33(5):253–6.
85. Manzoni GC, Micieli G, Granella F, Tassorelli C, Zanferrari C, Cavallini A. Cluster headache-course over ten years in 189 patients. Cephalalgia. 1991;11(4):169–74.
86. Manzoni GC. Male preponderance of cluster headache is progressively decreasing over the years. Headache. 1997;37(9):588–9.
87. Torelli P, Cologno D, Cademartiri C, Manzoni GC. Possible predictive factors in the evolution of episodic to chronic cluster headache. Headache. 2000;40(10):798–808.
88. Jurgens TP, Gaul C, Lindwurm A, et al. Impairment in episodic and chronic cluster headache. Cephalalgia. 2011;31(6):671–82.
89. Robbins MS, Bronheim R, Lipton RB, et al. Depression and anxiety in episodic and chronic cluster headache: a pilot study. Headache. 2012;52(4):600–11.
90. Schytz HW, Barlose M, Guo S, et al. Experimental activation of the sphenopalatine ganglion provokes cluster-like attacks in humans. Cephalalgia. 2013;33(10):831–41.
91. May A, Bahra A, Buchel C, Frackowiak RS, Goadsby PJ. Hypothalamic activation in cluster headache attacks. Lancet. 1998;352(9124):275–8.
92. May A, Ashburner J, Buchel C, et al. Correlation between structural and functional changes in brain in an idiopathic headache syndrome. Nat Med. 1999;5(7):836–8.
93. Bartsch T, Levy MJ, Knight YE, Goadsby PJ. Differential modulation of nociceptive dural input to [hypocretin] orexin A and B receptor activation in the posterior hypothalamic area. Pain. 2004;109(3):367–78.
94. Charbit AR, Akerman S, Holland PR, Goadsby PJ. Neurons of the dopaminergic/calcitonin gene-related peptide A11 cell group modulate neuronal firing in the trigeminocervical complex: an electro-physiological and immunohistochemical study. J Neurosci. 2009;29(40):12532–41.
95. Hosoya Y, Matsushita M, Sugiura Y. A direct hypothalamic projection to the superior salivatory nucleus neurons in the rat. A study using anterograde autora-diographic and retrograde HRP methods. Brain Res. 1983;266(2):329–33.
96. Barloese M, Jennum P, Lund N, Knudsen S, Gammeltoft S, Jensen R. Reduced CSF hypocre-tin-1 levels are associated with cluster headache. Cephalalgia. 2015;35(10):869–76.
97. D'Andrea G, Leone M, Bussone G, et al. Abnormal tyrosine metabolism in chronic cluster headache. Cephalalgia. 2017;37(2):148–53.
98. Holle D, Zillessen S, Gaul C, et al. Habituation of the nociceptive blink reflex in episodic and chronic cluster headache. Cephalalgia. 2012;32(13):998–1004.
99. Holle D, Gaul C, Zillessen S, et al. Lateralized central facilitation of trigeminal nociception in cluster headache. Neurology. 2012;78(13):985–92.
100. Medina JL, Diamond S. Cluster headache variant. Spectrum of a new headache syndrome. Arch Neurol. 1981;38(11):705–9.
101. Sjaastad O, Spierings EL. "Hemicrania continua": another headache absolutely responsive to indo-methacin. Cephalalgia. 1984;4(1):65–70.
102. Spierings EL. Hemicrania continua should not be classified as a trigeminal autonomic cephalalgia. Headache. 2013;53(5):869–70.
103. Vincent MB. Hemicrania continua. Unquestionably a trigeminal autonomic cephalalgia. Headache. 2013;53(5):863–8.
104. Cittadini E, Goadsby PJ. Hemicrania continua: a clinical study of 39 patients with diagnostic implications. Brain. 2010;133(Pt 7):1973–86.
105. Prakash S, Golwala P. A proposal for revision of hemicrania continua diagnostic criteria based on critical analysis of 62 patients. Cephalalgia. 2012;32(11):860–8.
106. Newman LC, Lipton RB, Russell M, Solomon S. Hemicrania continua: attacks may alternate sides. Headache. 1992;32(5):237–8.
107. Southerland AM, Login IS. Rigorously defined hemicrania continua presenting bilaterally. Cephalalgia. 2011;31(14):1490–2.
108. Peres MF, Silberstein SD, Nahmias S, et al. Hemicrania continua is not that rare. Neurology. 2001;57(6):948–51.
109. Bigal ME, Lipton RB, Tepper SJ, Rapoport AM, Sheftell FD. Primary chronic daily headache and its subtypes in adolescents and adults. Neurology. 2004;63(5):843–7.
110. Prakash S, Patel P. Hemicrania continua: clinical review, diagnosis and management. J Pain Res. 2017;10:1493–509.
111. Rossi P, Faroni J, Tassorelli C, Nappi G. Diagnostic delay and suboptimal management in a referral population with hemicrania continua. Headache. 2009;49(2):227–34.
112. Lay CL, Newman LC. Posttraumatic hemicrania continua. Headache. 1999;39(4):275–9.
113. Spitz M, Peres MF. Hemicrania continua postpartum. Cephalalgia. 2004;24(7):603–4.
114. Gantenbein AR, Sarikaya H, Riederer F, Goadsby PJ. Postoperative hemicrania continua-like headache - a case series. J Headache Pain. 2015;16:526.
115. D'Alessio C, Ambrosini A, Colonnese C, et al. Indomethacin-responsive hemicrania associated with an extracranial vascular malformation: report of two cases. Cephalalgia. 2004;24(11):997–1000.
116. Valenca MM, Andrade-Valenca LP, da Silva WF, Dodick DW. Hemicrania continua secondary to an ipsilateral brainstem lesion. Headache. 2007;47(3):438–41.
117. Prakash S, Dholakia SY. Hemicrania continua-like headache with leprosy: casual or causal association? Headache. 2008;48(7):1132–4.

118. Wang SJ, Hung CW, Fuh JL, Lirng JF, Hwu CM. Cranial autonomic symptoms in patients with pituitary adenoma presenting with headaches. Acta Neurol Taiwanica. 2009;18(2):104–12.

119. Kim KS, Yang HS. A possible case of symptomatic hemicrania continua from an osteoid osteoma of the ethmoid sinus. Cephalalgia. 2010;30(2):242–8.

120. Evans RW. Hemicrania continua-like headache due to nonmetastatic lung cancer--a vagal cephalalgia. Headache. 2007;47(9):1349–51.

121. Eross EJ, Swanson JW, Dodick DW. Hemicrania continua: an indomethacin-responsive case with an underlying malignant etiology. Headache. 2002;42(6):527–9.

122. Ashkenazi A, Abbas MA, Sharma DK, Silberstein SD. Hemicrania continua-like headache associated with internal carotid artery dissection may respond to indomethacin. Headache. 2007;47(1):127–30.

123. Peres MF, Zukerman E, Porto PP, Brandt RA. Headaches and pineal cyst: a (more than) coincidental relationship? Headache. 2004;44(9):929–30.

124. Matharu MS, Cohen AS, McGonigle DJ, Ward N, Frackowiak RS, Goadsby PJ. Posterior hypothalamic and brainstem activation in hemicrania continua. Headache. 2004;44(8):747–61.

125. Pareja JA, Caminero AB, Franco E, Casado JL, Pascual J, Sanchez del Rio M. Dose, efficacy and tolerability of long-term indomethacin treatment of chronic paroxysmal hemicrania and hemicrania continua. Cephalalgia. 2001;21(9):906–10.

126. Vanast W. New daily persistent headaches: definition of a benign syndrome. Headache. 1986;26:317.

127. Goadsby PJ. New daily persistent headache: a syndrome, not a discrete disorder. Headache. 2011;51(4):650–3.

128. Grande RB, Aaseth K, Lundqvist C, Russell MB. Prevalence of new daily persistent headache in the general population. The Akershus study of chronic headache. Cephalalgia. 2009;29(11):1149–55.

129. Li D, Rozen TD. The clinical characteristics of new daily persistent headache. Cephalalgia. 2002;22(1):66–9.

130. Peng KP, Fuh JL, Yuan HK, Shia BC, Wang SJ. New daily persistent headache: should migrainous features be incorporated? Cephalalgia. 2011;31(15):1561–9.

131. Rozen TD. New daily persistent headache: an update. Curr Pain Headache Rep. 2014;18(7):431.

132. Robbins MS. New daily-persistent headache and anxiety. Cephalalgia. 2011;31(7):875–6.

133. Uniyal R, Paliwal VK, Tripathi A. Psychiatric comorbidity in new daily persistent headache: a cross-sectional study. Eur J Pain. 2017;21(6):1031–8.

134. Robbins MS, Grosberg BM, Napchan U, Crystal SC, Lipton RB. Clinical and prognostic subforms of new daily-persistent headache. Neurology. 2010;74(17):1358–64.

135. GBD 2015 Disease and Injury Incidence and Prevalence Collaborators. Global, regional, and national incidence, prevalence, and years lived with disability for 310 diseases and injuries, 1990–2015: a systematic analysis for the Global Burden of Disease Study 2015. Lancet. 2016;388(10053):1545–602.

136. Scher AI, Rizzoli PB, Loder EW. Medication overuse headache: an entrenched idea in need of scrutiny. Neurology. 2017;89(12):1296–304.

137. Silberstein SD, Olesen J, Bousser MG, et al. The international classification of headache disorders, 2nd edition (ICHD-II)--revision of criteria for 8.2 Medication-overuse headache. Cephalalgia. 2005;25(6):460–5.

138. Bahra A, Walsh M, Menon S, Goadsby PJ. Does chronic daily headache arise de novo in association with regular use of analgesics? Headache. 2003;43(3):179–90.

139. Colas R, Munoz P, Temprano R, Gomez C, Pascual J. Chronic daily headache with analgesic overuse: epidemiology and impact on quality of life. Neurology. 2004;62(8):1338–42.

140. Aaseth K, Grande RB, Kvaerner KJ, Gulbrandsen P, Lundqvist C, Russell MB. Prevalence of secondary chronic headaches in a population-based sample of 30–44-year-old persons. The Akershus study of chronic headache. Cephalalgia. 2008;28(7):705–13.

141. Jonsson P, Hedenrud T, Linde M. Epidemiology of medication overuse headache in the general Swedish population. Cephalalgia. 2011;31(9):1015–22.

142. Straube A, Pfaffenrath V, Ladwig KH, et al. Prevalence of chronic migraine and medication overuse headache in Germany--the German DMKG headache study. Cephalalgia. 2010;30(2):207–13.

143. De Felice M, Porreca F. Opiate-induced persistent pronociceptive trigeminal neural adaptations: potential relevance to opiate-induced medication overuse headache. Cephalalgia. 2009;29(12):1277–84.

144. De Felice M, Ossipov MH, Wang R, et al. Triptan-induced latent sensitization: a possible basis for medication overuse headache. Ann Neurol. 2010;67(3):325–37.

145. Fumal A, Laureys S, Di Clemente L, et al. Orbitofrontal cortex involvement in chronic analgesic-overuse headache evolving from episodic migraine. Brain. 2006;129(Pt 2):543–50.

146. Chanraud S, Di Scala G, Dilharreguy B, Schoenen J, Allard M, Radat F. Brain functional connectivity and morphology changes in medication-overuse headache: clue for dependence-related processes? Cephalalgia. 2014;34(8):605–15.

147. Wilkinson SM, Becker WJ, Heine JA. Opiate use to control bowel motility may induce chronic daily headache in patients with migraine. Headache. 2001;41(3):303–9.

148. Cargnin S, Viana M, Sances G, Tassorelli C, Terrazzino S. A systematic review and critical appraisal of gene polymorphism association studies in medication-overuse headache. Cephalalgia. 2017;333102417728244.

149. Katsarava Z, Limmroth V, Finke M, Diener HC, Fritsche G. Rates and predictors for relapse in medication overuse headache: a 1-year prospective study. Neurology. 2003;60(10):1682–3.

150. Grazzi L, Andrasik F, D'Amico D, Usai S, Kass S, Bussone G. Disability in chronic migraine patients

with medication overuse: treatment effects at 1-year follow-up. Headache. 2004;44(7):678–83.

151. Zidverc-Trajkovic J, Pekmezovic T, Jovanovic Z, et al. Medication overuse headache: clinical features predicting treatment outcome at 1-year follow-up. Cephalalgia. 2007;27(11):1219–25.

152. Hoffman JM, Lucas S, Dikmen S, et al. Natural history of headache after traumatic brain injury. J Neurotrauma. 2011;28(9):1719–25.

153. Lenaerts ME. Post-traumatic headache: from classification challenges to biological underpinnings. Cephalalgia. 2008;28(Suppl 1):12–5.

154. Lucas S, Hoffman JM, Bell KR, Dikmen S. A prospective study of prevalence and characterization of headache following mild traumatic brain injury. Cephalalgia. 2014;34(2):93–102.

155. Erickson JC. Treatment outcomes of chronic post-traumatic headaches after mild head trauma in US soldiers: an observational study. Headache. 2011;51(6):932–44.

156. Lucas S. Posttraumatic headache: clinical characterization and management. Curr Pain Headache Rep. 2015;19(10):48.

157. D'Onofrio F, Russo A, Conte F, Casucci G, Tessitore A, Tedeschi G. Post-traumatic headaches: an epidemiological overview. Neurol Sci. 2014;35(Suppl 1):203–6.

158. Walker WC, Marwitz JH, Wilk AR, et al. Prediction of headache severity (density and functional impact) after traumatic brain injury: a longitudinal multicenter study. Cephalalgia. 2013;33(12):998–1008.

159. Theeler B, Lucas S, Riechers RG II, Ruff RL. Posttraumatic headaches in civilians and military personnel: a comparative, clinical review. Headache. 2013;53(6):881–900.

160. Couch JR, Bearss C. Chronic daily headache in the posttrauma syndrome: relation to extent of head injury. Headache. 2001;41(6):559–64.

161. Yamaguchi M. Incidence of headache and severity of head injury. Headache. 1992;32(9):427–31.

162. De Benedittis G, De Santis A. Chronic posttraumatic headache: clinical, psychopathological features and outcome determinants. J Neurosurg Sci. 1983;27(3):177–86.

163. Chibnall JT, Duckro PN. Post-traumatic stress disorder in chronic post-traumatic headache patients. Headache. 1994;34(6):357–61.

164. Bryan CJ, Hernandez AM. Predictors of posttraumatic headache severity among deployed military personnel. Headache. 2011;51(6):945–53.

165. Minen MT, Boubour A, Walia H, Barr W. Post-concussive syndrome: a focus on post-traumatic headache and related cognitive, psychiatric, and sleep issues. Curr Neurol Neurosci Rep. 2016;16(11):100.

166. Wilk JE, Herrell RK, Wynn GH, Riviere LA, Hoge CW. Mild traumatic brain injury (concussion), posttraumatic stress disorder, and depression in U.S. soldiers involved in combat deployments: association with postdeployment symptoms. Psychosom Med. 2012;74(3):249–57.

167. Strich SJO. Shearing of nerve fibres as a cause of brain damage due to head injury: a pathological study of twenty cases. Lancet. 1961;2:2443–8.

168. Kumar R, Husain M, Gupta RK, et al. Serial changes in the white matter diffusion tensor imaging metrics in moderate traumatic brain injury and correlation with neuro-cognitive function. J Neurotrauma. 2009;26(4):481–95.

169. Ghodadra A, Alhilali L, Fakhran S. Principal component analysis of diffusion tensor images to determine white matter injury patterns underlying postconcussive headache. AJNR Am J Neuroradiol. 2016;37(2):274–8.

170. Signoretti S, Lazzarino G, Tavazzi B, Vagnozzi R. The pathophysiology of concussion. PM R. 2011;3(10 Suppl 2):S359–68.

171. Werner C, Engelhard K. Pathophysiology of traumatic brain injury. Br J Anaesth. 2007;99(1):4–9.

172. Albalawi T, Hamner JW, Lapointe M, Meehan WPR, Tan CO. The relationship between cerebral vasoreactivity and post-concussive symptom severity. J Neurotrauma. 2017;34:2700.

173. Defrin R, Gruener H, Schreiber S, Pick CG. Quantitative somatosensory testing of subjects with chronic post-traumatic headache: implications on its mechanisms. Eur J Pain. 2010;14(9):924–31.

174. Defrin R. Chronic post-traumatic headache: clinical findings and possible mechanisms. J Man Manip Ther. 2014;22(1):36–44.

175. Schwedt TJ, Chong CD, Peplinski J, Ross K, Berisha V. Persistent post-traumatic headache vs. migraine: an MRI study demonstrating differences in brain structure. J Headache Pain. 2017;18(1):87.

176. Stacey A, Lucas S, Dikmen S, et al. Natural history of headache five years after traumatic brain injury. J Neurotrauma. 2017;34(8):1558–64.

177. Wiendels NJ, van der Geest MC, Neven AK, Ferrari MD, Laan LA. Chronic daily headache in children and adolescents. Headache. 2005;45(6):678–83.

178. Colombo B, Dalla Libera D, De Feo D, Pavan G, Annovazzi PO, Comi G. Delayed diagnosis in pediatric headache: an outpatient Italian survey. Headache. 2011;51(8):1267–73.

179. Seshia SS, Phillips DF, von Baeyer CL. Childhood chronic daily headache: a biopsychosocial perspective. Dev Med Child Neurol. 2008;50(7):541–5.

180. Lipton RB, Manack A, Ricci JA, Chee E, Turkel CC, Winner P. Prevalence and burden of chronic migraine in adolescents: results of the chronic daily headache in adolescents study (C-dAS). Headache. 2011;51(5):693–706.

181. Arruda MA, Guidetti V, Galli F, Albuquerque RC, Bigal ME. Frequent headaches in the preadolescent pediatric population: a population-based study. Neurology. 2010;74(11):903–8.

182. Wang SJ, Fuh JL, Lu SR, Juang KD. Chronic daily headache in adolescents: prevalence, impact, and medication overuse. Neurology. 2006;66(2):193–7.

183. Pascual J, Berciano J. Experience in the diagnosis of headaches that start in elderly people. J Neurol Neurosurg Psychiatry. 1994;57(10):1255–7.

184. Prencipe M, Casini AR, Ferretti C, et al. Prevalence of headache in an elderly population: attack frequency, disability, and use of medication. J Neurol Neurosurg Psychiatry. 2001;70(3):377–81.

185. Wang SJ, Fuh JL, Lu SR, et al. Chronic daily headache in Chinese elderly: prevalence, risk factors, and biannual follow-up. Neurology. 2000;54(2):314–9.

186. Martins KM, Bordini CA, Bigal ME, Speciali JG. Migraine in the elderly: a comparison with migraine in young adults. Headache. 2006;46(2):312–6.

187. Fisher CM. Late-life migraine accompaniments-further experience. Stroke. 1986;17(5):1033–42.

188. Dodick DW, Mosek AC, Campbell JK. The hypnic ("alarm clock") headache syndrome. Cephalalgia. 1998;18(3):152–6.

189. Liang JF, Wang SJ. Hypnic headache: a review of clinical features, therapeutic options and outcomes. Cephalalgia. 2014;34(10):795–805.

190. Schulman EA, Lake AE III, Goadsby PJ, et al. Defining refractory migraine and refractory chronic migraine: proposed criteria from the Refractory Headache Special Interest Section of the American Headache Society. Headache. 2008;48(6):778–82.

191. Levin M. Refractory headache: classification and nomenclature. Headache. 2008;48(6):783–90.

Index

© Springer International Publishing AG, part of Springer Nature 2019
M. W. Green et al. (eds.), *Chronic Headache*, https://doi.org/10.1007/978-3-319-91491-6

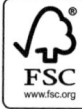